Bottom Line's

EXTREME HEALING

1,749 Innovative
**Treatments
and Techniques**
from Medicine's
New Frontiers

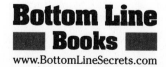

**Bottom Line
Books**
www.BottomLineSecrets.com

Contents

vi

Preface

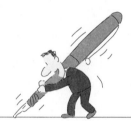

We are proud to bring you our brand-new book, *Bottom Line's Extreme Healing: 1,749 Innovative Treatments and Techniques from Medicine's New Frontiers*, with the latest health discoveries.

When you choose a Bottom Line Book, you are turning to a stellar group of experts in a wide range of specialties—medical doctors, alternative practitioners, nutrition experts, research scientists and consumer-health advocates, to name a few.

We go to great lengths to interview the foremost health experts. Whether it's cancer prevention, breakthrough arthritis treatments or cutting-edge nutritional advice, our editors talk to the true innovators in health care.

How do we find all these top-notch professionals? Over the past 20 years, we have built a network of thousands of leading physicians in both alternative and conventional medicine. They are affiliated with the world's premier medical institutions. We follow the latest research and we regularly talk to our advisors in major teaching hospitals, private practices and government health agencies.

Bottom Line's Extreme Healing is a result of our ongoing research and contact with these experts, and is a distillation of their latest findings and advice. We hope that you will enjoy the presentation and glean helpful information about the health topics that concern you and your family.

As a reader of a Bottom Line Book, please be assured that you are receiving reliable and well-researched information from a trusted source. But, please use prudence in health matters. Always speak to your physician before taking vitamins, supplements or over-the-counter medication…changing your diet…or beginning an exercise program. If you experience side effects from any regimen, contact your doctor immediately.

The Editors, Bottom Line Books, Stamford, CT.

1

Surprising Ways to Prevent Heart Disease and Stroke

Giving Blood Could Save *Your* Life

Giving blood helps safeguard the health of others, of course, but is it possible that giving blood might also enhance the donor's health? Controversy has swirled around this question for a number of years, but the "yeses" now seem to be adding up. Supporters say donating blood is good for the donor's health because the process removes iron from the body—and that is good, they believe, because stored body iron, even in the so-called normal range, may increase cardiovascular disease risk.

BLOOD DONATION— REDUCED CARDIAC EVENTS

One of the longtime leading proponents of reducing stored iron is Jerome L. Sullivan, MD, PhD, clinical assistant professor at the University of Florida College of Medicine in Gainesville. Dr. Sullivan points to a Yale University study published in 2005 as an important informational step forward. The study assessed two factors— the effects of blood donation frequency on body iron stores and several markers of vascular function.

It looked at two groups of blood donors: High-frequency donors, those who donated eight or more times in the past two years…and low-frequency donors, people who had donated only one or two times in the same period.

Researchers found that in comparison to the low-frequency group, people who were high-frequency donors had significantly better *flow-mediated dilation* (FMD) in the brachial artery—and FMD is an important indicator of vascular function. A second sign of better cardiovascular functioning in this group was the decrease in the presence of a particular marker (3-nitrotyrosine) of

Jerome L. Sullivan, MD, PhD, clinical assistant professor, University of Florida College of Medicine in Gainesville.

1

vascular oxidative stress, which is considered to be implicated in development of atherosclerosis. In conclusion, the study authors wrote that their findings support a potential link between high-frequency blood donation and reduced cardiovascular disease risk. This is in line with findings from several previous studies, but the Yale study design was the best designed one yet, according to Dr. Sullivan.

Evidence that supports this theory, says Dr. Sullivan, shows that menstruating women, who lose iron each and every month through their periods, seem to be highly protected from heart attacks. However, there are many scientists who disagree with this and point instead to the presence of estrogen as the reason for women's protection. But Dr. Sullivan argues that the Women's Health Initiative Study (done by the National Institutes of Health, National Heart, Lung, and Blood Institute) on hormone replacement therapy showed that taking estrogen, in fact, *increased* the likelihood of a cardiac event… this increase made the concept of estrogen as a protector of heart health much less credible, if credible at all.

IRON AND HOMOCYSTEINE

At this point, the iron issue starts to get a little more complicated. Homocysteine is an amino acid in the blood which, when elevated, is related to increased heart attack, stroke and peripheral artery disease risk. Further research, though, has shown that homocysteine may damage blood vessels in the presence of iron by working together in synergistic fashion to increase risk. Researchers determined this when they gave people a blast of homocysteine in conjunction with a chelating substance that would at the same time clear iron from their blood. The iron chelation seemed to offset the negative effects of homocysteine on endothelial function in blood vessels.

EFFECT ON OLDER WOMEN

How does this tie in with menstruation? Dr. Sullivan observes that in postmenopausal women, who no longer slough iron monthly through periods, homocysteine levels rise right along with their iron stores. And, as is well known, cardiovascular disease risk increases dramatically among postmenopausal women. Is there a connection? It's far from proven and there may be other contributing factors, but it is an observation worth noting.

STORED IRON AND SENIORS

Still, there is the deeply entrenched paradigm that stored iron is good, even necessary for health. Dr. Sullivan says that one reason for this belief is that studies among the elderly have shown that those who have iron depletion also have higher mortality rates. But this, he explains, is likely because iron depletion is a common indicator of many serious diseases, particularly colon cancer.

Or, as *Bottom Line's Daily Health News* consulting medical editor Andrew L. Rubman, ND, notes, seniors may have iron depletion due to decreased stomach acid and acid production, which impairs iron absorption. Whatever the reason, those with reduced iron stores may die earlier because they are sicker, not because the lower levels of iron are bad for them, says Dr. Rubman. He agrees that everyone needs sufficient iron to protect against anemia, but says stored iron levels that are labeled as "normal," may reflect an outdated way of thinking. When humans lived with chronic famines, in the occasional times of feast, the body built and held on to both fat and iron as protection against the next lean time, he explained. Today we live with an abundance of foods, including those that are iron-fortified. People usually do not need the protection of excess stored iron, he says, because we ingest it regularly in sufficient amounts to avoid anemia.

DO A DOUBLE GOOD DEED

As for blood donation, according to the Yale University study and other researchers, the key to obtaining health advantages from giving blood is frequency. To reduce iron depletion enough to contribute to health requires frequent giving—every two months as allowed. Certainly there is no reason to think frequent giving is dangerous. Potential donors must pass an anemia test every time, which assures that people are not iron deficient. Blood banks don't usually publicize the possible health benefits of frequent donations. But in fact, this may well be one of those rewarding opportunities to gain through giving.

Measuring PLAC in Your Plaque

Christie M. Ballantyne, MD, director, Center for Cardiovascular Disease Prevention, professor, department of medicine and associate chief, atherosclerosis and vascular medicine section, Baylor College of Medicine, Houston, Texas.

Ever since inflammation was identified as a key underlying factor in cardiovascular diseases, researchers have been on an aggressive hunt for new biomarkers of inflammation. One of the newest and most promising of these is an enzyme known as *lipoprotein-associated phospholipase A(2) (Lp-PLA2)*. The PLAC test, which measures levels of Lp-PLA2, was approved to detect heart disease and to ferret out stroke risk as well.

Christie M. Ballantyne, MD, director of the Center for Cardiovascular Disease Prevention at Baylor College of Medicine in Houston, Texas, says that along with more traditional tests, the PLAC test has proven very effective at helping to identify those at risk and encourage them to take proactive steps (such as better diet, more exercise and no smoking) to reduce their risk for heart attack and stroke. While PLAC screening does not replace cholesterol and homocysteine screening to measure risk, the enzyme it measures plays a part in the inflammatory process that correlates with cardiovascular risk.

RESEARCH BACKS UP CLAIMS

Lp-PLA2 is an enzyme in blood and arterial plaque buildup that studies have shown to be an important risk factor for heart disease and stroke—perhaps more important than high cholesterol levels. Scientists believe that this enzyme plays a key role in the formation and rupture of plaque that is most likely to lead to a heart attack or stroke.

Solid research backs up Lp-PLA2's role as a predictor of major cardiovascular events...

•**Over a 14-year period,** the MONICA (MONItoring of trends and determinants in CArdiovascular disease) study demonstrated that Lp-PLA2 was independently predictive of heart attacks in men who had only moderately elevated cholesterol. With each standard deviation increase in Lp-PLA2, there was a 37% increase in the risk of a coronary event.

•**In the Atherosclerosis Risk in Communities (ARIC) study,** Dr. Ballantyne and his colleagues found that Lp-PLA2 levels were associated with ischemic stroke. About eight out of 10 strokes are ischemic, caused by a clot or particle clogging a blood vessel and cutting off the blood supply to part of the brain. People with elevated Lp-PLA2 were twice as likely to experience a stroke as those with lower levels, independent of recognized risk factors such as body mass index and C-reactive protein (CRP).

GAUGE YOUR RISK

The PLAC test is good alone—but cardiovascular risk is even better understood when the PLAC test is used in conjunction with homocysteine screening. Talk to your doctor about the use of this diagnostic tool.

info The PLAC test is a blood test that must be ordered by your physician. It is available through many national laboratories, including Quest Diagnostics Inc. (*www.questdiagnostics.com*), Mayo Medical Laboratories (*www.mayomedicallaboratories.com*) and Berkeley HeartLab Inc. (*www.bhlinc.com*). To learn more, visit *www.plactest.com*.

Hidden Heart Attack Symptom Everyone Should Know About

Daniel S. Berman, MD, director of cardiac imaging, Cedars-Sinai Medical Center, Los Angeles.

I t's a chilling scenario. An older adult out for a walk experiences shortness of breath, serious enough that he/she decides to save the walk for a later day. However, all too often, the individual feels better once home and so lets the episode pass from memory. The problem is, for some people this story ends with a sudden heart attack—and death—not long after the ill-fated walk. In fact, shortness of breath, as a recent study makes clear, is as important a symptom of heart disease (and a possible heart attack) as chest pain and should prompt an immediate call to the doctor.

The study, conducted in part by Cedars-Sinai Medical Center in Los Angeles, investigated medical records of nearly 18,000 patients who came for cardiac stress testing and who were then followed for one to four years. It found that patients without known coronary artery disease (CAD) who had shortness of breath were twice as likely to suddenly die from a cardiac cause as patients who had typical angina (symptoms of pressure, fullness, squeezing or pain in center of the chest, sometimes also in neck, jaw, shoulder, back or arm after exertion). People don't realize that shortness of breath can signal danger and they don't seek help, says Daniel S. Berman, MD, chief of cardiac imaging at Cedars-Sinai, who is a coauthor of the study.

WHEN YOU EXERCISE...

Dr. Berman explains several important aspects of shortness of breath as a cardiac symptom. First, it is often associated with exertion, coming on during physical activity such as brisk walking. As a cardiac symptom it applies most commonly to older adults who could be considered for possible cardiac risk—usually having one or more of the cardiac risk factors, such as high blood pressure and cholesterol, excess abdominal weight, are over age 45, a smoking habit—usually not to a young person without risk factors who may become short of breath while at the peak of exercise. This type of shortness of breath that we are discussing here can be the first manifestation of a CAD symptom. Coronary artery disease can occur in both men and women, though it usually occurs about 10 years later in women.

If a person has unexplained exertional shortness of breath, he/she should see a physician. There are tests that can be done to determine if the symptom is from the heart and to assess the risk. "We have excellent treatments to prevent heart attacks and cardiac death as long as we identify who is at risk. The key is to be aware of the risk factors and the symptoms of CAD so that appropriate tests can be done and treatment begun before an event occurs," says Dr. Berman.

Bottom line: If you have known CAD or have risk factors, and experience unexplained exertional shortness of breath, stop the exercise. Think of this symptom in the same way you would think of exertional chest pain—and ask your doctor what to do.

New Study Shows Why Healthy People Have Heart Attacks

Sotirios Tsimikas, MD, director, vascular medicine, University of California, San Diego School of Medicine, La Jolla.

A lthough the medical profession knows a great deal about cardiac risk, many seemingly healthful people with healthy habits still have heart attacks, which means there is clearly much more to be learned. A new and exciting study, from researchers at the University of California, San Diego (UCSD) School of Medicine in La Jolla, may be providing fresh insight—a previously unrecognized but potentially crucial cardiac risk factor.

ABOUT THE STUDY

The study team analyzed blood samples from 500 patients who were being treated at the Mayo Clinic (Rochester, Minnesota) for heart problems and were referred there to have coronary angiography (an X-ray examination that uses a contrasting fluid to view the cardiac vessels and chambers). After taking into account known risk factors such as smoking, high cholesterol levels, elevated blood pressure, and diabetes, the team found that patients who had a high level of phospholipids (fats in the bloodstream) that had oxidized were highly likely to have coronary blockage.

There's more to the study findings, but first a brief explanation of cholesterol lipids. In addition to low-density lipoprotein (LDL) and high-density lipoprotein (HDL), there are several other cholesterol lipids. Among them is one called Lp(a) (lipoprotein [a]). Doctors have long known that Lp(a) attaches itself to coronary arteries and is a risk factor in developing plaque, but they haven't understood the process. This study shows that the oxidized phospholipids attach themselves to Lp(a) that is then transported from the liver around the body and into the coronary arteries.

THE RESEARCHER'S PERSPECTIVE

The lead researcher on the study was Sotirios Tsimikas, MD, director of vascular medicine at the UCSD Medical School. He discusses how this important study might change our understanding of cardiac risk. Dr. Tsimikas says that one of the key implications of this work is that it provides a new path to diagnosing cardiac risk—measuring Lp(a) and oxidized lipids.

Lp(a) is genetically determined, and about 25% of the population has elevated levels of it. (Elevated is considered to be greater than 30 milligrams [mg] per deciliter.) People with a strong family history of heart attack are likely to be in that 25% of the population and, he says, would do well to have their Lp(a) levels tested. This can be done with a simple fasting blood test. Unfortunately, at present, most doctors other than cardiovascular and lipid specialists are not familiar with Lp(a), so patients need to be prepared to educate their doctors on the subject. Also, the way results for this test are given have not been standardized, so they may vary somewhat from lab to lab. Even so, Dr. Tsimikas adds that the test and its results are routine enough, if not exact, to be valuable.

Finding out your level of oxidized lipids is more difficult, however. Thus far, the only test for it is at the lab at UCSD. Dr. Tsimikas says that it may become commercially available in the future, but it will take additional testing to further establish its predictive value.

We asked about testing for C-reactive protein (CRP), another marker for inflammation in the body, but he says CRP is completely independent of this problem. Dr. Tsimikas explains that elevated oxidized lipid and Lp(a) levels show up much earlier along the path to a cardiac event than does CRP, which elevates much later, after the disease has progressed considerably. Consequently, while a CRP test is useful, it does not have the value of a cholesterol screening of HDL and LDL levels.

LP(A) CAN BE LOWERED

But the purpose of testing for Lp(a) levels—and eventually for oxidized lipids—is to let you know if you need to take steps to lower them. The current treatment for lowering Lp(a) is niacin in high doses by prescription or, per *Bottom Line's Daily Health News* consulting medical editor Andrew L. Rubman, ND, in frequent doses of less than 1 mg. Low-dose niacin is available over the counter.

Side effects include uncomfortable flushing in some people, Dr. Tsimikas says, but that tends to go away.

Note: Use of niacin to reduce Lp(a) levels should be overseen by a physician or naturopathic physician trained in nutritional biochemistry. Improper use of niacin therapy—high doses in particular—can create system imbalances that affect brain and liver function. Dr. Rubman adds that people with diabetes should be especially careful to work with a trained professional. Improper use of niacin can make diabetes worse—there is a concern that it raises blood sugar levels—although taking niacin in conjunction with additional vitamin B can actually improve diabetes. Estrogen has also been shown to help lower Lp(a), but, again, that should be done with proper supervision.

Dr. Tsimikas recommends a diet rich in antioxidants, including colorful fruits and vegetables. Statin drugs, he says, seem to have some value, too. Dr. Rubman also suggests that you avoid fried foods and trans fats while eating plenty of fiber and healthful fats to aid digestion, and use natural alternatives to statins, such as red yeast rice.

Dr. Tsimikas and his team are conducting further studies on lipids and Lp(a) and are now looking at how the measures they found correlate with a special type of ultrasound test for coronary plaque, considered to be the gold standard. He expects to have results of their current studies in several years.

Skin Problem That Means Heart Trouble, Too

Hilal Maradit Kremers, MD, MSc, associate professor of epidemiology at the Mayo Clinic College of Medicine, Rochester, Minnesota.

Psoriasis is considered a chronic, lifelong disorder that usually begins before the age of 40. The sometimes painful, itchy, scaly patches or lesions can run from being mildly annoying to life-disrupting. But many people assume that this condition, which affects about five million Americans, is purely dermatological. Now, though, research is increasingly showing that psoriasis is a systemic inflammatory disorder that results from a disturbance in the immune response.

Contributing further evidence of a link with inflammation and immune-mediated disorders is a disturbing study recently released by the Mayo Clinic in Rochester, Minnesota. Researchers there found that having psoriasis puts people at a much greater risk of developing heart disease, similar to other immune-mediated disorders that are also highly associated with inflammation and immune system dysfunction. The longitudinal study followed a group of 622 people with psoriasis and matched each of them with two control subjects of the same age and gender. Researchers examined medical records of people starting at age 18 and tracked them until their death. This revealed the startling information that people with psoriasis were 42% more likely to have a heart attack than people without it.

We contacted Hilal Maradit Kremers, MD, MSc, one of the study's authors, about this troubling finding. Dr. Maradit Kremers says that the exact means by which the inflammation in psoriasis can be associated with heart disease is as yet unclear, but that research is ongoing concerning it and other aspects of this association. She also says that this study did not give insight into what specific preventive measures psoriasis patients should take to avoid heart disease. But she adds that they should be very aware of their increased risk and be on the alert for any cardiovascular disease symptoms. It is important for them to inform their doctors as well about this recently established association of cardiac risk and psoriasis since many doctors may not yet be familiar with it.

It is well known that certain lifestyle factors help decrease heart disease risk and inflammation—not smoking…keeping your weight down…eating a diet rich in fruits and vegetables, fish and whole grains, and high in omega-3 fatty acids…avoiding trans fats…and limiting saturated fats.

It would be good for everyone who wants to keep heart disease at bay to follow these rules of good health, but those with psoriasis should be especially vigilant.

The Heart-Healthiest Nighttime Activity

Joel E. Dimsdale, MD, professor of psychiatry, University of California, San Diego School of Medicine, La Jolla.

More and more research shows an important relationship between sleep quality and good health, which should be a wake-up call for our notoriously sleep-deprived population. Whether due to obstructive sleep apnea (a common and serious sleep disorder characterized by pauses in breathing during sleep that can be caused by excess weight, thick neck circumference or large tonsils or adenoids)…stress-induced insomnia…or the habit of staying awake for "The Tonight Show," few of us get the quality or quantity of sleep we need. That leads to all kinds of problems, says Joel E. Dimsdale, MD, a professor of psychiatry at the University of California, San Diego (UCSD) School of Medicine in La Jolla.

Tossing and turning at night has adverse effects on productivity, safety and quality of life. Now Dr. Dimsdale and his research colleagues have identified another negative effect—they've established a link between higher levels of sleep disruption and an increased risk for blood clotting, which is associated with a higher risk for heart disease.

SLEEP DISRUPTION— A SERIOUS HEALTH RISK

In full-night sleep studies, researchers recorded brain waves, and air flow at the nose and mouth, of 135 men and women with no history of sleep disorders. The mean age of the participants was 37. They were unmedicated men and women. Researchers accounted for age, gender, ethnicity, body mass index, blood pressure and smoking history. The researchers found that those with patterns of broken sleep had statistically significant higher blood markers for clotting. There are many reasons for not sleeping through the night, both physical and emotional. This study did not look at underlying reasons, however, only at the impact of sleep disturbances on cardiovascular health.

In earlier research, Dr. Dimsdale and his colleagues had already established that sleep disruption promoted clotting and increased cardiovascular risk in people with obstructive sleep apnea and those under extreme, long-term stress. But with this study, we now know that sleep disruption has the potential to raise cardiovascular risk even in normal, healthy individuals. The link between sleep disruption and clotting was similar whether or not the patient had apnea.

A WAKE-UP CALL

According to Dr. Dimsdale, there are simple steps to avoid sleep disruption and get the restful sleep the body needs. First, if you have extensive daytime fatigue and your bed partner reports that you snore loudly, schedule an appointment with a sleep specialist to see if you have obstructive sleep apnea. If you do suffer from this condition, there are several treatments for it.

Second, Dr. Dimsdale offers a few tips for improved sleep…

•**Exercise earlier in the day,** rather than just before bedtime.

•**Keep a regular sleep schedule.** Go to sleep at night and awaken at approximately the same time every day.

•**Reserve your bed for sleep and sex.** Regularly reading, watching TV, using your computer and/or doing paperwork in bed can make it more difficult to fall asleep there.

If you regularly have trouble sinking into or staying asleep, consider that this may indicate a need to reassess your life and choices, comments *Bottom Line's Daily Health News* consulting medical editor Andrew L. Rubman, ND. "If you simply try to manage the sleep disturbance pharmacologically, you may not consider other underlying problems that are obstructing the real solution." He also offered natural sleep aids, including *valeriana officinalis* (valerian), *humulus lupulus* (hops), *scutellaria lateriflora* (skullcap) and *lactuca virosa* (lactucarium) as useful alternatives. Naturopathic physicians have experience with these and other effective ways to help you fall asleep with ease.

Dancing Better for Your Heart than the Gym

Wayne Westcott, PhD, fitness research director and exercise physiologist, South Shore YMCA, Quincy, Massachusetts.

A weekly dance class can be fun, offer excellent aerobic exercise and provide a mental break from the hustle and bustle of life. Italian researchers have confirmed that waltzing is good for the heart as well. In fact, it is as good as—and in some respects may even be a little better than—conventional cycling and treadmill workouts.

Wayne Westcott, PhD, fitness research director and an exercise physiologist at the South Shore YMCA in Quincy, Massachusetts, believes in dancing's health benefits. He says that as long as exercise meets three important criteria—frequency (at least three days a week)...intensity (vigorous enough to raise the heart rate 60% to 80% of maximum, unless restricted by medication)...and duration (a minimum of 15- to 20-minute workouts)—it doesn't matter what type of activity you choose. If you find something you enjoy, you're more likely to stick with it. Warm up and cool down for five to 10 minutes with a lower-intensity exercise, such as walking or practicing dance steps, says Dr. Westcott.

ABOUT THE STUDY

In the study at the Lancisi Heart Institute in Ancona, Italy, researchers examined the impact of waltzing, cycling and treadmill workouts on people with chronic heart failure. In people with this long-term condition, the heart can no longer properly pump enough blood to other organs and tissues in the body. Consequently, the organs fail to receive sufficient oxygen and nutrients, which over time results in damage and loss of proper functioning. However, exercise may help improve functioning and quality of life.

The researchers divided heart failure patients into three groups. A group of 44 people exercised on a bicycle or treadmill three times a week for eight weeks...44 took waltzing classes for the same period...and 22 did not exercise at all. In those who waltzed or exercised, aerobic capacity improved. In people who did not work out, there was no change.

Specifically, researchers found that...

• **Oxygen uptake,** or the amount of oxygen reaching the tissues, rose 16% in exercisers and 18% in dancers.

• **The threshold of muscle fatigue,** or the time elapsed before muscles tire, increased 20% in exercisers and 21% in dancers.

• **While general fitness improvements in exercisers and dancers** were comparable, dancers showed greater improvements in quality of life—especially relating to emotions and mood.

These findings are in sync with earlier research showing that waltzing is beneficial in helping people recover the ability to function and improve quality of life following heart attacks.

PUT ON YOUR DANCING SHOES

Researchers speculate that the additional benefits of dancing stem from it's social nature and partnership. There's nothing magical about the waltz, of course.

Dr. Westcott advises that you choose any type of dance—or other aerobic exercise—that you enjoy...but check with your doctor first. Then simply channel your inner Ginger Rogers or Fred Astaire and get moving.

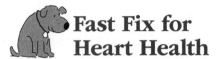 **Fast Fix for Heart Health**

Kathie Cole, RN, lead researcher of a study that evaluated the physical and psychological effects of introducing pet dogs to cardiac intensive care patients, is a cardiac care nurse at the University of California, Los Angeles (UCLA) Medical Center.

It's been said before, and now confirmed again...Spending time petting a dog can improve heart and lung function and relieve anxiety in heart patients—and it doesn't take long, according to a study presented at a meeting of the American Heart Association. A mere 12-minute visit with a dog resulted in measurable positive effects on patients' cardiac function and stress levels.

Seventy-six patients with heart failure at the University of California, Los Angeles (UCLA) Medical Center were randomly assigned to a 12-minute visit with either a dog and a human volunteer...a human volunteer only...or no visitors at all. In the dog and human volunteer group, specially trained dogs were placed on patients' beds so people could pet them during the observed study time.

The researchers showed significant results in three variables that characterize heart failure—changes in heart-lung pressures, stress hormone levels and anxiety.

HEART'S BEST FRIEND

In all three areas, those patients visited by a dog had superior results.

Cardiac-related improvements included a 5% drop in systolic pulmonary artery pressure during a dog visit and a 5% drop following the visit, as compared with rises in the other two groups. (Higher systolic pulmonary artery pressure—a measure of pressure in the lung—can make breathing more difficult in this group.)

Stress reduction occurred as levels of the stress hormone epinephrine dropped an average of 17% in those patients visited by a dog, as compared with a much lesser 2% drop in the human visitor only group and an average rise of 7% in those patients left alone.

And finally, those patients with a dog visitor had 24% less anxiety compared with a 10% drop in those visited by a human only and no drop in anxiety in those patients left alone.

Lead researcher Kathie Cole, RN, a cardiac care nurse at the UCLA Medical Center, says that the study shows that even short-term exposure to a dog can be extremely beneficial, both physiologically and psychologically. Perhaps more importantly, she says, studies like this one give animal-assisted therapy more credibility in the medical community. And, the positive effects from being around a dog are not limited to heart patients alone, but can be enjoyed by all people, in all conditions of health.

Is Your Attitude Hurting Your Heart?

Nalini Ranjit, PhD, research investigator, Center for Social Epidemiology and Population Health, University of Michigan, Ann Arbor.

A recent study is reminiscent of the "Type A" research of some years ago, that found that ambitious, achievement-oriented people with high levels of hostility were prone to heart disease. Now there's new affirmation that negativity affects our health from the University of Michigan in Ann Arbor, where researchers assessed 6,814 people, aged 45 to 84, to uncover potential health risks associated with three psychosocial factors—chronic stress, depression and cynical distrust. The

9

researchers took blood samples from the participants and tested for three inflammation markers—C-reactive protein (CRP), fibrinogen and interleukin-6 (IL-6), all three of which are associated with increased heart disease risk. The results showed that chronic stress was linked with higher levels of IL-6 and CRP, while depression was linked only with higher levels of IL-6. Cynical distrust, however, took the highest toll, showing the strongest and most consistent positive association with all three of the markers.

We talked with lead author Nalini Ranjit, PhD, research investigator at the University's Center for Social Epidemiology and Population Health. Her expectation was that depression would be the trait most highly associated with inflammation markers, so she was surprised to find the strong correlation between cynical distrust and inflammation markers. Dr. Ranjit describes "cynical distrust" as not only being cynical about life, but also having a deep-seated distrust and hostility toward other people. What was it about this attitude toward life that could change the body's chemistry? No one really knows conclusively how any of the three psychosocial factors connect physically to the raised measures of inflammation. Significantly, Dr. Ranjit says, the research team found a pattern of self-destructive behaviors including smoking, alcohol use and a lack of physical activity in people with cynical distrust. A higher body mass index was also associated with cynical distrust (and may be indicative of another self-destructive behavior—overeating) but the connection seems to be deeper than that, since there are obese people and smokers in the depression and chronic stress categories as well. She also notes that it is important not to confuse this trait with cynicism, since cynical distrust includes hostility toward others.

While it is a big challenge to alter such deep-seated attitudes, Dr. Ranjit says that people who know themselves to be cynical and untrusting should be aware that they are potentially at risk for heart disease. They should do what they can to resolve their emotional pains, but also take extra care of their bodies with healthy diet and exercise.

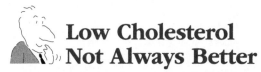 ## Low Cholesterol Not Always Better

Rodney Hayward, MD, director of the Veterans Administration Center for Practice Management and Outcomes Research, and professor of medicine and public health, University of Michigan Health System, both in Ann Arbor, Michigan.

L*ower, lower, lowest.* In 2004, an update of the 2001 recommendations from the National Cholesterol Education Program (NCEP) turned into a rallying cry against low-density lipoprotein (LDL) cholesterol, the type associated with coronary heart disease (CHD) risk. Today, doctors—and of course pharmaceutical companies—routinely push people at very high CHD risk to get their LDL down to 70 milligrams per deciliter (mg/dL) or lower, which may require taking multiple medications, following strict diets, careful monitoring and high cost. Is it worth it? Not necessarily, says a major recent study funded in part by the National Institutes of Health.

STATINS vs. LOW LDL

The researchers examined every study the NCEP used in the 2004 update as basis for its recommendations. They then evaluated other studies for cardiovascular outcomes of patients who had comparable CHD risks and LDL cholesterol under 130. They found that extremely low LDL may not matter, but that taking statins—powerful anti-CHD drugs with anti-inflammatory effects—benefited all high CHD-risk patients...whether their baseline (natural) LDL level was 100 or 200. In other words, the evidence proves that statins, not necessarily low LDL, improves outcome. Of all studies evaluated, the study's team could not identify any valid clinical evidence supporting low LDL (below 130 mg/dL) as an independent factor for decreased risk.

The study's chief author is Rodney Hayward, MD, director of the Veterans Administration Center for Practice Management and Outcomes Research and professor of medicine and public health at the University of Michigan Health System in Ann Arbor. He says that the low LDL push (below 70 mg/dL for very high risk people and below 100 mg/dL in high risk people) reflects a misguided interpretation of the clinical trials and their purpose. The trials investigated the effectiveness of statins for high-risk people. They did not correctly assess whether the amount that statins reduced LDL to low levels was independently protective...and statins do more than lower LDL, including impact inflammation, which is now known to be associated with CHD risk. According to Dr. Hayward, it is very possible that the total effect of statins is what makes the drugs valuable for people at high CHD risk. For the very few people with extremely high LDL—over 189—Dr. Hayward says it is worth considering multiple medications to lower it, but use of multiple drugs for others would be speculative treatment.

KNOW THE GUIDELINES

Dr. Hayward also says that there are many people taking statins today who should not be. Statins are recommended for high CHD risk people, and no one else.

And here is the reason: Say your 10-year CHD disease risk is only one in 100, and the drug reduces it to one in 250. But all drugs have risks, including statins, and if its 10-year risk affects even just one in 100 people, taking it puts you at more than twice the risk for serious side effects from the drug than it provides benefit against disease. Forget statins then, he says, and focus on maintaining your CHD risk as low as possible by keeping your weight down, eating healthily, exercising every day and not smoking.

However, if you are at high CHD risk, statins can dramatically reduce your risk of heart attacks, strokes and death.

info You can learn your 10-year risk for CHD with the Framingham risk scoring, which is based on the Framingham Heart Study (Massachusetts) and uses age, gender, smoking, total cholesterol, high-density lipoprotein (HDL) cholesterol, systolic blood pressure and blood pressure medication use to determine risk. To get yours, go to *http://hp2010.nhlbihin.net/at pjii/calculator.asp*.

See Your Chiropractor for Lower Blood Pressure

George Bakris, MD, director, Hypertension Center, and professor of medicine, University of Chicago.

Lots of people consider a chiropractor vital to their good health, but few would consider seeing one for treatment to lower blood pressure. So it was a real surprise when a new study from the University of Chicago's Medical Center demonstrated that a specific type of chiropractic manipulation of the first vertebra (Atlas) of the neck can do exactly that. The pilot study included 50 people with stage 1 high blood pressure—25 of them had an adjustment to this vertebra...while the 25 controls had a sham adjustment.

Results: Compared with the control group, those with the Atlas adjustment had, on average, a drop of 14 points in systolic (the upper) pressure and eight in the diastolic (lower) reading. Study authors concluded that the results were similar to the effectiveness of treatment with two blood pressure medications in combination.

MORE EVIDENCE

Study author George Bakris, MD, director of the Hypertension Center at the University of Chicago, said he'd heard about this particular treatment from a doctor in family practice who told him about patients who'd had the manipulation and significantly lowered their blood pressure. The adjustment had been to correct a very slight misalignment in the Atlas vertebra, which sits at the top of the spine and relies on muscle and ligaments for alignment. Their misalignments typically were the result of a head or neck injury at some point in their life—including some from long ago—such as falling off a bike, a sports injury or car accident. Dr. Bakris speculates that the resulting misalignment had likely created a kink or kinks in blood vessels in the area of the lower brain stem, either impeding blood flow to the brain or abrupting up against a particular area of the brain stem, changing the autonomic nervous system in ways affecting blood pressure. At the end of six months, 88% were still corrected without follow-up treatment.

BEFORE YOU GO TO
THE CHIROPRACTOR

Not everyone with high blood pressure is a candidate for an Atlas manipulation and not every chiropractor is qualified to do such manipulation. It may work for people with high blood pressure who have Atlas misalignment but that should be verified with imaging studies. There is now a large-scale study to validate the evaluation of Atlas misalignment so that it will have broader use in clinical practice. It is important to note that at this time the observations regarding changes in blood pressure need to be confirmed and should not be used routinely for this purpose.

Moreover, not only does the technique work only for a select population, but by no means are all (or even most) chiropractors able to perform this manipulation. Because it can be dangerous if improperly performed, it requires specific training and experience from a chiropractor associated with the National Upper Cervical Chiropractic Association (*www. nucca.org*).

Intriguing as this discovery is, Dr. Bakris says that for the moment, it is best to adopt a wait-and-see attitude. These single-center observations need to be confirmed with larger multicenter studies before a general recommendation for treatment can be made. To that end, two larger scale trials are being proposed to the National Institutes of Health, which is supportive of this work going forward.

Halt Climbing Blood Pressure Naturally

Louise Hawkley, PhD, senior research scientist, Center for Cognitive and Social Neuroscience at the University of Chicago.

C. Tissa Kappagoda, MD, PhD, director of the Coronary Disease Reversal Program, University of California, Davis School of Medicine, Sacramento.

Because it clearly is a risk factor for heart attack and stroke, high blood pressure (HBP) is typically treated aggressively with medication, which also means there is the potential for drug side effects and other risks. But researchers continue to cast a wider net in search of more ways to treat HBP or, better yet, keep it from developing. Two recent studies identified surprising factors that appear to affect HBP.

THE LONELY HEARTS CLUB

Focusing on the many ways loneliness leads to HBP, one study, from the Center for Cognitive and Social Neuroscience and the department of psychology at the University of Chicago, found that people who feel chronically lonely (more detail on that later in the article) had as much as a 30-point increase in their systolic blood pressure number (the upper figure in blood pressure measurement). The data was based on 229 randomly chosen people aged 50 to 68 of varied ethnicity. Each participant completed surveys and interviews and had their blood pressure (and other cardiovascular measures) tested over the course of the day they spent in the laboratory. Participants responded to questions about their lives and attitudes, including ones that revealed loneliness. After adjusting for known HBP risks, such as body mass index and smoking, the study found that loneliness was associated with increased systolic blood pressure.

Curious to know why researchers focused specifically on loneliness, we called Louise Hawkley, PhD, a senior researcher on the study. She says that this study, funded in part by the National Institute of Aging, emerged from a previous one the team did that showed young people who were lonely had increased vascular resistance—that is, their blood vessels over-constricted when they experienced stress. Younger adults can compensate for this constriction by slowing the output of blood—thus keeping pressure normal—but over time, the extra work involved in peripheral (vessels anywhere but the heart) vascular resistance decreases elasticity, starting a cascade of physiological changes. Dr. Hawkley explains that researchers wondered about the long-term effect of loneliness, theorizing that inflammation, atherosclerosis and HBP may result—hence, the study.

Dr. Hawkley points out that she and her colleagues aren't prepared to say that loneliness can cause HBP, but they are beginning to believe that loneliness itself—apart from depression or other factors that might accompany it—has a relationship to HBP. Knowing as we do that acute stress raises blood pressure, Dr. Hawkley says it is reasonable to assume prolonged stress (such as that experienced by lonely people) does as well.

DEFINING "LONELY"

It's important to remember that the kind of loneliness looked at in this study has nothing to do with being alone, emphasizes Dr. Hawkley. Researchers looked at how perceived loneliness affected people, rather than at their actual social support. Even while socializing, lonely people still perceive themselves as unconnected. They often find it difficult to form good relationships, either expecting too much of them or avoiding them in general, and they respond to life's challenges with stressful despair. She adds that the study team is continuing to collect and analyze the data, and in a few more years should know even more about the specific mechanisms of how loneliness contributes to HBP. But in the meantime, it seems evident that lonely people can benefit from therapy to learn how to get past their passive coping strategies and develop effective social skills. Overcoming loneliness, she says, is an important step, probably for blood pressure and definitely for life.

STUDY 2: GREAT "GRAPE" NEWS

In the second study, researchers in the division of cardiovascular medicine at the University of California, Davis, evaluated how grape seed extract might impact blood pressure. This study is part of a continuing investigation into the health properties of this extract, an antioxidant flavonoid useful in removing a harmful excess of free radicals from cells. The findings were impressive.

The study examined 24 people diagnosed with metabolic syndrome (having a constellation of symptoms including insulin resistance, abdominal obesity, elevated blood pressure and lipid abnormalities), and divided them into three groups. One group took 150 milligrams (mg) per day of the grape seed extract...another took double that dose (300 mg per day)...while the third group was given a placebo. Both groups taking grape seed extract had similar results—an average drop in systolic pressure of 12 points and in diastolic pressure of 8 points.

We spoke with C. Tissa Kappagoda, MD, PhD, University of California, Davis director of the Coronary Heart Disease Reversal Program at the School of Medicine in Sacramento, and author of the study, to learn more. Laboratory experiments had previously established that grape seed extract relaxes blood vessels, he says. Consequently, the study team is confident that this likely explains why it improves blood pressure in humans as well.

Note: The people studied belonged to a category of prehypertension (systolic blood pressure between 120 and 139 mmHg [a measure of pressure] and diastolic pressure between 80 and 89 mmHg). These people are not usually treated with medications. Instead, they are managed with lifestyle modifications (diet, exercise, stress management, etc.). Grape seed extract could be a part of such a regimen. It is not recommended for the treatment of hypertension. People with a diagnosis of hypertension should consult their physicians for appropriate treatment…and pregnant women and nursing mothers should consult their physicians for appropriate therapy.

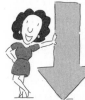

Supplement That Lowers Hypertension Risk by 46%

Michael Hirt, MD, former medical director, Center for Integrative Medicine, Encino-Tarzana Regional Medical Center, California, and associate clinical professor, University of California, Los Angeles (UCLA) School of Medicine. *www.drhirt.com.*

Folate, a B vitamin found in foods and also known as folic acid (the synthetic form used in supplements and fortified foods), has just earned another gold star. A study that evaluated the dietary habits of 150,000 women over an eight-year period showed that folic acid reduced their risk of developing high blood pressure.

The research, part of the ongoing Harvard Nurses' Health Study (Boston), evaluated women in two age groups—ages 43 to 70…and ages 23 to 44. Women in the younger group who consumed at least 1,000 micrograms (mcg) per day of folic acid in food and supplements had a 46% lower risk for hypertension (high blood pressure) compared with women whose daily intake was less than 200 mcg. In the older group, the risk was 18% lower. Women in both groups who consumed less than 200 mcg of folic acid in food per day but managed to increase the level to at least 800 mcg per day through supplements and foods showed a resulting decreased risk for high blood pressure of 45% in the younger group and 39% in the older group.

HOW FOLIC ACID WORKS

It's well-established that folic acid helps protect blood vessel health and that hypertension is most often a symptom of compromised vessel health. However, according to Michael Hirt, MD, medical director, Center for Integrative Medicine at Encino-Tarzana Regional Medical Center and associate clinical professor at the University of California, Los Angeles (UCLA) School of Medicine, folic acid's unique magic is in its ability to reduce dangerous *homocysteine levels.*

COPING WITH HIDDEN DANGERS

Nowhere do the study reports mention homocysteine, an amino acid in the bloodstream created by the liver. High levels of homocysteine may be related to genetic predisposition or to a deficiency in folic acid, B-12 or B-6. Homocysteine in elevated amounts damages blood vessel health and increases risk for stroke and heart attack. There are no symptoms that flag the presence of elevated homocysteine, and folic acid is the only thing that reduces homocysteine levels.

Consequently, to avoid the risks caused by elevated homocysteine levels and to lower your risk for high blood pressure, it is crucial to get plenty of folate on a regular basis. The good news is that even if you don't want to take a supplement, folate is easily available in foods, says Dr.

Hirt, especially in dark green, leafy vegetables such as spinach, kale, Swiss chard, romaine lettuce and others. It's also found in broccoli and cauliflower. Eat three or more servings a day of these. Many grain products are supplemented with folic acid, and virtually all multivitamins now contain 400 mcg of it.

Note: You should not take more than 1,000 mcg a day in supplements...however, you can eat any amount of it in foods without risk.

Men take note: Dr. Hirt says that men benefit equally from folic acid.

When you get your cholesterol checked, ask to have your homocysteine level tested as well. If you find that your level is high in spite of regular folate consumption, Dr. Hirt says this may reflect a problem with metabolizing it. Speak to a medical professional who is properly trained in nutritional supplementation about whether you need to supplement, and if so, by how much. High levels of folic acid supplementation have been linked to tumor growth, so you need proper guidance. Additionally, folic acid should be taken with B-12 and B-6 to be effective.

Prehypertension? What You Must Do Now

Adnan I. Qureshi, MD, director, cerebrovascular program, Stroke Center, University of Medicine and Dentistry of New Jersey, Newark.

In May 2003, a new medical condition was born. That's when the Joint National Committee on Prevention, Detection, Evaluation, and Treatment of High Blood Pressure issued its statement that blood pressure previously considered "high normal"—falling between normal at 120/80 to the start of high at 139/89—was now an official medical condition named *prehypertension*. At the time, doctors were not certain of how much of a health risk prehypertension might be, but they knew that it was important to monitor.

DEALING WITH THE NEW NORMAL

Now a new study reveals that prehypertension *dramatically* increases the risk of heart attack and heart disease. An analysis of data taken over 50 years from the long-term ongoing Framingham Study (Massachusetts) showed that participants with the condition were three times more likely to have a heart attack and 1.7 times more likely to have heart disease than people with normal blood pressure. The study's lead author, Adnan I. Qureshi, MD, director of the cerebrovascular program in the Zeenat Qureshi Stroke Research Center, University of Medicine and Dentistry of New Jersey in Newark, says that this finding undoubtedly lies behind many so-called "inexplicable" heart attacks suffered by seemingly healthy people. And it focuses on the possible need for more aggressive treatment for prehypertension than the previously advised lifestyle changes alone.

PREHYPERTENSION MEETS METABOLIC SYNDROME

However, it gets more complicated. Dr. Qureshi explains that the increased risk in the study may have to do not only with just prehypertension, but with a coming together of other early risk factors as well. During the 50 years of data this study analyzed, doctors had not identified metabolic syndrome—defined as having at least three of the five known cardiovascular risk factors (obesity, elevated blood pressure, elevated triglycerides, elevated blood sugar and low high-density lipoprotein [HDL] levels). It is probable that a number of prehypertensive participants likely had other early risks included in metabolic syndrome and that the grouping of early risk factors caused the heart problems. This study suggests that all prehypertension patients discuss their particular risk profile with their doctor for an overall evaluation. Those

15

with multiple risk factors may want to start a treatment program to normalize blood pressure as soon as possible.

Walk Away from High Blood Pressure

Janet P. Wallace, PhD, professor, department of kinesiology, Indiana University, Bloomington.

Surely everyone knows by now that regular exercise is vital in helping to prevent or control high blood pressure (hypertension). How much and how often, though, are questions that have been the subject of speculation and more than a few studies. Now comes one from the department of kinesiology at Indiana University and Indiana University Medical Center, Bloomington, with results that surprised even the study authors.

Researchers wanted to find out which is better for reducing prehypertension—continuous physical activity, in this case walking, or walking that totaled the same amount of time but was performed in short spurts.

Prehypertension is blood pressure that runs from 120 to 139 millimeters of mercury (mmHg/systolic) over 80 to 89 millimeters of mercury (mmHg/diastolic), which are under the official level of hypertension. They discovered that 40 minutes of walking, whether in one continuous outing or in frequent spurts for shorter periods of time, reduced blood pressure by a similar amount compared with control subjects (a 5.4 to 5.6 drop in systolic pressure, and a 3.1 to 3.4 drop in diastolic pressure). However, when the group took shorter, more frequent walks (four times a day, in this study) the effect lingered for 11 hours, versus only seven hours when the group performed continuous walking.

THE 45-MINUTE RULE

The study's co-author, Janet P. Wallace, PhD, says that both exercise groups did identical "work" (intensity)—whether it was continuous or broken up throughout the day. Participants walked at 50% of their capacity (or VO2 max, a measure of aerobic fitness), which is a moderate pace. "Brisk" walking is working at 70% of capacity, she says, but in treating blood pressure with exercise, the ideal is moderate intensity and longer duration—45 minutes is optimal and one hour is max, according to Dr. Wallace, since after an hour there is no further measured short-term benefit. (Anything over 60 minutes is affected by the law of diminishing returns...you do not get that much more out of working longer, she said).

Her advice, based on the study, is to do whatever fits best into your life—continuous or several briefer periods of activity in the day. And there's nothing magical about walking (other than how easily it can be done)...any kind of moderate intensity physical activity helps keep blood pressure down, she says. In a previous study her team discovered that even gardening and housework were helpful. The key is finding and doing activities that are easy for you to accomplish, and that you will do every day, be it 45 minutes on the treadmill at the gym or getting out of the house or the office every few hours for short walks outside.

Amazing Fresh Air Cures

Giuseppina Benincasa-Feingold, MD, Valley Health and Hyperbarics, Brewster, New York.

Harry T. Whelan, MD, professor of neurology, pediatrics and hyperbaric medicine at the Medical College of Wisconsin, Milwaukee.

Deep-sea divers have long known the benefits of hyperbaric oxygen treatment (HBOT)—a method for efficient delivery of pure oxygen—to treat those with the "bends," a condition that can occur when a diver rises to the surface too quickly. Changing pressure causes nitrogen gas bubbles to form in the lungs, tissues and bloodstream, leading to a potentially lethal blood flow blockage. Today, doctors use HBOT to treat a number of other conditions—carbon monoxide and cyanide poisoning, wounds that aren't healing properly, serious burns, soft tissue and bone infections, and certain complications from radiation therapy. While everyone agrees about the usefulness of HBOT for these conditions, there is another usage that is generating much debate—the practice of using HBOT to address neurological problems, including brain damage from strokes.

ABOUT HBOT

HBOT administers 100% oxygen (versus the 21% that is in the air we breathe) in a chamber with an air pressure considerably greater than the air around us. The pressure dramatically raises the number of oxygen molecules entering the bloodstream—by as much as 2,000%. The vastly increased oxygen level allows the oxygen to reach bone and tissue that it normally can't reach, where it may accelerate healing. The oxygen can also enhance functioning of white blood cells, the infection fighters, which may improve aspects of immune system function. It is the ability to heal tissue that has neurologists evaluating HBOT for use with stroke patients. Harry T. Whelan, MD, professor of neurology, pediatrics and hyperbaric medicine at the Medical College of Wisconsin, in Milwaukee, is leading a new study to determine the effectiveness of HBOT for acute stroke treatment.

OXYGEN AND STROKE

Dr. Whelan explains that an ischemic stroke—often caused by a blocked artery—kills some brain tissue that is deprived of oxygen. However, although the tissue in the surrounding area, which is called the ischemic penumbra, is starving for more blood, it continues to have at least some oxygen from nearby unblocked vessels, so this tissue continues to survive in an extremely delicate position. The

smallest change can kill it or, conversely, rescue it from destruction, potentially saving a great deal of the patient's future functioning. By using HBOT, concentrated levels of oxygen are rapidly delivered to the ischemic penumbra, helping to heal and improve blood flow to this precarious tissue as well as helping prompt formation of new blood vessels in the area. Dr. Whelan says that patients must receive therapy within 24 hours of the stroke and preferably within six to 10 hours. His institution has reviewed the medical literature and has started the pilot study.

HBOT FOR PREVIOUS STROKE DAMAGE

What about treatment for strokes that happened months or years ago? While logic would tell you otherwise, Giuseppina Benincasa-Feingold, MD, who has an HBOT center in Brewster, New York, has had success in treating these older injuries as well. The belief of those administering this HBOT is that the ischemic penumbra cells never die but remain idle, like Sleeping Beauty, waiting for something to revive them. (Dr. Whelan and others disagree, saying that the tissue cannot survive even days, to say nothing of months or years.) A pediatrician by training, Dr. Benincasa-Feingold became interested in HBOT when her then three-year-old daughter, who has cerebral palsy, took part in an HBOT study at New York-Cornell Medical Center. Her daughter showed rapid cognitive improvement, but when the study was completed, had no place to go for additional HBOT. Today, Dr. Benincasa-Feingold has a center in which she delivers HBOT to post-stroke patients as well as to children who have cerebral palsy or autism.

SURPRISING TIMING

When we spoke with Dr. Benincasa-Feingold, she explained that although common sense would indicate that using HBOT so long after the fact wouldn't work, she has seen real improvement with stroke patients —even six years post-stroke. Furthermore, she says that imaging techniques have shown the ischemic penumbra area of the brain light up when treated with hyperbaric oxygen many months and years later. Ideally, she agrees, treatment should take place immediately following the stroke, but that the possibility of improvement makes even later treatment worthwhile. She adds that it can't hurt (the only side effect seems to be popping in the ears, similar to take-off and landing in an airplane, and the main contraindication for treatment is for those on a few unusual medications) although it is admittedly costly and time consuming. Her protocol for stroke patients is 40 treatments given over four to eight weeks, and they run between $150 to $200 per treatment. As of now, insurance doesn't cover HBOT for stroke treatment.

info To discuss HBOT post-stroke therapy with a doctor, or for information about practitioners nationwide, go to *http://drcranton.com/hbo/find.htm.*

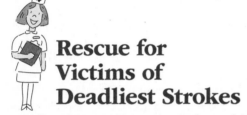

Rescue for Victims of Deadliest Strokes

Stephan M. Mayer, MD, associate professor of clinical neurology and neurological neurosurgery, Columbia University Medical Center, New York City.

Just 30 years ago, there was virtually no treatment for stroke. Those patients who didn't die often suffered great disability. Health-care professionals, having nothing to offer patients, took a what-can-you-do attitude. Since that time, numerous treatments for stroke, in particular ischemic stroke (by far the most common type and generally caused by blockages in the blood vessels), have developed and evolved. Awareness has also grown, and today, stroke victims who seek help immediately at the onset of symptoms often do quite well. But another type of stroke—one caused by intracerebral hemorrhage, or bleeding in the brain—has remained virtually untreatable.

While hemorrhagic strokes represent just 20% of all strokes (700,000 people suffer a stroke each year), about half the people who have one die from it. These are not to be confused with strokes caused by an aneurysm, a weakened artery wall that can eventually leak or even burst. Rather, they occur when a small blood vessel breaks and bleeds into the brain.

HOPE FOR THE DEADLIER STROKE

But at long last there is hope on the horizon for treating hemorrhagic stroke. It comes in the form of a product used to treat hemophilia, a blood clotting disorder. Hemophiliacs lack certain proteins in their blood called "factors" that are responsible for clotting. As a consequence, hemophiliacs do not form protective clots in response to internal or external triggers unless they are treated with the type of factor they are missing. One of the blood protein factors, *recombinant Factor VIIa* (referred to as rFVIIa), was dismissed for a long time by doctors because they thought it was unimportant in the clotting cascade. Ironically, it was discovered that rFVIIa is a *critical* initiator of clotting, and today it is the treatment protocol for hemophiliacs whose condition is particularly resistant.

HOW IT WORKS

This factor's key position in the clotting process, says neurologist Stephan Mayer, MD, at Columbia University Medical Center, gave him the idea that it might be an ideal agent for treating intracerebral hemorrhage. He thought that a dose of rFVIIa might supercharge a normal clotting system, and that the resulting clot would quickly staunch bleeding in the brain. Accordingly, he and his colleagues conducted a trial with 399 intracerebral hemorrhage victims at 73 sites in 20 countries. Some patients received placebos...others received varying strengths of the factor.

The results: In three months' time, patients receiving rFVIIa had a 38% drop in mortality compared with placebo patients. Survivors who took rFVIIa were three times more likely to avoid neurological damage as were placebo patients—24% versus 8%.

Although this has exciting implications for stroke treatment, the immediate concern is the risk for inducing clots elsewhere in the body, such as in a coronary artery. Dr. Mayer says that rFVIIa does indeed increase clot risk throughout the body, but the study showed only minor heart attacks and ischemic strokes from it—nothing compared with the catastrophic risk of the initiating stroke. In fact, he says, there are two much more important aspects to the treatment than the risk for thrombus (a clot forming in the bloodstream)—getting medical help in time, and obtaining optimum follow-up care.

PROPER CARE REQUIRED

To be effective, the patient must receive the dose of factor within four hours of the stroke's onset. Unlike ischemic strokes, which don't present with the same dramatic symptoms, hemorrhagic strokes come on quickly, generally with a ferocious headache followed by weakness, paralysis, numbness, loss of speech or vision and confusion. It is critical to be aware of these symptoms, call 911 immediately and be certain to describe the symptoms, says Dr. Mayer. Only that way can you get proper medical help quickly enough to possibly save your life and avoid disability.

But it gets tricky. Dr. Mayer explains that many emergency departments still do not have adequate equipment or trained staff for the initial treatment of stroke and for the follow-up care of those who survive the immediate danger. Bleeding in the brain, he says, is an incredible biological stressor. Although the factor stops the bleeding immediately and no follow-up is needed for that, the patient must have immediate intensive care, whether by a stroke team or a neurointensive team.

A number of hospitals have established themselves as stroke centers, with the necessary equipment, staff and ability to administer the latest forms of treatment. Call 911 immediately whenever a stroke is suspected, and insist that the ambulance go to the nearest major medical center to ensure the best care possible. Today, many stroke centers list themselves as such on the Internet, so familiarize yourself with those in your area.

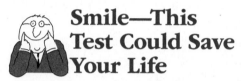

Smile—This Test Could Save Your Life

Gregory W. Albers, MD, professor of neurology and sciences, director of the Stanford University Stroke Center, Palo Alto, California.

American Stroke Association, *www.strokeassociation.org*.

American Heart Association, *www.americanheart.org*.

Time is everything when it comes to stroke. Following the onset of symptoms, there is a crucial three-hour window of opportunity in which the drug *alteplase* (Activase), a recombinant tissue plasminogen activator, can be administered to minimize damage to the brain. The problem is that few people actually receive this treatment because those around them do not always recognize what is happening, and the patient doesn't get to the hospital until after the window of time has closed.

RECOGNIZING THE SIGNS OF STROKE

Unfortunately, a lack of awareness can spell disaster. A stroke victim may suffer severe brain damage when warning signs aren't recognized.

Now a small study suggests that a simple three-part test can help bystanders determine if someone is having a stroke. *Here's how…*

S* Ask the individual to SMILE.

T* Ask the person to TALK...to speak a simple sentence coherently. (For example, "It is sunny out today.")

R* Ask him or her to RAISE both arms.

If he or she has trouble with any one of these tasks, call 911 immediately and describe the symptoms to the dispatcher.

A SIMPLE GUIDE

This test—which is also known as "The Smile Test"—is derived from study results presented at an International Stroke Conference by researchers from the University of North Carolina-Chapel Hill School of Medicine.

Gregory W. Albers, MD, professor of neurology and sciences and director of the Stanford University Stroke Center in Palo Alto, California, says that this is not "scientific" information, but rather "a simple guide" to help people remember how to test for several of the more common symptoms of stroke (facial weakness, speech problems and arm weakness).

EVERY SECOND COUNTS

Whether you choose to use the test or not, it is important to be aware of these common stroke warning signs, in yourself or in others...

•**Sudden numbness or weakness of the face,** arm or leg, especially on one side of the body.

•**Sudden confusion,** trouble speaking or understanding.

•**Sudden trouble seeing in one or both eyes.**

•**Sudden trouble walking, dizziness, loss of balance or coordination.**

•**Sudden, severe headache with no known cause.**

Review the Smile Test, remember it, and call 911 immediately if you or someone near you experiences any of the symptoms. As the American Stroke Association puts it, "Time lost is brain lost!"

Lower Your Risk of Stroke 26%

J. David Spence, MD, director, Stroke Prevention and Atherosclerosis Research Centre, Robarts Research Institute in London, Ontario, Canada and author of *How to Prevent Your Stroke* (Vanderbilt University).

Research is moving steadily forward on the challenge of rehabilitation after stroke—but it is much better to avoid a stroke altogether. Information on this has emerged from a report prepared at St. George's University in London. The report evaluated data from eight previous studies that tracked a total of 257,551 subjects for an average of 13 years.

The finding: People who ate three to five servings of fruits and vegetables each day had an 11% decreased risk for stroke. People who ate more than five servings each day had a 26% decreased risk.

J. David Spence, MD, director of the Stroke Prevention and Atherosclerosis Research Centre at the Robarts Research Institute in London, Ontario, notes that there are several important factors about fruits and vegetables as they relate to stroke prevention. First, eating a bounty of produce provides a high level of potassium—critical for regulating blood pressure as well as nerve and muscle activity—along with the numerous other important vitamins and minerals, especially calcium, magnesium and antioxidants. Dr. Spence reminds people to eat a variety of colored fruits and vegetables because the colors represent different antioxidants. As he says, Mother Nature is much better at combining antioxidants than any supplement could ever be. Various types of produce provide soluble fiber—part of what the body needs to properly manage cholesterol.

HEALTHFUL SUBSTITUTES

There is yet another consideration that Dr. Spence calls "the substitution issue." He points out that when you're eating five or more servings of fruits and vegetables each day, you are hopefully replacing fried and processed foods, trans fats and the like. Based on numerous studies, Dr. Spence recommends a Mediterranean diet, specifically from the Greek island of Crete. It includes olive oil, fish, beans and whole grains and, of course, lots of fresh fruits and vegetables. In fact, it's worth noting that in Crete people heap their plates with salad at lunch and dinner.

New Way to Regain Use of Limbs Affected By Stroke

Gitendra Uswatte, PhD, associate professor of psychology, associate director for research, Taub Therapy Clinic, University of Alabama at Birmingham.

I n a study at the Taub Therapy Clinic, University of Alabama at Birmingham, doctors restrained the good arm of 21 stroke patients ranging in age from 30 to over 85. The patients then participated in intensive therapy with the disabled arm six hours a day for 10 days over two weeks. At home during this period patients continued to keep their good arm restrained except for sleep. Amazingly, virtually all patients showed improvement in this short amount of time, some of them even regaining the ability to write with the affected hand. The therapy works for people who have suffered mild to moderate strokes even five or more years earlier.

MORE ABOUT THE RESEARCH

Gitendra Uswatte, PhD, associate director for research at the clinic and the study's coauthor, stresses that patients do not regain normal functioning, but he says that they do show a tremendous change from the therapy. Some who had started with their arm hanging uselessly at their side began to use it for spontaneous gestures as therapy progressed. In fact, Dr. Uswatte says that after the first week the patients were making so much progress they didn't seem to mind any frustration from the restraint. The object of the therapy is not muscle strength but neurological retraining to help recover motor skills, and researchers believe there are two reasons for its success. Data from neuroimaging studies support that the therapy rewires the brain. Additionally, Dr. Uswatte says it forces patients to break the habit of avoiding use of an impaired limb called "learned nonuse."

Would patients have even greater recovery with longer therapy? Dr. Uswatte says they haven't examined that thoroughly, but it appears this is all the time patients need to overcome nonuse of the limb and continued use of it is self-reinforcing. However, patients who can't use the affected limb for a time, for instance because of surgery, do lose the benefits and require retraining. "Use it or lose it," says Dr. Uswatte.

info For more information on restraint therapy at the Taub Therapy Clinic and for other clinics that offer it, go to *www.taubtherapy.com.*

New Brain Stents Help Prevent Strokes

Richard Klucznik, MD, director, Brain Aneurysm Center at the Methodist Neurological Institute, Houston.

W hile the statistics concerning stroke continue to be alarming—700,000 Americans a year have a stroke, and it is the country's leading cause of long-term disability—there are encouraging advancements in treatment and prevention. The most recent development concerns ischemic stroke, by far the most common type.

An ischemic stroke occurs when a carotid artery in the neck or an artery in the brain develops plaque buildup and a clot either breaks off or travels from another part of the body and cuts off blood flow into the brain. Plaque buildup in a brain artery is called intracranial disease, and until now, stroke-preventive treatment included aspirin or an anticoagulant medication to keep clots from forming...bypass on the affected artery...or opening the artery with a stent or an angioplasty balloon. The problem with the stent and balloon, though, was that the devices used were developed for coronary arteries and were therefore too stiff and large to work well in delicate brain arteries.

But the US Food and Drug Administration (FDA) has approved a stent that is specifically designed for the brain's fragile blood vessels. Called the Wingspan stent, it is both smaller and more flexible than coronary stents, and this enables interventional neuroradiologists to navigate it through the twists and turns of an artery, even deep within the brain, to position it to open the blockage. One of the doctors who has performed the delicate stent surgery is Richard Klucznik, MD, director of the Brain Aneurysm Center at the Methodist Neurological Institute in Houston.

CANDIDATES FOR WINGSPAN

Dr. Klucznik explains that people who are candidates for the Wingspan are those who have had a mini-stroke, called a TIA (transient ischemic attack). Symptoms of a TIA are similar to a full-blown stroke—numbness, confusion, and problems with speech, vision and balance—but they go away in minutes to hours. However, having a TIA is a red-flag warning of future stroke—one-third of TIA patients eventually have a major stroke. Dr. Klucznik says that anyone who suspects a TIA should go immediately to the hospital to be screened. If that shows plaque deposits in cranial arteries in the brain, the Wingspan may be the protection the patient needs from a future major stroke.

Implanting the Wingspan is no easy feat. Surgeons enter the femoral artery in the leg, just as they do for coronary angioplasty, to maneuver the device to the brain. Once the catheter has reached the blockage, a balloon attached to it cracks open the plaque formation, and the surgeon then puts the Wingspan in place to keep the artery open. Dr. Klucznik says it is theoretically possible that a piece from the cracked blockage could become a danger itself, but there has been no problem with it to date. In any case, he says the pieces would likely be too small to cause trouble.

RISKS VERSUS REWARD

While Dr. Klucznik is very confident of the effectiveness and safety of implanting the Wingspan, he stresses that using a doctor and hospital experienced with the procedure is critical to success. Going into the brain obviously requires highly skilled doctors, so be sure your surgeon has the experience required for the best outcome.

2

Amazing Breakthroughs in Cancer Care

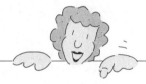

All Natural Cancer Helper Really Works

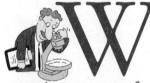**W**e are always on the lookout for new, interesting information on alternative or integrative treatments for health conditions, but something that sounds too good to be true can be a scam. That's why, when a report appeared in the highly respected newsletter *Alternatives* about a relatively new adjunct treatment for cancer called Avemar, we decided to check it out.

BACKGROUND ON AVEMAR

First, a bit of background. A defining characteristic of cancer is its uncontrolled metabolism and rampant cell division. Cancer cells really have only one function—proliferation. In the 1950s, a Nobel Prize-winning Hungarian scientist (named Albert Szent-Györgyi) made great strides in cancer research by examining how naturally occurring compounds could help control metabolism in cells, which in turn controls cell profileration.

Another Hungarian doctor built on Szent-Györgyi's work in the 1990s by showing that fermented wheat germ extract could achieve this effect. Avemar is a fermented wheat germ product.

AVEMAR'S EFFECTIVENESS

Avemar appears to have extraordinary abilities against cancer cells. "The pedigree on this stuff is pretty impressive," says *Bottom Line's Daily Health News* consulting medical editor Andrew L. Rubman, ND. "As of now there are more than 18 published studies in peer-reviewed journals, nearly all of them showing positive results. Research at the University of California, Los Angeles (UCLA) has demonstrated that Avemar reduces glucose flow

Andrew L. Rubman, ND, consulting medical editor for *Bottom Line's Daily Health News* and director of the Southbury Clinic for Traditional Medicines in Southbury, Connecticut.

into cancer cells, which inhibits their ability to reproduce."

Although no one is saying Avemar is a cure for cancer, it has been used as an adjunct to conventional therapies. It seems to be especially effective at reducing metastasis, or the spreading of the cancer to other sites throughout the body. "It seems that Avemar boosts immune system function sufficiently to allow the natural process of the body routinely killing cells to succeed much more effectively, " Dr. Rubman says. "It's conceivable that its ability to boost the immune system is the reason it is so effective at reducing the spread of cancer."

WHO SHOULD USE IT

Avemar is now being tested on patients with autoimmune conditions.

In Hungary, Avemar is an over-the-counter dietary supplement that is used by cancer patients in conjunction with other drugs. "In one pilot study in Budapest," Dr. Rubman notes, "a group of patients with advanced colorectal cancer were given Avemar and had no disease progression over nine months." And David Williams, MD, editor of *Alternatives*, has been quoted as saying, "There's absolutely no reason that Avemar shouldn't be used with every single cancer patient—particularly in those with severely impaired immune systems and those who are undergoing conventional therapies."

AVAILABILITY

Avemar isn't cheap, but its benefits seem substantial. It's available in this country under the name of Ave, and contains Avemar. It's sold through The Harmony Company, P.O. Box 93, Northvale, New Jersey 07447, at 888-809-1241 or on the Web at *www.theharmonyco.com*. It comes in packets and is taken as a drink once per day or as prescribed by your oncology team. Of course, don't take Avemar without your doctor's consent.

With such great immune-boosting benefits, can non-cancer patients benefit from Avemar, or even just plain wheat germ? Dr. Rubman says that eating wheat germ as a general immune booster can be good for many. As for taking Avemar prophylactically, if your health-care adviser believes that your immune system could stand improved function, Avemar may be a reasonable choice.

Antibody Works to Stop Cancer Before It Spreads

John J. Laterra, MD, PhD, research scientist, Kennedy Krieger Institute, Baltimore.

As therapy for many forms of cancer moves steadily forward, treatment for malignant gliomas, the most common primary brain tumor, has remained stubbornly complex and challenging. Standard therapy for cancerous gliomas includes one or all of the following, depending on tumor type—surgery, radiation and chemotherapy—and has a dismaying lack of success and can cause considerable brain damage, especially in children whose brains are particularly sensitive to these conventional therapies. Now, though, news comes of promising research that could profoundly affect treatment not only for gliomas but also for some more common cancers including breast, prostate and colon cancer.

ADAPTING CURRENT TECHNOLOGY FOR NEW USES

Monoclonal antibody (mAb) therapy for cancer involves administering a type of antibody that targets a specific growth factor protein responsible for stimulating certain kinds of cancer. The therapy is in use today to address a number of cancers including breast cancer. Recently, doctors at Kennedy Krieger Institute in Baltimore and Galaxy Biotech, LLC, in Mountain View, California, tested a new form of mAb—mAb L2G7. Researchers found mAb to be effective against hepatocyte growth factor protein (HGF), a trouble-making protein in gliomas.

Using live mice, the researchers administered L2G7 into the circulation and found that it induced tumor regression and dramatically increased survival. The animals in the control group receiving a similar but inactive type of mAb died within 41 days of starting the experiment…those treated with mAb L2G7 survived through day 70 with 80% of them remaining alive at day 90. To further test L2G7, researchers had waited to treat one group of mice until their tumors were advanced. Just three doses of L2G7 shrunk the large tumors to less than half their pre-treatment size.

Note: In pilot studies of this type, it is standard to monitor results at 90 days. If successful, the next step is then more expensive longitudinal studies. The difference in results between the control group and the test groups is very significant in this test and shows great promise for the future.

MORE RESEARCH NEEDED

We talked with the study's coauthor John J. Laterra, MD, PhD, a research scientist at Baltimore's Kennedy Krieger Institute, about this exciting development. Dr. Laterra says that in addition to attacking gliomas, mAb L2G7 will likely be useful to treat some breast, prostate and colon cancers because they, too, have the cancer-stimulating HGF protein. Furthermore, because HGF protects tumor cells in these cancers, adding L2G7 should enhance standard chemotherapy and radiation therapy as well. While the side-effect profile of L2G7 in patients is not yet known, it is expected to be well tolerated. Even if not completely side-effect free, it is anticipated that L2G7 will be a significantly better treatment for these cancer patients whether used alone or in conjunction with chemotherapy and/or radiation.

Results of human trials will determine if findings in mice hold up for people and provide answers to such questions as appropriate dosage and delivery methods.

Shedding Light on Blood Irradiation

Timothy C. Birdsall, ND, vice president, integrative medicine, Cancer Treatment Centers of America, Zion, Illinois.

Barrie R. Cassileth, PhD, Laurance S. Rockefeller Chair in Integrative Medicine, chief, integrative medicine service, Memorial Sloan-Kettering Cancer Center, New York City.

A technology that could potentially be an effective alternative treatment for cancer recently came to our attention. The technology in question is *photoluminescence* therapy, also known as ultraviolet blood irradiation.

WHAT IS PHOTOLUMINESCENCE?

Photoluminescence was first performed in the late 1920s. The basic procedure is similar today to what it was back then. Essentially, doctors withdraw a small sample of blood from a patient (the amount of blood is based on the weight of the individual), mix the blood with an anticoagulant and then expose the blood to ultraviolet light (a known way to kill viruses and bacteria). The blood, kept in an airtight container throughout the procedure, is then reinjected into the patient.

Early treatments were seen as a way to treat bacterial infections. (The first known use of photoluminescence was to treat a patient with a blood-borne bacterial infection—the infection reportedly cleared up within 24 hours.) Of course, the first antibiotic was being discovered at about the same time (penicillin was discovered in 1928), and, once further developed, those antibiotics quickly overtook photoluminescence as the treatment of choice. At that point, it seems that photoluminescence fell out of favor. The technology received little further scientific investigation.

CANCER READY?

So what about photoluminescence as a cancer treatment? Though there seem to be plenty of claims that photoluminescence is a viable treatment for cancer, our research turned up little to support the assertions.

One exception: In New Haven, Connecticut, Yale School of Medicine researchers have used UV exposure as part of a treatment called *transimmunization* for a certain type of lymphoma. This treatment is still being studied—and many photoluminescence-promoting Web sites mention this research as proof that photoluminescence works. However, transimmunization relies on UV light to activate a drug known as 8-MOP (which the patient has ingested) in a relatively complicated and time-consuming process—not the simple withdrawal and reinjection of the typical photoluminescence procedure. What's more, as mentioned above, transimmunization is noted as a potential treatment for cutaneous T-cell lymphoma, a relatively rare type of non-Hodgkin's lymphoma, and possibly other types of cancer.

A LACK OF EVIDENCE

Since we weren't having much luck finding solid photoluminescence research, we called some cancer experts to try to finally get some answers.

What we found: We were already on the right track.

"As a general rule, I'd say there's inadequate data to say that [photoluminescence] is an effective treatment for cancer," says Timothy C. Birdsall, ND, vice president of integrative medicine for Cancer Treatment Centers of America in Zion, Illinois. "Almost all of the data that was generated in the '30s and '40s really has to do with treating infectious processes, and it does appear that that approach would be very effective in that case." But, Dr. Birdsall adds, photoluminescence is invasive—blood has to be withdrawn and reinjected—plus it's not readily available, which means it has little chance of challenging the ease of taking an antibiotic pill three times a day.

According to Dr. Birdsall, the problem with photoluminescence as a cancer treatment is that, while the treatment can potentially boost the immune system, that boost would primarily be useful in a fight against bacteria and viruses, and wouldn't do much to fight cancer. Plus, it hasn't been studied in a clinical setting to see what, if any, kind of benefit it has.

"There's no such thing as a simple one-size-fits-all cure for cancer," Dr. Birdsall says, "and I get really concerned and more than a little suspicious when proponents of a particular therapy imply that it's the end-all, be-all therapy for all cancers."

Barrie R. Cassileth, PhD, chief of the integrative medicine service at the Memorial Sloan-Kettering Cancer Center in New York City, is even more skeptical. "These approaches spring up rather constantly, and there's just no data behind them," she says. "You can do a Google search on 'alternative' and 'cancer'—there are probably around 40 million hits these days—and you look at many of them and they're just selling absolute garbage. Patients need to be very vigilant."

OTHER OPTIONS

Of course, this shouldn't stop cancer patients from exploring their treatment options. Both Dr. Birdsall and Dr. Cassileth made recommendations in this regard.

One such recommendation, from Dr. Cassileth—clinical trials. "There are exciting new therapies that come along about every month," she says, "and some exciting advances that would have an infinitely better chance of doing something positive for the world, if not for that particular individual." Of course, clinical trials can be risky since the treatments are experimental, which means that information is not available regarding both effectiveness and risk. (For more on clinical trials, visit the National Cancer Institute's Web site, *www.cancer.gov,* and click on "Clinical Trials."

Another approach mentioned by Dr. Birdsall is called integrative oncology, which "utilizes the best of conventional treatment alongside intensive nutritional support, mind/body medicine, exercise and rehab, and intensive naturopathic remedies to enhance the effectiveness of the conventional treatment, reduce side effects and boost immune function."

"This requires a team approach to cancer care," warns Dr. Birdsall, "so that one therapy doesn't interfere with the efficacy of another therapy." Unfortunately, to be successful, it also requires an oncologist who is open to integrated treatments.

It seems like it's bad news concerning photoluminescence as a cancer treatment option, but luckily there are other possible avenues of help available.

Veggies Lower Risk For Non-Hodgkin's Lymphoma

Linda E. Kelemen, MSc, ScD, formerly with the department of health sciences research, Mayo Clinic College of Medicine, Rochester, Minnesota. She is currently with the Alberta Cancer Board in Calgary, Canada.

As if you needed one more reason to load up your plate with healthful veggies, a recent study indicates that a higher vegetable intake may lower the risk for non-Hodgkin's lymphoma (NHL). According to Linda E. Kelemen, MSc, ScD, formerly lead researcher and assistant professor of epidemiology at the Mayo Clinic College of Medicine in Rochester, Minnesota, disease-fighting antioxidants in foods such as broccoli and Brussels sprouts may have a protective effect against this dangerous lymphatic system cancer that will afflict 66,120 new people in 2008.

ABOUT THE STUDY

To determine the association between antioxidants in vegetables and fruits and the risk of developing this type of lymphoma, Dr. Kelemen and her Mayo Clinic colleagues examined the diets of more than 800 American adults with and without NHL. Normal, everyday living can create excess free radicals or oxidants that damage cells and may lead to cancer, explains Dr. Kelemen. She compares it with the development of rust on an unprotected car. Fortunately, eating antioxidant-packed vegetables and fruits protect against damage to cells—just like rust-proofing protects your car.

In the study, researchers found that...

• **People who ate the most vegetables a week** (20 or more servings) had a 42% lower risk for NHL than those who ate the fewest (eight or less servings).

• **Leafy greens such as spinach and green salad and cruciferous vegetables** (Brussels sprouts, broccoli, cauliflower, etc.) provided the greatest protection.

• **Two nutrients in particular, lutein and zeaxanthin** (high in leafy greens, spinach and broccoli), were singled out for their potent antioxidant action.

• **The mineral zinc** (common in certain nuts and seeds) also demonstrated a protective effect against NHL.

While researchers did not uncover any strong link between fruit intake and non-Hodgkin's lymphoma risk, Dr. Kelemen points out that the benefits of eating whole fruits to reduce the risk of other diseases is well known.

These findings were published in the *American Journal of Clinical Nutrition*.

EAT YOUR GREENS

When Dr. Kelemen was asked about dietary supplements, she responded that supplements do not contain the more than 100 antioxidants and phytochemicals found in fresh vegetables and fruit. If needed, they could be taken as an addition to—not as a replacement for—a healthy diet.

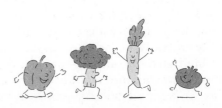

Too Much Bread Can Be Bad for the Kidneys

Francesca Bravi, ScD, a researcher at the Mario Negri Institute for Pharmacological Research in Milan, Italy. Dr. Bravi has published numerous research papers on the relation between cancer and diet.

I n 1981, epidemiologists estimated that "dietary factors" accounted for 35% of cancer deaths in the United States—roughly the same amount attributed to smoking at the time. In recent years, similar conclusions on diet and cancer have been reached by experts at the National Cancer Institute and the World Health Organization.

Now a new study from Italy adds another piece of data on the rapidly accumulating pile of evidence linking dietary choices with cancer risk. Researchers examined the food records of 2,301 Italians to see if they could uncover associations between certain foods and kidney cancer.

What they found was shocking: High bread consumption significantly raises renal cell carcinoma risk (kidney cancer).

"The association with bread consumption—which in Italy is mainly refined—may be due to the high glycemic index of refined cereals," Francesca Bravi, ScD, from the Mario Negri Institute for Pharmacological Research in Milan, Italy, and lead researcher on the study, says.

Note: In terms of this research, refined cereals mean pasta, rice and bread—not breakfast cereals. The glycemic index is a measure of how quickly blood sugar is raised after eating a food. When blood sugar is high, the body compensates by secreting a higher level of the hormone insulin, excess amounts of which may cause many problems. "It's possible that refined cereals may have affected the process of carcinogenesis by influencing the levels of insulin-like growth factors." Pasta and rice —other cereals that are known for having a high glycemic impact—also showed a relationship to kidney cancer, though not as strong a relationship as bread did.

"The highest quintile of bread eaters were consuming about 28 portions a week," Dr. Bravi explains. "At approximately four slices a day, these people had about twice the risk of getting renal cancer."

EAT YOUR FRUITS AND VEGGIES

While renal cell carcinoma accounts for only 2% of all cancers in adults, it's hardly the only cancer associated with diet...in particular, colon cancer has been shown in previous studies to have a major connection to diet. The Italian researchers also noted that vegetables had the strongest inverse association with the development of kidney cancer—the more vegetables you eat, the less risk of getting the disease. That correlation should come as no surprise to anyone. More than 200 studies have looked at the relation between diets high in fruits and vegetables, and the overwhelming bulk of them have found that eating plenty of them significantly lowers your chance of getting cancer.

There's a popular quote that is often repeated: "The whiter the bread, the quicker you're dead." It may be true.

Are You Getting Enough Sun?

Krispin Sullivan, CN, a Petaluma, California-based clinical nutritionist, has spent more than six years working with clients and researching the literature on vitamin D. She is the author of *Naked at Noon: Understanding the Importance of Sunlight and Vitamin D.* Basic Health.

Andrew L. Rubman, ND, consulting medical editor for *Bottom Line's Daily Health News* and director of the Southbury Clinic for Traditional Medicines in Southbury, Connecticut.

S ometimes it seems the more we learn, the more confused we get. Everyone "knows" you should avoid midday sun and always wear potent sunscreen. Or not? Numerous health experts are worried that we have turned into a nation (if not a world) of people suffering from deficiency of vitamin D—the sunshine vitamin. That's a serious issue because studies are emerging at a rapid rate that associate insufficient vitamin D with increased risk for many diseases.

The department of family and preventive medicine at the University of California, San Diego, published a study that showed a striking link between vitamin D deficiency and higher rates of cancer, specifically prostate, colon, breast and ovarian cancer. Another study from the Tufts-New England Medical Center in Boston, based on the long-term Nurses' Health Study (from Harvard in Boston), demonstrated that insufficient amounts of vitamin D and calcium may heighten the risk for type 2 diabetes. It also pointed out other studies that linked insufficient vitamin D to insulin resistance.

To find out more about this complex vitamin, we called nutritionist and writer Krispin Sullivan, CN, who has spent the last several years researching the literature on vitamin D, teaching clients how to get vitamin D safely, and has written a book about sunlight and vitamin D.

THE CHEMISTRY
OF VITAMIN D

Sullivan says that the vitamin D we make from sunlight or get from food and supplements is actually a prohormone from which our bodies produce *calcitriol*, the active form of vitamin D. The hormone calcitriol is one of the controllers of calcium in our bodies, which is why vitamin D is associated with rickets and osteoporosis. Recent research suggests this metabolite of vitamin D has other profound effects within our cells, regulating numerous cellular body functions, in processes in our skin, hair, muscles, bones and glands. Getting enough vitamin D is vital for good health—but there's a catch. Too much vitamin D is dangerous as well. Excess may cause bone loss, soft tissue calcification and other serious problems.

Deficiencies in children and adults can impair normal bone growth or strength (rickets, osteomalacia and osteoporosis). It is also associated with poor development or a decline in health of the jaw and teeth. In fact, getting enough vitamin D and calcium may prevent cavities and periodontal disease in young and old. Low levels of vitamin D are associated with many autoimmune diseases, obesity and many types of cancer, including breast and prostate. Getting enough vitamin D in later years has been shown to reduce fractures, maintain muscle mass, keep the immune system strong and improve memory and mood.

THE BEST SUN

The best and safest way to get vitamin D is through carefully regulated exposure to the sun, specifically to UVB rays, the rays of light that stimulate production of vitamin D in our skin. However, excess exposure to ultraviolet light, UVB or UVA is harmful. *Safe and effective sun exposure depends on the following factors...*

•**Location.** UVB decreases as latitude increases. Latitudes below 30 degrees (closer to the equator) have stronger UVB rays most of the day and most of the year. For example, Miami is 25 degrees North latitude, providing UVB most of the day and most of the year...New York is 40 degrees North latitude, with little UVB much of the day and year. Altitude also matters. The higher the altitude, the higher the intensity of UVB.

•**Time of year.** Vitamin D production in the skin requires the presence of sufficient UVB-containing sunlight. In most northern latitudes in the US, that's typically from late April or May until mid-August. Only Florida and some parts of Texas and Arizona, and some locations at higher altitudes have significant, nearly year-round, UVB. To make sunning for vitamin D worthwhile, the UV index really needs to reach 8 to 10. Lower UV index ratings require more exposure.

•**Time of day.** In most of the US the sun provides UVB primarily between the hours of 10:00 am and 2:00 pm, precisely the time most people are inside working or avoiding the sun for fear of sun damage. Yet this is when Sullivan recommends people be in the sun.

•**The amount of time exposed**—very fair-skinned people may need as little as five minutes (front and back), four or more times a week, without sunscreen. Melanin, the coloring agent in our skin, protects against UVB damage, but also increases the time needed to make vitamin D, so those with very dark skin or with suntans need more exposure to UVB to make adequate vitamin D (as much as 90 to 120 minutes a day), according to Sullivan. This could be nearly impossible for many busy people. How much is too much? If your skin turns pink, you've stayed too long.

•**The amount of skin exposed.** There is a substance in the skin, called pre-D, that is converted by UVB into cholecalciferol. The amount of pre-D is limited and genetically variable such that only so much vitamin D will be produced in any given skin area within a day. The more skin exposed, the more vitamin D produced. This means exposing small patches of skin for longer periods won't produce more vitamin D. Excess UV exposure, staying longer than you need to make your daily vitamin D, may actually begin degrading vitamin D that has already been produced. Sullivan advises exposing as much skin as possible, especially the back.

Vitamin A. It is also important for vitamin D to be in balance with vitamin A (which, like vitamin D, is converted into an active messenger, regulating cell functions), since the two work together in the body. Sunlight exposure depletes levels of vitamin A in the skin, a nutrient important for skin health and repair, so if you decide to sun it is especially important to get adequate vitamin A in your diet—in effect, sunning increases your need for vitamin A.

Sullivan advises eating liver—preferably beef, buffalo or venison liver—once a week to assure adequate vitamin A intake, but supplements can do the trick. According to *Bottom Line's Daily Health News* consulting medical editor Andrew L. Rubman, ND, typically, the 10,000 international units (IU) of vitamin A found in certain fish oil supplements will provide an adequate daily intake, if combined with sun exposure.

HOW MUCH VITAMIN D IS ENOUGH?

Ideally a person will get enough summer sun to meet vitamin D needs throughout the rest of the year simply by spending regular active time outdoors. Of course, in our decreasingly active society that spends an increasing amount of time in front of the computer or television, this is not the case for many. And, in reality, it is virtually impossible for most people to get enough vitamin D naturally.

Getting adequate levels of vitamin D is a particularly complex issue because the only food source with significant levels of vitamin D is the fat of fatty cold water fish and there is considerable disagreement among health professionals about how much vitamin D is safe, whether from supplements, food, the sun or in combination. The Dietary Reference Intakes (DRI) for vitamin D is 200 IU for people under age 50...400 IU for ages 51 to 70...and 600 IU for those over age 70. According to Sullivan's review of the literature, a number of medical professionals are now advocating a routine daily intake of 1,000 IUs of vitamin D for everyone except infants.

If supplementation is appropriate, there are several considerations...

How much is right? The highest safe amount (upper limit of safety, or UL, from the DRI group) is currently considered to be 2,000 IU a day. Sullivan firmly disagrees with the higher figure for most people. Vitamin D stores in fat and builds up over time. An initial high dose may be quite safe for many months, even a year or longer, but then rapidly increases blood levels of vitamin D to levels that may contribute to deposition of calcium in soft tissues, bone loss or heart disease. These changes may take place even when blood levels of calcium remain within normal range. She believes a safer dose would be between 800 and 1,200 IU daily.

Regular testing. Tracking levels of 25(OH)D (25-hydroxy vitamin D) should occur on a regular basis over a long period of time. The safest bet is to work with a trained, licensed health-care professional willing to monitor vitamin D and only supplement vitamin D under his/her watchful eye. The challenge is that vitamin D levels move up and down slowly, over time, and it takes having vitamin D levels tested every three or four months for a clear pattern to eventually emerge and give you information about whether your sun exposure or supplementation is producing the vitamin D level you need. Insurance may cover the cost of the first test, but will probably not cover subsequent tests.

Colon Cancer 90% Curable— So Get the Test!

Thomas F. Imperiale, MD, professor, department of medicine, Indiana University School of Medicine, Indianapolis.

When it comes to cancer—any type of cancer—early detection saves lives. Although colon cancer screening rates are on the rise, some sources estimate that nearly 41 million Americans age 50 (when screenings should generally start) and older have not been screened appropriately. That's a shame, because not only is colon cancer the third leading cause of cancer death in the US, it's also very easy to screen for and highly treatable. The disease is curable more than 90% of the time if caught in its early stages—meaning the number of deaths associated with the disease (an estimated 50,000 in 2008) could drop dramatically, if only more people would get screened.

NO PLEASANT OPTION

The problem is, of course, that screenings for colon cancer aren't exactly pleasant. Noninvasive screenings, such as the fecal occult blood test (FOBT), the immunochemical fecal occult blood test (I-FOBT, also called FIT) and the stool DNA test require that you collect a feces sample of varying sizes depending on the test. With the invasive screenings (either colonoscopy, which examines the entire colon, or sigmoidoscopy, to examine the last segment of the large intestine), a flexible tube containing a light, a small camera-like device and a means to remove lesions is inserted in your rectum so the doctor can visually examine the tissues of the colon and take biopsies or remove precancerous polyps. Typically, these procedures require unpleasant preparation, including a restricted diet and laxatives, in addition to sedation during the procedure (for colonoscopy). A relatively new option— "virtual colonoscopy"—is noninvasive, but still requires the unpleasant cleansing preparation. Plus, reports vary on the efficacy of the test itself, not to mention that if there are any findings at all, you will need to undergo a colonoscopy anyway. And finally, another option—the double contrast barium enema—enables visual examination of the entire colon with a series of x-ray images. This, too, requires an enema beforehand, and the test could potentially miss smaller polyps.

WHICH IS "BEST"?

The colonoscopy remains the gold standard test. However, according to Thomas F. Imperiale, MD, professor of medicine at the Indiana University School of Medicine in Indianapolis, of the available noninvasive tests, the I-FOBT is likely the best option for most people who are not considered at high risk for colon cancer, both because of its specificity (the test measures antibodies to human blood in the stool, not the presence of blood itself, so it isn't thrown off by red meat or tricky foods), as well as for its simplicity.

As many as 25% of colon cancers are thought to have a genetic basis, so genetic counseling (available at most major cancer centers) might be an option to consider if you have a family history of the disease. People with a higher than average risk of colon cancer should begin screening earlier than age 50 (discuss this with your doctor) and/or have more frequent screenings. *Here is a list of factors that put you at higher risk for colon cancer...*

•**Personal history of colorectal cancer or adenomatous polyps** (which probably means you have had a colonoscopy at least once before).

•**Personal history of chronic inflammatory bowel disease.**

•**Strong family history of colorectal cancer or polyps** (first-degree relative, which means a parent, sibling or child younger than age 60, or in two first-degree relatives at any age).

•**A known family history of hereditary colorectal cancer syndromes.**

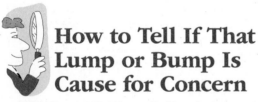

How to Tell If That Lump or Bump Is Cause for Concern

Ellen Warner, MD, MSc, medical oncologist, associate scientist, Odette Cancer Centre, Ontario, Canada.

Childhood is full of lumps and bumps as kids jump, climb, leap— and, yes, fall. But as people grow up and slow down, lumps and bumps become more unusual so any appearance of one can be cause for alarm. Why that peculiar lump on my arm? Why do the glands in my throat seem bigger today? What's the bump on the back of my neck? In truth, lumps and bumps are almost never anything to worry about. But that said, some are definite cause for concern and should prompt a call to the doctor because certain lumps and bumps might signal one of several types of cancer. How do you know what's what? When to worry and when to ignore it and wait for it to go away?

LYMPH NODES ARE KEY

Ellen Warner, MD, who is a medical oncologist and researcher at the Odette Cancer Centre in Ontario, Canada, says the type of lump or bump (or in this case actually a swelling) that is the most common cause for concern has to do with lymph nodes. These nodes exist throughout the body and in numerous locations—the head and neck, under the arms, in the chest and abdomen, in the groin area and in the legs. They also appear in approximately the same place on either side of the body. Lymph nodes are part of the body's immune system and swell in response to any type of infection and inflammation as part of their role in helping to fight it off or resolve it.

However, if a node swells and stays swollen on just one side or in several lymph nodes, and if there is seemingly no reason, such as a sore throat or other recent illness, Dr. Warner cautions that it must be checked out. Cancer of the lymph nodes (as opposed to cancer that metastasizes to nodes from another location) can be one of two types—Hodgkin's or non-Hodgkin's lymphoma. Dr. Warner explains that the difference between the two mostly has to do with cellular structure that shows up under the microscope. But they also have different survival rates. Hodgkin's is the more curable of the two with an 85% survival rate while the non-Hodgkin's rate is 60% after five years. This year it is estimated that there will be about 8,200 cases of Hodgkin's lymphoma diagnosed in this country as opposed to approximately 66,120 of non-Hodgkin's lymphoma diagnosed in the same year. Hodgkin's tends to be more common between ages 15 and 34 and at age 60 and over, though non-Hodgkin's is more common in older adults, 50 plus, and people who have compromised immune systems.

What to watch for: A considerable (not slight) swelling in a lymph node that may or may not be tender or possibly painful on one side, or in several lymph nodes, especially in the neck, and less commonly in the armpits or groin, when there has been no recent illness. Usually the swelling is under the chin, along the side of the neck. While there is no way to detect internal swelling of lymph nodes, there are symptoms such as itching, fatigue, coughing, fever, night sweats, weight loss and chest or abdominal pain, says Dr. Warner.

CANCEROUS BUMPS

Another frightening but even less common cause of dangerous lumps and bumps is cancer of connective tissue, a form of sarcoma called soft-tissue sarcoma. Fortunately, this type of cancer is extremely rare, accounting for less than 1% of malignancies diagnosed in this country each year. However, it can appear in numerous places in the body and is subclassified according to which soft tissue it develops. Do not confuse soft tissue sarcoma with fatty nodules called lipomas, which are benign. These are extremely common, usually appearing just under the skin in the arms, legs and trunk of the body.

Dr. Warner says lipomas are generally round and smooth with what she calls a roly-poly feel to them…they grow slowly and can become quite large, even several inches in diameter, and they are not malignant. Soft tissue sarcomas, on the other hand are almost always malignant and the tumor can grow quickly, most often appearing on the limb. But, it can show up on the abdomen or in other parts of the body as well, including the head, neck and trunk.

What to watch for: A sudden swelling that may or may not be tender or painful, beneath the surface of the skin, usually over a fairly large and diffuse area and a lump that does not have distinct borders. Do not hesitate to see a doctor immediately since the survival rate for soft tissue

sarcoma that is diagnosed while the tumor is still small and shallow is over 80%.

CANCER PATIENTS PAY ATTENTION

Finally, Dr. Warner says that anyone who already has cancer should be alert for any lump or bump that appears elsewhere on the body seemingly unrelated to the primary site. As is true with any mysterious lump or bump—one that cannot be explained for ordinary, everyday reasons such as a recent infection or fall—go to the doctor and insist on getting it checked, especially if it seems to grow quickly or change character, or becomes itchy.

No need to panic. Just be aware of your body and its changes. Careful observation can make a big difference in the long run.

Soothing the Side Effects of Chemotherapy

Matthew D. Bauer, LAc, has practiced acupuncture for more than 20 years. He is a regular contributing columnist to *Acupuncture Today*, and formerly served on the executive committee of the California Acupuncture Association. His practice is in La Verne, California.

Nausea and vomiting are two of the most dreaded side effects of chemotherapy. Considering that the cure can sometimes feel worse than the cancer it is meant to treat, some patients even elect to discontinue treatment. Although recent advances in antinausea and antivomiting medications have helped many cancer patients, the search for additional and more natural methods of relief for these hard-to-tolerate side effects continues. One method that was recently studied is acupuncture.

STUDY PINPOINTS WHAT WORKS

Can acupuncture reduce chemotherapy-induced nausea and vomiting? The Chinese healing method has been successfully used to treat a wide variety of ailments, including temporomandibular joint disorder (TMJ), drug addictions, alcoholism, allergies and back pain. It works by stimulating prescribed anatomical sites on the body.

In a review of 11 studies of acupuncture and its effects on chemotherapy-induced nausea and/or vomiting, the Cochrane Collaboration, an international organization that evaluates medical research, found a mixed bag of results, depending upon which acupuncture method was used and for which side effect.

A REVIEW OF THE FINDINGS

Electro-acupuncture (in which a small electrical current is passed through the needle) helped reduce vomiting during the first 24 hours after chemotherapy.

Traditional manual acupuncture using needles was not shown to be significantly effective for acute vomiting or nausea severity (within 24 hours of treatment).

Based on similar principles, but using (highly trained) fingertip pressure on acupuncture points, "acupressure" was looked at as well. This method showed no benefit for vomiting, but did reduce acute nausea—although it was ineffective for delayed nausea (after 24 hours of treatment).

It is unclear why electro-acupuncture reduced acute vomiting while needles-only acupuncture did not, or why one method was successful with nausea while another was successful for vomiting. Of note is that all participants in all the trials reviewed were taking antivomiting drugs, so additional research is needed to determine whether acupuncture alone is effective, or whether it should be considered an effective adjunct to medications.

EXPERT OPINION

Surprised by these findings, we asked acupuncturist Matthew D. Bauer, LAc, a former member of the Board of Directors for the California Acupuncture Association and a practicing acupuncturist in La Verne, California with more than 20 years experience, about these findings. In his view, it's hard to standardize this sort of study enough to make the findings meaningful. "So much depends on the practitioner's skill in placing needles at just the right angle in just the right place," he said. "In looking at this many trials, you're obviously dealing with many practitioners at varying levels of skill and experience, which, of course affects outcomes."

Acupuncture, he says, can be helpful in many ways for people undergoing treatment for cancer. It's worth a try since there's little risk and much potential benefit. It's important to work with a seasoned practitioner who has experience with oncology patients. And, of course, all cancer patients should check with their doctors before adding acupuncture or any other treatment to their cancer protocols.

3

Outstanding Techniques To Manage Your Diabetes

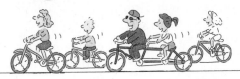

A Monster of a Diabetes Drug

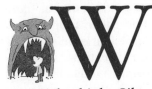

What in the world does a poisonous lizard have to do with diabetes? More than you might think. Gila monsters—one of the only two known venomous lizards in the world—produce a hormone in their saliva that has been a useful tool in the development of a new drug for the management of type 2 diabetes. Researchers isolated a hormone found in the saliva of the Gila monster and developed a new synthetic medication based on it called *exenatide injection* (Byetta).

But like all medications, it has its pros and cons.

First are the pros. "Byetta works similarly to a naturally produced substance in the body called GLP-1—glucagon-like peptide," says David M. Nathan, MD,

from Massachusetts General Hospital and Harvard Medical School (both in Boston). "GLP-1 increases insulin secretion and was discovered in the 1980s as a possible new way to help type 2 diabetics secrete more insulin. But the problem with GLP-1 was that they were degraded in the body so quickly that you had to give them intravenously."

HOW IT WORKS

Enter the gila monster. A hormone in the saliva of the gila monster was found to have a similar structure to GLP-1, and by producing a synthetic form of the hormone, researchers developed Byetta. "Byetta has a high degree of similarity to GLP-1," Dr. Nathan notes. "It increases insulin production and secretion."

David M. Nathan, MD, director of the General Clinical Research Center and of the Diabetes Center at Massachusetts General Hospital, and a professor of medicine at Harvard Medical School, both in Boston. He is also chairman of the Diabetes Prevention Program, a National Institutes of Health sponsored multicenter trial to prevent type 2 diabetes.

The type 2 diabetic has the ability to make insulin—but it isn't enough to lower blood sugar effectively because the cells are resistant to it. Doctors treat this with two main strategies—one is to increase insulin secretion or to give insulin by injection to meet the higher demands…and the second is to lower the resistance of the cells so that the amount of insulin produced is enough to get the job of lowering blood sugar accomplished. These two strategies are not mutually exclusive—some diabetic medications help lower glucose produced by the liver and reduce insulin resistance—*metformin* (Glucophage)—while others, a class called *sulfonylureas*, which includes Glucotrol and Micronase, help the body release more insulin. Byetta is in the latter category, stimulating insulin production and secretion. Byetta also appears to slow stomach contractions, delaying the absorption of food, which also helps to lower blood sugar levels.

THE WHOLE PICTURE

But there are also cons. "The problem is that you have to inject it twice a day and people are squeamish about doing that," Dr. Nathan says. "And compared with insulin, it's less effective at lowering blood sugar." Nonetheless, Byetta also modestly lowers weight, typically about five to eight pounds over six months, which is a big plus for a lot of people. "This is the opposite effect of insulin," Dr. Nathan points out, which usually increases weight.

The other problem with Byetta is nausea, diarrhea and vomiting. "About 40% of people experience nausea or diarrhea," Dr. Nathan explains. Byetta comes in only two doses—high and low. "The high dose is associated with greater weight loss," but it's also associated with more stomach upset.

"As an injectable drug we have to be careful not to confuse Byetta with insulin, which is far more effective at lowering blood sugar," Dr. Nathan concludes. "But there may be a population of patients for whom Byetta—or a combination of Byetta and other medications—may be useful."

Stop Diabetes Before It Starts

Michael Hirt, MD, former medical director, Center for Integrative Medicine, Encino-Tarzana Regional Medical Center, California and associate clinical professor, University of California, Los Angeles (UCLA). *www.drhirt.com.*

There are some illnesses that it seems you just "can't help." Then there are some that can be helped but require commitment on the part of the sufferer. Such is the case with type 2 diabetes. It is also the case with prediabetes, which affects nearly 60 million Americans, in which a person has elevated glucose levels but is not yet classified as diabetic. Much to the frustration of doctors, many people dismiss the impact of diabetes because some of its risks, including kidney failure, blindness, amputation and death, are felt in the long term, not in the short term.

While diabetes is definitely no fun to live with, it is often very manageable. There are a number of medications for diabetes, and many patients have progressed to the point that they must take them, but there are also vitamins and other supplements that address the particular problems. We reviewed the protocol for these with Michael Hirt, MD, former medical director of the Center for Integrative Medicine at Encino-Tarzana Regional Medical Center, California.

FREE RADICAL ATTACK

The main issue for people with diabetes is that high blood sugar levels cause dysregulated oxidative reactions in the body. This process can accelerate internal aging, resulting in such things as more rapidly hardening arteries and increased cardiovascular disease risk. To combat the free radicals contributing to this oxidation, it is necessary to take more antioxidants than diet alone commonly provides. Dr. Hirt recommends 1,000 milligrams (mg) a day of vitamin C (the long-acting one that lingers in the system) also known as Ester-C...and 200 mg to 300 mg a day of alpha-lipoic acid. This little known antioxidant is one of the most powerful, in part because it is the only one that can deactivate free radicals in both fat and water, giving much more bang for the buck. Studies show that alpha-lipoic acid has beneficial effects on the long-term nerve damage that often occurs in diabetes. Research also suggests that it helps improve insulin sensitivity.

EAT AND DRINK WISELY

A surprising aid to helping stabilize blood sugar is undoubtedly in your kitchen already—cinnamon. Dr. Hirt reports that researchers discovered this while testing people with diabetes to see how common foods affected their blood sugar levels. For some reason, patients' sugar levels didn't rise as anticipated when they ate apple pie. Ultimately, the researchers found that it was the cinnamon in the pie that helped prevent a rise. He recommends having one-half to one teaspoon a day, sprinkled over cereal, yogurt, fruit or other food or beverages of your choice.

Dr. Hirt adds that tea made from an ayurvedic herb called *Gymnema silvestre* seems to lower blood sugar and help pancreas cells work more efficiently.

MANAGING WEIGHT

An ongoing problem for diabetics is weight. One reason, of course, is that excess weight is a risk factor for developing the disease. In fact, 80% of people with diabetes are overweight. But as a double whammy, insulin—used to treat diabetes—can cause weight gain. Dr. Hirt says that he hasn't seen anything surefire to address this problem, but chromium picolinate may help. Being deficient in chromium, a trace element, can cause insulin resistance and increase blood glucose. According to the USDA Human Nutrition Research Center, diabetics who are chromium deficient significantly reduce fasting blood glucose levels by taking chromium picolinate. There are actually other more efficient delivery systems for chromium than the

picolinate salt used in research. Consult your naturopathic physician or pharmacologist for other options for you.

Always discuss every medicine you take or are considering with your physician. Doctors must have this overview information in general, and in the case of diabetes, it is especially critical.

The reason: One substance might offset or enhance the effectiveness of another and at the very least your doctor may want to alter the dosages of your medication or supplementation. Be aware that diabetics should also avoid taking unprescribed glucosamine, a popular supplement used as a remedy for osteoarthritis. According to a report from the National Institutes of Health National Center for Complementary and Alternative Medicine presented at the 2004 American Diabetes Association meeting, glucosamine can make insulin resistance worse.

Dr. Hirt also strongly urges those with diabetes to make any necessary changes in lifestyle to bring about better health. He explains that diabetes is a disease of poor nutrition and lack of exercise—both situations that people have the power to turn around. Eat well, exercise regularly, take your multivitamin once a day in addition to the other supplements you need and, he says, you should be able to greatly improve or even eliminate adult-onset, or type 2 diabetes.

Coffee Dramatically Drops Diabetes Risk

Rob M. van Dam, PhD, assistant professor, department of nutrition, Harvard School of Public Health, Boston.

Recently, coffee has been linked to a reduced risk for liver cancer. There is more good news for latte lovers from researchers at the Harvard School of Public Health (HSPH)—they found that people who drink coffee on a regular basis experience a substantially lower risk for type 2 diabetes.

These findings appeared in the *Journal of the American Medical Association* (JAMA).

ABOUT THE STUDY

In a retrospective review of nine studies of coffee consumption and type 2 diabetes risk, Harvard researcher Rob M. van Dam, PhD, and his colleagues in Boston looked at 193,473 regular coffee drinkers who experienced 8,394 cases of type 2 diabetes. They excluded from consideration studies that involved type 1 diabetes, animals or short-term exposure to coffee or caffeine.

Next, researchers calculated the relative risk of type 2 diabetes in relation to how many daily cups of coffee the participants consumed. *It turned out that the more coffee, the better...*

•**The risk for diabetes was lowest in people who consumed the most coffee each day (six or more cups).**

•**Those who drank four to six cups daily also faced a lower risk for diabetes** (about 30% reduction in risk) as compared with people drinking little or no coffee.

These numbers did not differ significantly according to sex, obesity or geographic region (which in this case meant the US and Europe). However, Dr. van Dam adds that the results were rather diverse in the lowest consumption category. He would not be surprised if future studies that are able to measure coffee consumption more precisely find a lower diabetes incidence for any amount of coffee.

MORE COFFEE, LESS DIABETES

These current findings serve to underscore the results of an earlier HSPH study in 2004, in which men who drank more than six cups of coffee a day reduced their risk of type 2 diabetes by more than 50% in comparison with men who did not drink coffee...and women by 30% in comparison with women who were not coffee drinkers. This beneficial effect was observed independent of lifestyle choices such as smoking, exercise and obesity.

Scientists don't know exactly how coffee cuts diabetes risk. Paradoxically, caffeine reduces insulin sensitivity and raises blood sugar in the short term—both no-nos for diabetes. However, Dr. van Dam emphasizes that coffee is a complex beverage that contains numerous chemical compounds and minerals, which may have both helpful and harmful impacts on the body. Components other than caffeine—such as the antioxidants chlorogenic acid and magnesium—actually improve sensitivity to insulin and thus help lower diabetes risk. In animal studies, *trigonelline* and *lignans*, also found in coffee, improved glucose levels. Dr. van Dam adds that additional studies on effects of coffee components in humans are clearly needed.

WHAT ABOUT DECAF?

For those of us who prefer decaf, coffee still packs some protection against type 2 diabetes. Although the effect appears to be more modest, some of this discrepancy may be attributed to study limitations. Decaffeinated coffee consumption was substantially lower than caffeinated coffee consumption, and this may have affected the estimates, explains Dr. van Dam. He points out that it is easier to detect larger contrasts in consumption than smaller differences. In addition, one can expect some misclassification when you ask for the amount of coffee people consume (change over time, differences in strength and cup size, etc.).

Dr. van Dam notes that in a recently published study on coffee consumption and C-peptide concentrations (a marker for insulin resistance), the association was actually similar for decaffeinated and caffeinated coffee consumption. He adds that it is currently unclear whether caffeine has detrimental effects on insulin sensitivity over the long term, because only short-term studies have been conducted. Nor is it clear if non-coffee sources of caffeine would have similar effects.

THE JOLT OF JAVA

Other trials have already lined up in coffee's favor, demonstrating that it can lower the risk of liver problems, gallstones, colon cancer and Parkinson's disease. Of course, there's also a downside to coffee (which pregnant women, children and people with colitis, hepatitis and other dietary challenges should not drink), such as jitteriness, insomnia and a rapid heartbeat. (Coffee stimulates liver function, which in healthy people is fine in moderation, but those with active liver disease may experience a worsening of symptoms when they consume coffee.)

Promising as it seems, Dr. van Dam and his colleagues do not go so far as to recommend drinking coffee to prevent type 2 diabetes. They emphasize that while coffee consumption may contribute to the reduction of risk for diabetes, it cannot replace the myriad health benefits of diet, exercise and weight management.

Many people stop drinking coffee because they think this is good for their health. Now coffee drinkers can take comfort in knowing that their daily jolt of java not only gets them up and moving, it also provides a health benefit.

Weight Loss a Big Help For Those With Diabetes

Mark H. Schutta, MD, medical director, Penn Rodebaugh Diabetes Center, University of Pennsylvania Health System, Philadelphia.

In study after study we learn more about how chronic diseases overlap and how one can lead to another. This is especially true of diabetes, which for many people is followed by kidney and/or cardiovascular disease and often other problems. While adequate control of diabetes requires careful monitoring of blood glucose levels to keep them as close to normal as possible, a new study indicates that the amount of fat people have in their cells may also be a key factor in preventing diseases related to diabetes.

FAT KILLS CELLS

One of the critical elements in scientific research of disease is the concept of cell death (apoptosis). All cells die but not all die as planned. This is especially evident in cancer cells, where cancerous cells do not die like "normal cells."

Scientists at Washington University School of Medicine in St. Louis investigated the role excess fat might have in the process of cell death. They discovered through studying cells in culture tissues and in rodents that cells can become overloaded with saturated fat and this situation results in an overproduction of the protein EF1A-1. This protein is abundant and normal in the body and indeed necessary for a number of cellular activities including protein synthesis and maintaining the cell's internal support structure.

However, when EF1A-1 increases substantially, as it does in the presence of excess cellular fat, it appears to turn on the cells and cause them to die.

The theory that has emerged from these studies is this: If insulin-producing cells in the pancreas are jammed with too much saturated fat (and so too much EF1A-1), these vital pancreatic cells end up dying. This likely contributes to the development of diabetes. Additionally, this study suggests that the same pattern of cell death takes place in cardiac muscle cells when they have a concentration of saturated fat and this might well contribute to the association of diabetes and cardiac disease.

NEED MORE RESEARCH

We called endocrinologist Mark H. Schutta, MD, medical director of the Penn Rodebaugh Diabetes Center at the University of Pennsylvania Health System in Philadelphia, to discuss the studies. He describes the information from them as interesting and intriguing, but he adds that until we have additional research to back this up, the theory of saturated fat-induced protein causing apoptosis remains speculative.

Of course, just because there is more research to be done, that doesn't mean it isn't a warning signal worthy of heeding. Dr. Schutta observes how this study underscores once again the ill effects of obesity and the dangers of the typical American diet. The study team used the saturated fatty acid palmitate in the research—the major component of palm oil and one of the most common saturated fats in processed foods.

Among his patients, Dr. Schutta says, there are some who are genetically predisposed to insulin problems, but there are many others whose diets are a strong contributory factor. He estimates that although his entire patient group receives extensive information and advice about weight loss and a healthful lifestyle, only 10% to 20% of patients actually go on to make these changes.

FEWER POUNDS, SO MANY BENEFITS

Admittedly, losing weight is especially difficult for people with diabetes—the disease itself predisposes people to excess weight because diabetes makes it more difficult to metabolize fats efficiently. Nevertheless, it is of the utmost importance for people with diabetes and those who have become insulin resistant to lose weight. Weighing less improves metabolism of fats, insulin sensitivity and can even lower blood pressure. Being lighter also increases energy, which in turn makes exercising easier.

Interestingly, it doesn't take a lot of weight loss to improve health among people with diabetes. Dr. Schutta says that his patients assume when he tells them they need to lose weight that he is recommending they get back to what they weighed in their youth. But in fact, this isn't so. A weight loss of just 5% to 7% of a person's current weight is all that is necessary to make a substantial difference. This holds true for both those considered obese, with a body

mass index (BMI) of 30 or above, and those with the all-too-typical extra 10 pounds to lose. This doesn't require any kind of dramatic dieting—just a healthful approach that includes protein, fruits (though no fruit juice because of its high sugar content), vegetables and whole grains—and getting rid of those saturated fats.

Statin Drugs Saving Lives for Diabetics

Jay S. Cohen, MD, associate professor (voluntary) of family and preventive medicine, University of California, San Diego. Dr. Cohen is author of *What You Must Know About Statin Drugs & Their Natural Alternatives* (Square One) and *Over Dose: The Case Against the Drug Companies* (Tarcher/Putman). Visit his Web site at *www.medicationsense.com*.

People with type 2 diabetes sometimes feel like they are between a rock and a hard place. They are at high risk for cardiovascular disease—four times more likely to develop it than people without diabetes—and 65% of people with diabetes will eventually suffer a stroke or heart attack. Many might be tempted to take statins such as *atorvastatin* (Lipitor) to reduce their cholesterol levels. However, because statins can impair liver function, a risk that diabetes also creates, doctors are concerned about the safety of statins for diabetics. Now a large study seems to show that the risk may be worth taking if you have diabetes.

ABOUT THE STUDY

The study, which took place in the UK and Ireland in collaboration with Pfizer and was called the Collaborative Atorvastatin Diabetes Study (CARDS), included more than 2,800 people with type 2 diabetes who were separated into two groups—one took a statin, in this case Lipitor by Pfizer, and the other took a placebo. The statin group had a 37% reduction in major cardiovascular events compared with those who took the placebo. Furthermore, the statin group's overall mortality rate was 27% lower than the placebo group. The study was stopped nearly two years earlier than planned because of the significant benefits to diabetic patients on the statin. The American Diabetes Association recommended that even for those with low low-density lipoprotein (LDL) levels (the "bad" cholesterol), all adults with type 2 diabetes should consider statin therapy.

Some medical professionals, however, are deeply disturbed by the current broad use of statins because all statins have side effects. Some are relatively minor, such as mild diarrhea or constipation, but some are much more serious. As mentioned earlier, statins can damage liver function—in fact, all people taking statins need to have regular liver enzyme checks, and people with diabetes must discuss their liver function before starting statins to be sure they are candidates for the drugs. Statins can cause muscle problems including statin myopathy, which if it becomes severe can lead to impaired kidney function. There is also considerable anecdotal evidence that statins can cause memory problems sometimes so severe they are perceived as Alzheimer's disease.

EXPERT OPINION

We called Jay S. Cohen, MD, a nationally recognized expert on medications and side effects, to get his advice on the statins front. Dr. Cohen first points out that he is definitely not "anti-statins." They are good drugs, he says, when prescribed correctly and for the right people, and because they are at high risk of cardiovascular disease, most people with type 2 diabetes are right to be taking them. But Dr. Cohen says he has strong reservations about how doctors are prescribing statins, to this population or others. He explains that many doctors today are routinely prescribing high doses of the most potent statins on the market —*atorvastatin* (Lipitor), *rosuvastatin* (Crestor) and *simvastatin* (Zocor)—without careful consideration of individual patients' needs. This problem results at least in part from the pressure our current medical system puts on doctors to rush patients in and

out. To counterbalance this trend, patients must be prepared to take a stand and demand what Dr. Cohen calls a start-low, go-slow approach.

AIM FOR FEWER SIDE EFFECTS

First, he says, review your risk factors, such as family history, diabetes and high blood pressure, with your doctor, and ask how much you actually need to lower your LDL level. Most people with a so-called cholesterol problem are only mildly elevated and simply do not need high doses of powerful drugs. People who have no or few risk factors for cardiovascular disease and who have only mildly or moderately elevated LDL levels for whom diet and nutritional supplements have been ineffective should start with low doses of less powerful drugs from the earlier generation of statins—*pravastatin* (Pravachol) and *lovastatin* (Mevacor), which are now available as generics, and *fluvastatin* (Lescol). These may well do the job and have fewer side effects. Even patients who are at high risk and need the new generation of statins should still demand to start low and go slow. Raise dosage levels only when it's clear that lower dosages are not working.

Dr. Cohen goes on to say that lifestyle changes—regular exercise, normal weight, a balanced diet full of healthful foods, not smoking and the like—are enough for many people to bring LDL levels under control (generally considered as under 130 mg/dL). Some natural supplements also have a proven track record of helping control LDLs and cardiovascular risk. He recommends fish oil in particular because of the omega-3 essential fatty acids it contains. (*Bottom Line's Daily Health News* consulting medical editor Andrew L. Rubman, ND, advises taking 1,000 milligrams [mg] a day of a fish oil that combines omega-3 EPA and DHA, and says he likes fish oils from Pharmax and Nordic Naturals.) There are other natural products as well, including niacin and plant sterols, that might help. Work with a medical professional knowledgeable about supplements to explore what is most effective for you. Everyone on statins, though, must take supplements of coenzyme Q10 (CoQ10), a powerful antioxidant, because statins destroy CoQ10 in the body. Dr. Cohen recommends taking 45 mg to 90 mg of softgel CoQ10 daily and more for people with cardiovascular disease.

REVIEW ALL FACTORS

Remember, too, that statins do not remove the risk of heart attack and stroke —they *reduce* risk. Dr. Cohen cautions everyone, including those whose LDL levels have plummeted because of statin therapy, that LDL levels are just one component of cardiac risk. Other factors, such as a low HDL level, high C-reactive protein level or other factors—triglycerides, homocysteine, lipoprotein A, etc.—may be just as important. Always remember that maintaining a healthful lifestyle (healthful diet, normal weight, moderate exercise) is as important as any medication in preventing heart disease and stroke.

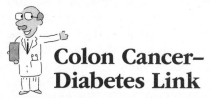

Colon Cancer–Diabetes Link

Donald Garrow, MD, MSc, fellow, gastroenterology and hepatology, Medical University of South Carolina, Charleston.

Diabetes for many people is much more than one disease. Having diabetes increases risk for heart disease, stroke, kidney failure and eye problems, among others. Now a new study has confirmed yet another increased risk—that of colon cancer. The study, from the Medical University of South Carolina, in Charleston, collected data from the National Health Interview Survey (an ongoing in-person collection of data on a wide variety of health-related matters) on more than 226,000 Americans. In analyzing the data from the 5.9% of respondents who had diabetes (mainly type 2 diabetes— which is approximately reflective of the national incidence of diabetes) the study

researchers discovered that they were 1.4 times more likely to develop colon cancer than people without diabetes. This was after the study team compensated for known colon cancer risk factors including age, gender, tobacco use and exercise.

STUDY DETAILS

We called lead author of the study, Donald Garrow, MD, MSc, a clinical instructor at the university, to find out more about this newly discovered risk. The increase in risk, he says, pertains to people who have type 2 diabetes rather than type 1. Type 1 diabetics do not produce any insulin, unlike the situation affecting those with type 2 diabetes, in which the body pumps out plenty of insulin but can't use it efficiently, resulting in soaring blood sugar levels. Dr. Garrow speculates that the increased cancer risk might have to do with how high levels of insulin in the blood—as happens with type 2 diabetes—affect cells in the mucosal lining of the colon. These cells contain insulin-like receptors, and lab experiments have shown that when high levels of insulin attach themselves to the receptors, the cells develop into cancer.

This study is clearly a cautionary message for everyone with type 2 diabetes to be especially careful about having colon cancer screenings. While there are several types of screening available, for this group of people Dr. Garrow recommends colonoscopy, in which the colon is viewed directly, because it has been shown repeatedly to be the most effective screener for colon cancer. As to when to start, he says he is currently evaluating data to determine if age has a role in the increased cancer risk. In the meantime, he supports the standard recommendation of starting at age 50.

The study team also plans to evaluate if spiking insulin and blood sugar levels impact risk. We should know this soon, he says, but it just makes good sense for all people with diabetes to tightly control their blood sugar and to eat the healthiest diet possible. In addition to perhaps helping lower their colon cancer risk, this approach likely offers better protection from all those other diseases as well.

___

Unbelievable! Pollutants Raise Risk of Diabetes

Duk-Hee Lee, MD, PhD, assistant professor of epidemeiology, School of Medicine, Kyungpook National University in South Korea. She has written extensively about the relationship of persistent organic pollutants (POPs) and diabetes.

Rick Relyea, PhD, ecologist, University of Pittsburgh, Pennsylvania.

___

The following almost reads like a detective story and sets the stage for what's to come…

A few years ago a story came out about how the population of gray tree frogs was being decimated by the use of a common pesticide, *carbaryl*. But the makers of carbaryl insisted it wasn't harming the frogs. They had numerous studies showing that if you take the little creatures and put them in a lab setting and expose them to the pesticide, nothing happens.

But still, the tree frogs were dying. And the environmentalists were positive it had something to do with their continued exposure to this pesticide.

FROGS RELEVANT TO DIABETES?

Rick Relyea, PhD, an ecologist from the University of Pittsburgh, in Pennsylvania, discovered that carbaryl was less harmful to frogs in the unnaturally tranquil setting of the lab (at least it was less likely to kill them). But most tree frogs don't live in a lab, they live in the wild. And in the wild there are constant dangers from predators. When tree frog tadpoles were exposed to a predator, the predator emitted a chemical cue that resulted in a stress response in the gray tree frog—a stress response just like we get when we're caught in traffic or miss a deadline. Expose a stressed frog to the pesticide and you've got a dead frog.

The combination of the two—physiological stress and a low-level pesticide, neither of which has a significant impact on survival alone—was lethal for a majority of the gray tree frog tadpoles.

"In other species such as bullfrog tadpoles, carbaryl became up to 46 times more deadly with the addition of predator cues. Moreover, this phenomenon has since been observed with both insecticides and herbicides, suggesting that it may be a quite common phenomenon," says Dr. Relyea.

The take-home point is that elements in the environment often interact with elements of our own physiology to cause serious problems. New research is emerging that suggests we may be seeing exactly the same phenomenon with diabetes.

AN INTERESTING TRAIL OF BREADCRUMBS

We've long known that obesity is a major risk factor for diabetes. But now it appears that exposure to pollutants can seriously aggravate the risk, and—in combination with obesity—may be associated with the increased risk of becoming diabetic. A recent study in the journal *Diabetes Care* looked at the connection between six persistent organic pollutants (known as POPs) and diabetes…and what they found was dramatic.

The prevalence of diabetes increased by 14- to 38-fold as the concentrations of the sum of the six POPs increased, irrespective of participants' weight, says lead researcher Duk-Hee Lee, MD, PhD, assistant professor of epidemiology at the School of Medicine, Kyungpook National University in South Korea. Her team divided the 2,016 subjects into groups comparing five levels of pollutants. Group 1 had the lowest levels and group 5 had the highest levels. Compared with group 1 (which had a .4% incidence of diabetes), group 2 had a 6.7% incidence of diabetes, while group 5 had an astonishing 25.6% incidence of the disease (groups 3 and 4 ranged in between). Dr. Lee notes that while obesity remains a risk factor for type 2 diabetes, the obese and overweight

43

people with very low concentrations of POPs had a much lower incidence of diabetes. Could obesity and pollutants interact to cause diabetes in much the way that the pesticide and stress interacted to cause the death of frogs?

"It's our hypothesis that obesity might be only weakly associated with diabetes among people with very low serum concentrations of POPs," Dr. Lee says. She explains that while her research concentrated on only six specific pollutants out of about 50 POPs identified in the National Health and Examination Survey, there was a striking connection between the blood concentrations of these six toxins and the prevalence of diabetes. This is not the first time that such a connection has been demonstrated. Earlier research from Sweden also found that exposure to POPs may contribute to the development of type 2 diabetes. And earlier research also demonstrated that exposure to at least one toxin—a dioxin called *TCDD*—increases the risk of diabetes and insulin resistance. It's believed that these toxins may interfere with glucose metabolism.

POPS ARE EVERYWHERE

POPs include certain chemical byproducts, PCBs and certain insecticides that have been linked to cancer, neurobehavioral impairment, endocrine problems and reproductive disorders. Previous researchers looked at special populations that are occupationally or accidentally exposed to high levels of these pollutants —for example, Vietnam veterans. (The US Department of Veterans Affairs includes type 2 diabetes in its list of presumptive diseases associated with exposure to the dioxin-containing Agent Orange.) But Dr. Lee's study is the first to examine the cumulative effect of most commonly detected POPs among a random low-level exposure in the general population. The six toxins in the study are found in the environment, and move through the air and water to accumulate in the environment.

Dr. Lee points out that pollutants by themselves do not necessarily cause diabetes, and expresses caution about jumping to strong conclusions based on one or two studies. "Plenty of people have exposure to these pollutants and don't get diabetes," she explains. "But the strong connection between high levels and increased incidence is very hard to ignore, as is the fact that there are such low levels of diabetes among those with low levels of exposure, even among the overweight and obese." Could genes be a factor? "It's prudent to act as if everyone is at risk, regardless of genetic makeup," she advises.

How do we get exposed to these chemicals in the first place? "Exposure to POPs comes mostly from fatty animal food consumption," Dr. Lee tells us.

When asked what protective measures people might take, Dr. Lee answers concisely: "A low intake of animal foods and a higher intake of plant foods may be beneficial. Aside from trying to avoid POPs, preventing obesity is still very important because the toxicity of POPs appeared to synergistically increase the risk of type 2 diabetes among obese persons."

4

Healing Secrets for Better Digestion

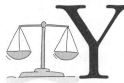

Simple Key to Better Digestion

You may have read a lot on the subject of vitamins and botanicals. But *enzymes* are critical to body function, and they are just starting to make headlines. Digestive enzymes are becoming more prominent as the dangers of long-term antacid use come to the attention of consumers and medical personnel. But, there are many other enzymes that make the body function. What do you need to know about them?

WHAT ARE ENZYMES?

Described as the "sparks of life" by Edward Howell, MD, an early and prominent enzyme researcher, enzymes are mostly protein molecules that act as catalysts for every single biochemical process in the body, from digestion to tissue regeneration. Without enzymes there would be no life...and when a person's supply of certain enzymes is inadequate, health problems follow. Because each bodily function needs a specific enzyme for activation—somewhat akin to the key that starts a car's engine—the body makes hundreds of thousands of them. *However, there are just three main categories...*

•**Metabolic enzymes**—manufactured by cells to carry out various functions.

•**Digestive enzymes**—primarily manufactured by the pancreas to digest foods and absorb nutrients.

•**Food enzymes**—*exogenous* (from outside the body) enzymes found in plants and animals, also necessary for aiding and accelerating digestion.

PANCREATIC IMPORTANCE

We asked chemist and enzyme therapist Lita Lee, PhD, why we hear so little about many enzymes. There is no reason

Lita Lee, PhD, chemist and enzyme therapist, and author of *The Enzyme Cure*. Ten Speed.

to worry about metabolic enzymes, she says, if digestion is functioning well. So the focus is on enzymes needed for digestion—those created by the pancreas and food enzymes. *Enzymes produced by the pancreas also fall into three categories…*

•**Amylase**—digests carbohydrates (a whole industry has grown up around the amylase enzyme lactase, a deficiency of which causes lactose intolerance).

•**Lipase**—splits fats and oils into fatty acids.

•**Protease**—breaks down protein into component amino acids.

ABOUT PLANT ENZYMES

Food enzymes are primarily plant enzymes (more about that later in the article), and include cellulase, another category of enzyme that is found only in plants and which digests soluble fiber.

To get the picture of what enzymes are about and why they are so important requires a brief review of digestion. Most digestion takes place in the small intestine, but the process of predigestion actually starts in the mouth. Saliva moistens the food, chewing releases enzymes from our food, and the stomach continues the enzyme release. The enzymes that do the work of predigestion are salivary amylase and plant enzymes and these, says Dr. Lee, are the key to a healthy digestive system. Pancreatic enzymes do not take over the job until food reaches the small intestine, and having adequate and appropriate plant enzymes for predigestion not only enhances digestion in general, it also greatly decreases the load that's put on the pancreas, a hardworking organ in the best of times. In fact, she says that enzymes in the mouth and stomach can predigest up to 60% of carbohydrates, 30% of protein and 10% of fat.

The catch: Few people have robust digestion—and so by definition few have adequate and effective plant enzymes. Many people point to age as the culprit here, with the belief that aging compromises enzyme function, but Dr. Lee disagrees

because children often have poor digestion as well. In addition, few people also eat adequate levels of plant enzymes at each meal, which contributes to digestive problems over time. Ideally, every meal should include fruits and fruit juices, she says.

REASONS FOR POOR ENZYME DIGESTION

Enzymes become less effective when heated above 140°F. Hence, much of the enzyme benefit is lost in highly cooked foods. The second factor for enzyme function has to do with pH balances in the digestive system. To be activated, an enzyme needs a highly specific and particular pH range. The popular antacid medications, both over-the-counter (OTC) and prescriptive, directly affect pH balance. A common misconception is that stomach acid is there to directly digest food. Rather, when a person eats, acid comes in to lower the pH balance of the stomach so that it will be the proper environment to activate the digestive enzyme pepsin. If there is too little stomach acid, the pH balance is incorrect and the digestive process is dramatically compromised.

BUILDING YOUR ENZYME PERFORMANCE

Virtually everyone benefits from improved plant enzyme ingestion. According to Dr. Lee, the place to start is with food. Dr. Lee advises eating all foods whole and usually organic—in other words, no processed foods (processing to create shelf life destroys enzymes), no "low-fat" items, no reconstituted and certainly, no fake foods such as artificial sweeteners. She staunchly advocates eating meat and fish because protein contributes to a healthy thyroid, and that contributes to healthy enzyme activity. She is strongly against estrogenic foods such as soy because she believes they affect thyroid function and may be carcinogenic.

MORE FOOD SPECIFICS

Look for grass-fed meats and poultry, and wild fish. Raw milk and cheeses, especially from goats or sheep, if you can find them, are full of healthy enzymes. Pasteurizing, however, destroys these enzymes—especially ultra-pasteurizing, the process used to make organic milk. Eat raw carrots and salads, of course, but avoid commercial salad dressings. Do not eat raw cruciferous vegetables such as cauliflower, broccoli, cabbage, kale and brussels sprouts, because they contain thyroid-inhibiting factors. Cooking these foods destroys the risk to the thyroid. It is best to steam them until brightly colored on the outside. This will preserve some enzyme activity while removing the *isothiocyanates* responsible for the antithyroid effect.

SUPPLEMENTING MAKES IT SIMPLE

Since most people don't eat a lot of raw food, Dr. Lee suggests taking plant enzyme supplements before each meal. The ones she recommends are those from leading enzyme practitioner Edward F. Loomis, Jr., DC (*www.naturalenzymes. com* or call 800-614-4400). *Bottom Line's Daily Health News* consulting medical editor Andrew L. Rubman, ND, also favors plant enzymes produced by Tyler, which are broadly available at health food stores and on the Internet.

Note: If you have digestive problems, work with a health-care professional who has been trained in enzyme therapy. This person can evaluate individual situations and prescribe a balanced formula of enzymes that will address your needs.

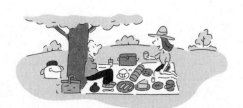

Achy Joints? Asthma? Rashes? It Could Be The Way You Chew Your Food

Trent Nichols, MD, board-certified internist, nutritionist and gastroenterologist, Center for Nutrition and Digestive Disorders, Hanover, Pennsylvania. He is lead editor of *Optimal Digestive Health* (Healing Arts) and has written and lectured extensively about digestive health topics.

Here's a quick question—what do bloating, gas, joint aches, muscle aches, worsened asthma and skin rashes have in common? You'd probably never guess that every one of those symptoms can be created—or made worse—by not chewing your food properly. But, according to Trent Nichols, MD, gastroenterologist at the Center for Nutrition and Digestive Disorders in Hanover, Pennsylvania, that's exactly the case.

"The smaller the particle of food, the easier it is to pass into the digestive system from the stomach," said Dr. Nichols. "If food isn't chewed properly, you're left with larger particles in the stomach and several things happen. One, stomach acid has to do a lot more work. And two, some of these larger particles get through the gut wall into the bloodstream," he explains.

FAMILIAR SYMPTOMS, DIFFERENT CAUSE

It's the latter situation that can cause real problems, according to Dr. Nichols. He explains that when these larger particles permeate the gut wall and enter the bloodstream, they trigger immune system responses. "The immune system gets mobilized by anything it doesn't recognize, and it doesn't recognize undigested food," says Dr. Nichols. "The result is that the immune system sends all its artillery to fight the strange substances, which creates a variety of symptoms that people don't always associate with food."

These symptoms aren't full-blown "food allergies" in the traditional sense, but rather what he calls "delayed food sensitivities." "You'll get these delayed sensitivity reactions from three to 72 hours after eating," said Dr. Nichols, "and they can include headaches, joint aches, bloating, muscle aches and other annoying symptoms."

What causes the gut wall to become increasingly permeable? "Nonsteroidal anti-inflammatories are a big factor," Dr. Nichols told us. "They cause all kinds of micro-perforations in the small intestine. Even aspirin on a daily basis can increase the permeability of the gut wall."

Dr. Nichols stresses that the best thing you can do to prevent this is to follow grandma's advice: "Slow down and sit down when you eat. Chew well and eat slowly. Target 30 chews per bite, which can be a real challenge for many bites. When you eat too quickly, more undigested food gets into the colon and results in more bloating."

The Mind–Body Solution for IBS That May Work Better than Drugs

Emeran A. Mayer, MD, director of the University of California, Los Angeles (UCLA) Center for Neurovisceral Sciences and Women's Health in the UCLA division of digestive diseases, chair of the UCLA Collaborative Centers for Integrative Medicine.

Irritable bowel syndrome (IBS) is what's called a "functional disorder," meaning there is no structural detectable abnormality, such as cancer or bowel inflammation, to explain the patient's symptoms. A functional disorder is unlikely to affect your long-term health. But don't tell anyone who suffers from IBS that the condition is "nothing to worry about." For them, IBS means near-constant anxiety about abdominal pain and discomfort, along with diarrhea, constipation or alternating bouts of both. In short, life is one endless worry. And being prone to worry, according to growing research, may be a big part of the problem.

PERSONALITY-TYPE AND IBS?

A recent study on this, from the University of Southampton in the United Kingdom and the University of Auckland in New Zealand, demonstrated that the people most likely to develop IBS were those whose temperament could be described as overly anxious and driven. Additionally, the study found that people at risk for IBS were also likely to be perfectionists who push themselves too far and, not surprisingly, were likely to be pessimistic about their illness, though not depressed.

A VICIOUS CYCLE

An expert on the impact of personality type on IBS is Emeran A. Mayer, MD, the director of the UCLA Center for Neurovisceral Sciences and Women's Health in the division of digestive diseases and the chair of the UCLA Collaborative Centers for Integrative Medicine. We spoke with Dr. Mayer about the role of anxiety in the disease and how these findings might be helpful to people with it. IBS often develops after bouts of gastroenteritis (an inflammation of the stomach and intestines caused by a virus, bacteria or parasites). In order to understand why this happens, it's important to remember that the gastrointestinal tract has its own nervous system called the enteric nervous system, says Dr. Mayer, which has been referred to as the third branch of the autonomic nervous system. This is an independent connection to the brain. It has as many neurons as the spinal cord and works like a continuous loop, with communication signals going both ways, from the gut up to the brain as well as from the brain down via parasympathetic and sympathetic nerve fibers in the body. This branch is one of the branches of the autonomic nervous system that mediates the effect of emotion on the body. We now know that how a person feels, thinks and copes influences those messages.

ANXIETY, THE BRAIN, AND THE GUT

There's some disagreement about exactly what IBS is, says Dr. Mayer, but some researchers believe that the condition develops only if there is an alteration in the normal way the digestive system and the nervous system interact. And studies suggest that chronic anxiety may play a role in biasing these brain/gut interactions. "In my experience virtually all IBS patients have at least mildly increased levels of anxiety," says Dr. Mayer. What remains to be studied is whether the IBS creates anxiety, anxiety creates IBS…or there are yet other factors at play.

Unfortunately, having IBS nearly always worsens anxiety in people who are already prone toward it, thereby setting up a vicious cycle in their brain/gut interactions, says Dr. Mayer. IBS patients become "hypervigilant" about the possible appearance of symptoms, which in turn causes the brain to send a message to the gut, telling it to become even more hyperresponsive and sensitive. The result is an elevation of symptoms and discomfort leading to heightened anxiety that leads to greater hypervigilance…and on and on.

A MIND–BODY SOLUTION FOR IBS

Although several different medications have been developed to treat IBS, with modest results, there is another road to healing that is at least as likely to succeed, and perhaps more so—by changing the nervous system messages IBS patients send between the brain and the digestive system. According to Dr. Mayer and many others, one way to do this is through cognitive behavioral therapy (CBT).

CBT is a brief period of therapy focused on teaching people to recognize their thought patterns more quickly and alter them in ways that calm the gut at symptom onset, rather than reacting with panic and anxiety. This can retrain the entire pathway between the brain and the digestive system, making it stronger and healthier, says Dr. Mayer. In his CBT program, IBS patients take part in five weekly sessions of two hours each. However, he says that even shorter programs produce positive results. In addition to CBT, patients learn how to control symptoms by breathing deeply from the diaphragm, using progressive muscle relaxation, and also by a form of self-hypnosis that replaces negative thoughts with reassuring ones that diminish symptoms.

HOPE FOR THE FUTURE

Research on IBS continues, says Dr. Mayer. He compares the disease to a jigsaw puzzle, predicting the pieces will all be in place within a few years. A new class of drugs that acts directly on the limbic system in the brain (which affects emotions and autonomic function), calming down hyperactive reactions such as those found in IBS, is being tested. However, natural solutions are always our favorite ones. Dr. Mayer encourages everyone with IBS symptoms to consider some type of CBT as one way to learn how to smooth out the dysfunctional brain/gut connection. Talk with your health-care provider about a referral to a CBT program in your area.

Why You May Need More Stomach Acid

Andrew L. Rubman, ND, consulting medical editor for *Bottom Line's Daily Health News* and director of the Southbury Clinic for Traditional Medicines in Southbury, Connecticut.

We already know that a diet full of too much sugary stuff—particularly the refined sugars found in candy and soda and refined grains like white rice and white flour—may lead to serious health problems such as obesity and diabetes. But many people are unaware that too much sugar in their diet can also cause another less talked-about condition—low stomach acid. This is because the byproducts of fermentation can impair proper levels of acid production in the stomach.

Relying on these foods for fuel is like putting low-grade gasoline in a car that requires mid-grade or premium, our consulting medical editor Andrew L. Rubman, ND, says. "Excess sugar may ferment, thereby feeding the growth of yeasts and bacteria. The result is poor digestion, which can lead to fatigue, mood imbalances, nausea and system-wide disease states consistent with malnutrition," he warns. Ultimately everything in the body—muscle, bone, central nervous system and cardiovascular function—is affected.

CRITICAL TO YOUR HEALTH

Stomach acid, or hydrochloric acid, activates digestive *pepsinogen* that helps your body break down food. Dr. Rubman explains that the stomach needs to maintain a very acidic mid-meal environment, with an average basal pH of 2.16 in men and 2.79 in women. "That's acidic enough to dissolve a pea-sized meatball in about 20 seconds," he says. Food doesn't digest properly if your stomach has insufficient acidity, or a pH that is too high. The results—gas, bloating, belching, diarrhea or constipation—are not pleasant.

WHEN YOUR DIET IS POOR

According to Dr. Rubman, approximately one-third of American adults over age 40 have less than optimal amounts of stomach acid, which many experts blame on poor diet, based on too many refined carbohydrates. These foods promote the unchecked growth of microorganisms in the gastrointestinal tract, triggering inflammation and excessive mucus secretion, and preventing the cells in the gut from producing acid in quantities adequate for digestion. Regular use of the many acid-suppressing medications or taking too many other medications (prescription and over-the-counter) can also hinder your stomach's ability to produce enough acid—as can aging. The result is an inability to absorb needed nutrients, and as explained above, a digestive system that can't control the growth of harmful bacteria and yeast.

REPLENISHING YOUR STOMACH ACID

If you experience gassiness and bloating, discomfort after eating, or notice that you have brittle nails, the root cause may be low stomach acid. While a conventional doctor would likely address each symptom separately, a naturopathic doctor, or ND, is more apt to recognize and successfully treat the condition of low stomach acid itself, says Dr. Rubman. Barring a medical condition such as stomach ulcer, he and others with his training and outlook will generally recommend a plant-based digestive enzyme to help restore the stomach's ability to produce acid. Limit refined sugars and include more moderate and low-glycemic index carbohydrates, such as most fruits and vegetables, and legumes, seeds, nuts and beans. Prescribing a probiotic to encourage the growth of healthy bacteria, if indicated from testing, may also be helpful. (This may involve taking a series of different beneficial bacteria supplements, but your physician will provide details.) And finally, try to eat three times a day, without snacking, and incorporate reasonable amounts of healthy fats and fiber into your diet, which will promote appropriately timed and more complete digestion.

Even a Few Extra Pounds Can Cause GERD

Brian C. Jacobson, MD, MPH, director, endoscopic ultrasonography, associate director of endoscopy services, Boston Medical Center, and assistant professor, Boston University School of Medicine.

Research has repeatedly found that overweight and obese people are particularly at risk for gastroesophageal reflux disease (GERD). But folks within the normal weight range also sometimes have bouts of GERD, when the tissue between the stomach and the esophagus does not function properly, causing heartburn and reflux. Now a study has investigated how modest gains of weight can trigger symptoms of GERD, even among people not considered overweight by the standard body mass index (BMI) measure of at least 25 in adults (For more information, go to the Centers for Disease Control and Prevention's Web site, *www.cdc.gov*, and search "healthy weight."

WOMEN'S WEIGHT AND GERD

This study, conducted in part by Boston University School of Medicine, was based on research data taken from 10,545 women involved in the long-range Nurses' Health Study (Harvard) concerning their weight history and GERD symptoms. The findings were startling, to say the least. The women with a BMI under 20 were 33% less likely to report symptoms of GERD than women with a BMI between 20 and 22.4. The women who had a BMI of between 22.5 and 24.9—still in the normal range by BMI standards—were nearly 40% more likely to have GERD symptoms than women with a BMI of 20 to 22.4. (Women who have a BMI over 25 to 29.9 have more than double the increased likelihood of GERD...those with BMI over 30 have close to three times the likelihood.) Furthermore, women who decreased their weight by at least 3.5 BMI points experienced a 40% decrease in risk of frequent symptoms compared with women whose BMI didn't change.

We spoke with lead study author and assistant professor at the school, Brian C. Jacobson, MD, MPH, who says that this study demonstrates the importance of avoiding even modest weight gains. For instance, a woman who is 5'4" has an ideal weight of 120 pounds with a BMI of 20.6. If she then gains 15 pounds, she raises her BMI to 23.2. This sounds inconsequential as a BMI, but it reflects a considerable increase in weight for her. Any excess weight can squeeze the stomach, he says, and much like squeezing a plastic bottle of soda, the contents will shoot up and out.

APPLIES TO MEN, TOO

Although this study looked at women, men likely have the same GERD increase with weight gain, says Dr. Jacobson. His advice to men and women, then, is to focus on maintaining your target weight and avoiding weight fluctuations. If you have GERD and have gained a few pounds, you may well benefit from getting rid of them. Watch your portions, exercise everyday and eat healthfully, advises Dr. Jacobson. It is hard to lose weight, but as he says, GERD is a hefty price to pay for a few extra pounds.

Surprising Problems That Start In Your Stomach

Andrew L. Rubman, ND, consulting medical editor for *Bottom Line's Daily Health News* and director of the Southbury Clinic for Traditional Medicines in Southbury, Connecticut.

By now we've all heard the warnings about common symptoms of gastroesophageal reflux disease (GERD). When acid from the stomach refluxes up into the esophagus, there may be heartburn, unexplained chest pain, inflammation of the esophagus and trouble swallowing. It's important to address these symptoms with your doctor rather than simply ignore them. However, there are a number of less common and seldom discussed side effects and complications of GERD, which range from chronic cough and sore throat to serious chronic respiratory problems, including non-allergic asthma, pneumonia and emphysema.

For information about the more surprising symptoms and complications of GERD, we turned to our own digestion guru, our consulting medical editor Andrew L. Rubman, ND. He tells us that there are many secondary symptoms and illnesses that are related to not only GERD, but also to the all-too-common conventional treatment of antacids, acid reducers and acid suppressants. Dr. Rubman described how GERD does its dirty work in the body, and what we can do about it.

THE RESPIRATORY SYSTEM: AN UPSIDE-DOWN TREE

Many of the more surprising symptoms and consequences of GERD are due to its effect on the respiratory system. You can think about the respiratory system as an upside-down tree, says Dr. Rubman. We breathe in through our noses, and air passes through the sinuses into the pharynx (home to the vocal cords), through the trachea or windpipe, which leads down the chest where it branches into the lungs. Problems arise when acid refluxes from the esophagus and penetrates the respiratory system. This acid progresses up from the stomach and esophagus and descends back down through the respiratory tree, explains Dr. Rubman. The farther down the acid seeps, the more damage it can cause. If the acid reaches the pharynx, you may experience hoarseness and a sore throat…symptoms you would ordinarily be more likely to associate with a cold or flu than with GERD. According to Dr. Rubman, if it penetrates all the way down into the lungs, you are more vulnerable to serious problems such as inflammation of the lungs, chronic obstructive pulmonary disease (COPD), asthma, pneumonia or emphysema. Since GERD may be overlooked as a contributing factor to these conditions, the opportunity to address and remedy the problem before it grows worse is often overlooked.

TRY TO GET IMMUNITY

Another commonly overlooked area of importance is the tonsillar ring, consisting of the tonsils and adenoids, notes Dr. Rubman. This ring is designed to alert the immune system about any unique challenges that are entering with the air we breathe. He warns that if the area is chronically irritated by the acid reflux from GERD, it will diminish the immune capacity of the respiratory tract and an individual may be more vulnerable to illness if he/she suffers from GERD.

All in all, with its negative impact on the respiratory system and immunity overall, GERD may result in surprising symptoms and complications, including…

- **Chronic cough**
- **Sore throat**
- **Difficulty breathing during the performance of exercise**
- **Non-allergic asthma**
- **Pneumonia**
- **Emphysema**
- **COPD, bronchitis**
- **Laryngitis or weaker voice**
- **Other respiratory inflammations and infections**

WHAT YOU CAN DO

The single most important thing—don't use antacids, acid suppressants (such as proton pump inhibitors) or acid reducers (such as H2 antagonists) says Dr. Rubman. Although these are heavily marketed as the solution to GERD, in fact their use can backfire and cause even more damage by making the stomach vulnerable to microbial penetration. Ignore all the marketing hype, encourages Dr. Rubman. It is a mistake to take antacids, acid suppressants or acid reducers and suppress stomach acid for any length of time, except when treating an acute ulcer (and that's for a maximum of 14 days). The truth is that we need stomach acid to digest the food we eat, and excess stomach acid is a rare condition, according to Dr. Rubman.

DOESN'T HAVE TO TAKE LONG

The good news is that a trained and qualified naturopathic physician can often cure GERD in three to four weeks, observes Dr. Rubman. Lifestyle modifications and detection and elimination of *H. pylori*-associated gastritis will help ensure the success of naturopathic treatments. *To send GERD symptoms packing, Dr. Rubman advises...*

•**Chew food thoroughly.** The better you break down food in the mouth, the less work you leave for the rest of the digestive system.

•**Monitor food combinations.** For optimal digestion, do not combine simple carbohydrates (such as processed and refined sugars) with saturated fats (red meat, dairy products, etc.)...eat fruits at least 30 minutes before or after meals...ease up on the sugary desserts, etc.

•**No grazing.** Your best bet to control stomach acid levels is to eat three square meals a day and let your stomach rest in-between.

•**Limited or preferably no water/fluids with meals.** Water and other fluids dilute stomach acid and render it less effective.

To prevent or control GERD symptoms, talk to your physician about healthier alternatives to antacids or any other acid reducing or suppressing drug. Dr. Rubman often prescribes natural digestive enzymes in products such as DuoZyme by Karuna to help break down foods into nutrients the body can more readily digest and decrease colonized microorganisms in the stomach. Other prescribed digestive aids may include hydrochloric acid supplements, *Gentiana lutea-L.* (yellow gentian), Glyconda, Compound Herbal Elixir (Eclectic Institute) and Gastri-Gest (Priority One).

To cope with the symptoms and complications of GERD, from the obvious to the subtle, once again the key is to support optimal function of the digestive tract. If you suffer from any of the less obvious symptoms of GERD, be sure to mention these to your physician.

The Dangers of Constipation

Andrew L. Rubman, ND, consulting medical editor for *Bottom Line's Daily Health News* and director of the Southbury Clinic for Traditional Medicines in Southbury, Connecticut.

Millions of Americans suffer from constipation on a daily basis. *Bottom Line's Daily Health News* consulting medical editor Andrew L. Rubman, ND, says that a digestive system that functions well is the core to a body that functions well. Conversely, a digestive system that is blocked impedes the flow of nutrients and removal of wastes. All that can result in symptoms ranging from headache and fatigue to immune system breakdown to doggy breath, according to Dr. Rubman.

How to treat constipation if you have it? And prevent it if you don't? Dr. Rubman shares his secrets for keeping the body's digestive system flowing. He points out that constipation has several very common causes. Once you figure out the reason for it you can take the necessary steps to reverse it and prevent it from occurring again.

WHAT IS CONSTIPATION?

First, let's take a look at what constipation is (and what it isn't). Constipation—infrequent or difficult bowel movements—is usually characterized by small, hard, dry stools that are difficult to pass. There may also be straining during elimination, abdominal discomfort or pain, bloating and an uncomfortable sensation of a full bowel.

But what constitutes irregular bowel movements? According to Dr. Rubman, "normal" is on average one bowel movement a day, usually in the morning. However, everyone is different, and consistency is the real test of normalcy. If you have roughly the same number of bowel movements day-to-day, no discomfort, and the size, texture and color of stool are consistent, then you're likely fine. If, on the other hand, you are not consistent on a regular basis, then there is a potential problem.

COMMON CULPRITS AND WHAT TO DO ABOUT THEM

Most people with constipation don't need strong medication. In fact, while Dr. Rubman considers it safe to take an occasional laxative, he warns that regular use of these drugs can be harmful. Over time, laxatives become habit-forming, as the body comes to rely on them in order to have a bowel movement.

Dr. Rubman outlines the four most common causes of constipation and what to do about them…

Problem 1: Dehydration. The large intestine plays a primary role in water balance and excretion, explains Dr. Rubman. As food makes its way through the large intestine, the intestine absorbs water from it and stools form. By the time the stool reaches the rectum, most of the water has been absorbed and the stool is harder. Drinking too much—or not enough—water can disrupt this process.

Solution: Make water your beverage of choice. Water is the most healthful beverage, and Dr. Rubman advises that you think of other beverages as occasional treats. He is not an advocate of the advice "drink eight eight-ounce glasses of water a day." Water needs vary from individual to individual, based on variables such as state of health, diet, medications, physical activity, environment, etc. If you're not sure whether you're drinking enough water, Dr. Rubman recommends asking your physician about a *urine specific gravity* test. The test will indicate the relative density of urine. If urine is too diluted or too dense, adjust your water intake accordingly.

Problem 2: Inadequate fiber intake. Fiber is the part of grains and produce that the body cannot digest. It adds bulk to stool and keeps it soft, making stools easier to pass. Fiber also stimulates the production of healthy flora in the gut, moves food efficiently through the digestive tract, and binds and transports bile acids and cholesterol for excretion out of the body. Most of us do not get enough fiber in our diets. The average American consumes 5 to 14 grams of fiber a day, even though experts recommend 20 to 35 grams.

Solution: Take in more fiber. Eat a well-balanced, high-fiber diet with plenty of oats, whole wheat bread, bran, brown rice, beans, fresh or dried fruits, nuts, seeds and steamed vegetables. Ideally, at least half the diet should consist of unprocessed foods, says Dr. Rubman. When you need extra help, his favorite fiber supplements are oat bran (which increases the bulk of stool and softens the stool) and glucomannan (which absorbs and binds components within the bowel movement). Both are available at most health food stores.

Problem 3: Inadequate peristalsis. Peristalsis consists of a series of smooth muscle contractions in the digestive tract. These contracting waves move food along through the large intestine. Inadequate levels of calcium and magnesium can lead to inadequate peristalsis and consequent constipation.

Solution: Take magnesium and calcium supplements. Dr. Rubman recommends calcium and magnesium in the combination dietary supplement Butyrex, made by T.E. Neesby. These capsules contain *butyric acid*, calcium and magnesium. Butyrex supports the lining of the gastrointestinal tract, allowing for optimal absorption of nutrients, and helps maintain a balanced microbial population in the gut. Take Butyrex with meals. A lack of bulk from low fiber can also lead to inadequate peristalsis since the bulk stimulates natural contractions.

Problem 4: Salt imbalance. People on low-sodium diets can have problems with constipation, observes Dr. Rubman. Sodium is an important mineral that helps regulate the body's fluid balance.

Solution: Adjust your salt intake. Discuss with your physician what your salt intake should be, advises Dr. Rubman. When considering salt intake, factors to take into account include overall health issues (such as salt-sensitive high blood pressure), blood tests and bowel movements.

FIND CONSTIPATION'S ROOT CAUSES

Of course, there can be other causes of constipation. For example, it may occur as a side effect of medications, or as a symptom of a disease such as a neurological disorder (multiple sclerosis) or metabolic or endocrine condition (diabetes or hypothyroidism). Most important is to work with a trained professional to resolve the underlying cause of the constipation and resolve it. Don't use laxatives to fix the symptom. Instead, identify and address the root cause. Exercise is an important measure to prevent constipation...and you should never ignore the urge to go. Constipation is about far more than inconvenience and discomfort. It can create even more problems down the road.

info For more information on constipation, contact the National Digestive Diseases Information Clearinghouse at *http://digestive.niddk.nih.gov.*

Natural Ways to Relieve Food Poisoning

Sonja Pettersen, NMD, naturopathic medical doctor. She is licensed to practice primary care medicine specializing in natural therapeutics in Arizona and is based in Scottsdale.

Although headlines sometimes describe food poisoning as the killer that lurks in your dinner, the problem rarely causes death. Food poisoning does, however, create extreme discomfort in as many as 76 million Americans every year with vomiting, diarrhea and abdominal pain that can last from a few hours to more than a week. Sometimes food poisoning is also accompanied by fever, severe dehydration and even shock—which can be life-threatening, so it's very important to take symptoms seriously. Though there are ways to decrease the incidence of food poisoning, it's nearly impossible to avoid ever facing it—so it is important to know how to handle the problem. With that in mind, we called naturopathic physician Sonja Pettersen, NMD, a naturopathic physician in private practice in Scottsdale, Arizona, for her treatment recommendations.

IT'S ALL IN THE BACTERIA

She told us that food poisoning in North America mostly comes from assorted naturally occurring bacteria, including *Salmonella*, *E. coli* and *Campylobacter*. *Listeria* is not common, but approximately 20% of patients die from it...and *Botulinum*, which causes botulism, is also rare. (Another kind called *Shigella* is found in tropical climates, especially where poor hygiene is present.) Botulism is far and away the most serious of these. It usually results from poor canning techniques, and fortunately occurs much less often than it once did. Nevertheless, when the live botulism organism is ingested, it can kill quickly, so it is crucial to act immediately. In the case of food poisoning, botulism has a paralyzing nerve toxin—so it can affect many bodily functions, including breathing, balance, speech and swallowing, notes Dr. Pettersen. The onset is rapid (incubation is six hours to 10 days) and unmistakable, characterized by paralysis in any or all of those functions. Effective antitoxin treatment is now available, and any sign of botulism requires a 9-1-1 call and a rush trip to the emergency room.

NATURAL LINE OF DEFENSE

Fortunately, most other cases of food poisoning can be handled at home. Although the vomiting and diarrhea are often intense and painful, Dr. Pettersen explains that this is the body's way of purging itself of the bacteria. "There is a turf war going on," she says, "between the body's natural immunity and protective intestinal flora, and the invading bacteria." The goal is to eliminate the bad bacteria promptly—if it is allowed to linger, toxins develop that can cause much more serious problems. The violent elimination is your body's natural defense against the organisms and their associated toxins. Therefore, you shouldn't take medications, such as Imodium A-D, to slow or stop the diarrhea. "Better out than in," says Dr. Pettersen. Also, don't take an antacid to quell the upset. Stomach acid is crucial as the first line of defense to diminish the toxins and keep the live bacteria from spreading through the rest of the gastrointestinal tract.

AT HOME

Even as your digestive system is turning inside out, there are ways to make yourself more comfortable. Dr. Pettersen advises taking a probiotic in the form of a high-quality acidophilus powder in capsules or mixed in a liquid per instructions on the container, and as prescribed by your physician. Often you'll be instructed to take a dose every half hour or so even when vomiting—it can't hurt you and will get more good bacteria into your system when it stays down. Other natural remedies include antimicrobial essential oils, herbs and/or supplements such as cilantro, ginger, tarragon, oregano, garlic, thyme or peppermint. Activated charcoal caps neutralize toxins to help stop symptoms quickly. (It is usually the bacterial toxins and not the bacteria itself that create the symptoms.) A homeopathic remedy often prescribed is *Arsenicum album*.

POST-ATTACK CARE

Within a few days, the attack begins to ebb and you will start to feel better. But understand that your digestive system has been under siege, and isn't ready for a normal diet. *Instead, Dr. Pettersen advises the following...*

•**Drink Pedialyte,** an electrolyte-replacement drink. (Avoid Gatorade, though, because it will make you feel worse, according to Dr. Pettersen. The high fructose corn syrup (anything sweet) can easily induce an osmotic diarrhea on top of gut troubles.)

•**Eat simple foods**—remember the acronym BRAT (bananas, rice, apple sauce, dry toast). Do not challenge your system.

•**Avoid sugar completely**—and this includes the 7-Up and ginger ale your mother probably gave you as a child after a bout (disruptive gut organisms tend to thrive on such sugary treats).

EMERGENCY MEASURES

Bleeding from the nose or mouth, or blood in your urine, feces or vomit are signs of an emergency. If this happens, go to an ER right away. Any neurological symptoms such as balance or visual problems, muscle weakening and the like also mean you need to get immediately to the hospital. Barring these symptoms, you'll need to stay in touch with your doctor if the debilitation from food poisoning is prolonged. "How bad this might get depends on your general health, but your recent experiences are a factor," says Dr. Pettersen. For example, if you've just completed a long, dehydrating flight, food poisoning will affect you much worse than it might if you are well rested and hydrated. Your physician will decide if IV fluid replacement is necessary and, in the case of *Salmonella*, if you need an antibiotic.

Note: Dr. Pettersen says that with many cases of food poisoning, the general prescription of antibiotics without a specific target can make the situation worse because they kill the friendly bacteria in the gut that would otherwise be warriors in the battle.

While much is known about how to avoid food contamination, it's a problem that remains very much with us today—as those scary headlines make all too clear. Knowing how to deal with it can minimize unpleasantness.

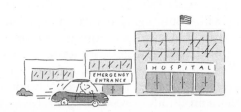

Eczema—the Problem Could Be More than Skin Deep

Mark A. Stengler, ND, naturopathic physician in private practice, La Jolla, California...adjunct associate clinical professor at the National College of Natural Medicine, Portland, Oregon...author of many books, including *The Natural Physician's Healing Therapies* and coauthor of *Prescription for Natural Cures* (both from Bottom Line Books)...and author of the *Bottom Line/Natural Healing* newsletter.

Living with eczema (dermatitis) is its own special torture. In many people, the chronic skin condition causes nearly incessant itching along with telltale unsightly red or sometimes brown rashes on the arms, face and neck, including in the folds of skin of knees and elbows. Worse, it is a lifelong condition—eczema has no known cure and the few treatments for it may only be marginally helpful. And so when a 53-year-old carpenter and painter called Mark A. Stengler, ND, a naturopathic physician in private practice in La Jolla, California, for a consultation about the eczema that he had had for more than two decades, he held out little hope.

The man's work exposed him to chemicals practically every day. It was hardly surprising that many of the specialists he saw over the years pointed to the patient's livelihood as the trigger for his eczema flare-ups and the reason why the condition became so intense at times. Indeed, the itching was often so bad that he got little sleep at night and the rash had grown to cover much of his body. He reported that his previous doctors had prescribed numerous different topical steroid ointments in an attempt to stem the chronic itching—but nothing really helped.

After meeting with him, Dr. Stengler figured that the man's toxicity was so deep, he needed some cleansing from the inside out. And so, to counteract any toxic residue that could result from frequent exposure to chemicals, Dr. Stengler put him through a detoxification program with liver-cleansing herbs, purified water and the like. Surprisingly, this didn't help much. Although the skin had the appearance of eczema, Dr. Stengler decided to look past the decades-long diagnosis to see what else it might be and what might possibly be an underlying cause.

A WHOLE DIFFERENT CAUSE

Eczema is sometimes associated with allergies or reactions to a variety of foods with milk, peanuts, soy, fish and tree nuts (walnuts, cashews) leading the pack. But there is another reaction to food that has been associated with a form of dermatitis as well—that is an intolerance to gluten, the protein found in many grains including wheat, barley and rye. (At one time oats were also on the gluten list, but some researchers now feel that oats may not produce a reaction.) Complicating the picture further, the gluten-associated rash is not actually eczema. This condition, which looks strikingly like eczema, bears the name *dermatitis herpetiformis*. In spite of the name, this has nothing at all to do with the herpes virus. It does, however, have everything to do with celiac disease, or gluten intolerance.

CONSIDER GLUTEN INTOLERANCE

Celiac disease is also a lifelong condition with symptoms that can surface in a number of different ways—from few symptoms at all to severe gastrointestinal distress, including diarrhea, abdominal pain, gas and bloating. In fact, celiac sufferers occasionally become seriously malnourished because the small intestine loses its ability to absorb nutrients, although many do not exhibit symptoms. Celiac disease can develop in childhood, but dermatitis herpetiformis is more apt to surface starting in the 20s or after. It occurs more frequently in men.

UNLOCKING THE PUZZLE

Dr. Stengler now tested his patient for antibodies to gluten in the digestive tract through a stool test. Having such antibodies reveals the presence of a gluten intolerance. The antibodies tested extremely high. Consequently, Dr. Stengler put his patient immediately on a strict gluten-free diet with no foods containing wheat, rye or barley and allowed him to eat oats only occasionally. After six weeks of faithfully following this diet the decades-old eczema-like disorder disappeared completely. In this particular case, diagnosed well over a year ago, Dr. Stengler's patient's skin remains clear and without any sign of a rash. It should stay like this as long as he adheres to his gluten-free diet. He sleeps peacefully without the itching that plagued him previously and he is able to continue his work around chemicals without any effect on his skin.

CONCLUSION

Dr. Stengler points out that although just less than 1% of the population is affected by celiac disease, some researchers estimate it is largely underdiagnosed and that many more people suffer from gluten intolerance. This disorder can cause a host of other problems including, as we have seen, skin rashes and digestive distress, but it might also be behind other chronic conditions including headaches, fatigue, mood swings, depression and joint pain.

Consequently, Dr. Stengler advises anyone struggling with problems such as these, who do not respond well to mainstream short-term treatment, to consider the possibility of gluten intolerance. The way to tell? Do not eat any foods containing wheat, barley or rye for a minimum of two weeks, he says, and see how you feel. In many cases, this small change in diet can make a big difference in how you feel. You can also visit a holistic doctor for gluten intolerance/sensitivity testing.

Surprise! Take Calcium to Prevent Kidney Stones

Andrew L. Rubman, ND, consulting medical editor for *Bottom Line's Daily Health News* and director of the Southbury Clinic for Traditional Medicines in Southbury, Connecticut.

People think of kidney stones as occurring in the kidneys. But, as our consulting medical editor Andrew L. Rubman, ND, is clear to convey, diet and digestion are significant contributors to this seemingly unrelated problem. Whether it's binge drinking or high-protein diets, how you fuel your body impacts its function. "Garbage in, garbage out," as the saying goes. Going overboard on what you eat and drink can make you more susceptible to these painful, hard masses. Conversely, making smart and consistent dietary choices can help prevent kidney stones.

To simplify, kidney stones are formed in large part as a result of incomplete or out-of-balance digestion where nutrients are not available to the body when and where it needs them. Most kidney stones are primarily made of calcium oxalate, although sometimes they also contain uric acid, cystine or struvite.

Once you have one stone, you are likely to develop more. *Fortunately, according to Dr. Rubman, there are a number of steps you can take to prevent formation of kidney stones...*

DRINK UP

The single most important thing you can do: Drink plenty of water, advises Dr. Rubman. Fluids make stone components such as calcium oxalate more soluble in the urine, so they are less likely to form into crystals. The standard recommendation is eight eight-ounce glasses of water daily. For a more precise calculation of how much water you should drink each day, divide your weight in half. That number in ounces is your recommended daily water intake.

What you drink matters, too. In one study, hard tap water increased urinary calcium concentration (a risk factor for calcium stones) by 50% compared with soft bottled water. If hard water is what's available in your community, it makes sense to invest in bottled water.

Other healthful drinks include mineral water with a splash of fresh lemon or lime juice. Mineral water contains calcium and magnesium that may reduce the risk of stone formation, while a half cup of lemon juice daily raises the intake level of stone-fighting citrate.

Note: Other citrus fruits, such as orange or grapefruit, do not have the same effect. In fact, as mentioned below, grapefruit can *increase* stone risk. Other studies have suggested that coffee and tea, both natural diuretics, have a beneficial impact by increasing urine volume.

Best to avoid: Cola and grapefruit juice. Cola reduces the level of citrate in urine… and multiple studies have suggested that grapefruit juice raises stone risk.

The jury is still out on beer. While some research indicates that beer acts as a natural diuretic to dilute urine and increase frequency of urination, Dr. Rubman points out that beer is packed with stone-prompting oxalates. If you do drink beer or other alcoholic beverages, do so in moderation (generally considered to be one drink a day for women and two for men). Binge drinking increases uric acid production and thus the risk of uric acid stones.

To monitor whether you're taking in sufficient fluids, keep an eye on the color of urine. If it's dark yellow, you're not drinking enough. Urine should ideally be pale in color.

UP YOUR CALCIUM CONSUMPTION

Nearly three out of four kidney stones are composed of calcium oxalate, so it stands to reason that restricting calcium should prevent stones, right? Wrong! There is an inverse relationship between consumption of calcium and stone formation, explains Dr. Rubman. He points out that many people with osteoporosis develop calcium stones not because of calcium in food or supplements, but because of the body's reabsorption of calcium. If the body is not supplied adequate amounts of calcium, it steals its own from the bone. This results in more calcium circulating in the blood and eventually passing into the urine.

To make sure you get enough calcium in your diet, eat foods such as broccoli, kale, collard greens, almonds, sesame seeds and canned salmon or sardines. (Although dairy is the most obvious source of calcium, Dr. Rubman says cow's milk is best left to the calves.) If you don't get enough calcium in your diet, consider taking a supplement. The generally recommended dosage is 1,200 milligrams (mg) daily in two or preferably three divided doses. According to Dr. Rubman, calcium citrate is the supplement form most readily utilized by the body, and for best absorption he recommends that you take calcium with magnesium. In particular, he recommends Butyrex, made by T.E. Neesby, which already combines calcium and magnesium for you.

Caution: Do not take larger-than-recommended dosages of calcium supplements, because it can backfire and lead to stone formation. There is also a subset of calcium stone sufferers who have supersaturated calcium in the urine and must restrict calcium consumption. Only your doctor can determine if you are in this group. Do not take magnesium without calcium to attempt to offset the excess calcium. Always take calcium and magnesium together unless specifically told otherwise by a properly trained physician.

WATCH PROTEIN AND SODIUM INTAKE

Diets high in protein (especially animal protein) have consistently been associated with kidney stones. Protein raises levels of stone-causing calcium, oxalates and uric acid in the urine, and reduces protective citrate. Does this mean that those on the protein-heavy Atkins diet are more prone to kidney stones? As a matter of fact, Dr. Rubman worked for Dr. Atkins early in his career and in his experience, yes, they are.

Your best bet: Keep meat portion sizes moderate (about the size of a deck of cards), and fill the rest of your plate with fresh vegetables and whole grains.

Vegetarians also at risk: One study found no difference in kidney stone risk between people who consumed equal amounts of beef and plant protein. Dr. Rubman theorizes that this may be because soybeans, a common source of protein eaten by vegetarians, contain high levels of oxalates.

Sodium increases the level of calcium in urine, so those with calcium stones are best off restricting their intake of salt (whether from sprinkling it on food or consuming sodium-packed processed or fast foods). How do you know the type of stone you have? Use a cup to catch it and give it to your doctor for analysis.

MORE STONE-FIGHTING FOODS: FISH OIL AND FIBER

As if their heart-healthy benefits were not enough, eating cold-water fish such as salmon, mackerel, herring and sardines may also help prevent the formation of kidney stones. Inflammation plays a role in kidney stone development, and fish oil is naturally anti-inflammatory.

Goal: Try to eat fish at least twice a week. If you're not a fish eater, consider a daily supplement of 2,000 mg fish oil.

Fiber-rich foods such as vegetables and whole grains are an integral part of any healthful diet, and a compound called phytate—in foods such as rice bran and wheat, which may inhibit formation of calcium oxalate crystals—may help prevent kidney stones.

MULTIPLE FACTORS— MULTIPLE CHOICES

Just as there are multiple causes of kidney stones, there is no one single thing you can do to prevent them, says Dr. Rubman. A multipronged approach is required, one that emphasizes more fluids, calcium, fiber and fish oil, and more moderate consumption of protein and (for those with calcium stones) sodium.

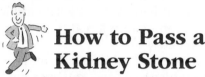

How to Pass a Kidney Stone

Andrew L. Rubman, ND, consulting medical editor for *Bottom Line's Daily Health News* and director of the Southbury Clinic for Traditional Medicines in Southbury, Connecticut.

Are there any secrets to success that can reduce the pain and suffering of trying to pass a kidney stone? Our consulting medical editor Andrew L. Rubman, ND, says that kidney stones generally do not constitute an emergency, and—if you have a good support system and sufficient stamina to tolerate the pain—in most cases you can pass a small stone in the relative comfort (if "comfort" can be used in the same sentence as kidney stones) of your own home.

A GOOD SUPPORT SYSTEM IS A MUST

If you're going to attempt to pass a kidney stone at home, the first thing you must have is a tolerant and understanding caregiver or partner, advises Dr. Rubman. He tells us that under no circumstances should you attempt to take on this task solo in the event that the pain becomes intolerable. If you live alone, enlist the help of a friend or neighbor. Why the need for company?

In case you say: I give up. I can't take it anymore. Take me to the nearest emergency room.

Fortunately, when Dr. Rubman had to pass a stone several years ago, his wife was there to help him through the process with unflagging support and good humor. Pleasant? No. Doable? Yes.

DRINK, DRINK, DRINK!

The single most important thing you can do to prevent kidney stones is to drink plenty of fluids, according to Dr. Rubman. This keeps the urine less concentrated and flowing freely. (A good benchmark: Aim for urine that is pale and watery, not dark yellow.) When it comes to passing a stone, fluids are even more critical, and Dr. Rubman recommends that you drink a minimum of two quarts a day. *Fluid choices include...*

•**Still water.** If the water out of your tap leaves something to be desired (for example, hard water is a risk factor for very common calcium oxalate kidney stones), reach for the bottled water.

•**Sparkling water.** Interestingly, sparkling water provides special benefits, as the carbonation—a combination of carbonic and phosphoric acids—decreases the tendency for spasm and allows for increased pain tolerance by buffering the acidic changes that accompany inflammation. Dr. Rubman's favorite sparkling water is San Pellegrino. He also recommends the carbonated spring water Gerolsteiner. Packed with electrolytes, this is an excellent water to help pass stones.

•**Soup and tea.** Dr. Rubman recommends egg drop soup, the Chinese penicillin. Mom's homemade chicken soup might also play a role here. In addition, tea (green is best) can help propel a stone out. All these beverages serve to increase urine volume.

Of course, not all fluids are created equal, and it's best to steer clear of sugar-packed products such as sodas and sports drinks. Sugar contributes to inflammation, which contributes to kidney stones. When in doubt, look closely at the list of ingredients. You'll be surprised to learn how much sugar lurks in even so-called health drinks. We asked Dr. Rubman about drinking juices as part of the two quarts a day.

His recommendation: Pomegranate juice diluted with water is best.

FEEL THE HEAT

Another important strategy is to apply heat. Heat can help relax muscles that are tense from pain and spasm, allowing for easier passage of a stone. In particular, Dr. Rubman recommends that you apply a thin layer of a highly aromatic, icy hot preparation such as capsaicin, menthol or eucalyptol over the painful flank (lower back). Once the cream or ointment soaks in, cover the area with a heating pad.

A variety of icy hot preparations is available at your local health food store.

Dr. Rubman's suggestion: Flex-A-Gesic (manufactured by Progressive Labs in Irving, Texas and available at *http://organicpharmacy.org*), which was originally developed for the Dallas Cowboys. This is a no-nonsense, industrial-strength remedy. You will need to don plastic gloves to apply it. (*Caution:* Icy hot preparations sting mightily at first, and some people cannot tolerate them. But if you can wait out the initial sting—about 10 minutes—the pain relief will soon begin to kick in. Be sure to wash your hands very well after application so you don't accidentally get it in your eyes.)

Another simple but effective option: Take a hot bath with Epsom salts. Alternatively, Dr. Rubman suggests that hydrotherapy—alternating hot and cold—is beneficial, but it may cause nausea. If you want to give it a try, make sure you have a strong caregiver nearby in case you feel dizzy or faint. If you do feel dizzy, get out of the water and lie down.

BOTANICAL OPTIONS

Botanicals that can be helpful at both easing the pain and passing the stone. These include corn silk, crampbark, gravel root, stone root, seven barks or khella to ease the discomfort of passing a stone. And wild lettuce, black hellebore, arnica and gelsemium can help ease the pain. Dr. Rubman warns that all of these medications should be prescribed and monitored by a professional. It is unwise to attempt to self-administer the pain remedies.

If you're prone to kidney stones, it's a good idea to have a naturopathic physician on board your health-care team, observes Dr. Rubman. He or she can help you develop and put into practice preventive strategies. If there is blood in the urine, severe pain, fever, an inability to urinate or a stone that fails to pass within 48 hours, go to a critical care facility or the hospital emergency room. In most cases (70% to 80% of the time) stones pass on their own with urine. If you have a good support system in place and know what you're in for, you may be more comfortable (or at least less uncomfortable) seeing the process out in your own home.

Drink to Your Health

Charles Bamforth, PhD, department chair, food science and technology, and Anheuser-Busch Endowed Professor of Malting and Brewing Sciences at University of California, Davis, and special professor in the school of biosciences at University of Nottingham, England. He is editor in chief of *Journal of the American Society of Brewing Chemists*. His most recent book is *Grape vs. Grain* (Cambridge University), a comparison of wine and beer.

Maybe you drink a glass or two of red wine every day because you have heard about its high levels of heart-protecting antioxidants, such as *resveratrol.*

What you may not know: The main heart-helping ingredient in alcoholic drinks is *ethanol*—alcohol itself.

MODERATION IS KEY

The health benefits from drinking alcoholic beverages depend on moderation— on average, no more than one drink a day for women and two drinks a day for men.

Example: A drink is five ounces of wine …12 ounces of beer…or 1½ ounces of distilled spirits or liquor, such as vodka or whiskey.

The benefits also depend on frequency. Studies show that it is healthier to have one or two daily drinks than one or two on just a few days a week. Of course, alcoholics and those with a family history of alcoholism should avoid alcohol.

Also, alcohol and many medications, including sedatives, don't mix. If you're taking a medication, ask your doctor if moderate drinking is okay.

DRINK TO YOUR HEALTH

Preventing heart disease may be the primary benefit of moderate alcohol intake, but studies show that moderate consumption of alcohol can benefit health in many other ways…

•**Diabetes.** Researchers at the Albert Einstein College of Medicine in New York City analyzed 32 studies on alcohol intake and diabetes and found that moderate consumption of alcohol (one to three drinks a day) lowered the risk for diabetes by 33% to 56% and the risk of developing diabetes-related heart disease by 34% to 55%.

•**Kidney stones.** Finnish researchers found that drinking a bottle of beer a day reduced the risk for developing kidney stones by 40%.

•**Gallstone disease.** Harvard researchers found that both wine and beer reduced the risk for gallstone disease (by speeding up the emptying of the gallbladder after eating a meal).

•**Osteoporosis.** Researchers have found that social drinking was associated with higher bone mineral density in older men and women.

•**Rheumatoid arthritis.** People who drink alcohol regularly are up to 50% less likely to develop rheumatoid arthritis than nondrinkers, say Scandinavian researchers in *Annals of the Rheumatic Diseases.* One possible reason is that alcohol reduces inflammation.

5

New Ways to Ease Allergy or Asthma Symptoms

Drug-Free Ways to Treat Fall Allergies

Many people associate fall allergies with piles of wet leaves. Truth is, the barrage of runny, stuffy and itchy noses and eyes, sneezing and wheezing that make millions of Americans miserable each fall begins at the end of summer when the ragweed blooms. Ragweed pollen is by far the most common autumnal culprit, although mold spores that grow in piles of wet leaves also prove troublesome for many. When plant growth is "supersized" by extra wet and rainy summers, the fall discomforts that follow are even worse.

While many people turn to the array of conventional treatments of prescription or over-the-counter antihistamines, there are growing numbers of allergy sufferers who would prefer to avoid the use of pharma-

ceutical drugs. For tips on how to cope with fall allergies pharmaceutical-free, we consulted Robert S. Ivker, DO, past president of the American Holistic Medical Association, who currently maintains a holistic medical practice in Denver. He shared a wealth of strategies for beating nasty allergy symptoms…

SUPPLEMENTS AND OTHER HERBAL REMEDIES

For those who want to avoid the uncomfortable side effects of antihistamines, Dr. Ivker recommends a wide variety of supplements that act as "natural antihistamines." Work with your doctor or someone properly trained in natural treatments to find the combination that works best for you. *According to Dr. Ivker, those that are most highly effective are…*

Robert S. Ivker, DO, maintains a holistic medical practice in Denver. *www.sinussurvival.com.* He is past president of the American Holistic Medical Association (AHMA), and cofounder and past president of the American Board of Holistic Medicine (ABHM).

•*Euphorbium* **nasal spray.** This homeopathic remedy may help reduce sinus pressure and allergy-related headaches while it improves breathing as part of a natural treatment plan. It is available at most health food stores.

•**Vitamin C.** Take as ester C or the ascorbate form at high levels (3,000 milligrams [mg] to 6,000 mg/day) to help reduce inflammation caused by allergies.

•**Grape seed extract.** This herb, with strong antioxidant and anti-inflammatory properties—should be taken in dosages of 100 mg to 300 mg daily, though sometimes more may be used depending on the individual. It is best taken first thing in the morning on an empty stomach.

•**Stinging nettle.** An average dose consists of 300 mg of the freeze-dried herb in capsule form three times daily.

•**Quercetin.** This bioflavonoid, which is usually found in red wine and onions, should ideally be started before the allergy season begins and continued throughout the season. For optimal absorption, take it with the digestive enzyme bromelain and on an empty stomach. The total daily dosage of quercetin is 1,000 mg to 2,000 mg divided into three to six doses.

•**Homeopathic remedies.** There are several homeopathic allergy remedies in tablet form that can be taken in conjunction with some or all of the above. These are also best taken on an empty stomach several times a day.

•**Nazanol and Sinupret.** These products are combinations of Chinese herbs that are highly effective in reducing inflammation of the mucous membranes, which lessens hypersensitivity and decreases allergy symptoms, explains Dr. Ivker. Both are available through health-care practitioners and should be used under their supervision.

Caution: Because these therapeutic doses often exceed standard recommendations, it is best to consult your health-care practitioner before taking them.

PRACTICE GOOD NASAL HYGIENE

Good nasal hygiene can also help reduce allergy symptoms by removing the pollen and reducing inflammation and hypersensitivity of the mucous membrane. *Dr. Ivker recommends the following daily practices...*

•**Saline spray.** Saline spray—preferably one containing aloe vera—can be used frequently throughout the day, especially in the early morning when the pollen counts are highest. Pollen particles rise during the heat of the day and allergy symptoms are generally not quite as severe.

•**Steam inhalation.** Steam acts as an effective decongestant and is best delivered with a device called a steam inhaler that can be found in most pharmacies. Adding a medicinal eucalyptus oil to the steam helps to reduce inflammation. Practice three or four times daily, preferably followed by nasal irrigation.

•**Nasal irrigation.** There are a wide variety of irrigation methods—Neti Pot, SinuCleanse and perhaps the most effective is the HydroPulse Nasal Irrigator. Irrigation is best after steaming, three to four times daily.

ADJUST YOUR DIET

A nutritious, hypoallergenic diet can be quite helpful in dealing with allergies of all kinds. Simply avoid the foods that you know or suspect you are sensitive to, along with foods that increase mucus and inflammation and reduce immune function. *Dr. Ivker makes the following suggestions...*

•**Reduce or eliminate milk and dairy products,** which can often increase mucus drainage.

•**Avoid sugar,** which Dr. Ivker believes can weaken immunity.

•**Eat a variety of fresh fruits and vegetables,** organic non-gluten whole grains (brown rice, quinoa, millet, amaranth), beans, legumes, nuts and seeds. Choose nondairy sources of protein such as fish and organic chicken or turkey.

•**Drink plenty of bottled or filtered water.** Increased water intake helps hydrate the mucous membranes and thin the mucus, making it easier to drain, explains Dr. Ivker. The average daily recommended amount for adults is a half-ounce per pound of body weight.

MORE LIFESTYLE CONSIDERATIONS

If you could only do one thing to control your allergies, it would be to avoid their triggers. *To that end, Dr. Ivker advises his patients to...*

•**Stay indoors on high pollen count days** (which your local TV or radio station will warn you about), with the windows closed and the air conditioner on. Dr. Ivker notes that it is especially important to avoid outdoor exercise on these days, particularly in the early morning hours when pollen counts are highest.

•**Use an air conditioner** rather than window fans to cool your home.

•**Invest in a negative-ion generator for the bedroom.** Choose one that does not emit ozone. These devices are highly effective in removing pollen from the air, notes Dr. Ivker.

•**Get seven to nine hours of sleep nightly.** This will help keep your immune system fully charged.

•**If you must mow the lawn or rake leaves, wear a mask.** Better yet, get someone else to take care of these chores.

•**Regularly clean moldy surfaces** (e.g., the AC, humidifier and dehumidifier).

•**Shower and wash your hair when you come in from outdoor activities.**

•**Wash clothing and bedding regularly in hot water.**

•**Be a good housekeeper** and keep your home as clean as possible.

IN CONCLUSION

All in all, when it comes to fall allergies, your best offense is usually a good defense. The best way to beat runny noses and itchy eyes is to maintain a balanced immune system with a few key supplements...eat a healthy, hypoallergenic diet...close the windows, etc. Using these simple strategies, chances are you'll breathe more easily this fall.

Hidden Causes of Allergy Symptoms

Andrew L. Rubman, ND, consulting medical editor for *Bottom Line's Daily Health News* and director of the Southbury Clinic for Traditional Medicines in Southbury, Connecticut.

When you think about controlling allergies or hay fever, you probably think about avoiding things like pollen or freshly mown grass or your friend's cat or a moldy basement. In many cases, this avoidance strategy is effective at controlling uncomfortable allergy symptoms. However, often the allergy triggers remain elusive and there's a possibility you may be overlooking an important one—what you eat and drink.

EAT, DRINK AND BE MISERABLE?

Since allergic sensitivities may be, in effect, cumulative, certain foods and beverages can make you more vulnerable to allergy symptoms such as sneezing, sniffling, congestion, skin irritations and red, watery eyes, confirms *Bottom Line's Daily Health News* consulting medical editor Andrew L. Rubman, ND. In his opinion, it's simplistic to just suppress these symptoms with medication. Instead, he advises looking deeper into dietary connections to potentially "cure" the problem rather than simply mask it. *Dr. Rubman shares more of his thoughts on so-called food allergies, along with advice on what you can do about them...*

In most cases, what we commonly refer to as food "allergies" would be more accurately described as food "sensitivities." On occasion, a person may experience a true food allergy—in the worst case, a life-threatening allergic reaction (anaphylaxis) to foods such as shellfish or peanuts. Far more commonly, however, a runny nose, sneezing, hives and other sorts of allergy symptoms reflect a sensitivity to certain foods that are difficult for the body to process, notes Dr. Rubman. The foods that typically are hardest to digest—cow's milk and gluten grains (wheat, barley, rye)—are the most likely to cause problems.

SURPRISING CAUSE AND EFFECT

We asked Dr. Rubman how a glass of milk and a sandwich on whole wheat bread—a meal you digest in the gut—can cause symptoms in the nose. He explains that the body has several mechanisms to deal with digestive challenges. Normally, food residues are effectively contained within the intestine, through which nutrients are absorbed while the remainder pass efficiently and completely from the body. However, when factors such as disease, stress, excessive alcohol, medication or foods containing dairy proteins/sugars or gluten cause inflammation, the intestinal wall may "leak," permitting tiny partially digested food particles to escape, causing the body to produce antibodies to attack the unknown particles (called antigens).

One surprising manifestation of these microscopic food particles is *rhinitis*, due to the body's powerful immune-modulating system. While nasal defenses normally handle airborne challenges, deftly filtering out and destroying millions of irritating pollutants, particles and chemicals in the air you breathe, at these times they also react to immune system responses due to intestinal permeability (or what's called "leaky gut"). This is asking a lot of the mucous membranes in the sinuses, which react by producing extra mucus (hence, the sniffles) to attempt, often ineffectively, to respond to antigens in the body.

STRATEGY TO REDUCE THE SYMPTOMS

While mainstream medicine generally treats allergy symptoms with antihistamines, decongestants or immunotherapy, far better, says Dr. Rubman, is to examine and change your diet as necessary. In general, he advises consumption of more whole foods—such as fresh vegetables and fruits and legumes, deep-water fish like salmon and tuna, and poultry without skin—and fewer processed foods laden with additives, saturated fats and sugar, all of which can worsen allergy symptoms and leaky gut. In particular, limit your intake of cow's milk, milk products and products with gluten because these have the greatest capacity to disrupt the gut lining, particularly the large intestine.

Specifically, Dr. Rubman makes these recommendations…

•**Leave cow's milk to baby cows.** This seemingly healthy drink has absolutely no place in the human diet, stresses Dr. Rubman. Every species of mammalian mother produces milk specially designed to be consumed by their young. Given that, it is not surprising that some people are allergic to the specific milk whey and casein proteins, since they are immunologically different from what humans naturally digest. Many people are also sensitive to lactose, a milk sugar. Among the unappealing symptoms cow's milk can cause are digestive disturbances, mucus buildup in the sinuses, immune system reactions and more. (*Note:* Cheese and yogurt are more easily tolerated in the lactose sensitive or intolerant. Start by cutting out cow's milk, and see whether you feel better.)

Because calcium is essential for healthy bones and teeth, not to mention numerous vital body functions, many people worry about giving up their daily glass of milk. However, there are many other rich—and more readily digestible—sources of calcium, including broccoli, kale and turnip greens, plus salmon and sardines canned with bones.

•**Cut back on gluten grain products.** Gluten—the complex protein in wheat, barley and rye—causes disturbances in the structural and functional performance of the intestine, explains Dr. Rubman. This can result in both intestinal (gas, bloating, diarrhea, for example) and nonintestinal symptoms (e.g., fatigue, irritability, and bone and joint pain in addition to the allergy symptoms), ranging from mild to severe.

Opt for gluten-free alternative grains such as quinoa, amaranth, buckwheat or brown rice. Look for gluten-free labels on processed foods (such as soy sauce, ketchup and salad dressings, which are among the surprising products that often contain gluten). Or, better yet, forego the processed foods altogether.

NOT SUCH AN "EXTREME" MAKEOVER

When you've explored the obvious causes—such as pollen and mold—and your allergy symptoms remain bothersome and unexplained, it's time to wonder whether your diet might be the real problem. Since dairy and gluten products are naturally challenging to the human digestive tract, it is likely that everyone is affected to varying degrees by a dairy and/or gluten sensitivity, says Dr. Rubman.

So the question is not "if," but "how much" milk or cereal it will take to trigger symptoms in you. Often, the answer depends on your overall health. *Dr. Rubman advises taking these factors into account...*

•**How pumped is your immune system?** The healthier you are, the better prepared your body will be to meet the challenge of processing hard-to-digest food and drink.

•**How old are you?** It's not always the case, but usually the older you get, the less robust immune protection you have, compared with younger counterparts.

•**Is your body busy meeting intermittent challenges such as seasonal airborne irritants (pollen, ragweed, etc.)?** If so, this can leave you especially vulnerable to the ill effects of digestive challenges, due to systemic inflammation that can affect intestinal permeability.

BACK TO BASICS

Dr. Rubman says that even in the absence of obvious allergy symptoms, everyone can benefit from eating more whole foods and fewer processed ones, cutting out cow's milk and limiting gluten. If you just can't live without the pasta, or milk on your cereal, have it as a treat one or two times a week. This allows your body to rid itself of the antigens before the next "attack." The more closely our diet resembles what we were meant to eat, back in the days before processing and manufacturing, the healthier we will be and the better we will feel.

Six Natural Asthma Relievers That Work!

Eliot W. Edwards, ND, a naturopathic physician with Upstate Naturopathic, Vestal, New York. www. dreliotedwards.com.

Most of the 20 million Americans with asthma (more than six million of whom are children) rely on medications such as corticosteroids, bronchodilators and sometimes a combination of the two. These medications work well to halt or fight attacks and can be lifesaving, so they should always be on hand for people with asthma. However, these drugs are not free of side effects, and long-term use of them can weaken the immune system, making the patient more susceptible to infection. The good news is that there are nonpharmaceutical options to help control asthma and reduce reliance on drugs.

WHEN ASTHMA ATTACKS

For information on natural options in asthma treatment, we spoke with Eliot W. Edwards, ND, a naturopathic physician with Upstate Naturopathic in Vestal, New York. The key, as with so many medical conditions, is to create a strong underlying system, which includes reducing irritants to the body and strengthening the immune system. Interestingly, most of Dr. Edwards' advice is for areas that are not the lungs.

DR. EDWARDS' ASTHMA STRATEGY

•**Avoid asthma triggers as much as possible.** Triggers vary from person to person and may include secondhand smoke, dust mites, mold, cockroaches, household pets and certain chemicals or foods. Food sensitivities may include dairy, wheat, eggs, citrus fruits and shellfish. Dr. Edwards suggests using an air purifier and avoiding forced air heating and wood stoves. While this seems obvious, there are two million emergency room visits each year caused by asthma attacks, many of which are a result of allergenic triggers.

•**Boost your immune system.** A strong immune system increases your body's resistance to irritants and decreases the likelihood you'll experience a reaction. Depending on the patient's needs, Dr. Edwards may use bioflavonoids and immune-supporting herbs such as echinacea, oregon grape and astragalus. Dosages for these herbs, as well as all others mentioned below, should be prescribed for a patient based on his/her size, severity of symptoms, potential interactions with the medications he is on and any possible sensitivities he may have. Dr. Edwards says that drinking more water, getting plenty of sleep and eating a diet rich in whole foods, fruits and vegetables can also help strengthen your immune system.

•**Support the detoxification pathways in the body.** The better your body's detoxification pathways are working, the better your body can deal with the irritants it comes in contact with. Dr. Edwards uses N-acetyl cysteine, essential fatty acids (fish oil), vitamin C and bromelain to support the detox system. Dr. Edwards also says that proper elimination is essential to the body getting rid of waste. Our consulting medical editor Andrew L. Rubman, ND, says his favorite elimination aid is a fiber called glucomannan.

•**Support your stomach.** Stomach acid aids in digestion and helps break down foreign proteins (irritants) before they get into the body. When not working properly, poor digestion can create inflammation and irritation in the pathways, which can in turn trigger asthma attacks. Controlling acid reflux and ensuring proper digestive function is critical to the control of asthma.

To help ensure healthy digestion, Dr. Edwards has patients with low stomach acid (hypochlorhydria) supplement with betaine HCl or take apple cider vinegar well before meals as a tonic. He also recommends probiotics to ensure a strong population of beneficial bacteria to support the gut and immune system.

•**Support your lungs.** To strengthen your respiratory system and reduce the chances of an attack, Dr. Edwards says a useful combination may include *tussilago* (coltsfoot), *lobelia*, *capsicum* (cayenne pepper), *verbascum thapsis* (wooly mullein), *elecampane*, *yerba santa*, milk vetch and nettles. *Ma huang*, also known as ephedra, was an effective antidote to breathing disorders but was banned by the US Food and Drug Administration.

•**Reduce stress.** Stress has an impact on asthma attacks and should be addressed, especially if anxiety issues are present. Deep breathing exercises are effective at reducing stress. Yoga, meditation and tai chi also may be helpful.

SEEK HELP

If you have asthma, see your doctor at least once a year, Dr. Edwards says. But if your asthma attacks become more severe or increase in frequency, schedule a medical checkup immediately. "Anytime you have an attack that doesn't respond quickly to treatment, get yourself to the emergency room, since asthma can be life-threatening without prompt, effective treatment," says Dr. Edwards.

And always seek the advice of a trained professional when using natural remedies so you are certain to be using them safely and at therapeutic dosages, Dr. Edwards stresses. "Bronchodilators can save the life of a person with asthma, but the degree to which an individual relies on them can be varied through naturopathic approaches."

info You can find a naturopathic physician in your area by visiting the American Association of Naturopathic Physicians' Web site *www.naturopathic.org.*

How to Get the Most From Steroidal Inhalers

Richard Firshein, DO, director of the Firshein Center for Comprehensive Medicine in New York City and author of *Reversing Asthma* (Warner) and *Your Asthma-Free Child* (Avery).

Currently, steroidal inhalers are a standard treatment for asthma in children. Yet a recent study in *The New England Journal of Medicine* reported that these drugs have no long-term impact on the progression of asthma or on lung function in preschoolers. While symptoms were controlled during treatment, benefits disappeared when treatment was halted. Additionally, steroids have many dangerous side effects, with children in the study experiencing slowed growth when using steroidal inhalers. Bad for children. Bad for adults.

FOR ACUTE SITUATIONS

To get an expert's take on steroids and learn about safer, natural alternatives, we spoke with Richard Firshein, DO, director of the Firshein Center for Comprehensive Medicine in New York City and author of *Reversing Asthma* (Warner) and *Your Asthma-Free Child* (Avery). He acknowledges that inhaled steroids are not a panacea, but they do play a helpful role when symptoms are particularly troublesome. For example, if a child is experiencing a high level of inflammation and/or wheezing and missing many school days, Dr. Firshein is apt to prescribe a corticosteroid

inhaler for short-term use. However, he does not recommend these drugs on a long-term basis, and emphasizes that his first line of defense is to prevent symptoms naturally. Patients with long-term asthma should consider Singulair or a bronchodilator on an "as needed" basis, he says.

BUILD A STRONG FOUNDATION

Asthma has many triggers. Among its possible triggers are airborne pollutants, secondhand smoke, allergens (dust mites, animal dander, mold, chemicals, foods, etc.) and cold air.

Also: Aspirin and NSAIDs can trigger an attack, as can a viral infection. To prevent asthma symptoms from occurring in the first place, rather than simply responding to them, Dr. Firshein stresses that you must make healthful changes—changes that reduce the exposure to the things that trigger asthma, and changes that strengthen the body's immune system to resist those triggers. That advice applies not only to children with asthma, but to asthma sufferers of all ages. Allergy shots have also been shown to reduce the sensitivity to allergy triggers such as dust, dust mites, pollen and pet dander.

To build a strong foundation, Dr. Firshein suggests that you…

•**Closely monitor your environment.** Go through your house carefully and remove possible triggers. For example, eliminate dust collectors such as wall-to-wall carpeting and heavy drapes…install an air filter to clean household air…frequently wash nonallergenic bedding and nonallergenic pillow and mattress covers…use a dehumidifier in damp basements and bathrooms and bedrooms…and avoid using air fresheners. Additionally, do not neglect school or work environments, where we spend so many hours of our lives. It's equally important to eliminate triggers here. Parents should speak directly to principals and teachers about a child's allergy triggers and have the necessary emergency procedures in place, should an attack occur.

•**Keep an eye on diet.** Dr. Firshein is particularly concerned with asthmatic children eating junk food, which he compares to an adult with heart disease eating fat-laden cheeseburgers and fries. He points out that junk foods promote inflammation, which promotes asthma. Instead, follow an anti-inflammatory diet rich in nutrient-dense whole foods such as fresh fruits and veggies (berries are especially rich in inflammation-fighting antioxidants), fish, nuts and seeds. Whenever possible, go with organic products.

•**Take immune-boosting supplements.** In particular, Dr. Firshein recommends vitamin C (1,000 milligrams [mg]), magnesium (500 mg), fish oil and a good multivitamin. When using inhaled steroids, which may compromise the bones, he also recommends a calcium-magnesium supplement (1,200 mg of calcium) for added protection.

Note: Dosages should be reduced in children by 50% to 75% of an adult dosage. In general, he finds that children respond much more rapidly to multivitamins than adults, allowing them to catch fewer colds and miss less schoolwork, and gain hardier immunity overall with relatively simple supplementation.

•**Learn to breathe easy.** Dr. Firshein discussed the Firshein Technique for Asthma Breathing, a series of exercises that teach children to stabilize their asthma. He finds that children above age five do particularly well with breathing exercises. Asthma sufferers often feel nervous and out of control when they approach a situation that they know brings on symptoms, such as exercise or cold air. These breathing exercises give individuals a sense of control over a situation, and also strengthen muscles in the diaphragm, which is crucial to controlling asthma.

EXERCISES HELP, TOO

Dr. Firshein offers these simple exercises when encountering potential triggers...

•**Breathe in through the nose for a count of five,** and breathe out through the mouth for a count of seven.

•**Next, breathe in deeply, and then blow out the air in a burst like you're blowing out a candle.** This strengthens the lungs and diaphragm, explains Dr. Firshein.

•**Use your stomach.** Lie down, and as you breathe in through the nose, consciously make your stomach expand. Breathe out and allow your stomach to deflate.

•**Try a rocking motion while standing,** breathing in and rocking to one side then breathing out while rocking to the other side. Then switch. Air gets trapped in the lungs of people with asthma, so they cannot take in enough new oxygen, observes Dr. Firshein. Rocking back and forth helps the body use the ribcage more to expel the stale air so there's more room in the lungs.

•**Get plenty of exercise.** Exercise is doubly important for the asthmatic child, says Dr. Firshein. Breathing exercises work by reducing stress, improving oxygen intake and by strengthening the muscles that are used in respiration. If exercise is a trigger of asthma symptoms, the physician should closely monitor the exercise program. In some cases, breathing exercises may ease and prevent attacks. Using a peak flow meter is the most effective way to monitor breathing at home.

HOW TO INHALE STEROIDS CORRECTLY

If you or your child must take steroids for a period of time, Dr. Firshein recommends a safer way to go about using them. Spacing devices provide an effective way of maximizing medication and minimizing deposits in the mouth. He cautions that steroids in dry powder form are difficult to inhale, with often as much as 90% of the powdered medication ending up in the mouth. When you swallow this, you are apt to experience greater side effects than with inhalation alone. To reduce side effects, following inhalation, rinse your mouth thoroughly.

A BETTER WAY

With side effects from steroids being so severe and their effectiveness being so limited, they should only be used when they are truly necessary. Using simple strategies that build a strong foundation for your health can lower risk of asthma attacks and cut back on the medication required to control them.

info For more information contact the American Academy of Allergy, Asthma and Immunology, *www.aaaai.org.*

Homeopathic Nasal Sprays that Work as Well as Drugs

Richard Mann, ND, chair of the homeopathy department, Bastyr Center for Natural Health, Seattle.

Ah, the joys of spring! The birds, the flowers, the greening trees, the warming weather. But for about 40 million Americans, the joy of the season is diminished by seasonal allergies, mainly hay fever. In the arsenal of conventional hay fever remedies, the over-the-counter (OTC) nasal sprays have been around for a while, but they can only be used safely a few days at a time. It's worth looking at natural alternatives.

At least one homeopathic nasal spray, Luffeel, has been found to be as equally effective as an OTC conventional nasal spray called *cromolyn nasal spray* (Nasalcrom). In a trial comparing the two, 146 participants (all of whom were hay fever sufferers), were either given Luffeel or Nasalcrom. The results? Both Luffeel and Nasalcrom worked equally well in reducing symptoms. Hay fever symptoms typically include sneezing, watery eyes and congestion.

Richard Mann, ND, chair of the homeopathy department at Seattle's Bastyr Center for Natural Health, says that the OTC homeopathic nasal sprays can certainly be effective. They are usually comprised of several homeopathic substances that have been known by homeopaths to have the effect of allergy symptom relief—temporary relief or modification of symptoms without permanently removing that symptom. Because the homeopathic nasal sprays are typically a combination of substances, it makes sense that patients will have a good chance of a response to one or more of these.

JUST USE SPARINGLY

As for risk? As long as the elements in the homeopathic sprays are low potency (30X or less) and are used occasionally when symptoms occur, there is minimal, if any, side-effect risk to the homeopathic sprays. Similarly, Nasalcrom provides minimal side-effects, if any, for short-term and occasional usage. According to Dr. Mann, "If one uses these products, he should use them for short-term management of symptoms only, and then be sure to follow up for deeper treatment, that will get to the cause of the symptoms."

In spite of the seeming success of Luffeel, Dr. Mann offers some caveats on using homeopathic products.

HOMEOPATHIC CAVEATS

At the core of homeopathy is the premise that homeopathic treatments for a "medical problem" have subtle differences, depending on the way the symptoms display in one person or another. The trained practitioner creates a personalized prescriptive plan for the treatment that best fits the patient's specific symptom pattern. The aim is not simply symptom suppression as an end in itself, but rather the discovery of the underlying causes of symptoms. In the homeopathic medical paradigm, symptoms represent the state of the whole organism, and not the cause of a medical problem. While a one-size-fits-all nasal spray sounds good, seeing a practitioner for a personalized perspective may be even more effective at eliminating the underlying cause.

In his practice, Dr. Mann has successfully treated people who presented with hay fever with homeopathic remedies tailored to that individual's unique physical condition. In people with hay fever, symptoms did indeed disappear—permanently—along with other symptoms, but it usually took a while, sometimes months or even a year or two, for the body to completely rebalance itself.

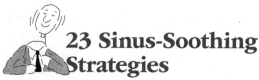

23 Sinus-Soothing Strategies

Robert S. Ivker, DO, maintains a holistic medical practice in Denver. *www.sinussurvival.com*. He is past president of the American Holistic Medical Association (AHMA), and cofounder and past president of the American Board of Holistic Medicine (ABHM).

Along with the cold and snow, winter months bring extra challenges for sinusitis sufferers. Dry air is tough on sensitive mucous membranes, and closed windows and poor ventilation can lead to the buildup of noxious particles (including fumes from harsh cleaning products, paint, perfumes, etc.), the enemies of sinusitis and allergy sufferers. Winter is also prime time for catching colds, which like allergies, often precede sinus infections.

To learn how to best cope with sinusitis during the winter and to more effectively treat ongoing chronic sinusitis in any season, we consulted Denver-based Robert S. Ivker, DO, past president of the American Holistic Medical Association, and who currently maintains a holistic medical practice in Denver. He shared a number of strategies to ease sinus suffering this winter and throughout the rest of the year.

KEEP AIR CLEAN AND MOIST

Whatever the season, a primary objective is always to create optimal air in your work and home environment, says Dr. Ivker. This means air that is clean (you can't see or smell it), moist (between 35% and 55% relative humidity), negative-ion and oxygen-filled and warm (between 65 and 75 degrees Fahrenheit). The nose and sinuses are the body's air filter and we breathe about 23,000 times a day. *He advises...*

•**When choosing a heating system, radiant heat/baseboard heating systems are preferable** to forced hot-air heating systems through ducts since it keeps the hot dry air and dust particles from flying through the house.

•**If you have a forced hot-air heating system, use an efficient furnace filter** (such as Filtrete made by 3M) and change it monthly or more often during the winter months.

•**Have your home's air ducts cleaned every three years.**

•**Fill your home with high oxygen producing and air filtering plants** (such as spider plants, chrysanthemums, striped dracaena and Boston ferns), which can remove toxins from the air and generate oxygen.

•**Place a warm mist humidifier in your bedroom.** This keeps air moist, preventing sinuses from becoming dry and irritated. In Dr. Ivker's opinion, two leading brands are Slant/Fin (*www.slantfin.com*) and Bionaire (*www.bionaire.com*).

•**Invest in a negative-ion generator.** These devices efficiently clean air by binding with dust particles, mold, animal dander, smoke, bacteria and viruses (all of which have a positive charge), with the subsequently heavier particle dropping out of the air and falling to tabletops, floors, etc. The end result is that the harmful particles are removed from your breathing space. There is also speculation within the scientific community that ion-filled air might have a beneficial effect on mucous membranes, lung function and even mood. Some psychological studies have shown negative ion-filled air, similar to the high ion content found by seacoasts, waterfalls, pine forests and mountaintops, can improve mood. Studies have also shown that ionized air has improved the lung capacity of asthmatics. Ionizers that do not emit ozone are best (ozone is an irritant to the mucous membrane), says Dr. Ivker.

•**Consider a HEPA (high-efficiency particulate arrestor) air cleaner.** According to Dr. Ivker, these are also highly efficient in their ability to purify air. However, they have none of the other beneficial effects of negative ions.

•**Avoid air pollutants, strong odors and fumes.** Secondhand smoke is the single, most harmful indoor air pollutant, warns Dr. Ivker. Others include radon, mold, dust, harsh cleaning products and air fresheners. Whenever possible keep chemical products out of your home, and instead use environment-friendly "green" cleaning products (baking soda, vinegar, borax, etc.), which are less irritating to the sinuses.

SOOTHE SINUSES, HEAL MUCOUS MEMBRANES

Dr. Ivker's regimen for healing mucous membranes includes saline spray, steam inhalation, irrigation, inhalation of medicinal eucalyptus oil and drinking lots of water, in addition to the air cleaning and moistening recommendations above. These strategies combine to reduce chronic inflammation, congestion, increased mucus secretion (postnasal drip), hypersensitivity and hyperreactivity of the mucous membranes. *His program includes...*

•**Use saline spray** to keep mucous membranes moist as well as to irrigate the particles that you may have inhaled. Ideally, use a saline spray containing aloe vera, for its healing properties on the mucous membrane. To help head off an infection, an ionic silver sinus spray is recommended, such as Peaceful Mountain's Sinus Rescue (*www.peacefulmountain.com*).

•**Steam sinus problems away.** Use a steam inhaler (available at most drugstores) three or four times daily. To reduce congestion and inflammation even further, add a medicinal eucalyptus oil to

it. It can also be applied to tissue and inhaled frequently throughout the day.

•**After steaming, irrigate your sinuses.** This can be done with a Neti pot, bulb syringe or SinuCleanse (also available at pharmacies). The SinuPulse Irrigator, utilizing the same pulsating technology as the Water-Pik device, is a very efficient method for irrigation (available at many pharmacies).

•**Drink plenty of bottled or filtered water.** The average daily recommended amount for adults is a half ounce per pound of body weight. If you weigh 160 pounds, you should drink 80 ounces a day.

PUMP UP YOUR IMMUNE SYSTEM

A strong immune system makes you better equipped to resist not only sinusitis, but the seasonal colds and flu that frequently lead to sinus infections in susceptible individuals. *For treating, preventing and often curing acute and chronic sinusitis, Dr. Ivker recommends...*

•**Get seven to nine hours of sleep nightly.** This will help keep your immune system operating at peak capacity.

•**Watch your diet.** Avoid inflammatory foods such as sugar, refined white flour, fried items, excess red meat, partially hydrogenated oils and additives. Also sharply reduce milk and dairy products, which can increase mucus drainage. Instead, fill your plate with fresh fruits and vegetables, organic nongluten whole grains (brown rice, quinoa, millet, amaranth, etc.), beans, legumes, nuts and seeds. Choose nondairy sources of protein such as fish and organic chicken or turkey.

•**Consider supplements.** Dr. Ivker often prescribes vitamin C (Ester-C), vitamin E, a good multivitamin, selenium, grape seed extract (take on an empty stomach), fish oil and flaxseed oil on a regular basis for preventive maintenance. With an active sinus infection, you should add echinacea, high-potency garlic (such as Allimax) and the homeopathic remedies *Kali sulphuricum* and *Kali bichromicum* (these homeopathics are most effective if taken right at the onset of an acute sinus infection).

•**For those who take antibiotics regularly or even intermittently…**an allergic reaction to fungal (including *Candida*) organisms was identified by the Mayo Clinic as a key contributing factor to the majority of cases of severe chronic sinusitis. This problem occurs most commonly as a result of the overuse of antibiotics. A naturopathic physician or DO can help diagnose and provide a treatment protocol to reduce the Candida overgrowth.

•**Get moving.** Regular moderate exercise will increase your energy level and help you build up your resistance to infections.

•**Feel your feelings,** especially repressed anger…find your passion and purpose in life…and connect with loved ones, yourself and your spiritual side. Unconditional love is life's most powerful healer, and the perceived loss of love is our greatest health risk. To create optimal health in all areas of your life, you must be committed to your mental, emotional, social and spiritual health.

MAKE YOUR ENVIRONMENT SINUS-FRIENDLY

If allergies act as a trigger of your sinus problems, as they do with nearly half of all sinus sufferers, it's important to keep them under control. *To make your environment sinus-friendly and inhospitable to allergies and sinusitis, Dr. Ivker recommends that you…*

•**Identify your triggers**—foods (most common trigger) and food additives, mold, dust mites, animal dander, chemicals, etc.—and reduce your exposure to them.

•**Keep your home and workspace clean and dust-free.**

•**Stay on top of mold.** For example, wash your humidifier's tank once a week with vinegar and water. Otherwise, it becomes home to mold and bacteria that are recirculated through the air.

•**Change pillow and mattress covers frequently,** and wash bedding and clothing in hot water.

•**Remove wall-to-wall carpeting and heavy drapes,** and invest in a vacuum cleaner with a HEPA filter.

This winter, don't let sinusitis keep you home from work or spoil your ski vacation. By paying attention to a few key strategies that address the causes of the problem—keeping air moist and clean, practicing good nasal hygiene, supporting your immune system, keeping Candida in check and controlling any allergies—you can face the cold and snow infection-free.

info For more information, contact the American Academy of Allergy, Asthma & Immunology, *www.aaaai.org.*

Breathe Easy— New Ways to Ease Or Avoid COPD

E. Neil Schachter, MD, medical director, respiratory care department, Mt. Sinai Medical Center, New York City and author of *The Good Doctor's Guide to Colds and Flu.* HarperCollins.

While breathing is something most of us take for granted, for those with lung problems, this simplest of physical tasks can become a formidable challenge. Some 12 million Americans suffer from a type of lung disease called chronic obstructive pulmonary disease (COPD), the inclusive term for chronic bronchitis and emphysema.

The information that follows is not related to asthma—although it too can be an obstructive disease. Chronic bronchitis, an inflammation of the airways, causes the glands to produce excess mucus which makes it more difficult to breathe. With emphysema, large air pockets develop in the lungs, which intrude on their ability to expand and contract for normal breathing.

The problems that COPD cause come about because the lungs can no longer exhale as much air as they need to. The stale air left in the lungs, called the residual volume, can leave patients gasping to breathe in enough oxygen-filled fresh air.

Most at risk for COPD: Smokers and ex-smokers.

Experts estimate that in addition to the 12 million known patients, another 12 million have early undiagnosed COPD. Although COPD in the early stages has no apparent symptoms, smokers in particular—and even ex-smokers—are at increased risk. By getting a diagnosis and acting on it before problems start, people can take steps that will help them avoid a future of seriously impaired breathing.

We called pulmonologist E. Neil Schachter, MD, to discuss the issues of lung function and what people can do to help themselves breathe better and avoid COPD. Dr. Schachter is medical director of the respiratory care department at Mt. Sinai Medical Center in New York City.

DETERIORATION WITH TIME

Everyone loses some lung function, says Dr. Schachter, starting at age 30. Over an average life span, people eventually lose up to about 20% of function, measured as the speed with which you can forcefully exhale. In the case of smokers, however, the percentage of lost lung function soars—smokers lose lung function twice as fast as nonsmokers. While COPD has other causes, such as air pollution (including secondhand smoke), genetics and sometimes a severe respiratory infection, smoking is by far the biggest culprit. In fact, Dr. Schachter estimates that about 90% of COPD patients are smokers or ex-smokers. Ex-smokers continue to have a residual risk. Doctors estimate how much risk by the amount and duration of a person's former habit. Because some 45 million people in this country currently smoke and another 45 million once did, cigarettes put a large segment of the population at risk for COPD.

SLOWING THE PROGRESS OF COPD

Although there is no cure for COPD, Dr. Schachter offers a number of ways to avoid COPD or slow the progression of the disease should you develop it. Of course, don't smoke. Quitting the habit may not mean you avoid COPD altogether, but if nothing else, it will reduce the severity of disease symptoms.

Next, if possible, prevent respiratory infections such as colds and flu. They can accelerate loss of function in those who already have COPD, and can increase risk for loss of function in healthy people, due to the resulting chronic inflammation and subsequent lung scarring. Dr. Schachter urges vaccination against flu and pneumonia, in particular for people over age 65 and for those with COPD who have chronic diseases such as diabetes, high blood pressure or cardiovascular problems.

HEALTHY DIET CAN HELP

Diet also plays a role in slowing disease progression and in creating healthier lungs in general. One theory concerning COPD is that much of its damage comes from excess oxidant activity that creates free radicals, which roam the body and, when found in excess, can cause many types of problems. Consequently, Dr. Schachter advises getting a lot of antioxidants, but through food rather than supplements. Research has shown that antioxidant supplements are not as effective concerning COPD and lung function without the cofactors found in food. Load up on ripe and colorful fruits and vegetables—these have higher amounts of antioxidants.

Exercise is also important for lung function—specifically, aerobic exercise. Because it strengthens the cardiovascular system, aerobic exercise takes some of the stress off the lungs. The lungs and heart are intimately tied in the way they function, says Dr. Schachter. A strong cardiovascular system delivers oxygen to the body more efficiently than a weaker one, and that relieves the lungs of having to work so hard. Exercise, however, cannot improve the lungs themselves, he says.

EARLY DETECTION CRITICAL

While there is no cure for COPD, early detection provides the means to slow its progression and even reverse it to some extent. COPD is most apt to develop in ex-smokers who have a history of smoking one to two packs a day for 10 years, says Dr. Schachter. He advises anyone who fits this criteria to be tested as early as age 45, which is when the first disease signs generally start to show up.

Testing is done with a machine called a spirometer that will measure vital lung capacity—the inspiratory vital capacity… expiratory vital capacity…and forced vital capacity. The FEV1 is the measure of the forced expiratory volume in the first second, which is how much air you can forcefully exhale in one second. If a spirometer reading shows that you have signs of early COPD, your doctor may refer you to a pulmonologist for more sophisticated tests and to determine treatment strategy.

If you test negative and smoke, talk to your doctor about how to quit and how frequently you should be tested. Better yet…quit! Former smokers who test negative should be tested again in five years, but unless they get a major respiratory infection, there's no rush, says Dr. Schachter.

TREATMENT OPTIONS

There are a number of effective medications for COPD, says Dr. Schachter, and they are very powerful. As is true with all drugs, they aren't without side effects, though most are well tolerated. Treatment generally includes a bronchodilator, now available in short- and long-acting types, and an anti-inflammatory drug such as an inhaled steroid. Our consulting medical editor Andrew L. Rubman, ND, adds that there are many natural therapeutics with fewer side effects that may work well to lessen the symptoms and slow the progression of COPD. These can be prescribed by a naturopathic physician working along with your pulmonologist. A combined regimen may improve results, usually lessens dependence on drugs and slows disease progression.

6

Latest News on Relieving Arthritis and Pain

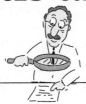

MSM—Should Stand For Miraculous

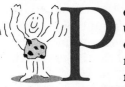

People who have been using a supplement called MSM claim it's nothing short of miraculous in alleviating arthritis pain. MSM (*methylsulfonylmethane*), an organic sulfur-containing compound that can be found naturally in food sources, plays many roles in the human body thanks to its sulfur content. Key among those roles is helping keep much of the body's tissues supple and flexible.

WHY IT'S A MIRACLE WORKER

Sulfur is the source of MSM's reputation as a miracle worker. It makes perfect sense when you consider that, for centuries, people have visited sulfur-rich hot springs to heal muscle aches and pains. Jacqueline Jacques, ND (naturopathic doctor), tells us that MSM has an important "structural role in maintaining connective tissues and joints" because sulfur is present in every cell of the human body. In a double-blind study of 50 men and women between the ages of 40 and 76, published in the journal *Osteoarthritis and Cartilage*, those who took 3 grams (g), equal to 3,000 milligrams (mg), of MSM twice daily for 12 weeks, significantly reduced their pain and improved physical functioning without any major adverse effects.

MSM USAGE

Dr. Jacques said that MSM could also be helpful in fighting allergies, particularly those affecting the skin—again, because of its high sulfur content—as well as for purposes of detoxification. Sulfur is important for phase II detoxification in the liver (processes called *sulfation* and

Jacqueline Jacques, ND, is a naturopathic doctor with more than a decade of experience in medical nutrition. Dr. Jacques is an expert on dietary supplements and frequently appears on television and radio. She is medical director for Catalina Lifesciences LLC, an Irvine, California company that provides nutritional care to weight loss surgery patients.

glucoronidation), which is how the body eliminates many drugs, hormones and environmental toxins. By supporting detoxification, MSM helps the body to eliminate irritants that can cause allergic reactions.

Dr. Jacques says that there is research supporting the use of MSM at doses from 1,500 mg to 6,000 mg, but she believes higher doses may be tolerated as well, if advised and overseen by a knowledgeable physician. Typically she prescribes about 1,500 mg for joint maintenance and pain prevention, and higher doses for patients suffering with arthritis. As with any supplement, however, it is important to be sure your physician knows you are taking MSM and supervises your use.

HOW IT'S MADE

Because MSM is only found in small amounts in nature, commercial MSM is created in a laboratory, not extracted from plants. There are two methods for extracting and purifying MSM from natural sources—crystallization, which is less expensive but also less effective and less reliably pure… and distillation. Do not buy supplements that contain additives or fillers.

GREAT RESULTS

"I've seen incredible results with MSM," Dr. Jacques recounts. She tells us the story of one patient with a rare connective tissue disorder (eosinophilic fasciitis), whose tissues were so swollen that she couldn't bend her knees or fingers. After treatment with high doses of MSM, she came in for a visit. "She walked in and said 'you have to see what I can do!' For the first time in six months, she could bend her fingers."

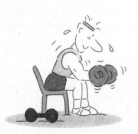

Studies Prove Exercise Eases Arthritis Pain

Carol Krucoff, founding editor, Health Section, *The Washington Post* and a registered yoga teacher.

Mitchell W. Krucoff, MD, professor of medicine/cardiology at Duke University Medical Center, Durham, North Carolina. He is also director of the Cardiovascular Devices Unit and the eECG Core Laboratory at the Duke Clinical Research Unit.

They are coauthors of *Healing Moves: How to Cure, Relieve and Prevent Common Ailments with Exercise.* Harmony Books. Visit their Web site at *www.healingmoves.com.*

When people have arthritis it often hurts to move, so many people with arthritis limit their movement. But inactivity can be crippling—literally—for people with any form of this ubiquitous disease.

Whereas a generation or so ago, people with arthritis were sent to bed in an effort to "save their joints," Mitchell W. Krucoff, MD, coauthor of *Healing Moves: How to Cure, Relieve and Prevent Common Ailments with Exercise* (Harmony), tells our editors scientific evidence now refutes that. "Study after study has shown that people with arthritis who exercise regularly report less pain and joint swelling, improved functioning and increased strength, endurance and flexibility—without harming their joints," he says.

EXERCISE ELEVATES MOOD

The psychological benefits are also dramatic. "The mind and body are not separate," adds coauthor and yoga instructor Carol Krucoff. "Exercisers experience less depression and anxiety, and greater feelings of control. When you can't function, it's very depressing. You can't walk stairs, or go places. And for seniors, the idea that they might fall down and not be able to get up is very frightening." Basic exercises give seniors a sense of control and the ability to do the functions of daily living. "They feel better about themselves and feel more capable," says Ms. Krucoff.

USE THESE FOR ACHING JOINTS

This is all well and good, but it still hurts to exercise with achy joints. *So, what kinds of exercise do the Krucoffs recommend for arthritis sufferers?*

1. Range-of-motion exercises. These are exercises that help reduce stiffness and keep the joints flexible. Dr. Krucoff explains that range of motion simply means the normal distance your joints can move in all directions. *There are five primary movements he recommends...*

•Shoulders. Slow easy arm circles. Starting with your arms at your sides, bring them all the way up toward the ceiling and then as far behind the body as comfortable in a huge circle. Repeat several times.

•Hips. Lie on your back with knees bent, feet on the floor and arms down along your sides. Bring one knee to the chest and rotate the knee in an easy gentle circle. Repeat with other knee.

•Wrists. Make circles with your wrists, rotating hands in both directions.

•Ankles. Draw big circles in the air with your big toe in both clockwise and counterclockwise motion.

•Knee. Lie on your back and bring one knee to the chest. Straighten your leg, pointing your foot toward the ceiling and bend a few times. Repeat with the other leg.

2. Endurance exercise (aerobics). "Like anyone interested in good health, people with arthritis need to accumulate 30 minutes a day of cardio activity," Dr. Krucoff tells us. He also notes that for people with arthritis it's especially important to strengthen large muscles, such as those of the legs, allowing more gentle and consistent compression of the sore joints, which in turn stimulates the healing process in the cartilage. When choosing an exercise, it's important to pick something that doesn't exacerbate arthritis. *Here's what the Krucoffs suggest...*

•Walk on a flat, even surface.

Good choice: A school track, using good supportive shoes. Or a mall or a sidewalk. Avoid bumpy fields or gravel roads.

•Water exercise. "For people who can't tolerate walking, water exercise is the gold standard," said Ms. Krucoff. "When you're in the water, it supports the body so there's less stress on hips and spine and knees. The Arthritis Foundation runs classes at YMCAs called PACE classes—People with Arthritis Can Exercise. These classes are great because they keep you in warm water at chest level. And they take you through a good range of motion and aerobic conditioning."

3. Strengthening exercises. The idea of people with arthritis pumping iron is quite new. "There are some very good studies showing that weight training for people with arthritis is very helpful," said Ms. Krucoff, "particularly for those with rheumatoid arthritis."

Important: Check with your physician before beginning any exercise program.

When starting, it's best to begin with light weights or even no weights and work up from there. "Your goal is to work out with a weight you can lift at least 10 times without being too tired," said Ms. Krucoff. "If you can't, it's too heavy."

•Chair extensions. Sit straight in a chair, knees bent 90 degrees, feet flat on floor. Then extend your leg straight out and bend it back down to starting position. "Do several of these leg extensions for each leg to strengthen the quadriceps muscle," said Ms. Krucoff. "When you can do eight to 12 repetitions, you can go to the next level and strap on light ankle weights."

•Toe raises. Work the calves by standing and raising your body up on your tiptoes and back down. Do eight to 10 repetitions.

•Chair squats. "These are probably the most useful exercises of all," said Ms. Krucoff. "You sit in a chair and practice standing straight up and sitting back down again, using the muscles of your legs. It strengthens the legs and gives you confidence that you can perform a basic daily task."

START EXERCISING NOW

The number one cause of nursing home admissions is not heart disease or Alzheimer's disease or diabetes. "It's weak joints and muscles," said Dr. Krucoff. These people can't do the activities of daily life. They can't get up or down, can't go to the bathroom. "You can prevent these problems with a good exercise program," said Dr. Krucoff. "And the time to start is right now." (After you get approval from your treating physician, of course.)

Exercise That Helps Arthritic Knees

Wayne Westcott, PhD, author of numerous books on fitness including *Strength Training Past 50.* Human Kinetics. He is a strength-training consultant for the American Council on Exercise and Fitness, and research director, Southshore YMCA in Quincy, Massachusetts.

Given the pain knee osteoarthritis (OA) can cause, patients are understandably reluctant to exercise the affected joint. Many people even fear that building strength in the quadriceps (the muscles in the front of the thighs) can actually harm the knee joint, especially when osteoarthritis occurs in people with malaligned knees. But it's time to rethink that—as a recent report makes clear. The study evaluated how having stronger quads impacts the knee and its cartilage, and the results tell us that strong quads help—a lot.

STUDY ON QUADRICEPS

The 30-month study, conducted in part by the Mayo Clinic in Rochester, Minnesota, followed 265 men and women, mean age of 67, who had symptomatic knee osteoarthritis. Researchers investigated how the strength of the quadriceps affected cartilage in the knee joint over time. The strength of the quadriceps was measured at the beginning of the study. Each person had an MRI of their knee at the beginning, middle and end of the study.

The results: Stronger quad muscles did not lead to an increased risk for cartilage loss in the knee joint, even in patients with malaligned knees. Furthermore, patients with stronger quads were less likely to have cartilage loss in the outer side of the knee joint behind the kneecap. In short, stronger quads, which help to stabilize the kneecap, help protect arthritic knees from getting worse.

STRENGTHENING STRATEGIES

We asked Massachusetts fitness expert Wayne Westcott, PhD, for advice on how people with OA could best improve their quads. He explains that strengthening the quads also improves the tendons and surrounding tissue of the knee and even the entire stretch of leg to hip.

According to Dr. Westcott, the best equipment for building quad strength is leg press equipment in which you push the weight away from you. Start slowly with abbreviated actions that do not cause pain. Find a weight that is light enough for you to comfortably do one to three sets of 10 repetitions. As you grow strong enough at the current level to move to the next, increase the weight by 5%—usually after at least several weeks of training with two or three workouts a week. Avoid leg extension equipment (the kind that bring knees from a fully bent to a straight position and back) because this puts too much pressure on the knees. Other helpful exercises include "half squats"...walking on a treadmill at an angle of 5 degrees or more ...elliptical machines...and stationary cycle machines. Dr. Westcott recommends that a licensed physical therapist (PT) or certified occupational therapist (OT) at the gym or the local YMCA guide you through a safe routine when you are first starting out. PTs and OTs are regulated by each state's licensing authority.

DAILY LIFE STRENGTHENS QUADS

Daily living activities also offer ways to improve the strength in your legs. In particular, plenty of walking improves general circulation as well as helps to keep legs strong. Stair climbing is also wonderful for quad strengthening. Always avoid any motion that brings your knee in front of your toes. The most frequent culprit is incorrect squatting. Most people go straight down so that the knee protrudes forward and the upper leg (thigh) and lower leg (calf) are touching.

Better: Hold shins straight toward the floor and lower hips into a squat so your "bottom" sticks out behind you like you are about to sit on a chair. Be careful to hold on to something for support until you are sure you can do this easily without losing your balance.

While these exercises will help, Dr. Westcott adds that "for people who are overweight, weight loss is a key factor in reducing the pain symptoms of osteoarthritis of the knee."

Make Arthritic Knees 50% Better

Susan J. Bartlett, PhD, assistant professor of medicine, division of rheumatology, Johns Hopkins University, Baltimore, specializes in weight management and weight loss effects on medical conditions.

Some believe that the knee is one of the most overworked, overstrained and under-appreciated parts of the human body. In our increasingly overweight world, that strain is becoming even greater. Did you know that being overweight by just 10 pounds increases the force on the knee by 30 to 60 pounds with each step? Because of the wear and tear this causes the knee, combined with other gender-related factors, overweight women have nearly four times the risk of developing osteoarthritis (OA) in the knees and overweight men have five times the risk as healthful-weight women and men. Once knees become arthritic, the pain makes ordinary activities difficult for some people and nearly impossible for others.

Susan J. Bartlett, PhD, assistant professor of medicine, division of rheumatology at Johns Hopkins University in Baltimore, specializes in weight management and how weight loss affects medical conditions. She recently concluded a study of people with mild to moderate OA in their knees, as diagnosed with X-rays, to determine how weight loss might affect knee pain from OA, and how much loss would be necessary to see a benefit. Study participants met regularly over four months to explore nutrition, physical activity, behaviors and attitudes that promote healthier living. At the same time they embarked on a gradually increasing exercise program. By the end of the four months all were walking for the equivalent of 30 minutes of walking daily—a total of 10,000 steps a day as tracked with a pedometer.

The final results were surprising: Participants—including even the most obese—improved their knee OA symptoms and pain by 50% after losing just 15 pounds. These results were based on self-reported answers to specific questions posed by validated standardized measures widely accepted in pain research—in this case the WOMAC (Western Ontario and McMaster Universities) Osteoarthritis Index. This is particularly impressive when compared with medications—the average improvement from drugs, including Vioxx when it was available, was only 20%–30%.

A LITTLE WEIGHT LOSS CAN MEAN A LOT

When we called Dr. Bartlett about the study, she said that overweight people with arthritis and the doctors who care for them have long assumed only a substantial weight loss would help them. For example, the average woman in her study, age 58, was 5' 4" tall and weighed 200 pounds. Typically this woman thought she would have to get back to the 120 pounds she weighed 30 years before to start feeling better, and that seemed just too overwhelming. Learning that a modest loss could make such a difference was invigorating for everyone.

While a few of the study participants did not show any improvement from weight loss, says Dr. Bartlett, this may have been because people with advanced knee OA have no cartilage left, have too much damage and need joint replacement at that point. Nonetheless, the study clearly indicates that there is an association between weight loss and happier knees.

Amazing! Shoes That Ease Knee Pain In 30 Days

Howard Hillstrom, PhD, director, The Leon Root, MD, Motion Analysis Lab, Hospital for Special Surgery, New York City.

Sufferers of arthritis in the knee (knee osteoarthritis, or OA) may find some uplifting news in the results of a recently release study. The study looked at whether full-length lateral-wedge shoes would diminish the joint pain and stiffness while improving the knee function of patients with medial compartment (bowlegged) knee OA.

The conclusion: After four weeks of wearing the insoles, study participants had significantly less pain, less stiffness and better function overall.

This study prompted us to call Howard Hillstrom, PhD, who is director of The Leon Root, MD, Motion Analysis Lab at the Hospital for Special Surgery in New York City, to learn more. He tells us there is a growing body of research that shows OA has a biomechanical involvement—meaning the structure of one's body (alignment) is related to the body's function (movement), which may, in some cases, even cause the disease. With medial knee OA (bowlegged alignment) there is an increase in pressure to the inner part of the knee called the medial compartment. Similarly, lateral knee OA (knock-kneed alignment) will place too much stress on the lateral compartment of the joint. As a result, the cartilage becomes overloaded and degraded, resulting in a knee that is quite sore. With specially designed shoe inserts, the extra weight load can be shifted and balanced over the entire joint, thus reducing pain and preserving what cartilage remains. Dr. Hillstrom adds that there are also specially designed knee braces, lightweight and comfortable, that can be helpful for knee OA as well.

BOW LEGS BEWARE

Biomechanical problems are common in people with bow legs, says Dr. Hillstrom. Leg length discrepancy can produce even more subtle biomechanical differences. In a study that involved 3,166 people in North Carolina (6.4% who had a leg length difference), researchers found that a leg length difference increased their risk for OA in both the knees and hips.

One way people notice this is because the legs on their pants hang differently, says Dr. Hillstrom. Knee OA patients may also feel pain while standing, walking or running. It is important to identify a possible body malalignment (bowlegged, knock-kneed, limb length discrepancy or excessive foot pronation where the arch tends to collapse) as early as possible in order to avoid problems down the road, says Dr. Hillstrom. If you suspect you have such a problem, perhaps because you are experiencing unexplained knee or hip pain, he advises seeing a health-care professional who is trained to detect and treat biomechanically related problems such as knee OA. These specialists include orthopedists, rheumatologists, physical therapists, podiatrists and orthotists.

SEE A PEDORTHIST IF NECESSARY

Dr. Hillstrom also stresses the importance of proper footwear, especially for people with OA in their knees. Find footwear that is comfortable, naturally, but also look for shoes that come in a variety of widths, to be sure yours fit properly. They should be shaped to the natural contours of your foot, and have good cushioning to absorb mechanical shock. He adds that fashion may have to come second, in this case, but the payoff in greater body comfort will be well worth it. A pedorthist can provide excellent advice for footwear needs, says Dr. Hillstrom.

Knee braces, foot orthoses and shoe gear can be "off-the-shelf" or custom molded. Again, appropriate health-care specialists can help you decide which are appropriate for your condition. Custom-molded technology generally fits better, but costs more.

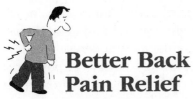

Better Back Pain Relief

Karl Knopf, PhD, executive director, Keep Fit Over 50, and author of five books including *Weights for 50+* and *Stretching for 50+* (both Ulysses). *www.keepfitover50.com.*

Eighty percent of Americans have some form of a back problem—leading to $24 billion spent in medical costs each year directly related to low-back pain. Is it possible to exercise with back pain? Which exercises are gentle on the back? For options, we spoke with Karl Knopf, PhD, a leading authority on exercise for baby boomers and author of *Weights for 50+* and *Stretching for 50+* (both Ulysses).

POSTURE FIRST

Poor posture is a major contributor to back pain. Dr. Knopf believes that the first order of business for strengthening and rehabilitating the back are posture exercises, which can be practiced absolutely anywhere. "Stand upright with your weight evenly distributed over the balls of your feet and heels, with legs slightly bent. Then tilt your pelvis slightly forward so your tailbone is slightly tucked under your hips. Make the distance from your belly button to your sternum as far as possible by letting the chest rise and open, countering

the "hunched over" effect. Your chin, sternum and belly button should be lined up from the front. From the side it should look like your earlobes are over your shoulders, which are over your hips." Practice that alignment whenever you are standing. When you sit, the alignment should be the same. Make sure you sit on the "sit bones" of the buttocks, not on the tailbone.

GUIDE WIRES FOR YOUR BACK

The back alone can't hold your body upright. "Think of standing a pencil upright on your desk balanced on the eraser," Dr. Knopf tells us. "You could make it stand—but it would take a lot of work and balance. How much more efficient to have guide wires? Well, the guide wires are the muscles that help keep the back aligned. These need strengthening to build a strong support system for the back.

The three basic "guide wire" muscle groups for the back are the abdominals, the gluteals (buttocks) and the perispinals (the muscles that run up and down the spine). "While many baby boomers are aware of the importance of training their abs, they often neglect the buttocks muscles, which are the other side of the guide wires. *To strengthen the abs, back and glutes, Dr. Knopf recommends the following exercises...*

1. Buttocks strengthener. Lie on your back with knees bent and feet flat on the floor. Tighten butt muscles and lift the butt off the floor slowly. Hold for a few seconds, return. Do 10 repetitions.

2. Hamstring stretch. Lie on your back, feet straight out. Pull your right knee into the chest and hold it there for a few seconds. Then gently extend the leg toward the ceiling until you feel a stretch in the hamstrings. Hold, return to start and repeat with the other leg. This stretches the hamstrings in the back of the thighs.

3. Mad cat. Get on your hands and knees. Arch your back like a cat. Keep your neck in a relaxed neutral position. Hold for ten seconds, then release. (*Note:* Don't do this if you have a ruptured disc.)

OTHER EXERCISES THAT
ARE GENTLE ON THE BACK

When choosing other exercises that are gentle on the back, Dr. Knopf recommends exercises that are done with the back supported and no "load" (or weight) on the spine.

Dr. Knopf has high praise for two specific forms of exercise. "The recumbent bike is my all-time favorite," he says. The recumbent bike, found in almost all gyms, is a bicycle (in either stationary or outdoor road versions) that allows you to sit on the bicycle as you would in a chair with your back supported, instead of upright or hunched over the way traditional bicycles do. Dr. Knopf also loves water exercise. "Vertical water exercise allows you to work all muscle groups without putting any stress or strain on the back whatsoever."

As for strength-training exercises, again, Dr. Knopf recommends those in which the back is supported and that avoid putting any "load" on it. *His favorites...*

1. Seated chest press

2. Lat pull downs to the front

3. Sit-to-stands (see opposite).

Avoid: Military or shoulder press... squats.

"You have to be careful with leg exercises," Dr. Knopf tells us. "If there's injury or pain, I'd prefer you do *sit-to-stands*. In this exercise, you sit on the edge of a chair, then stand up and sit down again. It's a "no load" version of the squat that works the front of the legs without putting any strain on the spine. You could work up to holding dumbbells in your hands to increase the resistance and build more strength.

BACK PAIN CHRONIC?
SEE A PHYSIATRIST

For anyone with chronic back pain who wants to exercise and eliminate pain, Dr. Knopf strongly suggests finding a physiatrist. "They are the most underused medical specialty I know of," he says. A physiatrist is a medical doctor who treats chronic pain and chronic conditions using a nonsurgical approach that often includes exercise. "They have no vested interest in doing surgery, and are usually very open-minded to alternative interventions such as chiropractic and acupuncture," said Dr. Knopf. "I've had back pain for years, and I always make the physiatrist the captain of my ship when it comes to back pain treatment."

7

Extraordinary Research on Aging Well

A Different Kind of Hormone Therapy

There are those who believe that they've discovered the fountain of youth in the form of the hormone DHEA... and then those who say that fountain is merely a mirage.

A RECENT STUDY

This popular antiaging supplement has been used for years by many naturopathic physicians to replenish the diminished supply in their patients. As we grow older and when we are stressed, the body's natural supply of this hormone is depleted, resulting in problems such as fatigue, decline in cognitive function (mood, memory and learning) and lowered immunity. Natural DHEA supplements help to counteract these processes by essentially "restocking" the body's deficient supply. However, a study conducted in part by the Mayo Clinic

(Rochester, Minnesota), and published in an issue of *The New England Journal of Medicine* (NEJM), concluded that DHEA had no proven beneficial effect in elderly people on body composition, physical performance, insulin sensitivity or quality of life—all of which are adversely affected by aging...a finding that leaves many who've had success with DHEA feeling confused.

We asked Susan Gordon, PhD, and *Bottom Line's Daily Health News* consulting medical editor, Andrew L. Rubman, ND, both of the Southbury Clinic for Traditional Medicines in Southbury, Connecticut, for their views. According to Drs. Rubman and Gordon, this study should not be considered reliable because there were methodological flaws in the research. Used appropriately, DHEA remains a valuable

---

Susan Gordon, PhD, Southbury Clinic for Traditional Medicines, Southbury, Connecticut.

Andrew L. Rubman, ND, consulting medical editor for *Bottom Line's Daily Health News* and director of the Southbury Clinic for Traditional Medicines in Southbury, Connecticut.

supplement which Dr. Rubman continues to prescribe frequently in his practice.

WHAT IS DHEA?

DHEA (or *dehydroepiandrosterone*) is a naturally occurring steroid hormone secreted primarily by the adrenal glands. It begins to decline naturally in the late twenties, often accompanied by a loss of muscle mass and bone mineral density and greater susceptibility to the chronic diseases and conditions associated with aging (depression, heart disease, dementia, etc.).

DHEA supplementation can safely and effectively slow the aging process and compensate for deficiencies, says Dr. Rubman. In his practice, patients who take this hormone have experienced improvements in energy level, mood, cognitive function and bone mineral density. While he most commonly prescribes DHEA for people at midlife and older, Dr. Rubman has also had excellent results with people of all ages—from early teens to the elderly with a myriad of health complaints—who are under high levels of stress.

DHEA is widely available over the counter in health food stores, but it should only be taken with proper medical oversight since too little will have no impact, while too much can lead to negative side effects. Only an experienced health-care professional, trained and skilled in natural hormone supplementation, can safely determine and monitor the correct individual dosage.

NEJM REPORT—
FLAWS IN THE STUDY

Dr. Rubman's experience differs from the findings published in the NEJM report. Dr. Gordon, who has studied steroidal biochemistry for 10 years, reviewed the NEJM study and found the methodology problematic and the results, therefore, inconclusive. *Here are some key points in her critique of the study...*

•**In attempting to bring the DHEA levels of people age 60+ to those of healthy 18- to 31-year-olds,** the study found no sustained favorable effects. But, Dr. Gordon points out, circadian rhythm (the 24-hour cycle of physiological processes in the body) is known to change as we age. Also, while it may be possible to restore a senior citizen's individual biorhythms to match those of a 20-something it's not necessarily safe.

•**The method and timing of dosage negatively impacted efficacy.** To achieve better results, twice-daily transdermal dosages would have been preferable. The oral tablets which were used in the study were chosen to ensure dosing uniformity and compliance. However, this form of DHEA is inefficient since tablets must be broken down by the intestines and liver—and only a fraction, usually about 15%, of the original dose is absorbed.

•**By taking blood tests to measure serum DHEA levels only every three months,** results were distorted, says Dr. Gordon. She compares it with taking a single snapshot when a movie of the "gestalt" of hormones is what's needed. One blood sample can't capture the changing nature of hormones and their metabolites over the course of the day, since DHEA levels rise and fall across a 24-hour period. A 24-hour urine sample would have provided a more representative measure of the hormone levels.

•**Not only was sample size smaller than optimal,** but even more detrimental for reliability was that for analysis of some outcome measures, groups of male and female patients were combined. Since gender is a factor in how steroid hormones are metabolized, this study design may not be ideal.

•**Researchers did not account for individual differences in diet, exercise and genetic factors**, which also affect the synthesis and metabolism of steroid hormones like DHEA. In particular, Dr. Gordon notes that diet has a major effect on how we process and excrete the metabolites of DHEA. For example, fiber may decrease DHEA levels and metabolites, while alcohol may increase the conversion of DHEA to estrogens in women.

NOW WHAT?

Dr. Rubman says that the naturopathic community continues to stand behind the efficacy of DHEA—when used under a trained and experienced physician's care. This particular study is not unlike other negative studies on natural modalities, including beta carotene and vitamins E and C. In this study on DHEA, the conclusions did not account for individual differences in biochemistry, age, gender, diet and lifestyle habits that are vitally important in understanding how hormones in general—and DHEA in particular—are used by the human body. All these studies failed to take into account that natural products in a natural environment operate in unison with other elements of the body, and therefore cannot be reduced to single, variable analysis.

CORRECT METHODOLOGY IS ESSENTIAL

While it is notable that the mainstream medical community is beginning to research such protocols, it's clear they may benefit from basing their findings on studies using more comprehensive methodology. As Dr. Rubman concludes, it's important to look closely at how research is constructed (not to mention, funded) in order to ensure the right methodology was used for evaluating the efficacy of a given product—or we may otherwise end up inadvertently eliminating valuable treatments such as DHEA from our medical arsenal.

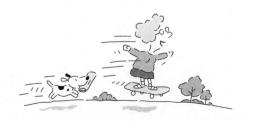

Beyond Cholesterol— Lowering Triglycerides For Better Health

Helene Glassberg, MD, assistant professor of cardiovascular medicine, University of Pennsylvania Health System, Philadelphia.

Mark A. Stengler, ND, naturopathic physician in private practice, La Jolla, California…adjunct associate clinical professor at the National College of Natural Medicine, Portland, Oregon…author of many books, including *The Natural Physician's Healing Therapies* and coauthor of *Prescription for Natural Cures* (both from Bottom Line Books)…and author of the *Bottom Line/Natural Healing* newsletter.

The medical mantra for people age 50 or over is to "know your numbers," which is to say, your cholesterol, blood pressure and blood sugar levels as they relate to cardiac risk, so that you can take action to address potential problems. While many people pay attention to this advice, and because there is enduring truth to this medical sound bite, it is important to mention that there is one number that eludes even the savviest health consumers…it is tested right along with cholesterol and blood sugar and is becoming increasingly respected as a marker for cardiac risk—triglycerides.

A TRIGLYCERIDES PRIMER

Like cholesterol, triglycerides are a type of fat in the blood, but they are quite different from their more famous cousin. Triglycerides are produced by the body and ingested through food, as is cholesterol, but they serve a different purpose. If the body's energy needs are exceeded by food intake, the body converts the excess calories into triglycerides and stores them to provide extra energy when called for.

However, for a variety of reasons, triglycerides can rise to unhealthy levels in the blood, sometimes along with a rise in cholesterol, sometimes independently of that. Normal fasting levels of triglycerides are less than 150 milligrams per deciliter (mg/dL) and when triglycerides rise to a fasting level of 200 mg/dL or over it's considered high. Occasionally levels go to even 500 mg/dL or higher, though this is usually because of genetic disorders or an underlying disease.

A good deal of controversy exists about the exact role of high triglycerides and atherosclerosis, but there is definitely an association between high levels of them and heart disease. People who have triglycerides over 150 mg/dL and HDL cholesterol under 40 mg/dL, have a higher risk for heart disease. And high triglycerides are also associated with a number of other diseases as well.

HIGH LEVELS AND DISEASE

Helene Glassberg, MD, assistant professor of cardiovascular medicine at the University of Pennsylvania Health System in Philadelphia, says that high triglycerides are especially associated with insulin resistance—a prediabetic state—and diabetes, in particular when it is poorly controlled. In fact, high levels of triglycerides signal the need to check for the presence of diabetes. Other problems that are sometimes associated with high levels are hypothyroidism or kidney disease. Pancreatitis is also associated with high triglycerides, which Dr. Glassberg says can exacerbate or even cause this disease.

LOWERING YOUR TRIGLYCERIDES

The good news is that this is one problem that lifestyle changes can often turn around. *Dr. Glassberg recommends...*

•**Normalize your weight**—obesity is a risk factor for elevated levels, especially if you carry excess abdominal weight.

•**Reduce or eliminate alcohol**—excessive drinking has been directly associated with elevated triglycerides...in some people even modest amounts of alcohol can affect the level.

•**Eat a nutritious diet**—pay special attention to getting plenty of omega-3s and eliminate excess carbohydrates, saturated fat and all trans fat.

•**Exercise at least 30 minutes each day**—push away from the table before dessert and go for a walk instead.

•**Avoid smoking.**

When lifestyle changes are not enough to lower levels sufficiently, Dr. Glassberg says that there are excellent medications patients can take that address the problem in addition to lifestyle changes. Of course pharmaceutical treatments often come with associated risks as well.

THE NATURAL APPROACH

There are also supplements that can manage triglycerides. Mark Stengler, ND, naturopathic physician in private practice in La Jolla, California, advises all individuals with high triglycerides to talk with a trained professional first. His favorites include aged garlic extract (AGE)—the most commonly available brand is Kyolic—with the caveat that people on blood-thinning medications clear it with their doctor first. Those on the muscle-relaxant drug *chlorzoxazone* (Paraflex and others) or the antiplatelet drug *ticlopidine* (Ticlid) must not take garlic supplements. Pantethine has also been shown to lower triglycerides.

Dr. Stengler adds his advice to Dr. Glassberg's in emphasizing how important it is to treat insulin resistance and diabetes, since triglycerides tend to be high in these people. In addition to a careful diet and regular exercise, Dr. Stengler suggests taking *chromium picolinate*, which research has shown may lower triglyceride levels significantly. And to end on a tasty note, a recent study in Norway showed that eating two or three kiwi fruits each day lowered triglyceride levels by as much as 15%.

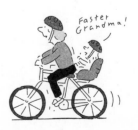

Seven Secrets to Healthy Aging

Mark Hyman, MD, founder and medical director of The UltraWellness Center in Lenox, Massachusetts, and author of *UltraMetabolism*, (Scribner), and *The UltraSimple Diet*, (Pocket). Dr. Hyman is the former co-medical director of Canyon Ranch, and editor-in-chief of *Alternative Therapies in Health and Medicine*, a peer-reviewed journal on alternative medicine. For more information about the books, go to *www.ultrametabolism.com* or *www.ultrasimplediet.com*.

As the years roll by and a generation of baby boomers searches for ways to turn back the clock, finding antiaging remedies has risen to the top of the "to do" list for many. Wine lovers may toast to the news that among the most promising of these is *resveratrol*, a disease-fighting antioxidant found abundantly in the skin of red and purple grapes and in red wine. At Harvard Medical School, researchers found that resveratrol slowed aging in mice fed a high-calorie diet, allowing them to remain healthy and disease-free for longer.

It's intriguing research, says Mark Hyman, MD, medical director of The UltraWellness Center in Lenox, Massachusetts—but, he points out, you'd have to drink hundreds of bottles of wine *a day* to achieve the equivalent intake of the mice in the study. And, he adds, no remedy can ever counteract the negative impact of poor lifestyle choices as we age. Still, Dr. Hyman was happy to discuss these findings, and offer advice on natural choices we can make to help ward off the degeneration and diseases of aging and remain healthy in our sunset years.

ABOUT THE STUDY

First, let's take a closer look at the study. Researchers put two groups of middle-aged mice on a high-fat diet (60% of calories from fat). One group was given high doses of resveratrol, and the other was not. When comparing the mice on high-fat diets, the resveratrol group fared much better. They had lower levels of blood glucose (blood sugar) and insulin, livers that were smaller and healthier, and also lived months longer.

In another study published in the journal *Cell*, mice given high levels of resveratrol doubled their exercise endurance in comparison to mice that were not.

Researchers found that resveratrol...

• **Improved insulin sensitivity,** contributing to more efficient blood sugar control.

• **Increased the number and function of mitochondria (the key power and energy producers in cells),** increasing the body's capacity to convert food into energy and burn calories.

• **Improved motor function,** making even older mice more agile.

WHAT THESE RESULTS MEAN

Dr. Hyman says these findings reinforce that glucose control, insulin sensitivity and mitochondrial function are key factors in aging. He said that scientists are excited about resveratrol because it appears to have a positive effect on these functions—which, when they don't operate optimally, make us more susceptible to inflammation, obesity and age-related diseases such as cardiovascular disease, dementia, etc. In Dr. Hyman's view, however, while some degree of antiaging benefits might theoretically be achieved with resveratrol (at least in mice), the perfect solution will never come in a bottle of wine, or a bottle of pills for that matter.

THE NATURAL PATH TO HEALTHY AGING

Taking positive steps toward a healthy lifestyle will naturally help protect us from degenerative aging and age-related diseases. *To accomplish this, Dr. Hyman recommends strategies such as...*

• **Make whole foods the focus of your diet,** and cut back on processed products. Fresh vegetables, fruits, beans, whole grains, nuts and seeds are dense in fiber and rich in nutrients. Conversely, processed foods are typically packed with sugar and/or refined white flour. These wreak havoc on blood sugar levels, initially sending them sky-high, only to crash a few hours later.

•**Increase your intake of healthy fats.** These have been demonstrated to reduce inflammation, and lower the risk of heart attack, stroke and depression. Rich sources of omega-3 fatty acids include deep water fish (such as salmon, black cod and tuna), walnuts, pumpkin seeds, flaxseed and flaxseed oil.

•**Eat protein with every meal.** In particular, consume protein (e.g., eggs, poultry, fish, lean meat, nuts, legumes or tofu) at breakfast each morning to regulate insulin levels, curb appetite and start the day on an even keel.

•**Consider supplements that support one or more of the following**—insulin function, blood sugar control and mitochondria. In particular, Dr. Hyman recommends coenzyme Q10 (CoQ10), which benefits mitochondrial function...chromium (such as chromium polynicotinate), which improves glucose control...acetyl-l-carnitine, alpha-lipoic acid, magnesium and fish oil, which benefit both glucose and mitochondrial function. Consult your health-care practitioner for dosages.

•**Get moving.** To fine-tune the mitochondria, you need to exercise and build muscle. Each week, make it a point to schedule two to three 20-minute strength-training sessions, and at least three 30-minute periods of aerobic conditioning. In particular, Dr. Hyman recommends interval training, in which you alternate fast (or intense) and moderate (or lighter) exercise (e.g., a series of short sprints followed by walking).

•**Practice effective stress management.** Whether you achieve this through meditation, exercise or a long walk on the beach is up to you, but it's essential to keep stress under control. Anxiety increases the body's level of cortisol, a hormone that disturbs blood sugar levels.

•**Reduce your exposure to toxins.** Our bodies are regularly bombarded with environmental insults, including pesticides, smog, heavy metals and other pollutants. These trigger inflammation, which is at the root of many of the diseases and conditions we associate with aging, and damage the mitochondria. Limit your exposure by choosing organic foods, fish raised in the wild instead of on fish farms, "green" cleaning products, and so on.

The "secret" to healthful aging is not really such a secret, notes Dr. Hyman. Just commit to living healthfully. Get back to basics, watch your diet, exercise, control your weight and stress levels—and, if you like, toast the good life from time to time with a glass of red wine, too.

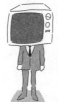

Turn Off Your TV to Live Longer And Better!

David A. Lipschitz, MD, PhD, senior advisor, Donald W. Reynolds Institute of Aging, chair of the department of geriatrics, and director of the Center on Aging, all at the University of Arkansas for Medical Sciences, Little Rock, and author of *Breaking the Rules of Aging*. LifeLine.

So you're home alone and you have nothing to do. You turn on the TV. It passes the time. It keeps you company. And it's killing you.

Loneliness is bad for your health. Television may not be the cause of loneliness, but it is often used to avoid facing and dealing with loneliness. "TV is a marker of how alone we are," says David A. Lipschitz, MD, PhD, author of *Breaking the Rules of Aging* (LifeLine). Dr. Lipschitz is affectionately known to the viewers of Arkansas Education Television Network (AETN) as Dr. David. He is also the chair of the department of geriatrics and director of the Center on Aging, all at the University of Arkansas for Medical Sciences in Little Rock. "When older people become isolated and lonely, they experience a dramatic increase in risk of heart attack and stroke."

TV IS ANTISOCIAL

It turns out that the things that keep us healthy, vital and independent are the exact opposite of television. "Love, faith, purpose and self-esteem are the keys to a long and healthy life." And these are exactly what television is replacing. "It might be a different story if people were gathering in big groups to watch television together. But in most cases, people are watching television because they are not with friends and loved ones," Dr. David notes. "TV distracts them from their loneliness."

He also warns that for older people, a fear of moving away from the ancestral home will contribute to excess TV watching. "Older people, usually women, who are afraid of losing their independence, will stay in a home that is too big for them and that might have stairs that they cannot maneuver." While these people think they are being independent, they have in fact become trapped in their home. "They end up eating poorly and watching television since they have nothing else to do and no where else to go. Their health will decline in very little time."

But Dr. David says that you are never too young to start building habits to prepare you for the future. Put some practices into place now that will contribute to a long and healthy life.

TELEVISION SUBSTITUTES

What should you be doing instead of watching your television? *If you want to stay healthy, here are some strategies...*

•**Fall in love—and stay that way.** Married people live longer and experience a better quality of life than single, widowed or divorced people. They are less likely to be depressed or abuse substances, and are more likely to eat breakfast, wear a seatbelt and go to the doctor. Married men live eight years longer than single men...and married women three years longer than single women. Faithful married people live longer than those who are not faithful.

•**Exercise.** Walking is good, but consider other fun and exciting ways to move and get going. Try swimming, biking or taking a dance class. "Obesity is one of the greatest health risks we face today, and TV is one activity that puts people at high risk for obesity, more so than other sedentary activities such as being on the computer or reading," says Dr. David.

•**Spend time with loved ones—every day,** seven days a week. You need to be around people that you love and who love you. Spending time with your parents, children, friends and neighbors is good for you. In fact, love is one of the strongest contributors to health and well-being. Older parents should not be left alone all day long. If you are older and have a big loving community, reach out to the people you know who are lonely or far from their children and friends. "We would never leave a baby or a small child unattended, but we do so with our older members of society all the time. It is dangerous for both their safety and their health," says Dr. David.

•**Participate in your spiritual community.** Faith is a great way to stay young and healthy. Go to your place of worship and find out what kinds of social programs they offer.

•**Take up a fun and active hobby—not stamp collecting or knitting.** Try running or kayaking. You're too old you say? Dr. David has a patient that started riding a Harley in her 80s, and one that started marathon training at 64. And there are many seniors who take ballroom dancing classes.

•**Volunteer.** Having a purpose is one of the best ways to keep yourself vital. It is also a great way to remind yourself of the blessings you have. It will get you out of the house and into your community. And doing something for others will boost your self-esteem.

OTHER CHOICES

What if you really are housebound? Perhaps creating a community on-line is right for you. There are many chat rooms on all sorts of subjects that consist of like-minded people. Or, you can play games on-line such as chess against distant opponents.

Television has its place. Unfortunately, its place is spreading in our homes like an out-of-control vine that needs pruning. Nip your excessive viewing in the bud.

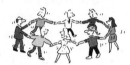

Good Friends Add Great Years To Your Life

Mary Sano, PhD, professor of psychiatry, director of the Alzheimer's Disease Research Center, Mount Sinai Medical Center, New York City.

You gotta have friends," Bette Midler's song tells us, and it's advice that's been dramatically underscored by a recent Australian study on longevity. The study, called the Australian Longitudinal Study of Ageing, involved regularly scheduled interviews over a 10-year period with more than 1,500 people aged 70 or older about their contact with different social networks, including family members, friends and other confidantes. After controlling for economic, environmental and lifestyle variables that impact health, the researchers discovered that study participants with extensive networks of good *friends* and confidantes outlived the others in the study by 22%. Oddly, family contact did not have the same impact on longevity.

STUDY IMPLICATIONS

We spoke with Mary Sano, PhD, professor of psychiatry at Mount Sinai Medical Center in New York City and the director of its Alzheimer's Disease Research Center, about the implications of the study.

Although we wondered if the stress that seems to frequent family relationships plays a role in this, Dr. Sano says the lowered impact of family support likely comes about for other reasons. She points out that many families are no longer geographically close and distance may make family support less important than that of local friends. Also, she notes that there is a chicken-and-egg aspect to the study—if you're well and hardy, you're more apt to be social and spend time with friends and live long. But, if you are frail, your social life is probably limited and because your health isn't good, you probably won't live as long.

VALUE OF SOCIAL NETWORKING

In spite of her caveats, Dr. Sano says she feels the study is worthwhile in general. It has, she says, several important messages that should speak to younger and older people. Research has long shown that, for older people, not only is a strong social network important for longevity, quality of life is as well. *Her advice...*

•**Stay involved as long as possible in as many activities as you can.**

•**Recognize that age will probably curb your physical activities to some degree,** so be sure to have nonphysical pursuits in your repertoire as well.

•**Look for and develop the traits and values that make it easy to create friendships.**

•**Be flexible,** be open to other people and different ideas and be willing to initiate social activities—including with people you don't know well but might like to.

Start valuing and building your network early in life, she says, because eventually you will be dependent on others even if just for friendship and comfort. If you learn this lesson well when younger, you will have a network in place for the future with the skills it takes to keep expanding it.

Have You Heard? HT Can Harm Your Hearing

D. Robert Frisina, PhD, director, International Center for Hearing and Speech Research, a joint program between the Rochester Institute of Technology and the University of Rochester Medical Center, in New York State.

Hormones and hearing are two words that aren't generally linked. But recent studies show that hormones play a definite role in how well we hear. The surprising new findings should be of interest to everyone with "aging" hearing, but especially to women who were or are on synthetic hormone therapy (HT).

The reason: Normal hormonal changes caused by aging—in women and men—plus the specific hormones used by women appear to affect hearing acuity.

HT AND STUDY FINDINGS

The scientist responsible for linking hearing to hormones is D. Robert Frisina, PhD, director of the International Center for Hearing and Speech Research in Rochester, New York. He had been working for many years to unravel the mystery of age-related hearing loss. He wondered if hearing might be affected by hormones (like conjugated estrogen) and progestin (a synthetic progesterone), both used in HT. He put together a study with 124 healthy women, ages 60 to 86—32 women had taken the combination therapy with conjugated estrogen and progestin...30 had taken conjugated estrogen alone... and 62 of them did not take HT. He gave each woman various hearing tests, plus one that is a sophisticated measure of the brain's ability to process the ear's signals or nerve impulses. The results were not good for the women who had taken combination HT—this group suffered a 10% to 30% hearing loss compared with the women who had used synthetic estrogen-only HT or who had never been on HT.

NEED FOR HEARING CHECKUPS

Our editors asked Dr. Frisina about his study findings and how hormones in general relate to hearing. He says that prior to the study he had assumed synthetic estrogen might actually improve hearing, since other researchers had demonstrated it to be good for nerve cells and also that women's hearing shows a slight improvement during the high-estrogen part of their menstrual cycle. Consequently, he was surprised to find that conjugated estrogen had no improvement on hearing in this study compared with those not taking HT. However, he says that he wasn't surprised by the finding that progestin had a negative impact on hearing. It was previously established that women's hearing in general ebbs, also very slightly, during the luteal phase of their cycle—the phase when progesterone peaks. We asked whether the hearing loss due to having once been on HT was permanent. Dr. Frisina says he is putting together a study to find the answer to that question. In the meantime, he advises women taking combination HT to have their hearing checked every six months, and if a problem shows up, talk to their doctor about changing HT dosage or duration.

MORE ON HORMONES AND HEARING

That isn't the end of the hormone–hearing story. Another hormone, called aldosterone, affects hearing acuity in both men and women. Levels of aldosterone decline with age. Indeed, in previous studies Dr. Frisina had found that older adults with severe hearing loss had, on average, about half the aldosterone as those with normal hearing. Aldosterone regulates potassium and sodium, which are both crucial chemicals that the inner ear needs to convert sounds into nerve impulses the brain can understand. Consequently, low levels of aldosterone—or an imbalance of potassium and sodium—can affect the inner ear's ability to signal correctly and the brain's ability to process in real time.

IT'S ALL IN THE PROCESSING

Here is what happens when that occurs. When sounds are made, the inner ear sends many rapid-fire nerve impulses to the brain. For a person to "hear" the sounds, the brain must process them at the same rate. If signaling gaps occur, the person thinks he/she didn't hear the sound, but the glitch was not in the sound, it was in the processing. This is why speaking louder may not help older adults "hear" better. More helpful, says Dr. Frisina, is to speak clearly and a bit more slowly, thereby giving the inner ear and the brain more time for signal processing.

HOW TO RECONNECT

The good news is that there are things you can do to help prevent or even improve age-related hearing loss, since the brain's nerve cells have the ability to reconnect. You can encourage this process in a number of ways, including studying a new language or undertaking any other challenging activity that stimulates thinking. You may have seen commercials for training programs that supposedly improve these skills, but Dr. Frisina says they provide only temporary improvement in the short run, not lasting prevention of age-related hearing loss.

THE VALUE OF SUPPLEMENTS

Antioxidants are probably helpful for hearing, as studies increasingly demonstrate, including vitamins C, E and alpha-lipoic acid. The use of bioidentical hormone therapy may be a further solution. The other reminder concerns potassium, which you need to balance properly with sodium. Potassium deficiency is not uncommon, but is easily correctable. Eat a banana a day or make other high-potassium foods, such as potatoes, a regular part of your daily diet.

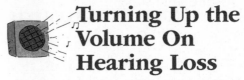

Turning Up the Volume On Hearing Loss

Barbara McLay, MA, audiologist, clinical associate professor of communication science and disorders, head of a hearing conservation program, University of Missouri, Columbia.

For about one in three people, aging brings with it the problem of hearing loss. This loss is generally gradual and difficult for many to recognize, but by age 75, about half of all people clearly miss elements of conversation, asking much too often, "What did she say?" Those with aging eyes know their abilities are waning and require corrective measures, but it is not as cut-and-dried when it comes to hearing loss.

To find more about age-related hearing loss—called *presbycusis*—and if there is anything we can do to minimize or delay its onset, we spoke with audiologist Barbara McLay, MA, clinical associate professor of communication science and disorders, and the head of a hearing conservation program at the University of Missouri, in Columbia.

THE HIGHS AND LOWS OF HEARING LOSS

McLay explains that age-related hearing loss occurs when the *cilia*, or tiny internal hairs, normally moved by different frequencies of sound, age and become less responsive. Once the cilia are impaired, hearing loss manifests itself in two different patterns or sometimes a combination of both. The first and most common one is loss of high-frequency sounds. Vowels and nasal sounds, such as m's and n's, are low-frequency sounds and as such are easier to hear. On the other hand, p, f, t and the other letters that require us to say on the phone, "…'v' as in Virginia, …'b' as in boy," are high-frequency sounds. Women's voices are usually in a higher frequency as well. As the ability to hear higher frequency wanes, parts of words disappear and the resulting sound is unintelligible, as if the person speaking is indeed mumbling. The second pattern has nothing to do with frequency. This loss shows up across the board—all sounds are muffled, not just those in particular frequencies.

CAUSES OF PRESBYCUSIS

Some people develop hearing loss as a result of specific diseases, such as Ménière's disease, or due to traumatic events, such as a blow to the head or the rupture of an ear drum by a cotton swab (the reason doctors caution against using them for ear cleaning). Presbycusis, however, generally develops over time for a variety of reasons...

• **Genetics.** According to McLay, anyone whose older family members tend toward hearing loss is more vulnerable to presbycusis as well.

• **Oxygen flow.** The auditory system is extremely sensitive to oxygen. Newborns who are oxygen deprived, for example, often develop hearing loss as a result. Anything, then, that interferes with a healthy oxygen circulation puts stress on the system. Smokers, for example, won't necessarily lose their hearing, says McLay, but they are nevertheless more likely than nonsmokers to suffer some loss.

• **Noise is a prominent cause of presbycusis.** For most people, occasional exposure to high-decibel experiences won't make a difference. Although these can cause temporary hearing loss, presbycusis usually results from a lifetime accumulation of noise exposure, says McLay. As evidence, in a decades' old study on an African bush tribe with especially healthy living and a quiet environment, researchers discovered that these natives had much better hearing in old age than people in noisier, developed societies.

• **Nutritional deficiencies.** *Bottom Line's Daily Health News* consulting medical editor Andrew L. Rubman, ND, adds that nutritional factors can also contribute to presbycusis, especially the general sound-muffling type of hearing loss. Deficiencies in B-vitamins, calcium and omega-3 fatty acids are known to have an affect on hearing.

SELF-PROTECTION

While you can't take back errors of youth and the impact of those rock concerts from past years, you can make healthy changes to reduce your risk for hearing loss.

Dr. Rubman adds that there are certain nutritional steps you can take to protect your hearing, such as avoiding trans fats and supplementing with B-12, multi-B vitamins, omega-3 oils and octacosanol. These supplements serve to improve neurological transmission.

TAKE ACTION

If it seems to you that more people are mumbling lately, see an audiologist for a hearing test right away. The first reason is to determine the cause of a hearing problem—it might be something that needs addressing, says McLay. For instance, a condition called otosclerosis, a bony growth in the ear, causes hearing loss and is correctable with surgery. If the problem is presbycusis, there are still ways to hear better, including a number of cutting-edge electronic hearing aids on the market today.

Additionally, consider these common sense measures: Face the other person in a conversation whenever possible...limit background noise as much as you can...and seek out good lighting so you can use visual cues to help understand what a person is saying. Finally, letting others know you have hearing loss makes it possible for them to make appropriate accommodations so that you don't have to miss out on the conversation.

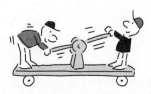

Best Ways to Stay Steady on Your Feet

Neil Alexander, MD, director, Mobility Research Center, University of Michigan Geriatrics Center, Ann Arbor, Michigan.

Sometimes a fall is just a minor annoyance, that results in minor abrasions. But not always. Falls can break bones and tear tendons. Even more worrisome, statistics show that falls are the leading cause of injury-related death among people age 65 and over. This unhappy statistic is partly because older people often have changes in muscle strength, reflexes and coordination. In addition, those with chronic conditions are more susceptible to falling—balance can be affected by the conditions as well as the drugs that treat them. But plenty of healthy folks fall as well. So, how can you "fall-proof" yourself?

RECENT RESEARCH

In a recent study from the University of Michigan in Ann Arbor, about a program called Combined Balance and Step Training (CBST), researchers gathered results from 162 people age 65 and older who were divided into two groups. One group was in a tai chi program, the ancient Chinese mind–body practice that is known to help practitioners avoid falls…and the other group took CBST. Both groups practiced their particular method three times a week in one-hour sessions over a period of 10 weeks. The CBST group performed slightly better than those who practiced tai chi (which has a long learning curve) in tests that measured specific abilities that promote fall avoidance.

The senior author of the study, Neil B. Alexander, MD, director of the Mobility Research Center at the University of Michigan Geriatrics Center in Ann Arbor, talks about CBST and how it helps people develop fall resistance. Dr. Alexander first explains that falls generally occur because of a confluence of factors, both internal and external.

To explain: You are talking on your cell phone having a heated debate about something and you cross a busy street. You are watching the traffic, but fail to notice the cracked cement on the other side of the street and over you go. A young healthy person might be able to right himself before falling, but that ability decreases with age and not just because of slowed reflexes, says Dr. Alexander. Falling often has to do with not just *what* you see, but also how you *process* what you see. Cognitive decline—even if mild—can interfere with visual processing, but so can everyday stress and fatigue whatever your age.

The reason: When stressed, your brain may fail to process visual cues, such as something in your peripheral vision that ordinarily you would take note of. Adding to the problem, 9% of people over age 65 have a balance problem that makes them more apt to tip. Dr. Alexander says this is often because of drugs side effects, or conditions such as peripheral nerve problems or silent strokes that cause no immediately noticeable symptoms, but rather affect the nervous system over time.

WALK THIS WAY

The *way* people walk—their gait—has a great deal to do with how stable they are in motion, too. With age, many people start to take shorter and slower steps. (This is also true of people affected by certain disorders such as Parkinson's or osteoarthritis.) But slower steps that are not long enough can make people more vulnerable to falling, says Dr. Alexander. Furthermore, one of the best ways to overcome an imminent fall is to make a rapid step of sufficient length in the direction of the fall, an ability many people lose. Consequently, CBST focuses on teaching participants to take longer steps at a faster speed, exactly the opposite of the shuffle walk associated with some older adults. It's also worth noting that long, fast steps require lifting the feet slightly higher. This provides better toe clearance, which in turn helps prevent a trip over small, near-to-the-ground bumps and curbs.

BALANCE RESPONSES

Fall prevention also includes having good balance responses, which means being able to right yourself quickly when you are thrown off balance. To develop these responses, the CBST study group practiced a series of exercises to train them in what Dr. Alexander calls "dynamic balance." *The following are some examples...*

• **Responding to a balance challenge while standing**—for instance, moving the upper body while bouncing and catching a ball.

• **Changing direction while walking,** such as walking backward or laterally.

• **Moving from a symmetrical (side by side)** to asymmetrical (one foot in front of the other) stance.

• **Maintaining balance while walking on a reduced base of support,** such as on a narrowing plank.

• **Braiding/grapevine stepping**—foot in front, foot in back while continuing to move sideways.

• **Stepping over small hurdles the height of an average step (about six inches).**

The group also did modest exercises to increase ankle, knee and hip strength.

PRACTICING AT HOME

Although a CBST program is relatively simple, Dr. Alexander recommends starting such training following a screening by a professional, such as a physical therapist. (You can get more information on CBST by calling the Mobility Research Center at 734-998-7424. Or visit the center's Web site, *www.med.umich.edu/geriatrics/moblab/.*) These professionals are trained to recognize weak spots and help people achieve their physical goals without causing themselves any injury in the process. He adds that everyone can and should integrate some balance training into an exercise regimen. These need to be more challenging than simply standing on one foot. He advises practicing doing two things at once (catching a ball as you move, for example), walking on something with decreasing support and teaching yourself to take longer, faster steps.

Caution: Do not practice any of this without holding on to something stable for support. The idea is learning to prevent falls, not to promote them. Remember, too, that when you are tired, stressed or distracted, your ability to move properly may be hindered—be especially careful at those times wherever you are.

Even better: Be sure you get plenty of rest so your mind and bodily responses are fresh.

THE RIGHT SHOES

One last contributing factor: What you wear on your feet plays a huge role in whether or not you are vulnerable to falls, says Dr. Alexander. Some soles, such as on sneakers, tend to grip. This is especially noticeable when you change surfaces, say from carpeting to linoleum, or when the surface rises slightly. Wearing sneakers, then, calls for extra awareness. Watch out for the lip (the tip of the shoe where the shoe front meets the sole) of the shoe, and how far it extends in front of your foot. An extended lip easily catches on steps or small hurdles along the way. The worst offenders are sandals and thick-soled shoes. As for high heels, Dr. Alexander says, one error and you topple. The shoes to look for, then, are those without much lip but with a good fit to provide adequate support to the foot and ankle. This makes slippers a no-no. Soles should not be so thick that they decrease the sensory input to your foot. If shoes have a slippery sole, scratch them up with a metal brush or the like before you wear them. Shoes without laces (fixation) or slip-ons without a back can also increase the risk of falling. Finding the right shoes may take some sleuthing, but fortunately there are many that fit the bill and are even fashionable enough to have you looking good while keeping you safe.

Being Too Thin Isn't Good for Your Health

Rosanne M. Leipzig, MD, PhD, professor of geriatrics and adult development and professor of health policy at the Mount Sinai School of Medicine in New York City.

The person who some people believe coined the now-famous maxim, "you can never be too rich or too thin," was the late Babe Paley, a society doyenne who was very thin indeed and, as the wife of CBS founder Bill Paley, extremely rich. Few of us can vouch for the too rich part...and despite the popular saying, you can indeed be too thin for good health. The physical dangers of the eating disorders anorexia and bulimia are quite well known. Less well known, however, is the fact that being underweight can also be harmful to your health, especially as you age. With nearly two-thirds of the country being too fat, it sounds peculiar to worry about being underweight. But, according to Rosanne M. Leipzig, MD, PhD, professor of geriatrics and adult development and professor of health policy at the Mount Sinai School of Medicine in New York City, a little padding can protect you in a number of ways.

BONE HEALTH

When we spoke with Dr. Leipzig, she agreed that these days it is almost an oddity to talk about being too thin. She tells us that, for a number of reasons, being underweight over time can in fact cause health problems, especially as people grow older. Probably the simplest issues of being underweight have to do with bone health. How many times have you heard the advice that to retain bone strength you need to perform regular weight-bearing exercises? If you are extremely thin, the inclusion of strength training in your regular exercise routine is vital. Fat produces estrogen and it is well established that estrogen helps insure adequate bone density. This is a safety net the very thin don't have. And there is yet another bone issue, says Dr. Leipzig. A little padding over the hips serves as a cushion for your hip bones in the event of a fall. Hip fractures are a common, serious problem for older adults. Hip protectors, garments that provide padding over the hips, have been shown to reduce the likelihood of fracture if worn when an older person falls. People who are underweight and have bone density problems should consult a doctor about the best exercise program for them.

NUTRITIONAL DEFICIENCIES

Of course, the reason most people are too thin is that they ingest too little food— or the wrong foods. On a regular basis, this can lead to nutritional deficiencies. An inadequate diet will not provide sufficient water-soluble vitamins (B complex and C) and with so little fat on your body, there is less space in which to store fat-soluble vitamins (A, D, E and K), says Dr. Leipzig. Complicating the situation further is the body's need for fuel to create its energy. The first place the body looks for fuel is blood glucose or glycogen stored in the liver and muscles. When that runs out, the body begins to burn energy from fat stores.

According to Dr. Leipzig, being underweight alone doesn't burn muscle tissue. That happens when the need exceeds the demand—that is, you're overexercising or, more likely, you're ill and trying to fight off a disease or heal a wound. At that point, you need additional sources of calories (energy)—and since very thin people don't have adequate stores of glucose, glycogen and fat, muscle tissue is the next to go. Having enough energy stores allows you to exercise longer, thus increasing muscle mass more.

SARCOPENIA

Another problem associated with age is a state called *sarcopenia*, which means a loss of muscle mass. It leads to frailty and that's real trouble. Experts in the matter often refer to sarcopenia as osteoporosis of the muscles, and the consequences of severely weakened muscles can become as serious as those of osteoporosis.

Sarcopenia becomes a threat to all of us as we age, but it is put into motion long before the so-called golden years. By the age of 45 the body naturally starts to lose muscle mass and accumulate fat. Exercising, in particular strength training, helps prevent loss of muscle mass. It is vital to have and maintain a healthy reserve of lean muscle mass throughout life along with a normal amount of body fat. You achieve both by making sure your long-term diet is adequate and rich in nutrients, especially protein, as well as exercising regularly over the years.

Beware—Many Seniors Have Eating Disorders

David J. Rissmiller, DO, associate professor, department of psychiatry, University of Medicine and Dentistry of New Jersey–School of Osteopathic Medicine, Stratford, New Jersey.

When most people hear the word "anorexia" they picture a young, previously healthy woman who has starved herself into a skeletal state. Seldom, if ever, do people think about an eating disorder among the elderly population. But as new research is coming to light, it shows a definite and growing problem in this group.

A full quarter of nursing home residents refuse to eat and are malnourished. The figure is expected to rise in the near future as the homes become more crowded and staffing becomes even more inadequate. Of course, there are a number of reasons why nursing home residents refuse to eat. Some have difficulty swallowing. Others suffer from diseases such as dementia that render them disinterested in food or un-

able to eat. They can even forget to eat. But there are also a number of people, previously healthy, who, for no apparent reason, refuse to eat and so they die.

TRIGGERING FOOD RESISTANCE

David Rissmiller, DO, is an associate professor in the department of psychiatry at the University of Medicine and Dentistry of New Jersey–School of Osteopathic Medicine in Stratford, New Jersey. He has been working with a population of older adults who give up on food, helping them overcome their resistance and regain their health. Dr. Rissmiller says that these are rational people who had been previously enjoying a good life. Then suddenly, something happens and they need to go into a nursing home. For sometimes unexplained reasons, they refuse to eat and this starts a horrible downward cycle. Dr. Rissmiller explains that "passive self-harm from not eating is one of the major risk factors for death in nursing home patients."

When a person rapidly loses 5% of his/her body weight, it begins to affect protein stores...a rapid loss of 10% of body weight can make a person lose the ability to fight infections or heal wounds. Malnourished individuals also lack the ability to utilize, react appropriately to, and successfully metabolize medications, which makes treatment with conventional means even more difficult. And yet the problem remains a hidden one, largely because the causes of death listed on the death certificates are the complications of malnutrition, not starvation itself.

WHO BECOMES ANOREXIC?

While many elderly people stop eating due to depression, there is a sub-group of older anorexics that stop eating because of a traumatic event that has to do with food. This generally has three aspects to it, he says. It happens in people who tend toward problems with anxiety...who are fastidious about their personal habits...and who had a bad reaction to something they ate. They might have choked on a piece of food...or were humiliated by an episode of unexpected, uncontrolled vomiting or a sudden onset of fecal incontinence and the resultant mess. At other times they fear a reoccurrence of severe constipation or impaction. Their fear of a repeat event turns into a food phobia, known as sitophobia, that is stronger than their natural impetus to feed their body.

FAMILY INVOLVEMENT

If this happens to a person in a nursing home or living independently, his/her physical and mental health can deteriorate quickly. This downward failure to thrive can frighten family members, but most are frustrated by the fact that there is nothing they can do about it. Sometimes a psychiatrist will misdiagnose depression when the elderly person is really phobic of eating. In such cases, Dr. Rissmiller urges family members to meet with the psychiatrist. He says that often the family can give the history of events that will bring the situation to light because the patient now is either too frightened to remember the incident or too embarrassed to talk about it. Inevitably, he says, once the catalyst event has been identified, the family will recognize that the anorexia started immediately afterward.

OVERCOMING THE FEARS

Food phobia is a difficult challenge, says Dr. Rissmiller. It requires reversing patients' nutritional patterns as well as their anxiety about what they perceived as a catastrophic event. In these patients, even the approach of food will be repugnant or cause panic, he adds. It is key, at this point, for family and staff to take a completely nonjudgmental attitude. Instead, the patient and his/her doctors should explore the details of the event, including what the patient was eating at the time, where it took place, etc. Doctors should give reassurance that this kind of thing isn't uncommon. Working with a nutritionist, doctors can then begin to introduce foods that are safe such as a little yogurt (as well as nutritional supplements). Many patients also take low-dose

medications that enhance appetite while decreasing anxiety.

Dr. Rissmiller has found that about one-third of the sitophobic elderly patients he has worked with resumed eating and recovered their health. Others require further work, but he says that he and his staff continue to explore ways to resolve this problem.

The first step, though, remains: To recognize anorexia for what it is and treat it accordingly. This is true whether the patient is 25 or 75.

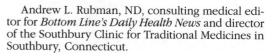

Making Sure Your Medicines Work Right

Andrew L. Rubman, ND, consulting medical editor for *Bottom Line's Daily Health News* and director of the Southbury Clinic for Traditional Medicines in Southbury, Connecticut.

It's one of the great ironies of the medical world. While older people are some of the most frequent consumers of medications, accounting for approximately one-third of national prescription and over-the-counter drug consumption, they also are among the least effective processors and potential beneficiaries of drugs due to the decline of their body functions. With increasingly diminished digestive and liver function, higher concentrations of drugs and their metabolites accumulate in the blood and tissues, leading to more frequent side effects and adverse reactions. The degree to which this occurs depends on overall health, digestive effectiveness, specific health problems and other drugs used.

However, according to *Bottom Line's Daily Health News* consulting medical editor Andrew L. Rubman, ND, while this problem is indeed common in seniors, it need not be so. Dr. Rubman has successfully helped many of his patients to overcome—or vastly improve—this problem in seven to 10 days.

Here's how...

PROPER DIGESTIVE AND LIVER FUNCTION—KEY TO PROCESSING DRUGS

Before getting down to the details of his treatment plan, we asked Dr. Rubman to explain exactly what digestive and liver function have to do with processing medicines. He says that the liver and the digestive tract work closely together to process almost everything that enters the body, including medications. *There are three important elements involved...*

•**Absorption of the drug from the gut into the liver.** The liver acts as the interface between the gastrointestinal (GI) tract and the rest of the body, explains Dr. Rubman. He points out that 98% of what you ingest goes into the liver, an important warehouse and processing hub for the transportation of nutrients.

•**Delivery of the drug from the liver to the rest of the body.** Next the medicine must be transported to the target tissues. Some drugs diffuse out, while others are transported out by protein and/or carbohydrate vehicles.

•**Elimination of the post-target residue of the drug.** Dr. Rubman tells us that most side effects occur because of potentially hazardous metabolites that result from a drug's breakdown. Drugs and their metabolites are bound onto bile, which is made from cholesterol, for transport into the intestines for excretion, explains Dr. Rubman. He points out that this means that other drugs may not be properly processed if you're taking a cholesterol-lowering statin drug.

WHAT YOU CAN DO

It's essential to provide your gut and liver with the right raw materials—i.e., healthful foods and adequate nutrients—in order to properly process drugs, Dr. Rubman emphasized. Efficient transport of a drug from the GI tract to the liver to

the rest of the body depends on these raw materials, as does the ability of tissue at the target site to absorb a drug and use it the way it is intended.

To keep your digestive tract and liver functioning at peak capacity, whatever your age, Dr. Rubman recommends...

•**Check your B-12 level.** For those 40 and older, with the typical American diet, you can almost assume a B-12 deficiency, especially in older people, observes Dr. Rubman. He encourages you to ask your health-care professional to assess your level of B-12 with a blood test. The liver requires this vitamin for optimal function. If a deficiency is confirmed, Dr. Rubman recommends sublingual B-12 pills, either *hydroxocobalamin* or *methylcobalamin*, which are equally as effective as and less expensive than B-12 shots. (Avoid *cyanocobalamin*, which is less well absorbed.) B-12 should be taken under a doctor's supervision. Too much can be dangerous.

Take a multiple B vitamin supplement at least twice daily. The typical dose prescribed is a B-50, two or three times a day. B-12 requires the presence of other B vitamins to function properly in the body, so your doctor will probably recommend this multi-B vitamin. The pills must be taken twice daily since they do not last 24 hours in circulation. Dr. Rubman adds that a good way to determine if you're taking in sufficient B is to keep an eye on the color of your urine...it should be bright yellow.

•**Consume plenty of fiber.** Good sources of fiber are whole grains such as oats, wheat bran and brown rice, followed by steamed vegetables, ripe fruits, nuts and seeds. Fiber promotes healthy flora in the gut and keeps food moving efficiently through the digestive tract. Ideally, at least half the diet should be composed of fiber-rich unprocessed foods.

•**Consider glucomannan.** If you don't get enough fiber in your diet, this supplement can help. It's made from konjac flour, consists of a soluble dietary fiber that stimulates the conversion of cholesterol to bile and decreases the intestinal absorption of cholesterol, thus potentially lowering excessive LDL or "bad" cholesterol.

•**Optimize your digestion.** Chew food thoroughly, avoid liquids with meals, vary your diet and eat real meals, advises Dr. Rubman. These simple strategies will maintain optimal stomach acid levels for efficient food breakdown and digestion. Proper digestion ensures proper drug uptake, says Dr. Rubman. If digestion is abnormal, uptake will be abnormal.

SEE YOUR
NATUROPATHIC PHYSICIAN

The GI tract and the liver can be quick to show the benefit of these recommendations. While you can adopt some of these healthy strategies on your own, for best results Dr. Rubman highly recommends that you see a licensed naturopathic doctor. He/she will soon have your body processing drugs as efficiently as it once did on its own many years ago.

Vaccine Lowers Shingles Risk By Over 50%

Michael N. Oxman, MD, professor, medicine and pathology, University of California, San Diego School of Medicine, chairman of the Shingles Prevention Study.

W hy is the recent US Food and Drug Administration (FDA) approval of a vaccine to prevent shingles (*herpes zoster*) so important? After all, chicken pox (*varicella*)—the precursor of shingles—is usually a relatively mild illness. But it turns out that shingles isn't the same as chicken pox, although both are caused by the same virus. During chicken pox, the virus enters nerve endings in the skin, travels up the nerves and establishes a silent infection in the nerve cells that lasts for life. Shingles occurs when the latent virus is reactivated.

This happens because of lowered immune function, which can be caused by such factors as cancer, advanced age or severe stress. Typically the virus travels from the root of the nerve near the spine, where it has been dormant, to the area of the skin connected to that nerve. A painful skin rash can result, which is usually limited to a small area on one side of the body. Less commonly, the infection travels to the eye, where it sometimes causes blindness. In individuals who are immunocompromised—due to AIDS, for example—widespread infection of the skin and internal organs can result.

SHINGLES AND PHN

About 20% of people get shingles in their lifetime (more than a million cases a year in the US), and shingles is more common and more severe in adults over 60 whose immunity to the virus has declined. What's more, anyone who has had chicken pox is at risk for shingles, and shingles pain can last for months or even years—a complication called *postherpetic neuralgia* (PHN). The pain of PHN can be excruciating and debilitating, especially in older people. Suddenly the vaccine's ability to lower the incidence of shingles in people age 60 and over by 51.3%, and to lower the risk of PHN by two-thirds, takes on new meaning.

To shed light on the situation, we called infectious disease specialist Michael N. Oxman, MD, professor of medicine and pathology at the University of California, San Diego and chairman of the Shingles Prevention Study Group, which conducted a double-blind clinical study of the zoster vaccine involving more than 38,000 participants age 60 and over. Dr. Oxman says that concern about PHN was the primary motivation for the study. PHN affects about 20% of people overall who get shingles, but the percentage rises dramatically with age. It is believed to result from damage to certain nerves and sometimes results in unbearable pain that can ruin the quality of life, says Dr. Oxman. The skin can become so tender that even air blowing on it creates pain. Patients may have to give up their normal daily activities as well as travel, sports and just about everything else that contributes to an enjoyable life.

AVAILABLE TREATMENT

There is no way to know who will develop PHN, except that risk increases markedly with age, above the age of 60. Once shingles occurs, no treatment is very effective in preventing PHN...and treatment of PHN is difficult, especially in older people. Moreover, PHN can last for months, years, even a lifetime. The most effective way to avoid PHN is to prevent shingles. This is where the new shingles vaccine, Zostavax, comes in.

Dr. Oxman points out that the most robust finding of the study was that the zoster vaccine decreased incidence of PHN by 66.5% in vaccine recipients compared with placebo recipients. That adds up to many people who never have to experience the debilitating pain of PHN.

It is important not to confuse Zostavax with the vaccine against chicken pox, Varivax, which has been widely used to prevent chicken pox in susceptible children and adults since 1995. Although the virus in the two vaccines is the same, Zostavax is much more potent.

MORE ABOUT THE VACCINE

Dr. Oxman says that side effects of the Zostavax vaccine consist primarily of redness, pain and tenderness, and swelling at the injection site, as well as occasional headaches. These are generally mild and resemble those associated with other vaccines given to older adults, such as vaccines against influenza. He urges anyone over the age of 60 who is not immunocompromised to be vaccinated. Although at this time the literature states that Zostavax is effective for four years, that is because study participants were only followed for about four years, so we do not know how long the vaccine's effectiveness will last. Studies to confirm this are currently under way. Nevertheless, Dr. Oxman says people

may eventually need vaccine boosters as with the vaccine for pneumonia, but we don't know yet.

Editor's note: Given the relative newness of the vaccine, you may want to wait and watch a little while longer to ensure its safety and effectiveness.

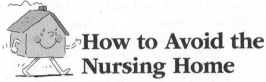

How to Avoid the Nursing Home

Louise B. Russell, PhD, research professor, Institute for Health, Health Care Policy and Aging Research at Rutgers, the State University of New Jersey, New Brunswick.

With the huge numbers of baby boomers entering their 60s—and plenty more on the way—insurance companies are pushing policies that will cover nursing home care. Sellers claim these will free parents of anxiety about becoming a burden and free children from having to care for a doddering mom and dad. Nevertheless, the idea of being in a nursing home is a grim thought for many. The good news is that a new study, based on 20 years of follow-up data and published in the *Archives of Internal Medicine*, shows that there are many actions people can take now to stack the odds in their favor in the future.

RISK FACTORS

The study analyzed data from two groups of people—3,526 who were middle-aged (45 to 64) when the study started and 2,936 who were older (65 to 74). All were participants in the first National Health and Nutrition Examination Survey and its two-decade Epidemiologic Follow-up Study. The purpose of this study was to determine if modifiable lifestyle factors impact who ends up in a nursing home—and who does not. Researchers investigated six health factors—smoking, physical inactivity, obesity, high blood pressure, diabetes and elevated cholesterol levels. Because many of these appear in clusters among people—e.g. smoking, obesity and inactivity are risk factors for diabetes—the study evaluated each factor independently as well as collectively in both groups. Diabetes, with or without its associated risk factors, was the most dramatic risk for nursing home admission over the next 20 years. Those who developed it in the younger group tripled their risk of admission compared with others in the group who did not have diabetes...those in the older group increased their risk by 50% compared with the group members without diabetes. All other health factors except elevated cholesterol showed increased risk of nursing home admission in both groups as well.

HEALTHY LIFESTYLE
BEST PRECAUTION

Smoking increased risk somewhat less —by 56% for those in the middle-aged group but just 32% for the older ones. But we spoke with one of the study's authors, Louise B. Russell, PhD, research professor at the Institute for Health, Health Care Policy and Aging Research at Rutgers, the State University of New Jersey in New Brunswick, and she points out that smokers tend to be thinner—and they die younger. Dr. Russell adds that the data demonstrate that the biggest benefits come to people who have established a healthy lifestyle by middle age...but oldsters, too, saw a reduction in nursing home admission. The study once again shows that living a healthy lifestyle is the best insurance you can have—not only to avoid nursing home care, but also illness and frailty, however long you live.

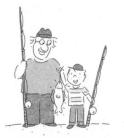

Supplement Helps You "Think" Five Years Younger

Ray Sahelian, MD, author, *Bottom Line's Mind Boosting Secrets: A Guide to Natural Supplements that Enhance Your Mind, Memory and Mood.* Bottom Line Books. *www.raysahelian.com.*

One of the most annoying aspects of aging is the "I can't think of it..." syndrome, when everyday names and words become maddeningly elusive. Any help in the memory department is worth heeding. Now, there is a study from the Wageningen University in the Netherlands that gives high marks to folic acid as a memory and cognition booster.

The study took place over three years and involved 818 cognitively healthy people ages 50 to 75 divided into two groups. One group took 800 micrograms (mcg) of folic acid each day, the other group took a placebo pill.

Results of the folic acid group were impressive: On memory tests, scores were comparable to people who were 5.5 years younger, and on cognitive speed, participants performed as well as people almost two years younger.

MORE FOLIC ACID BENEFITS

Ray Sahelian, MD, author of *Bottom Line's Mind Boosting Secrets: A Guide to Natural Supplements that Enhance Your Mind, Memory and Mood* (Bottom Line Books), explains that the folic acid–brain link is a simple one. Folic acid, part of the B vitamin family, reduces blood levels of homocysteine, an inflammatory amino acid. Homocysteine is toxic to brain cells, says Dr. Sahelian. He says that people who already get a lot of folate (the version found in food) in their diet will not notice any cognitive difference after taking a supplement. For those people who don't get enough folate from food, he recommends taking a B-complex supplement.

The supplement should include 400 mcg to 800 mcg of folic acid (check the label on your multivitamin before you supplement further because virtually all of them today contain folic acid). Some B supplements have much higher amounts of folic acid than that and, although there doesn't appear to be any short-term risk involved, Dr. Sahelian is concerned that large doses may cause an imbalance of some sort in the long run.

Of course, a diet rich in green vegetables can provide plenty of folate. Some of the best are spinach, kale, Swiss chard, romaine lettuce, as well as broccoli and even cauliflower. Many grain-based products are also fortified with folic acid. While the fortification is mostly trivial amounts, something is better than nothing.

Keep Your Memory Sharp for Life

Gary W. Small, MD, director, UCLA Center on Aging, Parlow-Solomon Professor on Aging, University of California, Los Angeles (UCLA), author of *The Memory Prescription: Dr. Gary Small's 14-Day Plan to Keep Your Brain and Body Young* and *The Memory Bible*. Hyperion.

Alzheimer's Association, *www.alz.org*.

National Institute on Aging Information Center, *www.nia.nih.gov*.

UCLA Center on Aging, *www.aging.ucla.edu*.

Many people experience some degree of memory loss by age 35, and by the time we're 65, it affects half of us. To get perspective on middle-age forgetfulness we spoke with leading psychiatrist and neuroscientist Gary W. Small, MD, director of the UCLA Center on Aging and author of *The Memory Prescription: Dr. Gary Small's 14-Day Plan to Keep Your Brain and Body Young* (Hyperion), among others.

Dr. Small says that lifestyle choices are a much bigger component of the equation than many people realize. He notes that even one small lifestyle change—for example, eating salmon once a week or walking 10 minutes a day—can help boost your memory and increase your resistance to Alzheimer's disease (AD).

THE HEALTHY BRAIN DIET

What's good for the heart is good for the brain, says Dr. Small. Keeping the blood flowing through the brain as well as the heart keeps us mentally sharp.

Dr. Small's recommendations to improve brain health...

•**Control your caloric intake.** This will help you maintain a proper weight and ward off the risk factors for heart and brain troubles (high blood pressure, diabetes, obesity, etc.). Many people munch their way through the day, loading up on calories without even thinking about it. Dr. Small encourages you to be mindful of how you feel, and eat only when you're hungry.

•**Consume plenty of antioxidant-rich foods** such as broccoli, berries, cherries, prunes, raisins, berry juice concentrates and green tea. As we age, our cells experience wear and tear from free radicals. This oxidative stress can damage DNA, accelerating the aging process and contributing to age-related diseases, including AD, cataracts and cancer. Antioxidants help protect cells from this damage.

•**Eat foods that are high in omega-3 fatty acids.** These include cold-water fish such as salmon, tuna, herring and mackerel ...flaxseeds and nuts (walnuts are especially good).

According to *Bottom Line's Daily Health News* consulting medical editor Andrew L. Rubman, ND, some of the top omega-3 supplement sources are PharMax, Nordic Naturals, Udo's Choice Oil Blend (*www.udoerasmus.com/products/oil_blend_en.htm*), and Barlean's (*www.barleans.com*).

•**Eat good carbohydrates such as fruits and vegetables and low-glycemic choices** such as sweet potatoes, yams, seeds and beans. Steer clear of simple carbs such as white flour, white potatoes and sugary treats that send blood sugar soaring (and then crashing).

STAY PHYSICALLY ACTIVE

According to two recent studies published in *Journal of the American Medical Association*, simply walking regularly is linked with better mental ability and a lower risk of developing dementia in older men and women. In one of the studies, women who walked for one and a half hours or more a week at an easy pace (a mile in about 21 to 30 minute) scored better in mental ability tests than women who walked for less than 38 minutes per week. Dr. Small suggests taking a nightly after-dinner walk with a family member or a friend. Not only does this increase physical and mental fitness, it will help you unwind from the day and give you the opportunity to connect with others in a relaxed state.

PRACTICE MENTAL AEROBICS

Engaging in social and stimulating activities keeps the brain in better condition. Good brain strengtheners include reading, doing crossword puzzles, knitting, taking up a foreign language and playing chess or bridge. A helpful brain-teasing exercise is to write with your left hand if you're a righty, and vice versa.

CONTROL STRESS

Chronic stress triggers the release of cortisol, a hormone that damages brain cells. By taking positive steps to control stress in your life, you can stave off both memory loss and AD, says Dr. Small. He recommends relaxing modalities, such as Pilates and yoga. And, since much stress is in the eye of the beholder, try to maintain a sensible perspective about your life. Don't have unreasonable expectations of yourself.

A WORD ABOUT SUPPLEMENTS

Dr. Small recommends taking a multivitamin every day, since as we grow older we don't absorb nutrients as efficiently as we used to. *Following is a roundup of the latest information on supplements that are commonly promoted for memory enhancement and AD prevention…*

• **Omega-3 fatty acids.** In September 2004, the US Food and Drug Administration (FDA) allowed qualified health claims to be made for omega-3 fatty acids, acknowledging evidence that they may lower the risk of cardiovascular disease. What's good for getting the blood flowing to the heart is good for getting the blood flowing to the brain. The FDA recommends that you consume a maximum of 3 grams (g) of fish oil daily, no more than 2 g of which is from supplements.

• **Coenzyme Q10.** This antioxidant occurs naturally in the body, and its synthetic version has become a popular treatment for age-related memory loss.

• **Ginkgo biloba.** In a study published in the *Journal of the American Medical Association*, ginkgo was shown to have a slight effect on improving memory in people with AD. Be sure to use freeze-dried ginkgo biloba produced by high-end suppliers such as Eclectic Institute. (*Note:* Ginkgo may reduce the ability of the blood to clot, so it should not be taken by people with bleeding disorders or in combination with anticoagulant drugs, such as warfarin or aspirin, without medical clearance.)

• **Huperzine A.** This herbal supplement is derived from the club moss *Huperzia serrata.* Clinical trials in China suggest that it may help protect nerve cells and thus may be beneficial in treating AD. Recently, the National Institute on Aging launched a trial of huperzine A as a treatment for mild to moderate AD. (*Note:* Huperzine A is similar to Alzheimer's medications known as cholinesterase inhibitors. Under no circumstances should these be taken together.)

Reminder: While natural, these items can interact with products you are currently taking and can affect people differently depending on individual health. Be sure to speak with a trained professional before taking any of these supplements.

As always, your best bet to prevent the chronic diseases of aging lies in a healthy lifestyle—eat a well-balanced diet, remain physically and mentally active, and stay on top of any underlying health problems.

 For more information on AD prevention, the Alzheimer's Association is sponsoring a series of workshops around the country called "Maintain Your Brain." Visit *www.alz.org* or call 1-800-272-3900 to learn when and where.

Single Most Important Way To Feel Younger

Edward L. Schneider, MD, dean emeritus, professor of medicine and gerontology, Leonard Davis School of Gerontology, University of Southern California, Los Angeles, and author of *AgeLess: Take Control of Your Age and Stay Youthful for Life*. Rodale.

You've heard people say it—today's 50 is yesterday's 40...60 is now more like 50. Yes, some of that's because life expectancy is rising. But that's not all. It's also because the social revolution of the 1960s and 1970s opened a path to timelessness. The baby boomers have taught the world a lesson with regard to defying aging through a youth-focused mind-set and health-conscious lifestyle. Anyone of any generation can choose to live youthfully—it's not just for baby boomers.

CHOOSE YOUR AGE

One example of youth-focused living is a group of seniors who tour in their own rock show, belting out witty takes on aging like "Stairway to Heaven," "Every Breath You Take" and "Forever Young." These seniors and many like them choose to live, not by the calendar or number of candles on their birthday cake, but from their heart—and to enjoy *all* their time on earth.

To learn more about "aging gracefully," we spoke to Edward L. Schneider, MD, dean emeritus and professor of medicine

and gerontology at the University of Southern California (USC) in Los Angeles, and author of *AgeLess: Take Control of Your Age and Stay Youthful for Life* (Rodale).

Dr. Schneider told us that there are two secrets to taking control of your aging...

•**Keep living.** If you drop out of life and just watch TV all day, you're going to feel your age (and more). Staying active and engaged is the real key to aging well.

•**Stay healthy.** Even if your spirit says, "I'm young," your body won't keep up if you don't take good care of it.

To maintain youthful zeal, Dr. Schneider recommends a number of building blocks for good health. They sound simple—no high-tech treatments or high-priced medications. That's the beauty of it.

GET MOVING

Physical activity is the single most important thing you can do. This doesn't have to mean intense workouts at the gym, stresses Dr. Schneider. Just get off the couch.

Dr. Schneider recommends: Put on your walking shoes, and join a few friends for a daily morning trek through the park. It's never too late to start moving, and exercise will make you feel better all around, mind and body. According to one study, walking 30 minutes five or more times a week at a rate of two to three miles an hour reduces your risk for cardiovascular disease by a big 30%.

WEIGHT TRAINING, TOO

Important as it is to get moving, that's not enough. You also need to pay attention to bone density. Falling down and breaking a hip is just about the worst thing that can happen to an older person.

Dr. Schneider recommends: Invest $10 in a set of hand weights, and use them every day. Weight training keeps bones strong and intact as you age.

GET YOUR SLEEP

Older people often find it difficult to get to sleep at all, let alone get a good night's sleep. But getting sufficient sleep

107

is essential to remaining active, cheerful and alert.

Dr. Schneider recommends: Take a hot bath or shower about an hour before bed, and then slip in between cool sheets in a cool, dark room.

WATCH WHAT YOU EAT

Good nutrition is the secret to preventing the degenerative diseases of old age, yet for one reason or another—social isolation, dental problems, reduced taste or smell, or physical or mental health issues—many older people fail to eat properly.

Dr. Schneider recommends: Sprinkle antioxidant-packed berries on whole grain cereal for breakfast...have a salad garnished with a few chicken strips or shrimp for lunch...or opt for the salmon instead of the prime rib the next time you go out for dinner. Try to eat omega 3–rich cold-water fish (such as salmon, tuna or sea bass) at least twice a week, and aim to eat five or more daily servings of fruits and veggies. If you live alone, make an effort to get together with friends for at least a few meals each week.

TAKE SUPPLEMENTS

According to *Bottom Line's Daily Health News* consulting medical editor Andrew L. Rubman, ND, even a good daily multivitamin cannot provide all the nutrients you need, so talk to a trained physician about supplementation. (*Caution:* Many older people have chronic health concerns for which they take multiple medications. This makes consulting an expert before taking supplements an absolute must.) *Dr. Schneider recommends...*

• **Calcium.** If you're age 50 or older, take 1,500 mg daily. For maximum calcium absorption, be sure your supplement includes magnesium.

• **Fish oil.** Take 1,000 mg daily of fish oil containing DHA and EPA. This is one of the best things you can do for your heart, notes Dr. Schneider.

Note: Do not take fish oil if you have a bleeding disorder or if you are taking blood-thinners, such as *warfarin* (Coumadin) or aspirin.

• **Folic acid.** Take 800 mcg daily. Folic acid is a B vitamin that lowers levels of homocysteine, an amino acid in the blood that damages blood vessel walls and contributes to cardiovascular disease.

LEARN TO LIVE WITH STRESS

Stress is not going to go away, so the best thing you can do is learn how to cope with it.

Dr. Schneider recommends: Develop your own coping mechanisms, such as exercise, meditation or talking things over with a friend. Try to keep a perspective on what's really important, and don't sweat the small stuff.

THE POWER OF PREVENTION

Of course, there's lots more you can do to stay healthy as you age—get regular checkups, control chronic conditions such as high blood pressure or diabetes, stay sharp by reading books and doing crossword puzzles, keep up with your friends and community connections and steer clear of unhealthy habits such as drinking too much alcohol or smoking.

The ageless truth? Treat yourself well and maintain a healthy attitude inside and out—and the future is yours to enjoy.

Study Shows Italian Food Lowers Alzheimer's Risk Up to 40%

Nikolaos Scarmeas, MD, assistant professor of neurology, Columbia University Medical Center, New York City.

The health benefits of the Mediterranean diet, which include a lower risk for cardiovascular disease, cancer and overall mortality, have been acknowledged for a long time. Now there's more good news. A recent study reveals that a Mediterranean diet—rich in fruits, vegetables, whole grains, beans, nuts, olive oil...moderate portions of fish and alcohol (especially wine), and limited dairy, meat, poultry and saturated fat—may also lower the risk of Alzheimer's disease (AD).

To learn more about these findings, we contacted lead researcher Nikolaos Scarmeas, MD, assistant professor of neurology at the Columbia University Medical Center in New York City. Dr. Scarmeas says that this is the first research to examine the link between the Mediterranean diet and Alzheimer's disease, and it is too early to make recommendations based on a single study. However, he adds that because of the proven effect that this diet has for other diseases, it doesn't hurt, and may help, to follow it.

ABOUT THE STUDY

Over a four-year period, Dr. Scarmeas and his colleagues looked at the diet and health of 2,258 individuals. Their food intake was rated on a Mediterranean diet scale between zero and nine, with higher scores indicating higher adherence to the diet. During this time, 262 people developed Alzheimer's.

Researchers found that the more closely participants followed a Mediterranean diet, the less likely they were to develop Alzheimer's. *According to Dr. Scarmeas, they discovered that...*

•**For every point increase on the scale,** there was nearly a 10% drop in the risk of AD.

•**In comparison to the people who scored lowest on the Mediterranean diet scale,** those who scored in the middle range experienced a 15% to 21% lower risk of AD.

•**Those with the highest scores had a 39% to 40% lower risk than those with the lowest scores.**

•**Results remained the same even when adjusted for age,** gender, ethnicity, education, calorie intake and body mass index.

These findings were published in the *Annals of Neurology.*

A SIMPLE FORMULA

It's a simple formula, and anyone who has ever traveled to Greece or Italy can assure you that it's also a very tasty one. Just eat more of the healthful stuff—legumes, fruits, veggies, olive oil, etc. ...and less of the bad stuff—meat, dairy, saturated fat. Bon appetit!

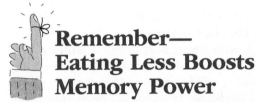

Remember— Eating Less Boosts Memory Power

Giulio Maria Pasinetti, MD, PhD, director of Neuro-inflammation Research Laboratories, and professor of psychiatry, neuroscience and geriatrics, Mount Sinai School of Medicine, New York City.

Much of the newest research on Alzheimer's disease (AD) has shown that lifestyle choices—exercise, eating a nutritious diet, not smoking and the like—may directly impact our risk for developing the disease, just as they do with cardiovascular disease. Now, researchers at Mount Sinai School of Medicine in New York City have shifted their focus slightly, and are investigating if how much people eat might impact AD risk.

LEARNING FROM MICE AND MONKEYS

Previously, the Mount Sinai researchers put mice that had been specially bred to develop Alzheimer's on a diet that was 30% lower in calories than normal. Surprisingly, the mice following this dietary regimen revealed at death a significant reduction of AD brain plaques.

In a follow-up study, the research team used squirrel monkeys—whose responses are that much closer to those of humans—and again put one group on a similar calorie-restricted diet. This time, monkeys were restricted to one macronutrient in addition to their reduced-calorie diet. When the monkeys died, the researchers discovered that the ones in the low-calorie groups were much less likely to have developed AD-type brain changes than those in the group eating a normal diet. Most interestingly, the researchers found that the calorie-restricted monkeys also had higher levels of SIRT1, a protein that has been linked to longer life spans and better health in old age and is receiving major attention because of being a target molecule involved in the treatment of AD plaques.

NEW EVIDENCE

One of the lead researchers of this latest study is Giulio Maria Pasinetti, MD, PhD, director of Neuroinflammation Research Laboratories at Mount Sinai School of Medicine. He says that he is amazed by how even a minor change in what we eat seems to result in major changes in metabolic pathways and cognitive deterioration. He adds that there is now evidence that calorie restriction may influence the way the brain utilizes glucose and consumes energy, and this might have a fundamental role in helping prevent Alzheimer's.

15% REDUCTION HELPFUL

But most people would find a 30% reduction in calories from a normal diet draconian and impossible to maintain. Fortunately, it appears we won't have to—Dr. Pasinetti says that another mouse study still underway is showing that even a 15% reduction would be sufficient to lower AD risk. And in yet another mouse study, the researchers found that a modest amount of red wine daily also has a positive effect. According to Dr. Pasinetti, the effect is likely due to the grape seeds used in making red wine and the fermentation process itself.

While his dietary studies continue, Dr. Pasinetti says they have enough findings now to advise healthy people to cut down by 15% less calories each day (after consulting with your doctor, of course—especially if you are on a low-calorie diet). For example on a 2,000-calorie-a-day diet, that would equal 300 calories. That's only one

serving of ice cream, as he points out, and a small sacrifice for keeping your brain healthy as well as your body.

An Apple a Day Keeps Alzheimer's Away

Thomas B. Shea, PhD, professor and director of the University of Massachusetts Lowell Center for Cellular Neurobiology and Neurodegeneration Research, in Lowell, Massachusetts.

Until recently, it was generally assumed that fate determined who developed Alzheimer's disease (AD) and there was no way to change it. But evidence is mounting that, as with so many other illnesses, healthful life choices can improve the odds against AD. New research from the University of Massachusetts in Lowell focuses on the impact of antioxidants and that yummy childhood standby—apple juice.

A USEFUL STUDY

In the study, mice—some of which were susceptible to cognitive decline—were given one of three diets. The first was a nutritious diet, while both the second and third were nutritionally deficient diets. But the third diet was supplemented with apple juice—the equivalent of two 8-ounce glasses of pure apple juice or two to three apples daily. Thomas B. Shea, PhD, the study's lead author, explains that the poor diet was meant to create oxidative stress because this would better isolate the subjects' response to apple juice. Dr. Shea, who is the director of the University of Massachusetts Lowell Center for Cellular Neurobiology and Neurodegeneration Research, describes the sub-standard diet the mice had as akin to the way most people eat.

JUICE MAKES A DIFFERENCE

After a month (equivalent to a year in human life), the mice were put into a maze to test their cognitive performance. The mice on a nutritious diet tested in the 70% to 75% correct range. Mice on a deficient diet without apple juice performed at just 50%, but the mice that had a poor diet and apple juice rose to the 75% level, demonstrating the value of the juice.

Further evidence: Dr. Shea says when they tested mice on apple juice and a nutritious diet, they achieved a 90% level, higher than any he had seen before. The researchers also found that *acetylcholine*, a brain chemical, increased in mice that had apple juice compared with those on a deficient diet without the juice. This is critical because acetylcholine plummets in people with AD. In fact, the activity of several current AD medications is to prevent the breakdown of acetylcholine.

ANTIOXIDANTS TO THE FORE

Dr. Shea says that the value here is definitely the antioxidants in apples, not a boost from the fruit's natural sugar. But most of these antioxidants aren't specific to apples, he says. You can also get them from blueberries, spinach and probably cranberries as well (though not from diluted or sugar-sweetened cranberry juice cocktail). If you prefer apple juice, though, be sure to get pure apple juice, not apple juice cocktail, which is loaded with sugar and contains less juice. For those who prefer the fruit, any kind is fine, but always eat the skin, the richest store of antioxidants. Be sure you wash it thoroughly before eating to reduce pesticides.

This is valuable research. It underscores the probable role of a nutritious diet in combating the risk of AD. As Dr. Shea points out, having a weakened form of certain genes likely increases the risk of AD in a person. Antioxidants alone aren't powerful enough to strengthen those genes, but having antioxidant-rich foods as part of a sound diet appears to make a big difference in reducing the risk of AD.

Delicious Ways to Prevent Memory Loss

David Winston, registered herbalist and founder and director, David Winston's Center for Herbal Studies, Broadway, New Jersey.

Researchers looking for ways to fight Alzheimer's disease are hopeful that one answer might be found in a simple bowl of curry. That's because *curcumin*, a compound found in the curry spice *turmeric*, may reduce the buildup of amyloid protein plaque that is associated with the disease.

That could explain why rates of Alzheimer's, which robs people of their memory and their ability to live independently, are among the lowest in the world in India, where the spice is a dietary staple.

In a recent study on rats, scientists found that curcumin significantly reduced the buildup of beta-amyloid protein in the synapses, or gaps, between brain cells. These synapses connect nerve cells and are critical for memory.

CURCUMIN AT WORK

Curcumin, and turmeric itself, have powerful antioxidant and anti-inflammatory properties, says David Winston, a registered herbalist and director of David Winston's Center for Herbal Studies in Broadway, New Jersey. According to Winston, scientists already found that nonsteroidal anti-inflammatory drugs (NSAIDs) such as *ibuprofen* (like Advil, Motrin) reduce the risk for Alzheimer's, but can cause side effects such as gastric bleeding.

Studies on rats and mice show that curcumin works similarly to NSAIDs but with fewer side effects, reducing brain inflammation and decreasing the oxidized proteins that form harmful plaque. Researchers think the compound may have similar effects in humans.

VARIETY OF ANTIOXIDANTS

Dietary antioxidants protect against problems such as chronic inflammation and oxidative diseases, says Winston. He recommends that people incorporate a variety of antioxidants into their diet, including turmeric, rosemary and blueberries. Additionally, ginkgo biloba increases circulation and reduces oxidative processes in the brain.

Eating curcumin or turmeric on a regular basis seems to be helpful, but if you don't like it, don't worry. You can take a curcumin or turmeric supplement, says Winston. He prefers turmeric, since it may provide more antioxidant constituents than curcumin alone. Plus, curcumin can cause stomach irritation in some people, he cautions.

Winston suggests three different ways to get your curcumin...

•**Turmeric capsules.** Take two capsules, two to three times a day.

•**Curcumin tincture.** Take 3 milliliters (ml) to 4 ml, three times a day.

•**Supplemental curcumin.** Take between 1,200 milligrams (mg) and 1,800 mg a day, in three divided doses.

Caution: Individuals prone to bleeding or on blood thinners should not take turmeric. Remember to stop using 10 to 14 days before any dental or surgical procedure.

While you're keeping your neural pathways clean, don't forget to keep your mind active. Research has shown that your brain creates new pathways when you learn something new.

Pick Up Powerful Dementia Prevention In the Vitamin Aisle

Andrew L. Rubman, ND, consulting medical editor for *Bottom Line's Daily Health News* and director of the Southbury Clinic for Traditional Medicines in Southbury, Connecticut.

Many aging baby boomers are deathly afraid that they will fall victim to the rising rates of Alzheimer's disease and dementia. The good news is that prevention may be as close as the vitamin aisle, thanks to research that suggests that vitamin B-12 (*cobalamin*) may help. When we mentioned this to *Bottom Line's Daily Health News* consulting medical editor Andrew L. Rubman, ND, he said that naturopathic physicians have long used B-12 as a treatment for dementia. While the mainstreamers are just catching on, once again naturopaths have been aware of its benefits for many years.

B-12 DEFICIENCY: MORE COMMON AS WE AGE

Vitamin B-12 is a central player in brain and nervous system processes, observes Dr. Rubman. In addition, a B-12 deficiency can lead to a wide variety of neurological problems. In mild cases, these might pass unnoticed—subtle changes in memory, depression, irritability and the like. But in extreme cases, B-12 deficiency may contribute to more serious disorders such as dementia.

Unfortunately, B-12 deficiency is very common among older adults, especially those over 60. Americans get plenty of B-12 in their diet through foods such as shellfish and beef. Yet older people have problems digesting B-12-rich foods and absorbing B-12, so its deficiency commonly increases as we age, explains Dr. Rubman. Given how important B-12 is to brain and nervous system function, along with the body's reduced digesting ability, it is easy to see why dementia may result.

WHAT YOU CAN DO

Even though we have broad government guidelines as to how much B-12 we should take in, Dr. Rubman points out that we must also take into account individual differences in how it is absorbed and utilized. Dr. Rubman encourages people to get a serum B-12 blood test through their doctor to assess their level of B-12. If there is a deficiency—contrary to the emphasis on B-12 shots in conventional medical practice—he says that certain oral forms work equally well. In particular, Dr. Rubman often prescribes sublingual B-12 pills, either *hydroxocobalamin* or *methylcobalamin*, which dissolve under the tongue. (Avoid *cyanocobalamin*, which may be poorly absorbed.) B-12 should be taken under a doctor's supervision. In order for it to function properly, other B vitamins are also required. One B-50 multivitamin, taken twice daily, is quite often prescribed along with the B-12, as they do not last 24 hours in circulation. If you're taking in sufficient B vitamins, urine should remain yellow.

WORK ON DIGESTION

Dr. Rubman adds that B-12 works best as a catalyst with other nutrients. He notes that if you have a poor diet or have digestive challenges that inhibit proper absorption and utilization of nutrients, B-12 can't function efficiently. He also warns that when you take acid-reducing or acid-suppressing drugs, the level of B-12 absorption can drop. To properly absorb nutrients, you need to work on digestion. In most cases, a naturopathic physician can get impaired digestion back on track within just a few weeks.

Beware These Fats that Zap Your Memory

Martha Clare Morris, ScD, associate professor and assistant provost for community research, Rush University Medical Center, Chicago. Dr. Morris is funded by the National Institute on Aging to investigate dietary risk factors for Alzheimer's disease and cognitive decline in a large population-based study of more than 9,000 older Chicago residents.

Long ago, many health-conscious home cooks replaced their aluminum pots and pans due to the reported connection between aluminum and an increased risk of Alzheimer's disease (AD). Now it seems that cooks across the country may need to go shopping again—this time to replace their copper cookware, thanks to a study that found a connection between copper and AD.

THE RESEARCH PROCESS

We spoke with Martha Morris, ScD, associate professor and assistant provost for community research, Rush University Medical Center in Chicago, and lead researcher for the study. Dr. Morris shared with us that they actually started out investigating if people's intake of dietary fat was related to their general health and cognitive decline in old age. "We also wanted to see if it was related to their risk for Alzheimer's," says Dr. Morris. It was. Early research by Dr. Morris' group showed that people with the highest saturated fat intake had about two times the risk of developing AD as those consuming the lowest amount. "People consuming the highest amount of trans fat had two to three times the risk," she adds.

THE COPPER CONNECTION

So where is the copper connection? "Among those with the highest intake of saturated fat and trans fat, copper made things a lot worse," she explains. Among people whose diets were higher in saturated and trans fat, copper intake was associated with a faster rate of cognitive decline. The association was most pronounced with vitamin supplements, although there was also a small association with copper from food sources such as nuts, whole grains and shellfish.

Copper cookware is often coated with another metal that prevents food from coming into contact with copper, but that coating can dissolve or wear off.

The good news for healthy eaters: Copper intake was not associated with cognitive change among people whose diets were not high in saturated or trans fat.

"I'd never suggest to people that they cut back on the foods that are high in copper," Dr. Morris tells us, "since those are among the most healthful foods in the world." Instead, Dr. Morris says, the take-home point is to cut back on the fats known to increase the risk for cognitive problems—trans fat and excessive saturated fat.

"Copper is essential for brain function," she told me. "But like a lot of substances, both too little or too much can be problematic. In the US, we're not in much danger of copper deficiency."

KNOW YOUR FATS

Dr. Morris is adamant in saying that it's not a no-fat diet that is the answer but rather the selection of fats that are known to be healthful. "We found lower rates of declines with diets higher in polyunsaturated and monounsaturated fats than saturated fat...and a significantly lower rate of decline with diets high in omega-3s," she says, echoing advice from many other experts.

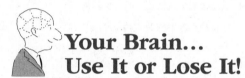

Your Brain...
Use It or Lose It!

Huntington Potter, PhD, senior scientist, Johnnie B. Byrd Sr. Alzheimer's Center & Research Institute, Tampa.

National Institutes on Aging, Alzheimer's Disease Education and Referral Center, *www.nia.nih.gov/Alzheimers*.

Alzheimer's Association, *www.alz.org*.

To lower your risk for Alzheimer's disease (AD), keep challenging your mind—a lot. That may not seem like startling news if you've been paying attention to research on AD. But mental stimulation was given an enthusiastic thumbs up recently following a study on AD involving genetically susceptible mice.

MIGHTY MICE

Huntington Potter, PhD, a study investigator and senior scientist at the Johnnie B. Byrd Sr. Alzheimer's Center & Research Institute, in Tampa, which performed the study in collaboration with the University of South Florida, says that, "Normally, these mice would develop Alzheimer's

by the time they're a year old. By putting them in an intensely enriched environment with toys, wheels, tunnels, mazes and other mice, they developed improved cognitive abilities and performed as well as healthy mice." Despite having brains similar to mice with AD—with evidence of amyloid plaque, plaques that contain a protein characteristic of the disease—the mentally stimulated mice suffered no mental impairment.

While past studies have shown that mental stimulation appears to reduce AD risk, these findings suggest an enriched environment may stabilize and even improve the memory of people genetically inclined to develop AD, enabling them to live more productive and rewarding lives. How this works is not clear. "Environmental enrichment partially reduces amyloid plaque," Dr. Potter says. "But it helps cognitive ability far more than can be explained by amyloid plaque reduction."

TRAIN YOUR BRAIN

A mentally challenging job that requires you to think and use your decision-making abilities may help stave off AD, Dr. Potter points out. But if your job involves little or no mental challenge, you may be able to reap similar benefits by getting a second job that does...or by enjoying mentally stimulating leisure activities (for a few hours each weekday and more on the weekends). Crossword puzzles and other brainteasers are good. Watching TV, for the most part, is not good. Reading can be active and stimulating, depending on the book and the person reading it, Dr. Potter says. Playing a musical instrument may help but doesn't involve the same memory functions as puzzles or mental tests. And retirement, if it means an end to mental stimulation, is not good.

WHAT YOUR BRAIN NEEDS

In addition to mental stimulation, Dr. Potter says that keeping your brain healthy requires...

•**Getting daily exercise.**

- **Being socially active, enjoying a variety of relationships.**
- **Eating a healthful diet.**
- **Avoiding smoking or the abuse of alcohol.**
- **Controlling your cholesterol, blood pressure and blood sugar levels.**

About 4.5 million Americans currently have AD, and by 2050, it's estimated that 11.3 million to 16 million will suffer from the disease. While scientists have not yet found a cure, you can take these preventive measures to stay healthier and functioning as long as possible until effective drugs and treatments to prevent the disease or halt its progression are developed.

Research Holds New Hope For Alzheimer's

Robert Brendza, PhD, research instructor in neurology, Washington University School of Medicine, St. Louis.

Alzheimer's disease (AD) now affects up to half of all people over the age of 85. It requires a two-pronged strategy for prevention and damage control for those who have it. Until now, AD research has mostly centered on slowing the progress of the disease, and without a whole lot of success. Now a recent study published in *The Journal of Clinical Investigation* demonstrates that the day actually may come when AD can be reversed.

No one knows what causes AD—the manifestation of it, though, is clear: Formation of *amyloid* (a protein) plaques in the brain in the areas that control memory and thinking. These plaques exist outside of the brain cells (neurons), not in them. They take over the area and, in the process, the plaques damage and push neurons out of the way. The primary protein making up the amyloid plaques is *A-beta*

peptide, which is normally in the body in soluble form but becomes insoluble and toxic in this form. Much AD research has been centered on finding ways to keep the A-beta peptide from taking this destructive path.

PROMISING RESEARCH

It's important to note that this study, from the Washington University School of Medicine (St. Louis) department of neurology, was conducted on mice, not on human beings, and it is impossible to know if what happens in mice can be duplicated in the human system. Still, it offers exciting potential for continued research and possibly future treatment.

One of the lead members of the research team on the study was Robert Brendza, PhD. He explains that this was a "proof-in-principle" study, one that is designed to establish the validity of a theory. The researchers placed an antibody (an immune protein) that specifically targets A-beta protein directly into the brains of mice modeled to have amyloid plaques. They knew that the antibody would clear the A-beta protein, but they wanted to see what would happen once that occurred. Would it be possible to slow or halt the progress of injury occurring in the brain? Much to the research team's astonishment, in just three days, the antibody did much more than the scientists had hoped to see. It succeeded in *reducing* the number and size of the amyloid plaques by 20% to 25%, and the swelling around the damage in those areas disappeared.

The implication of this, of course, is that in the absence of plaques, the brain might heal itself—at least in part. But how realistic is this for the 4.5 million Americans who currently have AD?

OF MICE, NOT MEN

Dr. Brendza says that while the systems of mice and of human beings, oddly enough, have many similarities, there are also a lot of differences. This is why scientists are so careful about predicting how the results of their mice studies will translate for use in human beings and why Dr. Brendza is cautiously optimistic about the results. However, Dr. Brendza says that the team is now working on several new mice studies concerning A-beta peptide antibody, including the manipulation of dosages and schedules to see the impact on the brain. They also are looking for ways to address and improve the damage that takes place within the neurons, to see if something will improve the cell itself. They expect to have much more information about what happens in mice brains within a few years, and they would like to think that they will also soon know more about human AD, but they remain wary about predicting this.

MORE RESEARCH TO COME

At this point, there is simply no way to anticipate what will happen with AD research as it progresses, but there is reason to hope. Dr. Brendza says that there are a number of early-stage trials now underway that are looking for ways to reduce A-beta production in the brain...and there is further research on ways to improve agents that enhance neuron activity, the current form of treatment. Ultimately, he says, effective treatment of this heartbreaking disease will probably combine a variety of approaches being developed in various laboratories today.

Astounding! Alzheimer's May Be A Type of Diabetes

Suzanne de la Monte, MD, MPH, associate professor of pathology and medicine and clinical neuroscience, Alpert Medical School at Brown University, and neuropathologist at Rhode Island Hospital, both in Providence, Rhode Island.

New research into the causes of Alzheimer's disease (AD) is showing an intriguing new direction in formal treatment—one that might lead to successful treatment in the early stages of the disease. Two recent studies from the Alpert Medical School at Brown University in Providence, Rhode Island, identified diminished insulin availability as well as insulin resistance in the brain, as a possible trigger for the brain deterioration, loss of cognitive function and buildup of plaques (protein fragments between brain neurons) and tangles (twisted fibers inside brain cells) that characterize AD.

"We've found AD to be a form of diabetes," says Suzanne de la Monte, MD, MPH, senior researcher on the study.

CAUSE AND EFFECT

In one study, researchers depleted insulin and at the same time produced insulin resistance in the brains of rats by injecting them with *Streptozotocin* (STZ), a compound known to destroy insulin-producing cells in the pancreas. As they had hypothesized, the result was overall brain deterioration in the rats.

Even more exciting: In a subsequent study using the same rats—who now exhibited symptoms resembling AD—researchers then reversed the insulin resistance in their brains by administering three classes of drugs called PPAR (*peroxisome-proliferator activated receptor*) agonists. (The agonists are drugs but the receptors are normally present in the brain.)

Following this treatment, the AD-like brain abnormalities and degeneration that the rats had displayed were either reduced or nearly absent. Of the three classes of agonists used, one—PPAR *delta*—had the most benefit in preserving brain tissues and improving learning memory. PPAR *alpha* was less effective. Another PPAR agonist—PPAR *gamma*—that is already being prescribed as a treatment in type 2 diabetes to modulate insulin response, was least effective. This research has yet to be applied to humans, notes Dr. de la Monte. But she is definitely thinking ahead.

BRAIN DIABETES

"We've seen the incidence of both type 2 diabetes and AD grow in epidemic proportions, and researchers now recognize both the overlap of the two conditions and the increased risk for developing AD in patients with type 2 diabetes." Dr. de la Monte refers to this as a separate process, a "type 3" diabetes or "diabetes of the brain."

CAN WE PREVENT ALZHEIMER'S?

Obviously, a great deal of research needs to be done before these findings lead to a solid connection between AD and diabetes, and even more until possible treatment is available.

Dr. de la Monte shares her thoughts on how this information might be useful in the short term: "When we think about type 2 diabetes and how much it is mediated by lifestyle and environmental factors—and that we know the same is true for insulin resistance in the liver—you can't help but wonder to what extent this is also true for insulin resistance in the brain, which our research showed often results in AD symptoms."

And, she concludes, when you start thinking like that, the next question is— "What are the specific lifestyle features that contribute to this? *Now*, you're talking about prevention, which almost certainly would involve lifestyle choices."

Dangerous Link Between Alzheimer's And Excess Weight

Samuel Gandy, MD, PhD, director, Farber Institute for Neurosciences, Thomas Jefferson University, Philadelphia, and former vice chairman, Alzheimer's Association's Medical and Scientific Advisory Council.

Recent research on Alzheimer's disease (AD) has opened the door to a key realization—it appears that conditions known to increase risk for cardiovascular disease also increase risk for AD. In particular obesity, uncontrolled diabetes, hypertension and elevated cholesterol have been linked. However, the way these conditions connect to AD has thus far been a mystery. Now, though, a new study may have the answer—and the connection is obesity.

The study, conducted at the Farber Institute for Neurosciences at Thomas Jefferson University in Philadelphia in connection with Edith Cowan University (Western Australia), measured body mass index (BMI) of 18 healthy adults as well as the blood levels of a sticky protein called *beta-amyloid*. The researchers found that people who were overweight or obese also had high levels of blood-borne beta-amyloid. That is disturbing because beta-amyloid is highly associated with development of AD.

The reason: The brain plaques that severely disrupt functioning in people with AD are made up of beta-amyloid.

THE MYSTERY OF BETA-AMYLOID

We called the study's lead author, Samuel Gandy, MD, PhD, to discuss the implications of the study. Dr. Gandy was formerly vice chairman of the Alzheimer's Association's Medical and Scientific Advisory Council. He says that beta-amyloid, produced from improperly metabolized "amyloid precursor protein," as of yet has no known purpose in the body, but that it can congregate and build up in the brains of people with AD. Doctors also don't know *why* it congregates nor do they know how the body rids itself of excess levels of it, though they theorize that it travels from the brain through the spinal fluid and into the blood for clearing. When the excess is excreted from the body, all is fine. The concern, though, is about the beta-amyloid that travels from the blood into the brain. There is a test that shows the amyloids levels in the blood, but at this time, the test is not used clinically.

GET THE WEIGHT OFF

While there is more to learn as a result of this study, the warning signs are clear. Risk of AD is yet one more reason for those who are overweight to get the weight off. Participants in the study all had a BMI of 30 or below, which means those with the high beta-amyloid scores were "merely" overweight or barely obese—none were morbidly obese. Research has not yet been done on the morbidly obese.

In yet another recent study concerning AD, researchers found that people who exercised even just 15 minutes at least three times a week reduced the risk of developing AD by 32%.

Start getting the weight off now before it's too late. Every little bit will help.

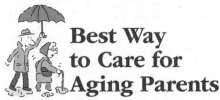

Best Way to Care for Aging Parents

Sandra W. Haymon, PhD, a psychologist in private practice, Thomasville, Georgia. She is author of *My Turn: Caring for Aging Parents & Other Elderly Loved Ones: A Daughter's Perspective*. Magnolia Productions.

As life expectancy rises, families increasingly face the challenge of caring for sick or elderly relatives. The diagnosis may be dementia in an aging parent, or multiple sclerosis or cancer in a formerly robust spouse or sibling, but the question remains the same—How do I find the strength to rise to the occasion and meet this challenge?

NO EASY ANSWERS

Caregivers face a multiplicity of complex issues, in which family beliefs, cultural values and spirituality all come into play. For example,

•**Which family member is the designated caregiver when a parent is ill?**

•**Is the responsibility to be shared?**

•**How long can you or should you care for a loved one at home?**

•**When is it time to consider institutional or hospice care?**

•**Is death to be embraced as a spiritual release,** or is it something you don't discuss in your family?

•**How do you juggle raising young children while caring for older parents?**

There are no easy answers to questions like these, and over time each family comes around to its own way of thinking and coping. But whatever path you choose, there is no doubt that caring for a seriously ill family member means riding an emotional roller coaster, with sensations veering from anger to denial to fear to guilt to hopelessness to grief. According to a study in the *American Journal of Geriatric Psychiatry*, one in three caregivers ends up developing symptoms of depression under all this pressure.

To learn how to summon the strength to care for an ill loved one, we spoke with Sandra W. Haymon, PhD, a psychologist in private practice in Thomasville, Georgia. She is also author of *My Turn: Caring for Aging Parents & Other Elderly Loved Ones: A Daughter's Perspective* (Magnolia Productions).

HOW TO STAY STRONG

Dr. Haymon suggests a number of things to do, including…

•**Develop a support network.** Involve other family members and friends in caring for your loved one. Chances are they're anxious to help but don't know how. Your best bet is to assign specific tasks—for example, doing yard work, feeding the pets, assisting with doctor visits or vacuuming the house. Don't be too proud to accept help from any and all who offer. They really want to help and you don't have to do it all alone.

•**Prioritize.** Dr. Haymon has seen too many caregivers try to do everything they did previously, on top of their new responsibilities. She suggests making a list of what's important and, keeping in mind that time and energy are finite, forgiving yourself for not being able to do it all.

•**Think outside the box.** Dr. Haymon recommends that instead of saying that things "should" be done a certain way, open the door to thinking they "could" be done in an altogether different manner. For instance, the yard "should" be tended to, but it "could" be done by someone else. Or, it "could" remain less than perfectly groomed, and that's all right, too.

•**Set aside time for yourself.** Make it a point to get out and do other things, even if it's just once or twice a week. For example, join a friend for dinner or a walk. Nature can be especially comforting, so catch up with one another as you stroll through the park or along the beach. Don't feel like you are deserting the person in need by taking time for yourself. Otherwise, you won't have energy and emotion to care for others in a loving way.

•**Join a support group for caregivers.** Here you can freely share your emotions with others who have faced or are facing similar challenges. Dr. Haymon adds that this is a great opportunity to pick up practical tips that will save you time and energy, learning from those who have already been there, done that. If you're uncomfortable with groups, consider one-on-one counseling.

•**Explore your spirituality.** If religion has played a big part in your or your loved one's life, now is the time to embrace it all the more. Attend religious services, arrange for clergy to visit, pray together and sing familiar hymns. On a practical level, church or temple members can play a valuable role in your support network.

•**Keep an eye on your own health.** In focusing on the needs of someone who is very ill, it's easy to forget to take care of yourself, warns Dr. Haymon. To stay strong, eat well, exercise and get enough sleep. Also, don't neglect regular checkups.

•**Don't use alcohol or cigarettes as crutches.** Drinking and smoking are not uncommon responses to caregiver stress. Be aware of this, and instead choose positive coping mechanisms. For example, set aside 15 minutes each morning to practice yoga, tai chi, meditation or deep breathing.

•**Consider respite care.** Advocacy groups such as the Multiple Sclerosis Society (*www.nationalmssociety.org*) and the Alzheimer's Association (*www.alz.org*) offer this service, in which trained individuals take care of the afflicted person while you take a breather. You can find respite care in your community at *www.respitelocator.org*. Other resources to tap into include local YMCAs, hospitals and civic organizations.

GIVE YOURSELF A BREAK

As many positive steps as you take to stay strong during this challenging period, there will be inevitable moments when you feel angry or upset or frustrated or disappointed, notes Dr. Haymon. You may even feel anger toward your loved one, and experience guilt about that. She advises that, above all, you allow yourself to freely experience these feelings.

Don't try to suppress what are completely natural reactions and emotions. Let the tears flow, or pour out your feelings in a journal...then move on, gathering comfort and strength from the fact that you're far from alone in your struggle, and there are concrete steps you can take to meet the challenge.

8

Super Healers for Your Eyes, Teeth and Skin

Five Simple Secrets For Keeping Your Eyes Young

A sure sign of middle age creeping in is the day you discover that you can no longer read a menu or use the phone book without eyeglasses. Blurred letters make *presbyopia*, the technical name for the problem, impossible to ignore, but other conditions can develop down the road that have potentially much more troubling consequences, including blindness. Especially serious problems include age-related macular degeneration (AMD), cataracts, glaucoma and diabetic retinopathy. Aging eyes are also prone to some annoying problems, such as dry eyes or excess tearing.

KEEPING EYES YOUNG

Lylas G. Mogk, MD, founding director of the Visual Rehabilitation and Research Center at the Henry Ford Health System in Grosse Point Park, Michigan, and coauthor of *Macular Degeneration: The Complete Guide to Saving and Maximizing Your Sight* (Ballantine), has two across-the-board rules for keeping your eyes young. The first is to eat well and take care of your whole self (more on that in a minute), and the second is to wear sunglasses.

DON'T FORGET YOUR SUNGLASSES

She explains that wearing sunglasses on a regular basis is a crucial preventive measure against both AMD and cataracts. Any kind of lenses that have a good ultraviolet (UV) filter are effective, unless you are at

Lylas G. Mogk, MD, founding director, Visual Rehabilitation and Research Center, Henry Ford Health System in Grosse Point Park, Michigan and coauthor, *Macular Degeneration: The Complete Guide to Saving and Maximizing Your Sight*. Ballantine.

Marc R. Grossman, OD, coauthor, *Natural Eye Care: An Encyclopedia*, McGraw-Hill. He is an international speaker on natural eyecare, nutrition and Chinese medicine, based in New Paltz, New York. Visit his Web site at *www.naturaleyecare.com*.

high risk for AMD (you are a smoker, are fair-skinned, have a family history of AMD or have had high exposure to sun without protection) in which case you should get amber/orange lenses with UV protection to more effectively block the blue end of the light spectrum. Polarized lenses will help further by reducing glare, or reflected low-angle light, which can cause eyestrain.

Wearing sunglasses also helps prevent wrinkles around your eyes caused by squinting…and prevents yellowing from *pinguecula*. Pinguecula are lesions—caused by UV rays—in the eye near the cornea that turn the white of the eye in the affected area yellow.

OMEGA-3s AND YOUR EYES

As for diet, Dr. Mogk is adamant about getting sufficient omega-3 fatty acids, which are abundant in cold-water fish and fish oil supplements. Omega-3s are important in preventing AMD and are valuable for keeping eyes properly lubricated, she says. The eyeball contains three layers—a mucus layer, a water layer and over these, an oil slick. A healthy oil slick is necessary for the eyes' comfort because it prevents evaporation from the water layer.

Without a healthy oil layer, the eyes become dry (not to be confused with the disease *Sjögren's Syndrome*, which affects all of the mucous membranes in the body) or, conversely, they can water too much.

The reason: In response to overly dry conditions, the eyes put the accessory tear glands—the ones employed in crying—into motion, and the result is too many tears. The oil slick contains fatty acids and depends heavily on omega-3s to do its job properly as well as to maintain the proper consistency of its oil.

DIABETICS TAKE NOTE

Dr. Mogk's other strong message concerns people who have diabetes of either type: Keep sugar levels under control. Over time, she says, uncontrolled sugar levels will lead to diabetic retinopathy, which occurs when the small vessels no longer feed the retina properly, resulting in vision loss and blindness.

INSIDE OUT EYE CARE

For more information concerning nutrients and eye health, we spoke with Marc R. Grossman, OD, coauthor of *Natural Eye Care: An Encyclopedia* (McGraw-Hill) and an international speaker on natural eye care and nutrition, from New Paltz, New York. In addition to omega-3 fatty acids (1,000 milligrams [mg] for prevention), he advises lutein (6 mg a day in supplements and plenty of dark green vegetables, such as kale and collard greens) and *zeaxantin*, the nutrient that contains the carotenoid believed to filter out UV blue rays and provide antioxidant protection to the center of the *macula*. Health food stores now carry pharmaceutical-grade zeaxantin (take 2 mg to 3 mg a day). It is also abundant in orange peppers and other brightly colored vegetables. Fresh, naturally ripened foods transmit the greatest flavonoid/carotenoid activity to the body.

In addition, he advises taking 2,000 mg of vitamin C in divided doses throughout the day, between meals. Dr. Grossman also recommends 300 mg of grape seed extract and 120 mg of bilberry, both of which help maintain the integrity of the blood vessels in the eyes. Be sure to review these recommendations with a trained professional, since individual needs vary.

ALL ABOUT CHECKUPS

Dr. Mogk recommends eye checkups every two years after age 40. Besides being able to monitor for any sign of glaucoma, an eye checkup allows viewing of the blood vessels behind the eyes, and it is the only place in the body where doctors can see blood vessels without the protective tissue of the skin over them. This provides the doctor with an excellent opportunity to review your blood vessel health in general and to see if their condition indicates the presence of high blood pressure, diabetes or coronary artery disease.

Natural Ways to "Get the Red Out"

E. Michael Geiger, OD, optometrist and natural eye-care specialist in private practice, New York City. He is the author of *Eye Care Naturally*. Safe Goods.

In comic-book land, one sure sign that a character is a bad guy is that he has bloodshot eyes. It's not true, of course, but sometimes it can be a challenge to get the whites of the eyes, technically called the *sclera*, bright and white, as nature intended. For help on the best ways to meet the challenge, we spoke with optometrist E. Michael Geiger, OD, optometrist and natural eye-care specialist in New York City, and author of *Eye Care Naturally* (Safe Goods).

DR. GEIGER'S RULES

Dr. Geiger's first rule for clear eyes is to get enough rest. He says that virtually everyone needs seven or eight hours of sleep a night—even those who claim they need less. Without those hours, red eyes are likely to result.

The second rule is to avoid irritants. This is difficult, indeed probably impossible, according to Dr. Geiger, because there are 60,000 different chemicals produced in our world, and 2,000 to 3,000 of them are irritants. These crop up in every corner of daily life.

Smoke, whether from your own smoking habit or secondhand, is also a key irritant. Obviously, while you can almost always stay away from smoke, you can't avoid many other irritants, which brings us to Dr. Geiger's third rule for clear eyes—wash out those irritants.

The way to rinse your eyes is with over-the-counter eyewashes. Be sure to choose one that is free of preservatives (he likes one called OcuFresh, for instance). Wash your eyes when you are exposed to an irritant and before you go to bed at night. Washing every night is okay if chronic red eye is a problem. A presleep wash will prevent toxins from sitting in your eyes

throughout the night and intensifying the problem.

Important: Never use eyedrops that are intended to remove the red in your eye. The sclera gets red because the eyes bring in extra blood to fight an irritant and nourish the eyeball. The drops stop this action, cancelling out its helpfulness. Eventually, regular use of them can cause infection, says Dr. Geiger. So, no Visine or other drops to "get the red out."

SPECIAL FOR CONTACT LENS WEARERS

Contact-lens wearers have a few extra rules to remember. Be sure that contacts are fitted properly, and get rid of them when their time is up. Dr. Geiger explains that extending the amount of time you wear them will not only irritate your eyes, it can also make them prone to infection.

However, if your eyes ever get the seriously bloodshot look of comic-book villains, says Dr. Geiger, call your eye doctor right away. Severely bloodshot eyes can be a sign of a disease such as glaucoma, a corneal ulcer or other serious eye problem. Immediate evaluation is indicated.

Powerful New Eye Test Helps Detect Diseases In Seconds

Barbara Manion, OD, optometrist in private practice in Westport, Connecticut.

Traditionally, eye exams have included dilating drops, rolling your eyes up, down, across and across again as the doctor peers with a bright light into them, and then sitting in the office for some period of time until the drops wear off enough that you can safely leave the office. Part of the reason for this eyeball workout is so that doctors can see deep into the eye in order to detect possible eye disease. In fact, this is critical.

If caught early enough, doctors can treat most conditions of the eye, including glaucoma and diabetic retinopathy, and save the patient's vision.

WHAT BACK OF THE EYE REVEALS

What many people don't realize, though, is that evaluating the back of the eye (the retina) also allows doctors to detect some diseases and conditions that may lurk elsewhere in the body. The condition of retinal blood vessels, for instance, can inform the doctor if the patient has unchecked high blood pressure, if diabetes is present or not being controlled adequately, as well as the rare possibility of certain tumors. Changes in the appearance of the optic nerve can indicate certain brain diseases or systemic conditions that can also affect vision.

DIGITAL RETINAL DISPLAYS

The good news is that the inconvenience of the drops may not always be necessary, with a new and powerful tool for investigating the retina. It is called the Optomap Retinal Exam and it is the first device that produces a comprehensive digital view of the eye. We spoke with optometrist Barbara Manion, OD, who is in private practice in Westport, Connecticut, about the value of this technology. She explains that it takes just seconds to take this digital picture, but the result is an astonishingly detailed display of 180 to 200 degrees of the retina. This compares with the approximate 45 degrees that is typically seen in an undilated exam. In addition, the red and green low-power laser beams have different wavelengths that display different retinal depths, thereby allowing doctors to determine at what layer a problem, if present, exists.

She says the technology makes in-depth analysis of the retina possible. The resulting picture also has advantages in patient education and compliance...because patients can actually see what is going on in their retina, and, says Dr. Manion, they understand much better why they need to address problems.

Note that as of yet, insurance doesn't cover the Optomap Retinal Exam, but it is not prohibitively expensive.

Dr. Manion recommends annual eye exams for all patients...those with diabetes should have an exam at least every six months.

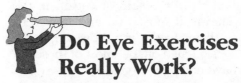

Do Eye Exercises Really Work?

E. Michael Geiger, OD, optometrist and natural eye-care specialist in private practice, New York City. He is the author of Eye Care Naturally. *Safe Goods.*

It's an unavoidable fact of life for just about everyone over age 40. Eventually you'll hear yourself saying seven inevitable words. "I can't read it without my glasses." It may start in a restaurant when a menu looks blurry, or when you pick up the phone book to find a telephone number. Eventually, most of us surrender to the inevitable and realize we need reading glasses. It's a natural consequence of aging.

OR IS IT?

Exercise programs for the eyes have been around since the early 1900s. They occupy a nebulous space somewhere between medical science and folk remedy. Most ophthalmologists and optometrists are dismissive of them, yet these programs abound. They include *Dr. Friedman's Vision Training Program* (Bantam)...Lisette Scholl's *Visionetics: The Holistic Way to Better Eyesight* (Dolphin)...and Taber's Eye-Robics (*www.eyerobics.net*)

Can these or any of the new crop of "natural" self-help vision programs being hawked on the Internet and late-night television actually help baby boomers throw away their reading glasses?

NOT FOR PRESBYOPIA

Not very likely. "The need for reading glasses is caused by a condition known as *presbyopia*," says E. Michael Geiger, OD, an optometrist and natural eye-care specialist from New York City, and author of *Eye Care Naturally* (Safe Goods). "You have a lens in your eye called the crystalline lens. It continually changes shape so you can focus. That's how you see from far to near," he explains. "When most cells die, they are either carried away by the bloodstream, sloughed off in the skin or cut off in the hair. They're disposed of, and new cells replace them. In the eye, however, some cells are sloughed off, but most of these old cells have nowhere to go. The lens is in a capsule, with no way out. So the old cells stay within the capsule and the capsule starts to get more and more encapsulated. By the time men are 45 and women are 40, the lens can be so 'crowded' that it simply can't flex enough for close reading. Hence the need for reading glasses."

MAYBE FOR OTHER CONDITIONS

While eye exercises—also known as vision therapy—may not help for presbyopia, they may be helpful for some other conditions. There is a proven segment of vision therapy known as *orthoptics* that can help with symptoms of visual strain or fatigue in individuals with mild eye coordination or focus problems, double vision or even *strabismus* ("crossed" or "turned" eyes) and *amblyopia* ("lazy eye"). A fundamental premise of vision therapy is that refractive disorders, such as *myopia* (nearsightedness) and *hyperopia* (farsightedness), have both hereditary and environmental causes, such as near point stress (excessive and prolonged focusing on objects close at hand) from reading. Certain eye exercises are designed to relieve so-called spasms of accommodation, which are disruptions of the eye's ability to focus due to eyestrain from the environment. Other exercises are said to improve the eyes' coordination or to straighten misaligned eyes.

EXERCISE TO SEE MORE CLEARLY?

Both mainstream optometrists as well as eye surgeons are critical of eye exercises because there is no reliable evidence that they help to eliminate or even reduce reliance on corrective lenses. Many doctors remain skeptical of the need for such programs. "The eye muscles never atrophy," Dr. Geiger says.

The best advice may be to keep your expectations in check. Maybe you will have visual improvement with the eye exercise programs, though many experts doubt it. As Dr. Geiger says, "While diet and lifestyle may be able to help keep some elements of vision beyond the lens' focus in check, there's nothing that can be done to change the dying of the cells."

Amazing! Exercise Lowers Risk of Macular Degeneration Up to 70%

Lylas Mogk, MD, founding director, Visual Rehabilitation and Research Center, Henry Ford Health System in Grosse Pointe Park, Michigan and coauthor, *Macular Degeneration: The Complete Guide to Saving and Maximizing Your Sight*. Ballantine.

Exercise is proving itself to be absolutely instrumental in achieving and maintaining optimum health—and not just for cardiovascular reasons, but for a wide array of health benefits.

The latest benefit of exercise: It helps safeguard against one of the leading causes of vision loss in people age 60 and over. Findings of the Beaver Dam Eye Study suggest that regular exercise lowers risk of one type of *age-related macular degeneration* (AMD) by as much as 70%.

EXERCISE AND AMD

AMD, a progressive disease, erodes vision in the central part of the eye leaving people primarily with peripheral vision. Currently 1.75 million Americans have significant vision loss from AMD and that number is expected to increase by 50%

by the year 2020. The long-term study, funded in part by the National Institutes of Health, involved nearly 4,000 men and women living in Beaver Dam, Wisconsin, and investigated development and progression of AMD. It showed that over the 15 years of the study, people who were the most active had a 70% lower risk of developing AMD and that even just regular walking lowered risk by 30%.

Note: Risk reduction applied only to the "wet" form of AMD rather than the other type, the "dry" form. In wet AMD, abnormal, delicate new blood vessels form in the back of the eye that are vulnerable to leaking and hemorrhaging into the eye. In the dry form of AMD (which precedes wet AMD) the light sensitive cells in the macula break down without the development of new blood vessels. This also leads to central vision loss. Although wet AMD affects only about 10% of people with AMD, it progresses more rapidly and more often leads to severe vision loss.

LOWERING RISK

We asked ophthalmologist Lylas Mogk, MD, founding director of the Visual Rehabilitation and Research Center at the Henry Ford Health System in Grosse Pointe Park, Michigan, and coauthor of *Macular Degeneration: The Complete Guide to Saving and Maximizing Your Sight* (Ballantine), about the study. She says that the probable reason exercise has more impact on wet AMD risk is because circulation and blood pressure may play a greater role in that type than in dry.

It may also help that exercise decreases inflammation and inflammation is increasingly recognized as a factor in promoting macular degeneration, says Dr. Mogk. But to reduce risk the most, you'll need to do really brisk walking, cycling or other aerobic exercise (which directly affects circulation) for 30 minutes at least three times a week. Dr. Mogk also reminds people that having a nutritious diet, including a lot of fish (or fish oil) and green leafy vegetables, has been shown to decrease risk,

and that not smoking is another important part of the equation.

Natural Ways To Prevent and Treat Macular Degeneration

E. Michael Geiger, OD, optometrist and natural eye-care specialist in private practice in New York City. He is the author of *Eye Care Naturally*. Safe Goods.

If your eyesight is fading from the middle of your focal area, you may be suffering from macular degeneration, the leading cause of vision loss and blindness in Americans aged 60 and older. One in four Americans aged 64 to 74 is suffering from it, as is one in three of those over 75. Is macular degeneration the visual version of age-related hearing loss? Is it preventable? Reversible?

MACULAR DEGENERATION DEFINED

The *macula* is the central area of the retina, where most of the cones are located, and it is responsible for focus and color vision. In macular degeneration, this area of the eye deteriorates, taking with it aspects of visual function. The cause of macular degeneration is not really known, though smoking, poor diet and obesity all increase the risk. Other associated factors include high blood pressure, light eye color, farsightedness, family history of the disease and being over age 60. The condition tends to affect whites and females in particular.

One theory on the cause of macular degeneration is that there is insufficient disposal of waste materials from the cells of the eye. Cellular metabolites are normally carried off, but in this case some are left behind, obscuring light and impairing cell function, which in turn impairs vision.

DRY AND WET

There are two types of macular degeneration—dry and wet. In the wet form, new blood vessels grow beneath the retina that leak blood and fluid, causing retinal cells to die and creating blind spots in central vision. The wet form of the disease clouds the tissue, usually leading to more serious vision loss. The dry form is more common than the wet—85% to 95% of patients with macular degeneration have the dry form—and it typically occurs gradually over a long period of time. Vision loss from macular degeneration is generally a slow, painless loss of vision. Symptoms include seeing shadowy areas in your central vision or experiencing unusually fuzzy or distorted vision.

Note: Viewing an Amsler grid is one way to tell if you are having these vision problems. You can view an Amsler grid at *www. allaboutvision.com/conditions/amsler-grid.htm.*

REGENERATION STRATEGIES

In the National Eye Institute's Age-Related Eye Disease Study (AREDS)—involving more than 4,757 people who were 55 to 80 years of age and who either did not have the disease or had the disease in one eye—the researchers found that supplementation with certain nutrients reduced the risk of progressing to advanced macular degeneration by 28%. What you eat affects the macula and many experts feel that diet and supplements can be used to treat or prevent the condition. To map out the best natural action plan for preventing or treating this age-related vision robber, we interviewed E. Michael Geiger, OD, a New York optometrist who specializes in natural eye care and wrote *Eye Care Naturally* (Safe Goods).

Here are Dr. Geiger's choices for preventing and treating macular degeneration…

1. Vitamin C. "Vitamin C helps prevent blood vessels from breaking and prevents the growth of excess blood vessels in the macular area," Dr. Geiger says. The ARED study recommended 500 milligrams (mg) per day.

2. Garlic. "Garlic helps with circulation," Dr. Geiger points out. "One of the problems with macular degeneration is the buildup of waste products, so you want to stimulate circulation." Fresh garlic seems to work as well as garlic tablets, available over the counter.

3. Lutein and zeaxanthin. "These members of the carotenoid family were not used in the original ARED study, but have since been found to be among the most effective supplements for eye health," Dr. Geiger says. Lutein, present in the macula of the eye's retina, appears to filter harmful, high-energy blue wavelengths of visible light from both natural sunlight and indoor light. Dr. Geiger recommends from 6 mg to 15 mg of lutein for general prevention, but 20 mg to 40 mg of lutein for someone who already has macular degeneration.

Note: Lutein and zeaxanthin come together in supplements and food sources, so if you purchase a formula with lutein, you're usually getting the right amount of zeaxanthin as well. There are no known risks or side effects from this level of lutein.

MORE HELPFUL IDEAS

Other supplements that have been found to be helpful include beta-carotene, zinc and especially omega-3 fatty acids. The *Archives of Ophthalmology* has reported that omega-3 fatty acids have a protective effect against advanced macular degeneration. Meanwhile, consumption of omega-6 fatty acids (prevalent in vegetable oils) not balanced with omega-3s is associated with an *increased* risk of developing macular degeneration. Most nutritionists recommend at least a gram a day of fish oil for its many health benefits and omega-3s. The original study also recommends 400 IUs of vitamin E a day (mixed tocopherols are the best kind).

Finally, Dr. Geiger likes *genistein*, a soy isoflavone that he believes to be particularly good for those with the wet form of MD. "It inhibits the formation of these undesirable blood vessels," he says. "Since the dry form turns into the wet form, genistein is not a bad idea for anyone." Follow the label directions on the supplement bottle.

Dr. Geiger also recommends aerobic exercise for increased circulation...and brown sunglass lenses. Brown lenses block blue light, which can be harmful to the macular area," he says.

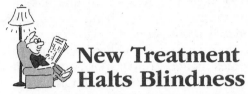

New Treatment Halts Blindness

Lylas Mogk, MD, founding director, Visual Rehabilitation and Research Center, Henry Ford Health System, Grosse Pointe Park, Michigan and coauthor, *Macular Degeneration: The Complete Guide to Saving and Maximizing Your Sight.* Ballantine.

Age-related macular degeneration (AMD) affects about 1.75 million Americans each year, typically over age 60. It is a leading cause of vision loss. Until recently, treatment for this dreaded condition was limited to potentially preventive measures, various forms of laser for the wet type and rehab that teaches how to better handle vision loss. But recently that bleak picture brightened for those with wet AMD when the FDA approved the drug *ranibizumab* (Lucentis). In two clinical trials, nearly all AMD patients treated with Lucentis demonstrated that vision did not severely deteriorate further...and in one study 11% to 15% showed their vision actually improved to 20/40. The drug's success lasted in patients throughout the yearlong trial, which was very encouraging for long-term prospects.

For more information, we called ophthalmologist Lylas Mogk, MD, founding director of the Visual Rehabilitation and Research Center of the Henry Ford Health System in Grosse Pointe Park, Michigan, and coauthor of *Macular Degeneration: The Complete Guide to Saving and Maximizing Your Sight* (Ballantine). Dr. Mogk says she is genuinely excited but cautions that the drug has its limitations. First and foremost is the fact that Lucentis treats only the wet type of AMD, which affects approximately 15% of AMD patients, not the more common dry AMD. Wet AMD occurs when abnormal blood vessels that break easily (causing hemorrhages, swelling and retinal scarring) begin to form in the back of the eye. Lucentis reduces formation of these blood vessels. However, it must be started in the early stages of the disease. Once scarring sets in, the drug can no longer help because it can't reverse scar tissue.

KNOW THE WARNING SIGNS

Dr. Mogk says that the early signs of wet AMD are small and medium-sized yellow or white spots (*drusen*) in the retina, seen during an eye exam. Drusen are common with age, but in normal eyes they are round and small, much like salt crystals, while AMD-related drusen are soft and cloud-like. When such drusen are spotted, the doctor guides patients in how to monitor any changes. If wet AMD does start, treatment with Lucentis should be considered. The drug is administered through regular injections, preferably once a month, into the eyeball. This sounds unpleasant, but Dr. Mogk explains that a very fine needle is passed through the white of the eye, which has few pain-sensing nerve fibers. Thus the injection causes little or no pain. The drug is expensive, approximately $2,000 per injection, with 80% of the cost covered by Medicare.

Another drug called Avastin (*bevacizumab*) that is chemically related to Lucentis and manufactured by the same drug company has been used off label to treat wet AMD. It is much less expensive and is thought to remain in the eye longer than Lucentis, allowing for fewer injections. The National Eye Institute of the National Institutes of Health has announced the start of a multicenter clinical trial to compare the safety and effectiveness of both Lucentis and Avastin.

SUPPLEMENTS AND DRY AMD

For the millions of patients with dry AMD, no proven treatment beyond nutritional supplements exists. However, a study has established that antioxidants and zinc significantly delays its progression. The combination of antioxidants in the study included vitamin C (500 milligrams [mg])...vitamin E (400 International Units [IU])...beta-carotene (15 mg, or 25,000 IU) ...zinc (80 mg zinc oxide)...and copper (2 mg cupric oxide). Also, remember to wear UV-blocking sunglasses outside and above all, don't smoke—whether you have wet or dry AMD.

Silent Sight Stealer

Gregory K. Harmon, MD, ophthalmologist, director of glaucoma fellowship program, New York-Presbyterian Hospital/Weill Cornell Medical Center, New York City, and chairman, Board of Directors, the Glaucoma Foundation. Dr. Harmon is also coauthor of *What Your Doctor May Not Tell You about Glaucoma—The Essential Treatments and Advances That Could Save Your Sight.* Warner Books.

At this moment, experts estimate that several million Americans are on the road to blindness and don't know it. The disease that wreaks this visual havoc is glaucoma and it has no symptoms—at first. Eventually, patients begin to lose peripheral vision, but by the time they notice, damage is already considerable and permanent. Everyone over age 40 needs to be aware of the disease to prevent suffering needless loss of sight. How can you reduce your risk?

Ophthalmologist Gregory K. Harmon, MD, is director of the glaucoma fellowship program at the New York-Presbyterian Hospital/Weill Cornell Medical Center and coauthor of *What Your Doctor May Not Tell You about Glaucoma—The Essential Treatments and Advances That Could Save Your Sight* (Warner Books). We spoke with him about the latest findings regarding glaucoma.

Dr. Harmon explains that the condition isn't a single disease, but rather several different ones that have a common denominator—they damage the optic nerve (a bundle of fibers in the back of the eye).

By far the most common type of glaucoma in the western world—and the focus of our discussion—is one called *open-angle glaucoma* with its slow, early asymptomatic progression. (The other principal type is *narrow-angle glaucoma*—which is most likely to affect Asians and has an acute, dramatic onset.) African Americans are much more prone to glaucoma than are Caucasians—their risk of it is four to six times higher, says Dr. Harmon. And, it appears that Hispanics probably have the same vulnerability as African Americans.

EYES UNDER PRESSURE

Until recently, doctors believed that the common factor for all conditions leading to glaucoma was pressure from a build-up of fluid in the eyeball. They have now discovered that people with a normal pressure reading can still have the disease—a condition called "normal-tension glaucoma." This makes the old-fashioned eye pressure test, routinely administered to patients after age 40, insufficient for diagnosis. Rather, the best way to diagnose glaucoma is to have an eye doctor measure eye pressure (tonometry) and examine the optic nerve to see if there is nerve damage.

RISK FACTORS

The most important risk factor for open-angle glaucoma is pressure in the eye, says Dr. Harmon. However, you can have elevated eye pressure and not have glaucoma (a condition called *ocular hypertension*.) *Other risks include...*

• **Being 45 or older** (although even babies can have the disease).

• **Having a personal family history of the eye disease,** and/or of diabetes.

• **Being substantially nearsighted**— farsighted folks are more vulnerable to narrow-angle glaucoma.

• **Having high or low blood pressure.**

• **Having experienced trauma to the eye.**

• **Use of corticosteroids,** such as prednisone, whether taken internally, inhaled or used topically in the eyes.

•**Doctors also evaluate the thickness of the cornea in glaucoma exams** because people with thin central corneas are at much greater risk than others.

TREATMENT STRATEGIES

The goal of treatment is to reduce eye pressure, including in those patients with normal-tension glaucoma. Even in people with normal pressure, reducing it further prevents disease progression just as it does for patients with elevated pressure. Eye drops—either to reduce the fluid in the eyeball or improve the efficiency of its drainage—are the first line of treatment. The side effects of the most commonly used drops are few—lashes get longer and thicker and blue-green eyes may turn brown—and patients generally use drops for life. However, drops are not effective enough for everyone. In that case, the next step is laser surgery.

There is a new laser, Dr. Harmon explains, that creates a small amount of inflammation within the eye's drainage system. This, in turn, causes macrophages (infection-fighting white blood cells) to come into the eye's drain and chomp up the debris inside the drain, a sort of Liquid Plumber effect, and leave it flowing more smoothly. The surgery can be performed multiple times without any known harm as of now. Patients generally continue using drops after laser treatment and the surgery allows for much better success with the drops.

When all else fails, the last measure is to have traditional surgery that creates a new drain. Whatever the treatment, all patients require regular monitoring to be sure the glaucoma doesn't begin to progress once again. Should that happen, more aggressive treatment is called for (or in the case of post-surgery patients, a return to drops).

NO PREVENTION— RISK REDUCTION

Modern medicine cannot prevent glaucoma, says Dr. Harmon, but there are ways to lower your risk of vision loss. In particular, he recommends regular aerobic exercise—studies have shown it lowers eye pressure—and eating foods that contain lots of antioxidants, such as green leafy vegetables and brightly colored fruits. It is critical to be checked annually, either by an optometrist or an ophthalmologist. Should an optometrist find a problem, the patient is referred to the ophthalmologist for medical treatment.

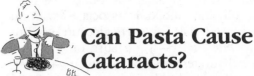

Can Pasta Cause Cataracts?

Chung-Jung Chiu, DDS, PhD, research scientist, Laboratory for Nutrition and Vision Research, Jean Mayer USDA Human Nutrition Research Center on Aging (HNRCA) and assistant professor, School of Medicine, Tufts University, Boston.

Visually significant cataracts, the clouding of the lens of the eye, affect approximately half of Americans age 75 and over. This creates vision problems for many people. According to recent research, what we eat can actually lower the risk—or increase the risk—for cataracts.

Cataracts, a form of age-related eye deterioration, occur in three types...

•**Nuclear.** The clouding occurs in the center of the lens. Seeing in dim light and driving at night can be a real problem.

•**Cortical.** Begins as whitish, wedge-shaped streaks that start on the outer edge of the lens, and as it progresses, extends to the center. Both distance and near vision can be impaired and focusing problems are common.

•**Posterior subcapsular.** The cataract starts as a small, opaque area in the back of the lens. These cataracts often interfere with reading vision and can cause halos around lights at night. They can occur in both eyes but tend to be more advanced in one rather than the other.

RESEARCH FINDINGS

This research shows that high carbohydrate foods actually increase the risk for cataracts. Chung-Jung Chiu, DDS, PhD, research scientist in the Laboratory for Nutrition and Vision Research at the Jean Mayer USDA Human Nutrition Research Center on Aging (HNRCA) and an assistant professor at Tufts University School of Medicine in Boston, says that "In the Age-Related Eye Disease Study (AREDS) of the National Eye Institute, which is the largest and most comprehensive intervention trial up to date, we found that total carbohydrate intake is associated with an increased risk for cortical cataracts but *glycemic index*—a measure of how fast carbohydrates raise blood sugar—is irrelevant for this kind of cataracts."

The glycemic index, however, may indeed matter when it comes to nuclear cataracts. "In the AREDS, consuming diets with a higher glycemic index was associated with a higher prevalence of nuclear cataracts," Dr. Chiu says. This research dovetails with other research showing that high carbohydrate foods in general and high glycemic index carbs specifically—may be linked to many other age-related diseases, including heart disease, diabetes, cancer and macular degeneration.

DEFINING "BAD CARBS" FOR YOUR EYES

Vegetables and fruits count as carbs, but they're loaded with protective antioxidants, phytochemicals and fiber—all substances you want more of, not less. Eating fruits and vegetables may even play a role in the prevention of cataracts. These are not the carbs focused on in the studies because they account for only a small part of our total carbohydrate intake. Rather, the dangerous carbs are from refined grains and sugars. "According to our research, we would suggest that you consume fewer high-glycemic carbs," says Dr. Chiu. These products (processed and refined carbs) provide virtually no additional nutritional value to your body and instead overload the body's metabolism and tax the body's disease-fighting systems.

However, more studies are needed to define the optimum level of dietary

carbohydrate for the prevention of cataracts and other age-related eye diseases, says Dr. Chiu.

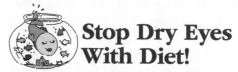 **Stop Dry Eyes With Diet!**

Biljana Miljanovic, MD, lead study author, divisions of preventive medicine and aging, Brigham and Women's Hospital, Boston.

Dry eye syndrome (DES) affects about eight million Americans, most of them women. It develops when there are either too many or too few tears or when the quality of them is poor. Results are a gritty sensation in the eyes, pain, itching or redness. Eventually, DES can harm vision.

Aging is a risk factor, with estimates of more than half of all people over age 65 suffering from DES. Other causes include *Sjögren's Syndrome*, an autoimmune disorder involving destruction of the gland that produces tears and saliva. It can appear as a side effect of asthma and diabetes, among other diseases. Now, recent research has identified another risk factor for DES—too little omega-3 essential fatty acid in the diet or too much omega-6.

LATEST FINDINGS

Researchers from Boston's Brigham and Women's Hospital (BWH) and Schepens Eye Research Institute (both affiliated with Harvard Medical School) tracked the eating habits and health of 32,470 women enrolled in the BWH-based Women's Health Study. Through data analysis, researchers discovered that the women with the highest consumption of omega-3 reduced their risk of DES by 20%. Conversely, there was a 2.5-fold increased risk for women whose ratio of omega-6 to omega-3 was more than 15:1. (Omega-6 and omega-3 are essential fatty acids that the body cannot make and so must get through diet. Ideally, omega-3 and omega-6 should be in an even balance or, at most, three to five omega-6 to one omega-3. However, omega-6 is abundant in processed foods, resulting in a typical ratio in today's American diet of about 15:1, omega-6 to omega-3.)

DIETARY REBALANCING

Our editors spoke with the lead study author, Biljana Miljanovic, MD. She says that although it is shocking how out of balance modern diets are in omega-3 and omega-6, people can correct the imbalance. For example, the study showed that women who ate tuna five times a week had a 68% reduced risk of developing DES compared with the women who ate it just once a week. While this solution is not optimal (tuna can have high concentrations of mercury), there are other sources to choose from. Salmon, sardines, mackerel and herring are rich in omega-3s, as are walnuts and flaxseeds. Supplements are an easy option, too. Fish oil supplements from Nordic Naturals or Pharmax are reliable brands.

At the same time, limit omega-6, found in most plant oils made of corn, soy, safflower and sunflower—in other words, virtually all baked goods and salad dressings.

Is Eye Surgery Right for You?

Deborah DiStefano, MD, board-certified ophthalmologist with a practice in Chattanooga, Tennessee and assistant clinical instructor, University of Tennessee College of Medicine.

Amazing advances in corrective eye surgery have taken place in recent years, and they can make a big difference in your life. Imagine not having to deal with dry and gritty eyes from wearing contacts...or wondering for the umpteenth time where you left your glasses.

Still, these procedures are relatively new. What if something goes wrong? Do doctors know the long-term impact of the surgery? What are the risks? To learn more, we spoke with Deborah DiStefano, MD, a board certified ophthalmologist with a practice in Chattanooga, Tennessee, about two of the most common eye procedures—LASIK and PRK.

LASIK: LASER-ASSISTED IN-SITU KERATOMILEUSIS

LASIK is by far the most common type of corrective eye surgery—it corrects nearsightedness, farsightedness and astigmatism by correcting the shape of the cornea (the outer layer of the eyeball).

After administering numbing drops, an ophthalmologist uses one laser to make thin flaps in the corneas, and another to reshape the corneas so you can see better. According to Dr. DiStefano, the procedure is painless and takes only about 10 minutes per eye. The amount of tissue removed is less than the thickness of a human hair. (*Note:* In the past, the procedure was performed with a surgical instrument that was riskier than the current laser technology. Make certain that you have a trained surgeon who uses only lasers for LASIK.)

What to expect: LASIK can correct higher degrees of aberration than is possible with glasses or contacts, says Dr. DiStefano. Her patients have been delighted with their outcomes. They often walk into the office unable to see much of anything at all without glasses, and walk out with 20-20 (sometimes even 20-15 or 20-10) vision. LASIK does not correct "aging eyes." It will have no effect on inelasticity of the lens—the need for reading glasses will continue, as will the changes that come with aging.

Recovery consists primarily of checking in with the ophthalmologist to make certain the eyes are healing properly. This will take place within 24 hours of surgery, and at regular intervals over the following six months. Rarely is there any serious pain involved. You may experience sensitivity to light and your eyes might feel as if there is something in them—but don't touch! Wait one to three days to engage in any contact sports, and avoid swimming, hot tubs and whirlpools for one to two months. Serious complications are rare.

If you wear contacts, you must stop using them for up to several weeks before evaluation for LASIK, since contacts change the shape of the cornea.

PRK: PHOTOREACTIVE KERATECTOMY

Like LASIK, PRK corrects nearsightedness, farsightedness and astigmatism. However, this is an older procedure than LASIK, and laser is used only in part. Although effective, PRK is more painful and invasive than LASIK, observes Dr. DiStefano. As with any procedure that involves the cornea, you must stop wearing contact lenses for up to several weeks before evaluation. PRK or LASIK is a choice of the surgeon and depends on corneal topography and thickness. Generally, LASIK is done more often.

After administering numbing drops, the ophthalmologist scrapes away the surface corneal cells—that is, the outer layer or epithelium of the cornea. Next, he or she uses a laser to reshape the cornea and correct a person's degree of refractive or vision error. A bandage contact lens is placed over the eye for two or three days, and anti-inflammatory and antibiotic eye drops are administered.

What to expect: Results take time, and it may be days or even weeks before PRK patients experience improved vision after surgery. Because the outer layer of the cornea needs to regenerate gradually and grow back, there is a longer recovery period than with LASIK. You will need to be examined by your surgeon shortly after surgery, and at regular intervals over the next six months. Since healing takes longer, activities (contact sports, swimming, etc.) are likely to be limited for a longer period with PRK than with LASIK.

LASIK OR PRK?

The outcomes of PRK and LASIK are comparable after six months. However, whereas a tiny flap in the cornea is made with a laser in LASIK, the surgeon actually has to scrape away a layer of cells with PRK. This makes a big difference when it comes to pain, recovery time and safety considerations. *LASIK is by and large coming to replace PRK as the most commonly performed procedure because...*

•**PRK is more painful and invasive,** and there is a longer recovery time.

•**PRK entails more risk of scarring and requires healing of the cornea.**

•**The risk of infection is slightly higher with PRK,** although infection following either procedure is rare.

EXPERIENCE AND UP-TO-DATE TECHNOLOGY ARE PARAMOUNT

As with any medical procedure, there are risks as well as benefits associated with corrective eye surgery. In the worst cases, people experience double vision, dry eye syndrome or even vision loss. Fortunately, however, these outcomes are rare.

In order to have safe and successful surgery, your best bet is to find the most skilled and experienced surgeons and eye centers that feature a variety of the latest technologies, says Dr. DiStefano. You can find the most experienced people by researching on-line. Look at the qualifications of each individual.

Key: Have a conversation with your eye doctor about your particular problems and how they will be addressed. At that meeting you can also question him on his experience and find out if he has done a corneal fellowship.

Most medical insurance does not cover elective surgery. Do not price-shop this procedure. The technology can be expensive and you should be aware of bait-and-switch advertising. You generally get what you pay for, but the average price for LASIK surgery is about $1,575 per eye. However, Dr. DiStefano points out that the out-of-pocket costs may actually turn out to be less than the cost of buying and wearing eyeglasses or contacts for 20 years...not to mention the risk of infection that comes with contacts and contact lens solution.

Contact Lens Implants—Are They Right for Your Eyes?

Deborah DiStefano, MD, board-certified ophthalmologist with a practice in Chattanooga, Tennessee and assistant clinical instructor at the University of Tennessee, College of Medicine.

The US Food and Drug Administration (FDA) has approved the Visian Implantable Collamer Lens (ICL) for nearsightedness, and doctors anticipate that it will soon be FDA-approved for farsightedness, as well.

To learn more about this option, we spoke with board-certified ophthalmologist and assistant clinical instructor at the University of Tennessee College Medicine, Deborah DiStefano, MD, who already has performed a number of lens implants in her Chattanooga, Tennessee, practice. In her experience thus far, ICL is both safe and effective.

WHO IS IT FOR?

According to Dr. DiStefano, contact lens implants are an excellent alternative for people who are not good candidates for LASIK (*laser-assisted in situ keratomileusis*), the most common type of refractive eye surgery. When your vision is too poor you may not have the best results with LASIK (which works best in those with mild to moderate vision problems). When your cornea is too thin or not the right shape for LASIK, implantable contact lenses may be the answer.

WHAT TO EXPECT: THE WOW FACTOR

Implanting a contact lens takes only 10 to 15 minutes, says Dr. DiStefano. To begin, the surgeon numbs the eye with concentrated anesthetic drops. Next, a tiny incision is made in front of the eye's natural lens for the ICL. The contact lens is rolled up like a little cartridge, explains Dr. DiStefano. When the surgeon inserts it through the incision, it unfolds like a flower petal in the eye. The lens is made of a proprietary, highly biocompatible polymer made with collagen.

The procedure is not painful, and there is instant gratification. After years of visual impairment, patients almost immediately have 20-40 vision or better, which Dr. DiStefano refers to as "the wow factor." Within three years, more than half of people's vision improves to 20-20.

Another advantage: The lens lasts "forever," though the procedure is reversible and the lens can be replaced should the cornea change or you develop a cataract. Because there is only a tiny, microscopic incision involved, there is a correspondingly minute degree of scar tissue—even less than that of cataract surgery.

There is always a small risk for infection with any procedure, although infections were rare or nonexistant in clinical trials of the ICL. Another rare but potential complication is a nick to the eye. After a two-week recovery period, there are no activity limitations with the implanted lenses.

CHOOSE AN EXPERIENCED SURGEON

As with any procedure, it is best to have an experienced surgeon. Dr. DiStefano recommends that you choose an eye center that performs a variety of procedures, has the most up-to-date equipment and practices the latest technologies. Because ICL procedures are elective, there is little likelihood that your insurance will cover it. Depending on your geographical location, the out-of-pocket cost ranges on average from $2,900 to $5,000 per eye. Dr. DiStefano's patients think that the wow factor is worth it.

Better Than Bifocals

Marguerite McDonald, MD, FACS, cornea/refractive surgeon, Ophthalmic Consultants of Long Island, Lynbrook, New York.

Ben Franklin was the first person to put together two different lens halves to create glasses (bifocals) that allowed for seeing both near and far with the same glasses. Bifocals and tri-focals are used by about half of eyeglass wearers with *presbyopia*, the gradual loss (due to aging) of ability to see near ob-jects. Other lenses that simultaneously allow for more than one vision correc-tion are called progressive lenses (bifocal or multifocal lenses with no visible lines on the lens), but while the technology is newer, it is not problem-free. Complaints about progressives include their small and restrictive area for close vision, glare and the haloing of lights at night and, for some wearers, the slight feeling of nausea the lenses can induce, as well as headaches. It's about time for something better, and finally, that something has ap-peared—wavefront-optimized lenses.

TECHNOLOGY FROM OUTER SPACE

Wavefront technology for spectacles is similar to the technology used to build the Hubble telescope, and it is also now used for laser vision-correction surgery. Cur-rently, wavefront-based technology allows eye doctors to diagnose and measure re-fractive errors or irregularities of the eye, with 25 times more precision than previ-ously possible, and allows lab technicians to customize eyeglass lenses for crisp, clear vision both day and night.

CATCH THE WAVEFRONT

In 1987, New Orleans ophthalmologist Marguerite McDonald, MD, a cornea/re-fractive surgeon now with the Ophthalmic Consultants of Long Island in Lynbrook, New York, was the first surgeon in the world to perform excimer laser surgery to eliminate or reduce the need for glasses and contact lenses. Later, laser surgery was improved with wavefront-guided tech-nology, enhancing surgical precision and clinical outcomes.

Dr. McDonald is now a leading re-searcher in wavefront technology, includ-ing the use of this technology to develop promising new eyeglass lenses. Dr. Mc-Donald recently presented the results of her study of wavefront lenses that showed 67% of the 609 participants rated them as "better" or "clearly better" for distance vi-sion...65% rated them as better or clearly better for intermediate vision...and 72% better or clearly better for near vision than standard progressive lenses.

Dr. McDonald considers wavefront technology "extraordinary." It allows for the creation of lenses that optimize how light enters the eyes from all directions. With this technology, it is now possible to correct all parts of the lens, significantly decreasing (if not entirely eliminating) glaring and halos, and creating overall crisper vision with less blurring than tradi-tional progressives.

VARILUX PHYSIO LENSES

One type of wavefront lenses, varilux physio lenses from Essilor, has three times less distance distortion compared with standard progressive lenses. They also reduce induced astigmatism and provide a 30% wider field of sharp intermediate distance (computer distance) vision, cor-recting for near- and farsightedness and astigmatism, and provide greater stabili-zation of near power over a greater area of the lens. Standard progressive lenses also correct far, intermediate and near vision, but with much greater distortion and instability of the correction, and with a narrower "strip" of intermediate vision. Dr. McDonald says that people also find these wavefront-based lenses easier to get used to than standard progressives. Many people who hated the standard progres-sives are now able to wear the varilux physio lenses without problems.

WHERE TO GET THEM

These wavefront-based lenses do not re-quire a specialized prescription. Simply re-quest Essilor's varilux physio lenses when ordering new lenses. Dr. McDonald says that the Essilor lenses can be purchased at most local optical shops. Essilor's varilux physio lenses are more expensive, costing approximately 25% more than standard progressives.

Another type of wavefront lens (iZon from Ophthonix) requires your optician to have special diagnostic devices to generate the prescription—to date these devices have only been placed in a handful of optical shops nationwide—and then the lenses are made with special equipment in a central laboratory in California.

Simple Way to Protect Your Vision

Deborah DiStefano, MD, board-certified ophthalmologist with a practice in Chattanooga, Tennessee, and assistant clinical instructor at the University of Tennessee College of Medicine.

American Optometric Association Sunglass Shopping Guide, *www.aoa.org/x6385.xml*.

By now it's been successfully drummed into our heads that we need to protect our skin from overexposure to the ultraviolet (UV) rays of the sun, but sometimes we overlook the fact that eye protection is equally important, all year long. Not just in the summer. UVA and UVB rays—invisible parts of the light spectrum—can be harmful to both the skin and eyes, and may contribute to the development of ocular conditions such as cataracts, macular degeneration and even skin cancer around the eye lids.

For more insight into eye protection, we spoke with Deborah DiStefano, MD, a board-certified ophthalmologist with a practice in Chattanooga, Tennessee, and assistant clinical instructor at the University of Tennessee College of Medicine.

SHADES:
THE COOL SOLUTION

Fortunately, the formula for protecting eyes from the sun is very simple—wear sunglasses that protect your eyes from UVA and UVB rays. In the US, even inexpensive shades are usually manufactured to meet this standard. You can pay hundreds of dollars for high-end fashion or sports sunglasses or $10 at your local department store for generic sunglasses, and still achieve the same level of eye protection, observes Dr. DiStefano. She adds that you must check the labels to make certain that lenses are treated to block ultraviolet rays. Look for labels that say 100% UVA and UVB blockage. Tinted glasses do not block a lot of the visible light so they may not be as effective as sunglasses in bright light. The color of the lenses has nothing to do with the blockage of UV light. Therefore, you still need that protection with all colored glasses.

More safety tips from Dr. DiStefano...

• **Sunglasses with dark tints** generally offer the greatest protection against visible light, but UV protection is still needed.

• **For those who prefer a lighter tint,** consider polarized lenses. These are specifically formulated to eliminate reflective glare, even with a lighter lens tint. Brown and green tints and gray tints seem to work the best during outside sports.

Note: Polarization just reduces glare, so you must also make sure that sunglasses offer UV protection, too.

• **If you're a fan of water or winter sports,** polarized lenses are an especially good idea. As every sailor and skier knows all too well, water and snow significantly magnify reflected glare. They also increase UV exposure.

• **Athletes should also think about investing in impact resistant lenses,** such as those made from the light but rugged plastic, polycarbonate.

• **Wraparound sunglasses are best,** since they prevent UV rays from entering from the side.

• **Large lenses offer more protection than small ones.**

• **Sunglasses should fit properly (close to the face),** so rays can't sneak in and bounce back into the eye. An antireflective coating on the inside of the lens can help.

• **Consider coatings or special lenses.** For example, photochromic lenses automatically darken and lighten as light

135

changes…a flash or mirror coating reduces the amount of visible light that reaches your eyes.

•**A wide-brimmed hat** can offer additional protection from rays that beam down from overhead.

With or without the protection that sunglasses offer, it's important to never look directly into the sun, warns Dr. DiStefano. It is also very important to wear UV protection even when overcast. Smoke or gray tint is a neutral color that provides true to life contrast. Amber lenses dramatically increase the contrast in an overcast situation. Sunglasses not only add to your "cool" quotient, they'll also protect your sensitive eyes from harmful UV rays.

Conquering Strabismus In Adults

Steven E. Rosenberg, MD, ophthalmologist, pediatric and adult strabismus specialist, Maimonides Medical Center, Brooklyn, New York.

We all know young kids whose eyes don't track together. It is a condition called *strabismus*, which causes people to have a wandering eye or be wall- or cross-eyed. Often thought of as a childhood disorder, strabismus actually affects more adults than children—4% of all adults versus 3% of children.

Surprisingly, most people, including those who have the condition, assume that if their problem wasn't treated in childhood, it's too late for treatment—but that's not true. Much of the confusion around strabismus treatment apparently arises from a secondary disorder children with strabismus can develop called *amblyopia*. Although amblyopia is commonly called "lazy eye," this does not mean that the eye is crossed or wandering. Rather, the name refers to the fact that the brain and the eye are not working together—the eye has become "lazy." To achieve proper vision, doctors must treat amblyopia early.

Strabismus can also lead to social discomfort. The good news is that it is in fact treatable even in adults.

ABOUT ADULT STRABISMUS

Adult strabismus can result from a number of factors. Many adults with the condition are actually born with it or develop it in childhood, but are unaware of the problem because they seemingly have no symptoms. The brain is able to compensate for the misalignment, thus allowing the person to have apparently normal vision and eye tracking. But with age, other problems (such as the need for reading glasses) set in and begin to stress the visual system further, ultimately overwhelming the brain's ability to continue compensating. At this point, people's eyes may start to wander or cross, though not necessarily all the time. The misalignment is most likely to show up when affected people are tired or stressed and they often don't even realize their eyes are not tracking properly until someone else points it out. Strabismus can also develop later in life because of certain diseases such as Graves disease, or because of stroke or trauma to the brain or eye. It is also possible to develop temporary adult strabismus because of a correctable problem with the optic nerve, a situation associated with diabetes or having a tumor.

CONQUERING STRABISMUS

Ophthalmologist Steven E. Rosenberg, MD, pediatric and adult strabismus specialist at Mount Sinai Medical Center in New York City, says that there are two primary challenges for adults with strabismus. Double vision is the most common symptom. Although this is an indication that the brain has begun to decompensate after so many years, double vision is also typical of temporary strabismus. One treatment for the problem—especially in the case of temporary strabismus when a damaged nerve needs time to heal—is to place prisms into the patient's glasses.

Prisms, as you might remember from long-ago science classes, bend light, and it is possible for doctors to do this in such a way that it appears to a person with double vision that there is just one image.

BOTOX AND DOUBLE VISION

Another way of treating temporary double vision is with botox injections, into one or more of the extra-ocular muscles around the eye. (Dr. Rosenberg points out that originally botox was developed for medical use as a way to treat strabismus, not wrinkles.) An injection of it temporarily relaxes the ocular muscle, and that corrects double vision for about three months. By then, the condition should have corrected itself.

SURGICAL OPTION

In addition to double vision, the major challenge for strabismus sufferers is the splayed presentation of their eyes. With surgery for realignment, individuals can improve their vision as well as correct the socially awkward problem of crossed or wandering eyes. Dr. Rosenberg says that patients generally assume the surgery will be on just one eye, but often both eyes need realignment in much the way it is necessary to realign all four tires of a car. To do this, the surgeon tightens or relaxes one or more of the six muscles that hold each eyeball in place. The surgery is done on an outpatient basis, and patients can go back to work in a week or so. Patients find, though, that it is one to two weeks before they can resume driving because any sudden movement of their eyes generally causes pain.

It takes from six weeks to three months for the results of surgery to take hold, says Dr. Rosenberg, and the overall success rates for people having one surgery is from 75% to 80%. Some patients need a second surgery to completely resolve the problem, which brings the success rate close to 100%. It is possible, 20 or so years down the road, that the strabismus that motivated the original procedures will reappear, making it necessary to have another surgery at that time.

KNOW THE SURGICAL RISKS

As with any surgery, there are risks involved including, in very rare cases, loss of vision. Interestingly, double vision is another possible risk, but it can be treated with prisms or additional surgery. For those who are not ready for surgery, there are exercises that also may help strengthen the muscles and overcome the strabismus. A behavioral optometrist can help in this case.

Surprising Dangers Of Gum Disease

Alan A. Winter, DDS, periodontist in private practice and associate clinical professor of implant dentistry at the New York University College of Dentistry, both in New York City. Dr. Winter has published several medical journal articles on gum disease.

Tom McGuire, DDS, a holistic dentist based in Sebastopol, California. Dr. McGuire is president of The Dental Wellness Institute, founder of the International Association of Mercury Free Dentists (IAMFD), and author of *Mercury Detoxification: The Natural Way to Remove Mercury from Your Body* (The Dental Wellness Institute) and *Tooth Fitness: Your Guide to Healthy Teeth* (St. Michael's Press). Visit his Web sites at *www.dentalwellness4u.com* and *www.mercuryfreenow.com*.

American Dental Association, *www.ada.org*.

Research that demonstrates a connection between periodontal disease and serious health problems (such as heart disease, stroke, and diabetes) is growing. Symptoms of periodontal disease include inflamed or bleeding gums and sometimes even loose teeth.

To learn more about the connection between oral health and overall health, and to obtain advice on how to prevent or reverse periodontal disease, we consulted dental experts Alan A. Winter, DDS, a periodontist in private practice and associate clinical professor of implant dentistry at the New York University College of Dentistry in New York City, and Tom McGuire, DDS, a holistic dentist based in Sebastopol, California, and author of *Tooth*

Fitness: Your Guide to Healthy Teeth (St. Michael's Press).

INFLAMED GUMS = INFLAMED BODY

We asked our experts how periodontal disease leads to disease in other parts of the body. Dr. Winter explain that, as with many systemic problems, an inflammatory response is the underlying cause In people with serious gum disease, bacteria and their irritating toxins enter into the bloodstream, eliciting a systemic inflammatory response. The condition will do even more damage once the tissue that supports the tooth breaks down and the infection begins to destroy the bone.

Many health problems, such as heart disease, are related to advanced gum disease. Inflammation triggers the liver to make C-reactive protein (CRP), which is considered a "marker" of inflammatory activity. According to Dr. McGuire, elevated CRP levels are associated with an increased risk of more serious health problems such as heart attack and stroke. Periodontal disease is also associated with an increased risk for diabetes, low birth weight and pre-term births and respiratory ailments. Recent evidence also links pancreatic cancer with periodontal disease. In addition, when your body has to work extra hard to fight infection and inflammation, it puts significant stress on your immune system 24/7, which can dramatically lower your resistance to other diseases.

THE COST OF IGNORING THE PROBLEM

With gum disease, it's not unusual for people to allow the infection and inflammation to go unchecked for weeks, months or even years, notes Dr. McGuire. A big part of this is fear—approximately 30% of the population has fear or anxiety significant enough that they avoid going to the dentist until symptoms have progressed far along and caused disease. Cost is an impediment thanks to the lack of dental insurance for many people…and cost and fear can overlap. The third major factor, he says, is that far too many people aren't aware of the serious effect on their health from gum disease.

According to Dr. Winter, if you extrapolate current findings, here is what may be gained by improved oral care…

- **Fewer heart attacks.**
- **Fewer strokes.**
- **Better control of type 1 and type 2 diabetes.**
- **Less respiratory disease.**
- **Lower risk of pancreatic cancer.**
- **Reduced rate of premature births.**
- **Reduced rate of low birth-weight newborns.**

Prevention and treatment not only improve quality of life and life expectancy, they also save time and money, observes Dr. McGuire. More than 164 million work hours and 51 million school hours are lost each year due to dental disease and its effects, according to the US Department of Health and Human Services.

TROUBLE IS BREWING

How do you know if your gums are in trouble? Healthy gums are firm and pink. You know trouble is brewing when they grow red, tender, swollen and are prone to bleed when you brush. Bad breath can be an early symptom, too. This can be early-stage gum disease, or gingivitis, and you should bring these symptoms to the attention of your dentist.

Though your personal health history (including heredity) may also be a factor, gum disease often develops due to poor oral hygiene, when a lack of brushing and flossing causes a sticky layer of bacteria or plaque to coat the teeth, and inflammation develops along the gum lines. Certain medications, such as Dilantin for epilepsy, as well as smoking and chewing tobacco, definitely exacerbate gum disease. Left uncared for, the plaque hardens to become *tartar* or *calculus*, building up over time. If the plaque and calculus further irritate the gums and lead to pockets of infection, you have a serious problem—periodontal disease, characterized by infection and inflammation that now is destroying bone and supporting tissue.

SOMETHING TO SMILE ABOUT

The good news is that early periodontal disease can be treated and usually reversed. Once the infection has been cleared up, you can prevent any further gum disease with diligent home care and regular dental checkups.

Bottom Line's Daily Health New's consulting medical editor Andrew L. Rubman, ND, says gum hygiene should include antiseptic oral rinses such as Listerine, which is formulated to target oral bacteria. This can help prevent the plaque from further damaging the gums and leading to those pockets of infection. In many cases, the real culprit, he believes, is chronic oral yeast infection. The yeast predisposes the gum tissue to become secondarily colonized by bacteria, which can produce both plaque deposits and dissolve enamel, says Dr. Rubman. He adds that Listerine and other oral rinses also effectively treat yeast as well as other microorganisms.

AVOIDING PROBLEMS

To find out if you're facing potential problems, ask your dentist whether you have any periodontal pockets and how deep they are, advises Dr. Winter. One to three millimeters is considered normal. Once pockets reach a depth of four millimeters, you have a problem that must be attended to. Other factors your dentist may take into consideration are bleeding, loose teeth and bone loss. People with implants must be especially diligent about their oral hygiene as poor oral hygiene is a leading cause of failed implants.

In Dr. Winter's opinion, in addition to twice-yearly visits to your regular dentist, your best bet is to see a periodontist for periodic exams. The severity of the disease determines the course of treatment, which may range from a thorough cleaning all the way to gum surgery. In Dr. McGuire's view, a dentist and hygienist can take care of most gum disease, although he refers patients with advanced gum disease to a periodontist (especially when surgery is required). "I also recommend a checkup at least once per year to look for symptoms of other diseases that can show up in the mouth, particularly oral cancer," says Dr. McGuire.

AS MOM ALWAYS SAID...

For healthy teeth and gums, Dr. McGuire recommends...

• **Brush.** Use a soft-bristle brush to clean teeth and gums in the morning, after eating, and before you go to bed. Replace the brush every three to four months, and soak it in an antibacterial rinse like Listerine overnight after you've been sick with a cold or flu. The brand of toothbrush does not really matter, according to Dr. McGuire. Check with your hygienist, regardless of what type of toothbrush you use, and ask if you are getting the job done.

• **Floss.** Do this at least once a day, and always brush first.

• **Use mouthwash.** When you have gum disease, you should use an antimicrobial mouthwash, such as Listerine, after every brushing and flossing session. Once the infection has been eliminated, you can switch to a more natural product (anything you find in a health food store that contains natural ingredients). You can also use a warm, salt-water rinse.

• **Consider an oral irrigator.** These are especially effective at reaching between teeth to remove food. For people with severe disease, this is a must, along with brushing and flossing.

• **Stay away from sugar, and refined and processed foods as much as possible.** When you allow yourself the occasional indulgence, be sure to brush, floss or at least rinse well afterward.

• **See your dentist for an exam and cleaning every six months.**

• **Avoid smoking.** It is known to irritate gum tissue, stress the immune system and lowers the body's resistance to infection of any kind.

Oh, No! Smoking Makes Your Teeth Fall Out!

Michael P. Bonner, DDS, coauthor of *The Oral Health Bible*. Basic Health Publications. He is health and wellness coordinator for a group dental practice based in San Antonio, Texas.

The purely esthetic pitfalls of cigarette smoking—stained teeth and foul breath—should come as no surprise. But did you also know that smoking can make your teeth fall out? A study published in the *Journal of Clinical Periodontology* found that people who smoke are six times more likely than non-smokers to lose their teeth from periodontal disease. And periodontal disease can lead to generalized inflammation of the body. This dangerous because it is associated with an increased risk for heart disease, stroke and other chronic illnesses.

THE SMOKING GUMS

To learn more about the connection between gum disease and smoking, we spoke with Michael P. Bonner, DDS, from San Antonio, Texas, and coauthor of *The Oral Health Bible* (Basic Health Publications) with Earl L. Mindell, RPh, PhD. "Gums are meant to provide a barrier to disease-causing bacteria," Dr. Bonner explained. "When gums are diseased, microorganisms found normally in the mouth enter the bloodstream and wreak inflammatory mischief wherever the body is susceptible. If I have a patient with a sick mouth, I have a sick patient."

Each puff a smoker takes causes numerous toxins to enter the body, weakening the immune system and promoting the development of *calculus* ("tartar" or hardened plaque on the teeth that requires professional cleaning to be removed). The bacteria in calculus inflame the gums and cause them to pull away from teeth, forming pockets of bacteria. As pockets between the gums and teeth deepen, more bacteria enter the body, destroying the soft tissue

and bone that anchor teeth to the jawbone. In severe cases, teeth become loose or painful and either fall out or have to be extracted. Unfortunately, when smokers do get their diseased gums treated, they don't heal as quickly or as reliably, as a result of their weakened immune system.

TO MAINTAIN OR RECLAIM GOOD ORAL HEALTH

Nine out of 10 adults have some evidence of gum disease, says Dr. Bonner, so everyone needs to be proactive about oral hygiene. Smokers, he says, have even more reason to be vigilant since their risk for gum disease increases with every puff. *He suggests this gum-protecting protocol...*

• **Brush twice a day.** Use a soft brush or a powered toothbrush such as a Sonicare Ultrasonic.

• **Use nontoxic toothpastes and mouth rinses.** Check labels carefully and avoid products that contain potentially inflammatory ingredients such as *triclosan, propylene glycol, sodium hydroxide, sodium lauryl sulfate, sodium laureth sulfate, polyethylene glycol, ethanol* and FD & C color pigments.

• **Floss.** Daily flossing helps control tooth decay.

• **Scrape your tongue.** Your tongue harbors microorganisms that contribute to decay and gum disease.

• **Irrigate.** Using an oral irrigator reaches the *sulcus*, the area under the gums. Dr. Bonner says a pulsating irrigator is most effective at killing microorganisms, eliminating odors and reducing inflammation.

• **Get professional cleanings.** Your dentist can tell you how often you need to come in.

• **Supplement.** Certain nutrients can be taken to protect your gums. It's best to meet with a trained professional who can design a program specifically for your needs.

If you're a smoker and this information inspires you to quit today, go right ahead! New research shows that people who quit smoking on the spur of the moment are more successful at kicking the habit than those who formulate a "quit plan," a strategy generally recommended to smokers. Quitting right now enhances the chance you'll keep your teeth into your later years.

Eat Your Way to Beautiful Skin

Nancy Appleton, PhD, retired nutritional consultant now in San Diego, California and author of *Lick the Sugar Habit* (Avery) and *Stopping Inflammation* (Square One).

Diet and other lifestyle choices are clearly reflected in your face and skin, the body's largest and most protective organ. Take care of yourself, and your skin will show it. Eat poorly, smoke and skimp on sleep, and your skin will be worse for wear. Your skin's condition is, in some ways, a barometer of the health of your entire body.

RECIPE FOR HEALTHY SKIN

Proper nutrition will keep you glowing and rosy, as will getting enough sleep, regular exercise and fresh air (but not too much sun)...keeping your worries under control...and avoiding negative habits such as smoking and overindulgence in alcohol. While this sounds simple, it is important to keep in mind that your skin needs proper nourishment to ensure proper function. It is not just a shell that keeps your insides in. Your skin is a functioning body organ.

What you should eat and drink for healthy skin...

STAY AWAY FROM SUGAR

According to Nancy Appleton, PhD, retired nutritional consultant now in San Diego, California, and author of *Lick the Sugar Habit* (Avery) and *Stopping Inflammation* (Square One), sugar has a major impact on the skin. In young people, it upsets digestion, which can lead to inflammatory skin problems such as acne and rashes. In older people, sugar makes the skin age more rapidly by changing the structure of collagen, a protein that is the building block of skin. As the structure of the skin changes, wrinkles become increasingly apparent.

CUT BACK ON SATURATED FAT AND FRIED FOODS

A high-fat diet may contribute to the development of skin cancer, according to researchers at Baylor College of Medicine in Houston, Texas. In a two-year study of 76 skin cancer patients, half followed their usual diet (about 40% fat) while half adopted a low-fat diet (20% fat). In the months that followed, researchers found that low-fat dieters developed an average of only three new precancerous lesions (called *actinic keratoses*), while high-fat dieters developed an average of 10. To cut back on saturated fat in your diet, eat more fish instead of red meat, and remove the skin from poultry.

In Dr. Appleton's opinion, the problem is not so much in fatty foods but in how they are prepared. She says that the real culprits are *acrylamides*—the carcinogenic chemical by-products of cooking carbohydrates at high temperatures. Frying, barbecuing, baking and smoking foods leads to the formation of acrylamides. Highly processed foods, such as french fries and chips, are also high in these carcinogens and should be eaten very sparingly, if at all. It's easy to cut back on acrylamides by poaching rather than grilling fish and by eating boiled potatoes instead of fried.

IDENTIFY AND AVOID FOOD ALLERGENS

Foods that some people can handle with no problem can cause food sensitivities in others, observes Dr. Appleton. She explains that when the gut fails to fully digest hard-to-process foods, such as simple sugars, fried foods and hydrogenated fats, partially digested food particles enter the bloodstream. The body reacts to these particles as foreign invaders, with the immune system establishing inflammation around them in an effort to protect the body. When this reaction takes place on the skin, inflammatory skin problems such as pimples and rashes result. Inflammation can occur anywhere—and in multiple locations—in the body, where it manifests itself in different ways. In the case of acne, hair follicles become clogged with substances such as sebum (oil) and *P. acnes* bacteria. *P. acnes* produce large amounts of inflammatory enzymes called *porphyrins*, and white blood cells rush in to protect the body. The result is inflammatory acne, characterized by pimples, pustules, blackheads and whiteheads. According to Dr. Appleton, the good news is that when you stop eating reactive foods, such as sugary junk foods, fried foods and overly processed products, these symptoms will go away.

EAT MORE NUTRIENT-RICH FRUITS AND VEGETABLES

Your skin will benefit from eating a wide range of fruits and vegetables...especially, as Dr. Appleton points out, if you eat them instead of sugary and fried foods. For optimal skin health, plenty of nutrient-rich vitamins and minerals are a must, and a lack of A, B or C vitamins can lead to dry skin and rashes. Fruits and vegetables are also rich in antioxidants, which can prevent the oxidation of free radicals that leads to inflammatory skin problems.

DRINK PLENTY OF FLUIDS

To cleanse your body of toxins, it's important to drink plenty of fluids. The standard recommendation is eight glasses of water (or other healthy liquids such as herbal teas or fresh juices) daily. This flushes toxins out of the bowel, kidneys and liver, and keeps the skin supple and hydrated.

Note: Make sure that your drinking water is of high quality. Contaminants such as lead and bacteria can harm the skin and may even increase cancer risk. If you have concerns about water purity, install a filter.

MONITOR YOUR DAIRY INTAKE

Word comes from Boston's Harvard School of Public Health that milk—rather than greasy foods or chocolate—is the most likely dietary contributor to severe teenage acne. While researchers do not go so far as to recommend that teens eliminate dairy from their diets, they recommend moderating their consumption of milk. Also keep in mind that there are other rich sources of calcium, including canned salmon, sardines, tofu and green vegetables, such as broccoli and collard or turnip greens.

All in all, the same balanced diet that benefits your health overall will keep your skin in tip-top shape, too.

Shocking! Melanoma Patients May Need *More* Sun

Marianne Berwick, PhD, associate director for Population Health and coleader of the Program in Population Health and Cancer Control, University of New Mexico Cancer Center, Albuquerque.

Eugene Butcher, MD, professor, department of pathology, Stanford University Medical Center, Palo Alto, California.

Having had the skin cancer–causing dangers of sunlight drilled into us, we Americans have become sun-phobic. Many of us smear on sunscreen every time we venture outside. But as more and more research shows, the truth is that some unprotected sun exposure is not only all right but beneficial. Recent news comes from a lab study at Stanford University that builds upon earlier research from findings from the University of New Mexico regarding, survival rates in melanoma patients.

ABOUT THE STUDIES

Skin cancer researcher Marianne Berwick, PhD, associate director for Population Health and coleader of the Program in Population Health and Cancer Control at the University of New Mexico Cancer Center in Albuquerque, found that melanoma patients who had greater amounts of sun exposure had better rates of survival than those who had some sun exposure, but not enough to significantly affect the deep layers of the skin. According to Dr. Berwick, sun exposure was measured by recreational sun exposure (the number of times per year individuals engaged in outdoor recreation as well as vacations)...the number of sunburns (any versus none)... and *solar elastosis* (a measure of collagen damage around the area of the melanoma as assessed by a pathologist). She says that they are following up on individuals to find out whether they died from melanoma or another cause. "At the time the paper was published, we found that those who did have solar elastosis lived twice as long as those who did not," says Dr. Berwick.

The most useful form of vitamin D is produced when the skin is exposed to ultraviolet radiation, though it may also be absorbed from food sources. Dr. Berwick explained that the operational hypothesis with regard to the cancer survival rates is that when activated by sunlight, vitamin D in the bloodstream will also stimulate *apoptosis*, or cell death, in fast-growing cancer cells.

FUTURE ILLUMINATION

And now a recent study from Stanford University provides further insight into the subject, confirming the hypothesis from the study noted above regarding the impact of sunlight on the activation of vitamin D-3. Having triggered this process in the lab, the Stanford scientists found that the "activated" vitamin D signals T-cells to localize to the epidermis, the surface layers of the skin, more than when they were not stimulated by the vitamin D. According to Stanford University study coauthor, Eugene Butcher, MD, these T-cells may help protect against cancer and may target cancer cells to reduce their survival.

THE SUN AS FRIEND

Based on these studies, Drs. Berwick and Butcher say we should add the ability of sunlight to improve local vitamin D activity in the skin to the list of sunlight's

many healthful benefits. They may help target anticancer T-cells as well as protect against proliferation of cancer cells.

So, don't be afraid of the sun. Most experts say that how much sun you need depends on where you live and the color of your skin (dark skin is more protected and needs more). For most people, 15 minutes a few times a week between 10 am and 3 pm should do it. "We don't want people spending the day at the beach with no protection," Dr. Berwick said, "but neither do we want them to be completely afraid to get a little sun. In fact, we believe it may be good to do so."

Shedding Light On Drivers'-Side Cancer

Ellen Marmur, MD, chief, division of dermatologic and cosmetic surgery at the Mount Sinai Medical Center in New York City. She is skin health editor of *Your Health Now.*

You might think there's no reason to worry about the sun's harmful rays when you are driving. But you'd be wrong, as a recent study from Saint Louis University made clear. Researchers there evaluated data from 1,047 people with skin cancer and discovered that 53% of them had skin cancers on the left side of the body. When researchers looked at cancers that were only on the arms, hands, head and neck, they found more cancers on the left side (the side that is exposed while driving), especially in men. Researchers speculate that people who drive frequently may be more apt to have left-side cancers.

GLASS NOT A BARRIER FOR SKIN CANCER

Ellen Marmur, MD, chief of the division of dermatologic and cosmetic surgery at the Mount Sinai Medical Center in New York City, explains that for a long time, people assumed that the glass in cars blocked all ultraviolet (UV) rays. Now we know that while glass blocks most of UVB rays, it only filters less than half of UVA rays, leaving people vulnerable to damage from the sun. Until recently, it was believed that UVB rays were the main cause of skin cancer—but recent research proved that to be wrong as well, with UVA rays equally potent and dangerous, says Dr. Marmur.

All windshield glass is laminated to prevent shattering. As a result, it blocks more UVA rays than the glass in side windows, but still allows 20% of rays through. That plus the rays from the side windows adds up to a considerable amount of exposure. Convertible drivers—even those whose top-down days were years ago—have yet another skin cancer concern, says Dr. Marmur, which is skin cancer on the scalp. Hair offers some protection, but not much. Drivers who rest their left arm on the window ledge risk sun damage, too.

PROTECT YOURSELF

Tinted windows, popular in some areas of the country, have more protection than clear ones, says Dr. Marmur, but even better protection is available from special films that can be applied to clear or tinted glass to reduce UVA rays. Check with your car dealer or local garage for more information. Go to *www.skincancer.org* and type "UV film" in the search bar for a list of recommended products. However, she still advises everyone to wear sunblock or protective clothing when in the car for extended periods of time and, of course, keep the windows closed to avoid direct sun exposure. She reminds everyone to do a body check—including the scalp—each month, looking for any changes on the skin, and to see a dermatologist once a year for a full body check.

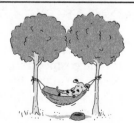

Spotting Hidden Melanomas

Ellen S. Marmur, MD, chief, division of dermatologic and cosmetic surgery, the Mount Sinai Medical Center, New York City. She is skin health editor of *Your Health Now.*

Melanoma used to be one of the scariest words in the English language...so dire was the expected outcome. But today, because of more research and better detection, melanoma skin cancer can—and often is—treated successfully. In fact, if caught early enough, it has a 95% cure rate. Still, the incidence of melanoma has soared. Complicating the problem further are so-called "hidden" melanomas, ones that are in hard-to-detect places or even within the body.

To find out what people can do for prevention and early detection of melanomas hidden or otherwise, our editors called Ellen S. Marmur, MD, chief of the division of dermatologic and cosmetic surgery at the Mount Sinai Medical Center in New York City. She explains that all melanomas form from *melanocytes*, cells that produce the body's pigment. Consequently, a melanoma can develop anyplace there is pigmentation in the body. Hidden melanomas are rare, but should not be ignored. One particular type, intraocular melanoma, is within the middle layer of the eye, called the *uvea*, which contains the iris. When Dr. Marmur does total body skin checks for her patients—a procedure she says should take place once a year—she looks into the eyes as well, but she also stresses the need to have regular eye exams as part of melanoma detection.

Also: Wear sunglasses that say 100% UV protection. Photochromic lenses with UV protection are best if you have a prescription. Higher end sunglasses have better quality lenses and protect you from headaches (due to bad quality lenses).

Other unusual areas where melanomas can appear are on the scalp, under the nails, the palms of the hands and soles of the feet and between the toes. Even more troubling, melanoma does not only develop on sun-exposed skin. It can also develop on the pink mucosal lining of the mouth, genitalia, anus, urinary tract and esophagus (*mucosal melanoma*). While not a hidden melanoma, a "*halo nevus*"— visible as a white halo effect around a brown spot or mole—can also be associated with melanoma. In these cases, the brown spot seems to be disappearing, but actually the body is attacking the mole or a more lethal process is actually under way—the melanoma is digging deeper, leaving less of it on the surface.

DETECTION

Dr. Marmur recommends doing a personal body skin check each month and a full check with a dermatologist annually. Look at all brown spots everywhere on your skin including between the toes, on the bottom of the feet and the palms. You are investigating to see if there are any new moles or growths…any which have changed or grown over a one- to three-month period…any that have asymmetrical, ragged borders, uneven color or signs of inflammation (redness, warmth, swelling, tenderness to the touch)…or are more than six millimeters in diameter. Another danger sign—brown spots that go away and reappear (unlike a halo nevus). Don't forget to check the scalp for the same lesions you would see elsewhere on your skin—new or persistent brown spots or red spots or anything that bleeds easily. To check your scalp, use a blow dryer to part your hair as you search and follow up with a finger check for new bumps, which, if found, should be evaluated and followed by a dermatologist, says Dr. Marmur. Melanomas in the nails are most often in the thumb or big toe nail and appear to be a brown or black colored streak, much like what you see after an accident that involves your nails or as a side effect of certain medications. However, trauma or drugs usually affect more than one nail while a melanoma is singular. Obviously you can't

see esophagus/mouth or mucosal melanoma, but there are signals. *They are…*

- **Unexplained bleeding from the nose, urinary tract or genitals.**
- **Isolated pain in the throat.**
- **Difficulty swallowing or trouble with regurgitation.**
- **A feeling of tightness in the esophageal area.**

Should you have any suspicious findings symptoms, call your regular doctor or dermatologist right away.

AT RISK

Everyone should be wary and aware of melanomas, but there are some people who are at higher risk. Having a family history of skin cancers or several abnormal-appearing moles called *dysplastic nevi* (the technical word for mole) puts people at risk. Having had a previous skin cancer of *any* type dramatically increases risk—even a simple basal cell skin cancer puts you at a 25 times greater risk for another type of skin cancer including melanoma. Fair-skinned people with light eyes and a history of sunburns (such as Caucasian golfers or sailors) are at higher risk. Blacks and other dark-skinned groups are at low risk of melanomas but not for under-the-nail melanomas (subungual) and mucosal melanoma. People of color develop these cancers much more often than do light-skinned people.

SELF-DEFENSE

Avoiding too much sun is the surest way to prevent melanoma, but there is other, encouraging research on possible ways to prevent this cancer. A recent mouse study, for instance, demonstrated that exercise was protective. Two groups of mice were exposed to UVB rays following which both groups developed skin cancer tumors. However, the mice that had access to an exercise wheel developed 32% fewer tumors than their non-exercising buddies. Researchers suggest that this might be because exercise enhances a process called *UVB-induced apoptosis*, in which the body kills sun-damaged cells. The lower body fat of the exercising mice might also play a role. Dr. Marmur says that further studies need to be conducted and the role fat plays in skin cancer is still unknown.

Other key preventive measures: Wearing sunscreen starting from infancy through maturity is the best way to prevent skin cancer. UV-protective fabrics are widely available. They offer an SPF (sun protection factor) of 30. Normal cotton T-shirts offer an SPF of 2 to 5.

Hope for Sun-Damaged Skin

Kenneth A. Arndt, MD, clinical professor of dermatology, Harvard Medical School, and editor, *Harvard Health Letter.*

Topical retinoids (creams and gels containing chemicals derived from vitamin A) first developed to treat acne and psoriasis have proved effective at repairing skin—beyond improving appearance—that's been damaged by long sun exposure.

How they work: Topical retinoids lighten freckles and spots and improve skin's appearance. They also increase collagen production to help make small wrinkles disappear. Retinoids improve the quality of skin growth and decrease the number of atypical skin cells.

Topical retinoids are a prescription drug, so consult your doctor. They are safe for everyone (except during pregnancy), but may cause skin irritation.

Hand Care for Men and Women

Barney J. Kenet, MD, dermatologist specializing in skin cancer, New York City, cofounder, American Melanoma Foundation, and author of *How to Wash Your Face* (Simon & Schuster).

Apply sunblock regularly to prevent sun damage, which causes brown spots, freckles and thinning skin that produces a skeletal look in later years. During the day, apply a rich lubricating lotion, especially after washing hands and while skin still is damp. Good choices include Neutrogena Norwegian Formula Hand Cream...Kiehl's Very Unusually Rich—But Not Greasy At All—Hand Cream with Sunscreen SPF 10...Curél Soothing Hand Lotion, an especially good product if you wash hands often during the day. All are available on-line and in stores. Give hands intensive nighttime treatment by soaking them for a minute or two in a mixture of half water and half whole milk—the lactic acid in milk helps remove dead cells and soften cuticles and the natural fats help replenish dry skin—then dry hands, apply Aquaphor ointment and wear gloves to bed, to keep ointment on hands and off sheets.

Alternative nighttime treatment: Apply pure honey to hands, and leave it on for five minutes—it is sticky but soothing as well as softening.

9

Nutrition Updates: News For a Healthier You

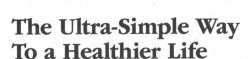

The Ultra-Simple Way To a Healthier Life

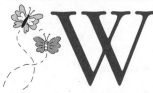

Whether you are trying to lose weight for health reasons or appearance, it's often easier said than done. Many people think that eating less and exercising more are the keys to weight loss. Lately, however, experts are beginning to recognize the important role inflammation—specifically, the body's physical and psychological response to stress and toxins—plays in the weight-loss equation. Mark Hyman, MD, the former comedical director at Canyon Ranch in Lenox, Massachusetts, has spent years studying the role of inflammation and its impact on body weight. In his book, *The UltraSimple Diet* (Pocket), he outlines a detailed, step-by-step, seven-day program to help people structure their eating habits and lifestyle to keep inflammation and its destructive role at bay. This isn't a "diet" in the traditional sense, Dr. Hyman notes, but an eating program for optimal wellness that he believes can benefit everyone, whatever his or her weight.

THE TWO KEY CULPRITS: TOXICITY AND INFLAMMATION

We are always surrounded with potentially "toxic" influences, and are bombarded daily by junk foods, poisonous pollutants, negative thoughts and destructive behavior. Normally, inflammation is the body's short-term healing response to such insults and injuries. But under continuous attack like this, your immune system shifts into constant high gear to protect you. The hormones and other chemical messengers

Mark Hyman, MD, founder and medical director of The UltraWellness Center in Lenox, Massachusetts, and author of *UltraMetabolism*, Scribner, and *The UltraSimple Diet*, Pocket. Dr. Hyman is the former co-medical director of Canyon Ranch, and editor-in-chief of *Alternative Therapies in Health and Medicine*, a peer-reviewed journal on alternative medicine. For more information about the books, go to *www.ultra metabolism.com* or *www.ultrasimplediet.com*.

it fires out are meant to defend the body but, because they are too abundant, they often cause chronic inflammation instead. Experts believe this chronic inflammation is what lies at the root of a multitude of diseases, including obesity, heart disease, cancer and Alzheimer's disease.

Although the body's natural state is a healthy weight, many of us have developed a "protective coating" (excess weight) as a by-product of our constant state of self-defense. In order to return to the optimal state, we must normalize the "environment." We need to rid our bodies of inflammatory influences. This is the thrust of Dr. Hyman's eating program.

STRATEGIES TO REDUCE TOXICITY AND COOL INFLAMMATION

Before starting Dr. Hyman's program, he recommends that you take his "Toxicity and Inflammation Quiz," so you can monitor your results. Go to *www.ultra simplediet.com/temp/preview.html* for the link to the quiz.

Once you have taken the quiz and have your baseline score, you're ready to begin the *UltraSimple* program. *Here are several key aspects...*

•**Eat an anti-inflammatory diet.** Focus on eating whole foods in the form nature intended. This means getting rid of bad foods that stimulate inflammation.

Beware: This long list includes white flour and sugar products, high-fructose corn syrup, trans fats, additives, preservatives, pesticides, hormones, alcohol, caffeine, fast and fried foods—and, for the first week at least, red meat, too. Dr. Hyman also has patients eliminate potential sensitizing foods such as dairy, gluten, eggs, corn, yeast and peanuts for the first seven days. While you may not be sensitive to *all* these foods, the only way to find out is to avoid them for a week and see how you respond.

UltraSimple tip: Make healthful substitutions. For example, replace your morning cup of coffee with anti-inflammatory green tea. In place of sugary soft drinks, treat your body to cool, clean, filtered water or sparkling water with a twist of lemon or lime. Whenever possible, avoid foods grown with hormones, antibiotics and petrochemical pesticides and eat those that have been organically grown. The idea is to make healthier choices, not deprive yourself.

•**Add good foods.** Next, feed your body the way nature intended by eating more nutrient-packed whole foods. A sample day's meal plan might include a cup of green tea, hot water with lemon, and a protein shake for breakfast (see sample recipe below)...2 cups of steamed or lightly sautéed veggies, one-half cup of brown rice and an (optional) protein shake for lunch...1 cup of vegetable broth, 2 cups of veggies, one-half cup of brown rice, and 4 to 6 ounces of fish or chicken for dinner.

ULTRASHAKE RECIPE

To make a tasty, healthful protein shake, in a blender, combine in a blender and purée...

½ cup of plain, unsweetened, gluten-free almond or hazelnut milk

1 to 2 tablespoons of nut butter (almond, macadamia, pecan) or ¼ cup of nuts (soaked overnight in water) such as almonds, walnuts, pecans or any combination of these

1 tablespoon organic combination flax and borage oil

2 tablespoons ground flaxseeds

½ cup fresh or frozen noncitrus organic fruit, such as cherries, blueberries, raspberries, strawberries, peaches, pears or frozen bananas

Ice (made from filtered water)

2 to 4 ounces of filtered water to desired consistency

Note: Use flaxseeds in no more than two shakes a day.

Dr. Hyman's tip: To reduce food cravings, eat protein for breakfast every day, and have a healthy snack (for example, a handful of walnuts, almonds or pumpkin seeds) when hungry. These strategies help keep your blood sugar—and thus your energy level—on an even keel.

Note: Bottom Line's Daily Health News consulting medical editor Andrew L. Rubman, ND, points out that for those with digestion challenges due to stomach acid levels, it may be better to stick with three solid meals a day in order to make optimal use of your stomach's acid.

•**Detoxify.** Dr. Hyman finds it helpful to kick-start the process of fighting inflammation with a cup of homemade detoxifying vegetable broth. This keeps hunger at bay while cleansing the system.

BROTH RECIPE

To make a homemade detox vegetable broth, combine...

10 cups filtered water

6 cups chopped mixed organic veggies

Fresh or dried herbs and spices, such as bay leaf, oregano, lemongrass, fennel and ginger, among others

A variety of vegetables that include at least four of the following—shiitake mushrooms, burdock root, sweet potatoes, carrots, onions, celery, sea vegetables, dark leafy greens, daikon and daikon leaf, and root vegetables such as turnips and parsnips. (In the case of less widely available vegetables such as burdock root and daikon, it may be necessary to visit a specialty or ethnic market or health food store.)

Add the herbs to the veggies and water, and bring to a boil in a large stockpot. Turn heat to low and simmer approximately 60 minutes. Strain and drink warm, at least 3 to 4 cups a day. The broth keeps in the fridge for two days; may be frozen.

Note: You may feel a bit foggy or fatigued the first day or two, as your body adjusts to your healthful new eating program. However, this should clear up quickly.

WHAT'S NEXT

After seven days, take the quiz again to see how far you've come. If you've eaten only those foods that are healthy for you and avoided foods that are toxic and cause inflammation, you will have lost weight and gained energy by the end of the week. Some people choose to reincorporate some eliminated foods back into their diets gradually, but be careful about what foods are reintroduced. Consider these the first seven days of your new life—one devoted to healthful eating and wellness. Also, be sure to check with your doctor before starting any diet program.

Even if you make only some of the changes Dr. Hyman recommends, he says it will improve your health and well-being.

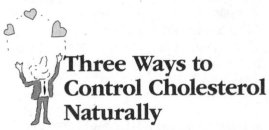

Three Ways to Control Cholesterol Naturally

Andrew L. Rubman, ND, consulting medical editor for *Bottom Line's Daily Health News* and director of the Southbury Clinic for Traditional Medicines in Southbury, Connecticut.

We spend an inordinate amount of time talking about how to raise good cholesterol and lower bad cholesterol. The body actually needs both kinds, and it's the balance between the two that is most important. We recently discussed this—how the media, along with all those "cholesterol lowering" drug manufacturers, are delivering the wrong message—with our consulting medical editor Andrew L. Rubman, ND.

BALANCE THEORY OF CHOLESTEROL MANAGEMENT

"Cholesterol is necessary for life," says Dr. Rubman, "*ergo* it can't really be 'bad.'" It only causes trouble when it gets out of proportion, with too much low-density lipoprotein (LDL) and too little high-density lipoprotein (HDL) relative to each other. When it comes to the total cholesterol/HDL ratio, the American Heart Association recommends a ratio of less than 5:1, optimally, 3.5:1. Dr. Rubman says the ratio is more useful than a fixed target number that people are prone to strive for. "The real focus with cholesterol is—or ought to be—how to manage it better," he notes. In order to accomplish that, we need to understand what cholesterol is and what it does.

PROTEIN BUILDING BLOCKS

What we commonly call "cholesterol"—both the "bad" (low-density lipoprotein or LDL) and the "good" (high-density lipoprotein or HDL)—is actually a little container of protein and fat synthesized together by the liver. These help your body produce cell membranes, create estrogen, testosterone and other vital hormones.

Ideally, the body should naturally balance HDL and LDL when properly nourished. But that doesn't often happen in modern times on modern diets. Since the body works with whatever elements it has on hand to produce HDL and LDL, a first step to achieving balance is to eat and digest the right forms of protein.

What kind of protein should you eat? "High-quality, minimally processed food," says Dr. Rubman, suggesting you strive to include one "good high-value protein" at every meal. Dr. Rubman's favorite sources of protein include lean organic chicken or beef, and wild, deep-water fish, as well as beans and other legumes.

ABSORBING THE PROTEIN

Equally important (and less often understood) is that we need to make sure the protein is adequately digested and absorbed. "There's a huge digestive link to the whole issue of cholesterol," Dr. Rubman says. The digestion process starts in your mouth. When you chew, the action triggers the production of saliva, which contains enzymes that start to break down your food. So the more you chew your food, the more you help the digestion process. Proper chewing can actually influence how much cholesterol your body will absorb and then synthesize. Depending on what's on your fork, aim for 30 or more chews per bite to insure optimal digestion.

Similarly, having adequate amounts of stomach acid will help ensure complete digestion of your proteins. This means that older people and regular users of acid-suppressing medications—both over-the-counter (OTC) and prescription—may be inhibiting their body's ability to fully digest protein.

B VITAMINS, GARLIC AND FIBER

In order to manufacture cholesterol optimally, the liver also needs B vitamins, Dr. Rubman explains. For his patients, he prescribes a good, high-potency B complex vitamin to be taken at least twice daily, and often a separate vitamin B-12. Second, he advises regularly eating dark green, cruciferous foods (one serving daily is ideal) like Brussels sprouts, broccoli and kale.

Garlic can also be helpful in balancing cholesterol. Even in the mainstream medical community, garlic is understood to be an agent for lowering LDL cholesterol, while some research has shown it to actually raise HDL as well. Garlic supplements are usually unnecessary, says Dr. Rubman. "For most people, cooking regularly with garlic is adequate and helpful."

Finally Dr. Rubman recommends fiber: "Many types of soluble fiber can bind cholesterol and carry it out of the body with the bowel movement," he explains. This is how the body eliminates excess cholesterol. He often prescribes supplemental glucomannan (Konjac fiber), taken a half hour before the largest meal of the day with a large glass of water.

One last recommendation from Dr. Rubman on achieving cholesterol balance—exercise. It increases the metabolic use of lipids, enabling your liver to make more high-density lipoproteins (HDL).

Forget Statins—Here's The Best and Safest Cholesterol Reducer

Sonja Pettersen, NMD, naturopathic medical doctor. She is licensed to practice primary care medicine specializing in natural therapeutics in Arizona and is based in Scottsdale.

Although it is important to keep cholesterol at a healthful ratio of total cholesterol to HDL (4 or under is ideal), all the focus on low-low cholesterol is not necessarily a good thing. You could keep cholesterol in check with the pop of a statin pill and consider the problem solved. Or, you could avoid the risk of side effects from statins, and instead go the natural route—red yeast rice…blueberries…or plant *sterols*. Plant sterols—and their cousins, plant *stanols*—are compounds that occur naturally in many fruits, vegetables, nuts, seeds, cereals, legumes, vegetable oils and other plant sources, and are both cheaper and safer than statins.

RESEARCH ABOUNDS

There's a considerable amount of research showing that plant sterols can lower cholesterol quite effectively. A study in the *European Journal of Clinical Nutrition* has shown that 2 grams (g) of plant sterols taken daily resulted in a 6.5% reduction in total cholesterol. In another study, 1.8 g taken daily, coupled with a fiber called glucomannan lowered total cholesterol. A third study in the *American Journal of Clinical Nutrition* got similar results. And an article in the *British Medical Journal* concluded that if 2 g a day of plant sterols (or stanols) were added to the diet, there would be a reduction in the risk of heart disease of about 25%, "larger than the effect that could be expected to be achieved by reducing…intake of saturated fat."

IT'S OFFICIAL

The cholesterol-lowering effects of plant sterols have been known for some time. The US Food and Drug Administration (FDA) has already authorized a coronary heart disease health claim for plant sterols and plant stanols. According to the "Talk Paper" released by the FDA to the press, this ruling was based on the FDA's conclusion that plant sterols "may reduce the risk of cardiovascular disease by lowering blood cholesterol levels."

GETTING YOUR STEROLS

Plant sterols can be incorporated into the diet by eating lots of plant foods. Vegetable oils including safflower, soybean and olive also are a good source, but be sure to buy cold-pressed—organic if possible—and balance your vegetable oil intake with nut oils and fish oil. Some margarines (such as Benecol) tout their cholesterol-lowering properties largely due to the addition of plant sterols. The best sources remain fruits and vegetables…however, supplements based on plant sterols also are becoming widely available (for example, CholestaPRO, CholestOff and Lipid Shield).

Some top sources of sterols include…

Rice bran oil

Corn oil

Sesame seeds

Safflower oil

Soybean oil

Olive oil

Peanuts

Italian salad dressing

Garbanzo beans

Bananas

Carrots

Tomatoes

By keeping your cholesterol in check with plant sterols you will also reap additional benefits. According to Sonja Pettersen, NMD, based in Arizona, "Plant foods—and the compounds they contain—improve immune function, have anti-cancer properties and seem to be helpful in a wide variety of health conditions, from eczema to chronic fatigue."

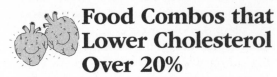

Food Combos that Lower Cholesterol Over 20%

David J. Jenkins, MD, PhD, professor in both the departments of medicine and nutritional sciences, Faculty of Medicine, University of Toronto, and director of the Clinical Nutrition and Risk Factor Modification Center, St. Michael's Hospital, Toronto, Canada.

According to Forbes magazine, the two biggest selling drugs in America are Lipitor and Zocor, which bring in billions of dollars in annual sales. Both are cholesterol-lowering medications, part of a group known as statin drugs. The problem is, statin drugs have potentially serious side effects...and they're expensive. So when we came across some research recently that indicated that certain combinations of foods may be as effective at lowering cholesterol as the statin drugs and may lower inflammation as well, we decided to find out more.

"Cholesterol is a good indicator for heart disease, though not the only one," says David Jenkins, MD, PhD, the lead investigator on a study published in the *American Journal of Clinical Nutrition*, professor at the University of Toronto and director of the Clinical Nutrition and Risk Factor Modification Center at St. Michael's Hospital in Toronto, Canada. "But my concern is that we're drugging ourselves so that we can survive the rather unhealthful lifestyle that we've designed for ourselves."

According to Dr. Jenkins, there is a very protective effect of certain foods, particularly eaten in combination, and for people who are at lower risk for heart disease, lifestyle changes—such as eating more of these foods—might be the way to go.

THE RESEARCH

In the research, Dr. Jenkins and his team combined plant sterol-enriched margarines with other foods known to have cholesterol lowering ability—soy protein (miso, tofu, soy burgers), almonds and fiber-high foods such as oats and barley—to create a kind of food "portfolio." For 12 months, 55 hyperlipidemic participants were prescribed diets high in plant sterols, soy protein, viscous fibers and almonds. They then measured the effect on cholesterol and found that this combination of foods reduced LDL ("bad") cholesterol by more than 20%, very similar to what would be achieved with some statin drugs, in 31.8% of the participants. "These foods also tend to be as good as statins in lowering C-reactive protein (CRP)—an important measure of inflammation," Dr. Jenkins notes.

DIET CHANGES VS. PILLS

Dr. Jenkins is not challenging the benefit of statins for those at high risk for cardiovascular disease. However, we don't know the long-term effects of these drugs when used as preventive medicine on a large section of the broader population who are at low risk. Taking a pill may give people the false impression that they have nothing further to do to protect their health and that they do not need to make any lifestyle changes. Emphasizing diet changes in general can help the many people at lower risk to improve their health without the need for medications.

Are Low Calorie Foods Making You Fat?

Leo Galland, MD, director of the Foundation for Integrative Medicine in New York City. He is author of *The Fat Resistance Diet.* Broadway. *www.fatresistancediet.com.* Dr. Galland is a recipient of the Linus Pauling award.

Obesity is rampant in America and is only getting worse. *The latest estimates are more far-reaching than anyone had imagined...*

• **Two hundred million Americans are overweight,** and half of them are obese.

• **The rate of extreme obesity** (body mass index/BMI greater than 40) is increasing twice as fast as obesity in general.

•**Forty percent of the population suffers from metabolic syndrome,** a group of symptoms (including high blood pressure, high triglyceride levels and high fasting blood sugar) that is a complication of obesity and a precursor of type 2 diabetes. Having metabolic syndrome also triples the risk of developing Alzheimer's disease.

•**Osteoarthritis,** which can be a complication of obesity, is the number one cause of chronic disability.

•**One out of three American children born in the year 2000** is predicted to develop type 2 diabetes during his/her lifetime, a devastating long-range effect of the obesity epidemic.

•**Despite excessive caloric consumption,** over three-quarters of the population has a deficient intake of one or more essential nutrients. Greater levels of obesity are actually associated with lower nutritional status.

A DIFFERENT THEORY

"A solution to the obesity crisis is the single most important thing that needs to happen in improving the health of Americans," Dr. Leo Galland says. Dr. Galland has developed a novel and provocative theory on how to control weight, based upon recent scientific insights into the way that levels of body fat are normally controlled. The foundation of his approach, which he calls the Fat Resistance Diet, is nutrient density and control of inflammation.

"We have inborn, natural regulatory systems that support a healthy weight, but our food choices and our lifestyle interfere with their functioning," Dr. Galland explains. *Leptin,* for example, is a compound that lets your brain and body know how much fat you are storing. When leptin level goes up, your appetite goes down. Leptin also speeds up your metabolism. "The problem is that overweight people have developed resistance to leptin," Dr. Galland says. "Their leptin levels are high but it's not depressing their appetite and it's not stimulating their metabolism."

INFLAMMATION FACTOR

According to Dr. Galland, inflammation is a large part of the reason why leptin doesn't work as it should in very overweight people. "Inflammation disables the leptin signal," he explains. "It also contributes to insulin resistance, a central feature of obesity and diabetes." In the presence of inflammation, the fat control mechanisms simply don't work.

NUTRIENT DENSITY

The other part of the equation has to do with what's called nutrient density. "What matters most about the calories in any food are the nutrients that accompany them," he said. No one in his right mind would recommend a calorie-controlled diet consisting of 12 100-calorie packs of Oreos. "Even though the calories are on target, you'd be completely screwed up by the lack of fiber, the lack of protein and other nutrients and the resulting blood-sugar roller coaster," says Dr. Galland. "That's why a weight reduction program that looks at calories only completely misses the boat."

"The way that Americans have been taught to think about food is to try to find lower calorie equivalents of foods we like to eat," Dr. Galland points out. "That hasn't worked. Some artificial sweeteners in low-calorie foods actually make you hungrier."

According to Dr. Galland, we need a new approach to the way people eat. "I think the American palate has been corrupted," he said. "We've lost the ability to really savor herbs and spices and all the subtle flavors that are so wonderful. Those herbs and spices have nutritional value—they're rich in antioxidants, rich in minerals and especially rich in anti-inflammatories."

FLAVORFUL, HEALTHFUL OPTIONS

Some of the best anti-inflammatory spices and herbs include cloves, ginger, parsley, tumeric, cinnamon and basil. "We need to reeducate our palate to learn to appreciate the wonders of these foods," Dr. Galland explains. *He has identified 12 core principles to eating for fat resistance...*

• **Choose foods that are loaded with nutrients such as colorful vegetables and fruits,** and lean, minimally processed protein. As much as possible, avoid food that has been processed.

• **Avoid trans fats.**

• **Consume foods with plenty of omega-3 content.**

• **Eat fish three times a week or more.**

• **Eat at least 25 grams of fiber per day.**

• **Eat at least nine servings of vegetables and fruits daily.**

• **Average one serving a day of alliums** (onions, scallions, garlic) and crucifers (broccoli, cabbage, kale, cauliflower).

• **No more than 10% of total calories should be from *saturated* fat.** This doesn't mean only 10% of total diet is from fats—it means to be careful about eating *saturated* fats. Animal foods (and some plant foods) are the main source of saturated fats.

• **If you eat eggs, don't scramble the yolk.**

• **Don't follow a "low-fat" diet.**

• **Eat two healthy snacks a day**—such as berries, tomatoes, string cheese, organic turkey slices.

• **Eat fruit instead of sugary sweets.**

The Easiest Weight Loss Secret Ever

Jonny Bowden, PhD, CNS, is a board-certified nutritionist, "Weight Loss Coach" on iVillage.com and author of the best-selling *Living the Low Carb Life* (Sterling) as well as *The 150 Healthiest Foods on Earth* (Fair Winds). Find out more at *www.jonny bowden.com.*

Are there things overweight people can do, without turning their lives upside down, that could make a real difference to their health? Small, simple things, perhaps, that they could do without feeling as if they were on a diet?

SALAD DAYS

"Absolutely," says nutritionist and life coach Jonny Bowden, PhD, CNS. "A salad before each meal can make a huge difference." Dr. Bowden explains that a small, simple salad eaten before the main course would accomplish three things—it would add to the body's stores of valuable antioxidants...increase the daily intake of fiber...and improve satiety, thus reducing overall calories, which could help you lose weight.

"Salads are natural appetite suppressants," Dr. Bowden says. "The soluble fiber helps to slow the entrance of glucose (blood sugar) into the bloodstream, making you less likely to be hungry after eating. And, according to one study published in the *Journal of the American Dietetic Association*, when 42 women ate a simple 100-calorie salad before dinner, they consumed 12% less calories during the meal, even without trying to diet or limit their intake." According to Dr. Bowden, attacking the bread box at dinner has the opposite effect. "It drives blood sugar up, making it more likely that you'll store calories as fat," he says.

EXTRA BENEFITS

"The trick is to consume a lot of colorful vegetables," says Dr. Bowden. "The cruciferous vegetables, such as broccoli, contain cancer-fighting substances like *indoles* and *sulforaphane*, and using a variety of colored vegetables—red peppers, carrots, spinach and red onions—guarantees a wide spectrum of antioxidants."

You get a triple whammy from the salad if you use oil and vinegar on it. "Research shows that vinegar helps lower both blood sugar and insulin," Dr. Bowden says. "According to research at Arizona State University, it also helps increase the feeling of fullness." Dr. Bowden says two or three tablespoons of vinegar on the salad along with high-quality olive oil ought to do the trick. The fat in olive oil actually helps the body make the most of many of the nutrients in the salad—such as fat-soluble vitamins and antioxidants. It also slows stomach emptying, thus preserving a full feeling and improving the quality of digestion.

And don't forget the fiber you'll be getting if you choose those vegetables wisely. "Several studies have shown a correlation between high-fiber diets and lowered rates of degenerative disease," Dr. Bowden says. "Even without the weight loss benefits, a salad before a meal is a nutritional bonanza."

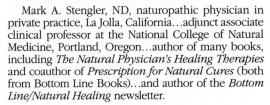

Natural Appetite Suppressors

Mark A. Stengler, ND, naturopathic physician in private practice, La Jolla, California…adjunct associate clinical professor at the National College of Natural Medicine, Portland, Oregon…author of many books, including *The Natural Physician's Healing Therapies* and coauthor of *Prescription for Natural Cures* (both from Bottom Line Books)…and author of the *Bottom Line/Natural Healing* newsletter.

For a fresh and healthful look at how to curb appetite, we consulted Mark Stengler, ND, a licensed naturopathic medical doctor in La Jolla, California and author of *Bottom Line Natural Healing* newsletter. He warns that standard over-the-counter (OTC) and prescription remedies are often ineffective in achieving weight loss, and many may cause dangerous side effects such as overstimulation and heart palpitations. Fortunately, there's another way. Dr. Stengler outlined a number of safer natural strategies to suppress the appetite.

FILL UP ON FIBER

This is old news, but bears repeating. One of the easiest and most inexpensive ways to suppress the appetite is to include fiber in every meal. Fiber, which is abundant in veggies (especially leafy greens like spinach) and fruits, makes you feel full, explains Dr. Stengler. For the greatest impact, he recommends that you eat a salad

or vegetables at the start of every meal. At breakfast, add one or two tablespoons of fiber-rich ground flaxseed, flax meal or oat bran to cereal, yogurt and fruit, or a protein shake. Read labels to make sure your cereal is packed with fiber and not sugar, and drink eight to 10 ounces of water after consuming ground flaxseed.

If you don't take in enough fiber through diet alone, fiber supplements are another option. In particular, Dr. Stengler recommends psyllium, which is often used to relieve constipation. To curb the appetite, take three to four grams before breakfast and dinner, with eight to 10 ounces of water. Do not take psyllium if you have difficulty swallowing. Also, be sure to take all fiber supplements two hours before or after vitamin/mineral supplements or drugs, as they may interfere with their absorption.

A favorite strategy of *Bottom Line's Daily Health News* consulting medical editor, Andrew L. Rubman, ND, is to up fiber intake with a natural fiber supplement called *glucomannan*. Take one capsule with eight to 10 ounces of water 30 to 45 minutes prior to meals.

CONSIDER NUTRITIONAL SUPPLEMENTS

For many people, especially those with a history of years of overeating, dietary fiber by itself may not be enough to turn the tide. For even greater appetite suppression, Dr. Stengler says you can try a nutritional supplement. Begin with the first one below, and if that doesn't do the trick, try the second. Take only one at a time. *Options include…*

CARALLUMA FIMBRIATA

For centuries, people in India have eaten this common vegetable in curries or raw to control hunger and thirst. Scientists believe that chemical constituents called *pregnane glycosides* are partly responsible for caralluma's natural appetite-suppressing effect. In his practice, Dr. Stengler finds that eight out of 10 patients experience effective appetite suppression with caralluma.

Side effects are rare, although some people experience minor digestive upset. If this is a problem, take caralluma with food. A significant benefit is that there is no stimulant effect with this supplement. Caralluma should not be used by pregnant or nursing women, and children should take it only under a physician's supervision.

PINOLENIC ACID

Another appetite tamer comes as an extract from the Korean pine nut (*Pinus koraiensis*). Pinolenic acid appears to work by modulating levels of hormones associated with hunger and satiety. In one trial, overweight women who took pinolenic acid reported a "desire to eat" that was 29% lower than their counterparts taking a placebo.

As with caralluma, side effects are rare, this supplement should not be used by pregnant or nursing women, and children should take it only under a physician's supervision. Also, there is no stimulant effect.

Note: Those with nut allergies should avoid taking it.

Natural appetite suppressants are still only part of the larger weight loss equation. To successfully shed excess pounds, you need to watch not only how much you eat, but also what you eat, and make sure you fit in regular exercise, too.

Taking the Hood Off Hoodia

Eric Yarnell, ND, RH, Northwest Naturopathic Urology. Dr. Yarnell is author of numerous books including *Clinical Botanical Medicine*. Mary Ann Liebert. He is president of Healing Mountain Publishing and vice president of Heron Botanicals. Visit his Web site at *www.dryarnell.com*.

The natural appetite suppressant *Hoodia gordonii* has been around for years, but recently, seems to be heavily advertised as a weight-loss wonder. A quick Internet search provides tales of primitive cultures surviving in the desert thanks to Hoodia. Natural—that's good. Used "forever"—also good. But, is it too good to be true?

For the lowdown on Hoodia, we contacted Eric Yarnell, ND, RH—a naturopathic physician in Seattle and American Herbalists Guild registered herbalist—and author of *Clinical Botanical Medicine*. Dr. Yarnell has a whole different spin on Hoodia than what the promotions would have you believe.

GOOD FOR THE BUSHMEN, BUT NOT FOR US

Although it is often referred to as a cactus, Hoodia is more accurately a succulent from the Kalahari Desert in Africa. According to Dr. Yarnell, it is indeed true that for centuries, the bushmen have turned to Hoodia to control hunger during long desert treks. It is believed to work by convincing the brain that you feel full even when you haven't eaten.

Now hucksters all over the Internet have hopped on the Hoodia bandwagon and are aggressively marketing it for weight loss. Unfortunately, while it may work just fine for the bushmen, the Hoodia sold in the US is usually not even Hoodia—it's more likely a mix of other herbs with a smattering of Hoodia.

ECOLOGICAL AND CLINICAL CONCERNS

Hoodia is a slow growing plant, found only in one small area, and it is not yet sustainable as a cash crop. Additionally, the plant is illegal to export or import without a permit from the US Department of the Interior. "I am of the strong opinion that Hoodia should absolutely not be used, on the basis of both ecological and clinical concerns," emphasizes Dr. Yarnell. "The number of products claiming to contain Hoodia far outstrip the supply, so most of what's on the market is garbage."

There is also little solid evidence that Hoodia works. According to Dr. Yarnell, if clinical trials ultimately confirm that it decreases appetite in dieters and a sustainable supply of the cultivated plant can develop, then we can take a second look. Since

Hoodia is neither available nor proven, he advises that we steer clear of it.

There's still just one formula that has proven to work time and again: Eat less and exercise more.

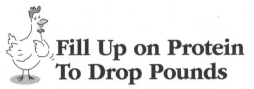

Fill Up on Protein To Drop Pounds

Nancy Appleton, PhD, retired nutritional consultant in San Diego, California, and author of *Stopping Inflammation* (Square One) and *Lick the Sugar Habit* (Avery).

While the Atkins Diet seems to have become yet another fad diet for many, there is a critical part of the diet that is a lesson to remember—in addition to its nutritional properties, protein is a critical component in helping to both lose weight and maintain weight loss. This is because protein is more satiating than carbohydrates, reducing cravings and appetite overall.

ALL PROTEINS ARE NOT CREATED EQUAL

Our bodies require protein for energy, growth and to build and repair muscles and bones. Because we cannot store protein, we need a new supply every day.

According to the Institute of Medicine (IOM), 10% to 35% of daily calorie intake should come from protein. Our consulting medical editor Andrew L. Rubman, ND, explains that the amount needed depends on your physical activity level. *Each protein is made up of 20 basic building blocks called amino acids...*

•**Complete proteins** (meat, poultry, fish, eggs, milk and cheese) contain all the essential amino acids your body requires each day.

•**Plant or vegetable proteins** (beans, soy, whole grains, nuts) are usually low in one or more essential amino acids. If you follow a vegetarian diet, make sure that you eat a variety of plant foods in order to take in all the protein you need.

HOW MUCH PROTEIN IS ENOUGH?

The average person requires 50 grams (g) to 65 g of protein daily, and it's easy to meet this requirement—for instance, with wholegrain breakfast cereal and low-fat milk...rice and beans for lunch...a snack of peanut butter on apple slices or a hard-boiled egg...and halibut or tuna for dinner.

To give you an idea of how quickly the numbers add up, protein contents of food include...

•**A four-ounce serving of meat, poultry or fish** (the size of a deck of cards) contains 25 g to 35 g of protein.

•**Two ounces of hard cheese contain 16 g.**

•**One cup of low-fat milk provides 8 g of protein.**

•**Two tablespoons of peanut butter contain 8 g.**

•**One cup of cooked lentils contains 18 g.**

•**Two slices of whole wheat bread provide 6 g.**

HOW MUCH PROTEIN IS TOO MUCH?

But can there be too much of a good thing? Yes. Those with liver or kidney disease are particularly vulnerable to trouble with larger-than-normal amounts of protein, or sudden increases in protein intake, due to difficulty disposing of the waste products of protein metabolism.

As for the general population, there is also increasing concern that too much protein long-term may affect healthy people, putting them at increased risk of kidney stones and bone-thinning osteoporosis. While a few weeks of high-protein dieting is not likely to do any harm, over time, processing excess protein may pull too much calcium from bone.

PROTEIN AND HEALTH

About those high-protein diet plans... obesity is a major health challenge in this country, and getting to an appropriate weight should be a goal for everyone. In the South Beach, Zone and Atkins diets, the idea is to replace empty carbohydrates such as white bread and pasta (which lead to booms and busts in your blood sugar and appetite) with protein, which is more satisfying and keeps the metabolism functioning on an even keel. Protein stimulates the digestive tract and lingers in the stomach, making you feel fuller longer.

Do high-protein diets work? Recent studies show that they are as effective as low-fat diets, and you may even lose a few more pounds in the first six months. Long-term they can be dangerous to your health. Your best bet for the long term is to eat less and exercise more, as always, and consult your physician before starting any diet.

PROTEIN CHOICES

Identifying protein-rich foods is not hard. But you must make the choice to include them in your diet. *Some suggestions to help you do it...*

•**Change your mindset.** Forget about traditional western notions of acceptable breakfast food. If you don't like eggs, consider soup for breakfast. It's warm and satisfying without being too heavy.

•**Look at the whole picture.** Keep in mind that beans, soy, whole grains and nuts supply healthy protein with fiber and nutrients, and without most of the saturated fat of meat. If you eat red meat, choose lean cuts.

•**Consume soy in moderation.** While soy is high in protein, there have been suggestions recently that it's not the nutritional superstar we once believed.

•**Rotate your proteins.** Eating a variety of protein-containing foods each day will ensure that you take in all the amino acids your body needs.

•**Go nuts for health.** A number of studies, including Harvard's Nurses' Health Study and the Brigham and Women's Hospital's Physicians' Health Study, have shown that eating protein-packed nuts several times a week helps lower cholesterol and cardiovascular risk. There are even suggestions that eating nuts might help prevent type 2 diabetes.

By incorporating a variety of healthy proteins into your diet, you will be providing more sustainable energy to your body—your body will run better and longer, without keeping you running to the pantry for more fuel.

Surprising Symptoms Causes by Too Much Bread

Andrew L. Rubman, ND, consulting medical editor for *Bottom Line's Daily Health News* and director of the Southbury Clinic for Traditional Medicines in Southbury, Connecticut.

National Digestive Diseases Information Clearinghouse, *http://digestive.niddk.nih.gov.*

It's often hard to pin down just what's causing common gastrointestinal complaints such as gas, bloating, diarrhea or abdominal pain. Add to that some fatigue and a vague sense of not feeling quite right, and what do you have? Possibly gluten intolerance—an intolerance of a protein (gluten) in wheat, barley and rye, suggests *Bottom Line's Daily Health News* consulting medical editor, Andrew L. Rubman, ND. A degree of gluten intolerance is common in the population and frequently under-diagnosed, he says.

GLUTEN SENSITIVITY RANGES FROM MILD TO SEVERE

Gluten intolerance is an autoimmune condition encompassing a variety of symptoms. In people with this condition, gluten causes some degree of change in the mucosal tissue lining the small intestine, says Dr. Rubman. When the severity of gluten intolerance progresses beyond a certain point of frequency, duration and intensity, it is called celiac disease.

Celiac disease affects one in 133 Americans, damaging their small intestine and causing lasting problems with nutrient absorption. Other reactions that may be associated with gluten intolerance include discomfort that is mild and fleeting, such as cramps or a feeling of uncomfortable fullness...sudden mid-meal bloat...chronic diarrhea. When people go to the doctor complaining of these problems—especially those on the milder end of the spectrum—it may be very difficult to diagnose the cause, since mild gluten sensitivities don't always show up on blood tests. Physicians may explain the symptoms away as a by-product of the passing years, anxiety or hereditary digestive difficulties. Typically medications are prescribed, including over-the-counter (OTC) remedies for gas or diarrhea—so the problem gets mistreated, and the cycle continues, usually getting worse.

INTESTINAL AND OTHER SYMPTOMS

Possible intestinal symptoms of gluten intolerance: Abdominal pain...bloating...gas...diarrhea...constipation...changes in appetite...nausea...vomiting...lactose intolerance...unexplained weight loss...and bloody, fatty or foul-smelling stools. As the problem persists, these symptoms may become chronic.

Possible nonintestinal symptoms include: Fatigue...depression...irritability... bone and joint pain...and behavioral changes. There may be skin problems, such as dermatitis herpetiformis, causing unattractive, uncomfortable rashes and water blister eruptions. Some hair loss is another possibility. Some suspect wheat proteins may be involved in degenerative diseases like MS, just as diet also plays a role in other autoimmune diseases such as diabetes. Many sufferers experience a sudden realization that the discomfort they've been living with is not necessarily "normal," leading them to look for the cause of their misery.

GOING AGAINST THE GRAIN

People diagnosed with celiac disease must maintain a gluten-free diet for the rest of their lives to allow the small intestine to heal and continue to function efficiently. For those with a mild form of gluten intolerance, total abstention isn't necessary, but moderating your intake is, says Dr. Rubman. People with mild gluten intolerance also suffer intestinal damage to a certain degree, and often times reducing gluten, rather than eliminating it, may be protective enough. However, this needs to be closely monitored by a physician.

Admittedly, this is easier said than done, since foods that contain gluten are all around us—in products such as bread, cereal, pasta, pizza, cookies, cakes and pies. Even more insidious is the fact that many processed foods—such as cold cuts, soy sauce, salad dressings, frozen yogurt and licorice—may also contain gluten. As yet, food labels are not required to identify gluten content, but the rules are being reconsidered. The US Food and Drug Administration (FDA) and the Codex Alimentarius, the international body responsible for setting food safety standards, are both proposing to standardize the definition of "gluten-free" for use on food labels. For now, a consumer's best bet may be to look for products that are specifically marked as "gluten-free." Gluten is also found in some medications (as an additive), so people should ask their pharmacist about any medications they are taking as well.

WHAT YOU CAN DO

If you frequently experience uncomfortable symptoms such as stomach upset, gas, irritability and fatigue, consider that the cause may be gluten intolerance. Stop eating all foods that contain wheat, barley, rye and oats for 10 days, advises Dr. Rubman. Instead, choose naturally gluten-free alternatives such as potatoes or rice, or grains such as amaranth, buckwheat and quinoa. Additionally, make it a point to consume more whole, fresh foods and fewer processed products.

If you don't have celiac disease, it's fine to slowly reincorporate two or three weekly servings of gluten back into the diet, enjoying foods such as pasta, cereal and sandwiches.

Note: People with severe symptoms that suggest celiac disease, including those with symptoms of irritable bowel syndrome (IBS), bloating, and appetite issues should consult their health-care providers before removing gluten from their diet. Otherwise, they may inadvertently cover up symptoms and further complicate later diagnosis by avoiding prompt medical care and diagnosis.

Secret to Strong Bones

Susan E. Brown, PhD, director of the Osteoporosis Education Project, Syracuse, New York, *www.betterbones.com*

Practically everyone knows how important calcium is to bone health, but there's another mineral that is equally critical, albeit in lesser amounts—potassium. In fact, a number of research studies recently focused on the connection between potassium and bone health, so word is getting out. One study, from the University of Basel, in Switzerland, showed that a group of postmenopausal women with low bone density had, on average, a 1% increase in density after a year of taking a particular potassium supplement.

BALANCING THE EQUATION

Susan E. Brown, PhD, director of the Osteoporosis Education Project in Syracuse, New York (*www.betterbones.com/* and *www.susanbrownphd.com*) says that "without question potassium is one of the most important bone nutrients." Exactly how potassium relates to bone health turns out to be fairly complicated.

Potassium is important in helping the body achieve a proper pH balance. In fact, when out of balance, you can die—really

fast—so our bodies make this process a high priority. How does it work? As part of its normal metabolic processing, the body creates acids, which exit our systems via the lungs and kidneys. To buffer the harshness of these acids and protect delicate kidney tissue, the body neutralizes them with alkaline (basic, as apposed to acidic) compounds derived from fruits and vegetables. These are stored in our blood, other fluids, in muscle tissue and above all in bones. Our skeleton, in fact, is our largest storehouse of alkaline mineral reserves.

The severe lack of fruits and vegetables in the modern American diet creates an acidic environment in many. To neutralize excess acid, we need alkaline compounds, which the body obtains first from easily available blood reserves, then from muscles, leading to muscle loss, and then by reaching into the bones. When and if that happens, we're left with bone breakdown and mineral loss—in other words, weakened bones.

NATURAL POTASSIUM CITRATE SOURCES

Now, back to potassium. The particular form of potassium that serves to buffer the acids is potassium citrate, generally found in fruits, vegetables and legumes. People who regularly consume enough potassium citrate through a diet rich in those foods assure their body sufficient alkaline compounds to avoid any need to call on emergency supplies for homeostasis. As Dr. Brown notes, "If you eat enough potassium-containing foods, which should not be a problem, you have the proper pH balance." However, people today load their diet with meat, poultry, dairy and grains, which are metabolized as acids, creating a greater need for offsetting alkalis. If the body can't find these in foods, it turns elsewhere, including body tissue and bones.

Though the US "Adequate Intake" (AI) potassium recommendation for adults is 4,700 milligrams (mg) per day, average consumption by adults in this country is around 2,200 mg for women and 3,200 mg for men.

Our lack of dietary potassium consumption looks to be a health crisis in the making, putting our bodies at risk for "consuming themselves," says Dr. Brown. In addition, potassium serves many other essential functions in the body. It contributes to nerve impulse transmission, muscle contraction and heart function, and also helps protect against stroke, kidney stones and high blood pressure.

GETTING IT RIGHT

Though we know too little potassium is a problem, too much can also be an issue. For example, a heart problem can arise if the kidney is weak and the potassium load is too great for the weakened kidneys to eliminate excesses. In fact, by law potassium supplements do not exceed 99 mg to discourage people from taking too much. Because excess potassium can accumulate in the blood when there is kidney weakness, potassium supplements should only be taken with care under proper supervision.

SUPPLEMENTS OR DIETARY HELP

The 1% increase in bone density achieved by the women in the Swiss study is considered significant, especially because it affected the hips and spine—two areas especially vulnerable to fracture. Though the study used potassium citrate supplements, it is possible, as Dr. Brown points out, to get what you need from dietary sources. You can achieve the AI of 4,700 mg per day by including 13 one-half cup servings of fruits, vegetables and legumes in your daily food intake. Admittedly, 13 sounds like a lot, but a large salad, for example, is four to six servings, a large apple is two. Those, plus a banana (440 mg, about one-and-a-half fruit servings) for an afternoon snack, and a baked potato at dinner along with a green vegetable and other vegetables, bring you easily to the goal of 4,700 mg.

If you decide to take potassium citrate supplements anyway, it is important to do so under the direction of a health-care professional who is well-versed in potassium needs and balance, such as a naturopathic physician or nutritionist.

Soda Is B-B-Bad For Your Bones

Katherine L. Tucker, PhD, a senior scientist at the USDA Jean Mayer Human Nutrition Research Center on Aging at Tufts University in Boston, where she is director of the Epidemiology and Dietary Assessment Program. She is also a professor at the Friedman School of Nutrition Science and Policy and an adjunct professor at Tufts Medical School. Dr. Tucker has contributed to more than 120 articles in nutrition and medical journals and is an associate editor for *The Journal of Nutrition.*

I s there anyone around who has a good word for sodas? Besides our kids? We already know that sugary soft drinks are one of the main culprits when it comes to obesity, and the ingredients in the diet versions have their own set of problems. Research from Tufts University in Boston provides even more fuel to the anti-soda fire.

Colas, in particular, have been connected to bone loss due to the phosphoric acid that gives them their tart flavor. The phosphoric acid is added to the colas as a flavoring agent and acts as a preservative. Researcher Katherine L. Tucker, PhD—director of the Epidemiology and Dietary Assessment Program at Tufts—explains that because not all soft drinks contain phosphoric acid they didn't see the bone loss with, for example, the lemon-lime or grape sodas used in the study. However, there are in fact quite a few non-colas that do contain phosphoric acid, including Dr. Pepper, root beer and cream sodas.

"The data are very strong," said Dr. Tucker. "Women drinking as few as three 12-ounce cans of cola a week showed significantly lower bone density." And this includes diet colas. "People drink huge amounts of diet cola thinking it can't possibly do any harm since it has no calories,"

Dr. Tucker warned. "But the research shows that diet soda is far from innocent when it comes to bones."

The reduction of bone mineral density was even greater with the consumption of caffeinated colas, since caffeine itself has a somewhat negative effect on bone density. "But even the decaf colas had an effect," says Dr. Tucker.

MEN, WOMEN AND COLA

Although the study only saw a pronounced effect of colas in women, Dr. Tucker believes that colas (and the phosphoric acid they contain) affect the bones of men as well. "Men usually have larger, denser bones, so it might take more cola to produce a measurable effect," she said. "However men who are smaller—and those who are worried about osteoporosis—should still be careful."

The American Beverage Association issued a press release in an attempt to cast doubts on the results of the Tufts University findings and assure people that colas had no significant negative effect on bone density. "Don't believe it," said Dr. Tucker.

Finding the Hidden Salt in Your Diet

Suzanne Havala Hobbs, DrPH, RD, author of *Get the Trans Fat Out*. Three Rivers. She is clinical assistant professor and director, Doctoral Program in Health Leadership, Department of Health Policy and Administration, School of Public Health, The University of North Carolina at Chapel Hill.

The US Food and Drug Administration (FDA) has made it mandatory to include information about trans fat on food labels, and recently experts have taken aim at another dietary ingredient. The American Medical Association (AMA) has called for new labeling about the salt content in foods. However, while there's nothing good to say about trans fat, it's a different story with sodium. Simply put, it is essential to our health.

It's just not healthy in the high quantities in which it appears in processed foods ranging from bread and cereal to canned soup, frozen snacks and prepared meals, and macaroni and cheese.

To look further into this matter, we consulted Suzanne Havala Hobbs, DrPH, RD, the author of *Get the Trans Fat Out* (Three Rivers). Dr. Havala Hobbs is a doctor of public health, and clinical assistant professor at the School of Public Health at The University of North Carolina at Chapel Hill. She says it's time to work on federal food policies that will support each American's efforts to cut down on sodium intake.

HIDDEN SODIUM IN PROCESSED FOODS

Reading labels is a good idea, especially for people who are salt-sensitive (individuals with high blood pressure that elevates or decreases with sodium intake or reduction) and must closely monitor their intake. Some people are more greatly affected by higher sodium intakes than others, but none of us need the extreme levels found in most processed foods, observes Dr. Havala Hobbs. However, reading all the labels in the world cannot protect your health if you continue to eat a diet high in processed foods and low in whole foods like fresh fruits and vegetables.

A BEHIND THE SCENES LOOK AT SALT REGULATION

Dr. Havala Hobbs shares some "behind the scenes" information about how salt is regulated. While the US government's Dietary Guidelines Advisory Committee discussed the Institute of Medicine's national sodium recommendation of 1,500 milligrams per day, the committee recommended a daily sodium level of less than 2,300 milligrams. Some experts speculate that it is because the food industry lobbied heavily against the lower level, arguing that salt is such an integral part of the food production system, used as a flavor enhancer, for texture, and as a preservative. The food industry also called the lower sodium level an unrealistic goal and suggested that the government not base its sodium recommendations on the 25% of population that is salt sensitive.

The government seemed to adopt the industry's position. The new salt guideline doesn't tell you what's really best for your health, says Dr. Havala Hobbs. Instead, it tells you what the government thinks is doable. Many people would likely benefit from reducing sodium intake considerably, and the sodium that naturally occurs in whole, unprocessed foods provides all the sodium we need, says Dr. Havala Hobbs.

GETTING THE SALT OUT

When it comes to sodium intake, the danger lies not so much in the salt shaker as in the hidden quantities of salt in processed foods. As a result, your best bet is to limit processed foods to the absolute minimum. For instance, sodium in canned beans, added as a preservative, can be easily rinsed away by placing beans in a colander and rinsing in running water, says Dr. Havala Hobbs. Unfortunately, there's often no practical way to remove excess sodium cooked into most processed food.

The take-home message is to spend the majority of your time in the outer aisles of supermarkets, where most whole foods, from fresh produce to meats and fish, are stocked.

The best recipe: Prepare more meals at home, using as many fresh ingredients as possible, and make foods in their natural state as large a part of your diet as you can, recommends Dr. Havala Hobbs. The greater the degree of processing and convenience of the prepared food, the lower the nutrient value and the greater the likelihood that the food is a health risk.

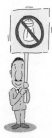

A Whole New Kind of Low-Calorie Sweetener

Garth Smith, PhD, plant physiologist, and co-founder, BioVittoria Limited, Hamilton, New Zealand.

Sometimes what's old is definitely new again. One of the latest rediscoveries is luo han guo (*siraitia grosvenori*), a Chinese fruit that has been used for more than 300 years in Asia in drinks and food and medicinally as a health enhancer. Luo han guo made its way to America more than 100 years ago when Cantonese immigrants, who helped build the transcontinental railroad, imported the dried fruit.

LATEST INCARNATION

Today, luo han guo is making its way back to our shores as a noncaloric, high-intensity sweetener for use in foods and other products. Luo han guo's sweet taste comes from compounds called *mogrosides*. They are 300 times sweeter than cane sugar, so a little bit goes a very long way.

Several companies are importing luo han guo, among them BioVittoria Limited, which is marketing its luo han guo product to manufacturers under the PureLo label as an ingredient in food, beverages and dietary supplements. We talked with one of BioVittoria's founders, plant physiologist Garth Smith, PhD, from New Zealand, to find out more about what we can expect from luo han guo sweeteners. The primary concern, of course, is about safety, given the continuing focus on the safety of low-calorie sweeteners.

TRACK RECORD OF SAFETY

Dr. Smith says that luo han guo has a proven history of safe use, as the fruit has been consumed as a food ingredient and healthful tea for hundreds of years. Toxicology studies in China and the US using animals have also taken place to evaluate PureLo's safety. According to Dr. Smith, the studies did not show any significant adverse effects on the health of the laboratory animals, even though they consumed very high levels of the PureLo product, much more than humans ever would. According to BioVittoria, PureLo has been declared GRAS (Generally Recognized As Safe) by an independent panel of experts. By attaining GRAS status, PureLo has met the US Food and Drug Administration (FDA) prescribed safety guidelines for food ingredients, and can legally be used as a sweetener in foods and beverages in the US.

HOW LUO HAN GUO WORKS

Some people speculate that PureLo satisfies taste bud sweet receptors (that tell the brain it is satisfied) as effectively as sugar and does not lead to increased sugar cravings. This means that luo han guo may truly be a low-calorie sweetener that helps people lose weight.

How it works: The unique structure of the mogroside molecule tastes sweet...the taste buds sense them, but the body can't digest them. This provides satisfaction without the bulge (artificial sweeteners can often create even more cravings since they physiologically don't satisfy the sweet craving).

Luo han guo is currently available in combination with other sweeteners both as an ingredient in foods and as a solo sweetener. Finally, a low-calorie sweetener that may truly be satisfying.

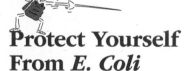

Protect Yourself From *E. Coli*

Ronald H. Schmidt, PhD, food science professor, University of Florida, Gainesville, Florida, and author of the *Food Safety Handbook*. Wiley.

US Food and Drug Administration, *www.fda.gov.*

In the wake of recent *E. coli* contaminated spinach and jalapeno scares, many consumers have become nervous about fresh produce in general. What can we do to protect ourselves and our families?

The truth is that the food supply is very safe, and these outbreaks are relatively uncommon. Still, there are many simple steps we can—and should—consistently take as consumers to ensure food safety. Ronald H. Schmidt, PhD, a food science professor at the University of Florida and author of the Food Safety Handbook (Wiley), offers a number of helpful tips...

AT THE STORE

•**Choose fresh fruits and veggies that are not bruised or damaged.** The bruises provide an environment that allows bacteria to grow.

•**When buying produce such as packaged salads or fresh-cut fruit cups,** make certain they are refrigerated or surrounded by ice.

•**Ask your grocer to bag fresh produce separately from meat, poultry or seafood** to avoid cross-contamination on the outside of the packaging.

IN YOUR KITCHEN

•**Store fresh fruits and vegetables that need refrigeration** (such as melons, berries, spinach, lettuce, etc.) in a clean, cold refrigerator.

•**Refrigerate precut or peeled produce within two hours of purchase.**

•**Always store raw foods separately from cooked foods.** Don't place cooked food on plates that held raw meat, poultry or seafood.

•**Wash your hands for 20 seconds with warm water and soap** before and after handling any fresh or raw food product, including produce.

•**Cut away damaged or bruised areas on fresh fruits and vegetables before preparing or eating.** When in doubt, throw it out.

•**Wash all produce under cold, running water.** Although some precut produce is prewashed (it should say so on the package), Dr. Schmidt still advises consumers to give it a quick rinse in the colander. Even if you plan to peel produce before eating, it is important to wash it first. Surprisingly, the US Food and Drug Administration (FDA) does not recommend washing fruits and vegetables with soap or detergent or using a commercial produce wash.

•**Scrub firm produce,** such as melons and cucumbers, with a produce brush. Dr. Schmidt cautions that the brush itself should be properly washed and sanitized, something which is often forgotten. Wash it in the dishwasher.

•**To further reduce the chance of bacterial contamination,** dry produce with a clean cloth towel or paper towel.

•**Use separate cutting boards for meat, seafood, poultry and produce.** Wash cutting boards, utensils, dishes and counter surfaces with hot water and soap after contact with raw meat, poultry or seafood.

•**Don't leave perishable, prepared or leftover foods at room temperature for more than two hours** (or more than one hour on a hot summer day—90° F and over).

•**Cook foods to a safe temperature.** Most harmful organisms are killed at temperatures between 145° F and 165° F, depending on whether you are cooking meat, seafood, poultry or with eggs.

•**Defrost food safely.** Thaw tightly wrapped (so it won't drip on other food items) meat, poultry or seafood in the refrigerator on the lowest shelf (again, to prevent dripping). You can also thaw frozen food in the microwave on the "defrost" setting or immerse it in cold water and change the water every 30 minutes. Do not defrost or marinate food on a kitchen counter.

•**If you are in a high-risk category (elderly, children, pregnant women, immunocompromised, etc.),** avoid foods such as raw or undercooked seafood, undercooked meat or poultry, raw sprouts, unpasteurized milk or juices and soft cheeses. Always avoid raw eggs as they could contain *Salmonella* bacteria, which is destroyed by brief heat exposure.

What to Eat for Better Sleep

Chin Moi Chow, PhD, researcher, Delta Sleep Research Unit, and senior lecturer, discipline of exercise and sport science, The University of Sydney in Australia. Coresearchers included Ahmad Afaghi and Helen O'Connor, PhD.

Don't you sometimes feel as if researchers spend a lot of time (and money) figuring out what everyone in the world already knows? That was the thought when we recently read about a pilot study that seemed to surmise that eating carbohydrates at bedtime may make you sleepy. Isn't that why moms always offer a snack of toast at bedtime? But the relationship between carbs and sleep is a little more complicated—and interesting—than it would initially appear.

First, some background: Researchers at The University of Sydney in Australia wanted to see if the glycemic index (GI) of a meal eaten before bed would have any effect on sleep. Remember that the glycemic index is a measure of how much your blood sugar goes up (and how quickly) after eating a particular food. Previous research has suggested that high-carb foods raise tryptophan, which then converts to serotonin and makes you sleepy.

"We hypothesized that a high glycemic index meal was going to be effective in inducing sleep," Chin Moi Chow, PhD, tells us. "We believed it would directly impact the increase of tryptophan." She and her colleagues gave 12 healthy men three meals on three separate occasions. One meal was a high glycemic meal one hour before bed…one was a high glycemic meal four hours before bed…and the third was a low glycemic meal of jasmine rice with just a little protein from vegetables four hours before bedtime.

HIGH GI MEALS AND INSOMNIA

Researchers found that the men who ate the high glycemic meal four hours before bedtime fell asleep the fastest, in only nine minutes on average. The low-glycemic diners who ate at the same time took almost twice as long to fall asleep, while the men who had the high glycemic meal one hour before bed fell asleep a little sooner than the low carb diners (about 15 minutes). Though the research leaves some questions unanswered, and therefore should not be considered "conclusive," Dr. Chow did sum up the findings, suggesting that "a high GI carb meal may help people with insomnia, both occasional and chronic."

But is that really a smart way to eat? We asked Dr. Chow about the wisdom of recommending high-carb meals at night, which increase insulin and may increase the amount of calories converted to fat. "We caution that it may not be appropriate for people who are obese or who have diabetes to use a high GI meal or snack to promote sleep, since these individuals are often advised to adopt a low glycemic eating plan," says Dr. Chow. And she is quick to point out that the men in the study were good sleepers, and the effect might be different with chronic insomniacs.

Stay tuned: "We are currently planning a study of that," she says.

"Getting a good night's sleep is about having good sleep habits," Dr. Chow reminds us. "That means regular bedtime and wake-up time, and avoiding caffeine and alcohol before bedtime. If you struggle to fall asleep even after paying attention to those things, you can discuss with your doctor if a high GI evening meal might help you."

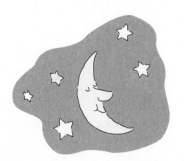

Drink Up to Lower Cancer Risk and More

Susan M. Kleiner, PhD, RD, CNS. Dr. Kleiner is owner of High Performance Nutrition, a consulting firm on Mercer Island, Washington, and author of several books, including *The Good Mood Diet: Feel Great While You Lose Weight* (Springboard), *Power Eating*, 3rd Edition (Human Kinetics) and *The Powerfood Nutrition Plan* (Rodale). Dr. Kleiner is cofounder of the International Society of Sports Nutrition.

A recent article in *The Wall Street Journal* stated how beverage companies are in search of drinks that will appeal to children. They mentioned Starbucks specifically, which is targeting kids with Banana Crème Frappuccino Blended Crème coffee-free beverages. With many schools banning sodas and sugar-sweetened drinks from their vending machines, and childhood obesity on the rise, it seems clear that there is only one drink that should really be given to children on a regular basis—water. That said, what's a parent to do? Children are constantly plied with unhealthy soft drinks. Even at special children's events, organizers don't think twice about offering Coke or Sprite as the main beverage choices. It seems we have a way to go. Susan M. Kleiner, PhD, RD, CNS (Certified Nutrition Specialist), owner of High Performance Nutrition, a consulting firm on Mercer Island, Washington, and cofounder of the International Society of Sports Nutrition, concurs.

THE SIMPLEST WAY TO REDUCE CANCER RISK

According to Dr. Kleiner, there is mounting data about the healthful benefits of drinking water, including the strong epidemiological evidence that average-sized people who drink as little as five or six glasses of water a day may have a significantly decreased risk of cancer of the bladder, colon cancer and fatal coronary heart disease. Other research shows that about eight glasses of water a day in healthy adults may contribute to weight loss. "The numbers are there," says Dr. Kleiner. "And this data on water—not just fluids, but regular water—keeps coming up, even when the studies control for other good health habits such as eating more fiber and vegetables. There's something about water that's really good for you. It's a benign, noncaloric beverage that clearly benefits you."

BUT...I DON'T LIKE WATER

Kids aren't the only ones who complain that they don't like water. Grown-ups complain too. Perhaps it's not that they don't like it...it's that they have been trained to like other things that are richer, sweeter, and of course, more profitable for manufacturers. For kids and grown-ups alike, it often just takes time to readjust your taste buds to water's lightness. "If your kids don't like the taste, do something about it," Dr. Kleiner advises. "If your tap water tastes 'funny,' get a filtration system (like Brita) or buy bottled water. If you don't like it warm, make sure it's cold." Dr. Kleiner suggested making your own "homemade" water drinks. "Start with sparkling water and add a splash of grape juice, or concentrated pomegranate, cherry or cranberry juice," she says. The berry concentrates provide an extra pinch of antioxidants as well.

"You have to educate your kids about this," Dr. Kleiner concludes. "Encouraging kids to drink water is really important—and if you haven't done that, it's time to start. Sit down with them and talk to them about their nutrition the way you do about drugs, smoking, school and everything else."

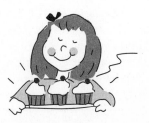

Sweet! Six Ways to Tame Sugar Addiction

Kathleen DesMaisons, PhD, author, *The Sugar Addict's Total Recovery Program*, Ballantine, and CEO and President, Radiant Recovery Addiction Center, Albuquerque, New Mexico. *www.radiantrecovery.com.*

We are born loving sugar—anyone who doubts this need only witness the way a baby's face lights up when her tongue connects with a sweet taste. But for some people this natural pleasure takes an unhealthy turn, triggering a craving that some experts call a "sugar addiction." That's strong language. The medical definition of "addiction" is a "habitual, physiological and psychological dependence on a substance or practice beyond one's voluntary control." While some feel more comfortable calling this a sugar "sensitivity," Kathleen DesMaisons, PhD, author of several books including *The Sugar Addict's Total Recovery Program* (Ballantine) and the head of Radiant Recovery in Albuquerque, New Mexico, a treatment program for recovering addicts including those hooked on sugar, says it is more complicated than that. Though less obviously destructive, she says that sugar, much the same as alcohol, nicotine or drugs, can produce addiction. In addition, Dr. DesMaisons says that excessive sugar is harmful to your health, due to sugar's association with inflammation in the body, along with numerous diseases.

SUGAR ADDICTION DEFINED: MORE THAN A SWEET TOOTH

Sugar addiction is not the same as enjoying desserts or an occasional afternoon sweet. What distinguishes sugar addicts is a lack (perhaps even inheritable) of the ability to walk away from sweet treats. Dr. DesMaisons explains that nonaddicted people—those who do not have the sugar sensitivity that sets them up for a sugar addiction—enjoy desserts, sodas and candy with a take-it-or-leave-it attitude. If they see they are consuming too many sugary foods, they simply cut back. Sugar addicts are amazed at this attitude and ability, she says, because they can't relate to either of them. They, too, may vow to eliminate sweets but within days they discover they can't say no. Literally finding themselves in physical withdrawal, they "give in" to sugar. Not only does it please their taste buds, sugar can act as a drug to heighten *beta-endorphin* levels in the brain. This is a "feel-good" opioid peptide neurotransmitter that the body uses to dull pain and enhance the body's sense of well-being.

THE REBOUND EFFECT

Though it's normal to have a rebound effect after a high-sugar snack, becoming edgy when blood glucose levels once again drop, in addicted people the rebound effect is much more dramatic. Dr. DesMaisons describes how, when the beta-endorphin levels crash, the sugar-addicted person ends up feeling awful both physically and emotionally.

SUGAR AND WEIGHT

Not surprisingly, many sugar addicts are overweight, says Dr. DesMaisons. She believes that most people who are heavy are likely sugar-addicted. Which comes first—the addiction or the excess weight? They actually seem to work together, she says. People of normal weight can also be sugar-addicted, and—most importantly—no matter what the scale says, all sugar addicts put their health at risk. By pouring so much sugar into their systems, they frequently end up with high blood glucose levels, a condition that can lead eventually to diabetes in susceptible people.

TAMING THE BEAST

The healing process consists of stabilizing your blood sugar while you make slow and planned changes to your lifestyle. Dr. DesMaisons advises not going cold turkey—it won't work. *She offers these strategies, as integral components of the healing process...*

•**Eat three meals a day,** including breakfast, every day, on a regular schedule. At every meal, be sure to have protein and some complex carbs—vegetables and whole-grain products.

•**As you feel more stable, wean yourself from sugary foods** including ice cream, cookies, pastries and all those really gooey, sugar-rich foods. Also target beverages with high fructose corn syrup, an insidious type of sugar that may also destabilize glucose metabolism.

•**Avoid snacking.** If you must eat between meals, stay away from sugar. Similarly, do not eat refined and processed carbohydrates such as white breads, bagels and other baked goods, as they can cause reactions in the body similar to sugar in a sugar sensitive person.

•**Do not drink soda, including diet soda.** In fact, do not consume any artificial sweeteners in foods or drinks, because their sweet taste actually triggers a desire for more sweets in some. Check labels for all ingredients ending in the letters "ose." They are all forms of sugar. If there are several, avoid this food—even if they are listed at the end.

•**Avoid all alcohol.** Alcohol and sugar activate the same neurochemicals. Also, beer and wine are made from sugars. Changing your diet can help with this task and make it easier.

•**Exercise regularly.** Do whatever kind you like best, but do it almost every day. In addition to being healthy and burning calories, exercise releases beta-endorphins, which is the natural and healthy way to access the neurotransmitters that lead to that wonderful sense of well-being we all crave.

You'll need to follow this regimen for several months to finally overcome your sugar addiction. If you occasionally fall off the wagon, get back on. Slip-ups are part of the learning process that will lead ultimately to ownership of your new skill—how to live sugar- and addiction-free.

Infectobesity— Can a Virus Make You Fat?

Nikhil Dhurandhar, PhD, associate professor in the department of infection and obesity at Pennington Biomedical Research Center, Louisiana State University System, Baton Rouge. He and his research team have been at the forefront in the investigation of obesity of infectious origin.

All is not fair in the obesity battle… some people gain weight easily and struggle to lose, while others who eat fairly freely and don't exercise much are able to maintain a trim and healthy figure. Though obesity is known to have multiple causes, researchers have tended to focus on the genetic and behavioral ones—with good reason, as those usually are the culprit. But some scientists have set out in a new direction, thanks to research spanning over 20 years that shows certain infections—specifically some viruses— may be associated with obesity.

It's an intriguing story that poses an interesting question: What if catching a virus makes you more vulnerable to developing obesity?

ONCE UPON A TIME…

In 1988 Nikhil Dhurandhar, PhD, a biochemist and young physician in India, happened to be chatting with a fellow researcher about a virus that was killing local chickens. Autopsies on the dead birds revealed, oddly, that the infected ones had excess abdominal fat. His curiosity piqued, Dr. Dhurandhar injected some healthy chickens with the virus, and they too grew chubby. On a hunch, Dr. Dhurandhar then examined human blood samples from a group of obese male and female patients for presence of the virus antibodies. He found that 20% of them had indeed been exposed to the virus. That percentage is not likely to be found by chance, so he hypothesized that there must be a connection. It was an important discovery for two reasons—first, that the SMAM-1 virus

was likely to have jumped to humans, which had not been thought possible back then…and second, that there could be a viral connection to obesity.

MORE THAN ONE VILLAIN

Fast forward a few decades. Now an associate professor of infection and obesity at Pennington Biomedical Research Center at Louisiana State University System in Baton Rouge, Dr. Dhurandhar has been fighting conventional wisdom in an attempt to pin down a pathogenic role in obesity—with considerable success. While researchers have isolated 10 different pathogens that are linked to obesity in animals or humans, his research team is currently investigating one of them intensely.

OBESITY CAUSING VIRUS

It's not the particular virus that is important, he says, so much as the concept of what he calls "infectobesity." "It's the idea that obesity might be caused—in some cases—by an infectious origin. We're currently investigating only one of the obesity-causing viruses, but imagine how many might be out there awaiting discovery?" The virus Dr. Dhurandhar's team is working with is not an animal virus or pathogen, but a human adenovirus known as *Adenovirus 36*, or AD-36. In one study, the researchers have detected AD-36 antibodies in 30% of obese people—and, interestingly, the antibodies were also present in 11% of nonobese people.

Dr. Dhurandhar stresses that he's not suggesting a virus is at the root of all obesity. However, he notes, "an interesting fact is that the 11% exposed to the virus who are not obese are significantly heavier than the nonobese people who haven't been exposed. This 11% is not technically obese— at least not yet—but the fact that they're significantly heavier than those with no antibodies shows that the exposure to the virus may be having an effect."

ALAS, NO MAGIC POTION

Dr. Dhurandhar warns that no one should be fooled into thinking a magic potion in the form of drugs or a pill to combat the problem will soon be available—though he does hope to someday develop a vaccine to protect against this particular cause of obesity.

According to their studies, AD-36 increases the number of fat cells and the amount of fat stored in them, which possibly contributes to obesity. Dr. Dhurandhar says, they are currently working on mapping out a detailed molecular mechanism. Yet even as pathogens that contribute to obesity are identified and treatments become available to fight them, he notes that people will still need to take responsibility for eating right and exercising regularly.

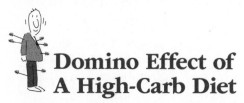

Domino Effect of A High-Carb Diet

David Leonardi, MD. Dr. Leonardi specializes in anti-aging medicine and was medical director of the Cenegenics Medical Institute before starting the Leonardi Executive Health Institute in Greenwood Village, Colorado. Visit his Web site at *www.go2Lehi.com.*

Many sugary foods are high glycemic foods, which trigger a rapid rise in blood sugar, triggering a rapid rise in insulin, which in turn triggers a rapid drop in blood sugar, creating hunger and cravings. Why? Because when blood sugar drops, we're supposed to burn glycogen and fat for energy. But the persistent high insulin level blocks those processes. We run out of energy and the cravings begin. So…we eat! It's the classic blood sugar roller coaster.

GLYCEMIC INDEX FOOD RANKING

One way to predict the effect a food has on your blood sugar is a measure of the speed at which it is digested and turned into glucose. To measure this, foods are ranked on something called the glycemic index (GI). This measures how fast a food raises blood sugar compared with glucose. But it's been controversial, because

nutritionists point out that it's only a measure of one food eaten alone…and that it doesn't take into account portion size as the glycemic load—the GI times the amount of carbohydrates consumed—does. Now, recent research is showing that the glycemic load actually does predict how your body will respond to food, even when it's eaten in combination with other foods. "So if 50% of your meal has a GI of 50, and 50% of your meal has a GI of 100, the overall glycemic impact of the meal will be approximately 75, though the calculation is far more complex than a simple average," explains David Leonardi, MD, of the Leonardi Executive Health Institute in Greenwich Village, Colorado. (A GI of 45 or more is considered "high" whereas a GI of 40 or below is considered "favorable," says Dr. Leonardi.)

THE CARRYOVER OF THE INDEX

Even more important, the glycemic impact of a meal can influence how your body digests, absorbs and processes the next meal, even if the next meal is 10 hours away (the typical time elapsed from a typical evening dinner to breakfast the next day).

Why do we care? Research suggests that continual meals with high net glycemic indices will put an undue burden on your pancreas, among other organs. The more things we can do to control blood sugar (and insulin) fluctuations, the better off we are. High blood sugar, insulin levels and blood sugar swings are linked to diabetes, obesity, heart disease and even some cancers.

Dr. Leonardi says that "It's been previously shown that the glycemic load—or impact—of breakfast can affect your blood sugar response to lunch four hours later by changing insulin sensitivity, which in turn impacts nutrient uptake and management." The significant finding in this latest study is that the time interval is even longer than was previously thought. What you eat at dinner can actually influence how your body will respond to breakfast.

How Eating Out Packs On The Pounds

Kathleen Keller, PhD, New York Obesity Research Center, Columbia University, New York City.

When you stop for lunch at a family-style restaurant, you assume—correctly—that the food will be piled high on your plate. Unfortunately, many health experts consider those giant portions one reason Americans have become so fat—logical enough, given that Americans consume one-third of their daily calories outside the home and have added, on average, 206 additional calories to their daily load. The US Food and Drug Administration (FDA) has been eyeing this problem as well. Consequently, it commissioned a report to address the nation's obesity problem in relation to "away-from-home" foods.

REPORTING THE OBVIOUS

The report has some excellent—and in some ways very obvious—ideas, particularly for the food service industry, including increasing the number of lower-calorie and healthier dishes...adding more fruit and vegetable ingredients in menu items... and giving customers calorie counts and nutrition information for foods. The problem is that providing this information may be too expensive for many restaurants. As for smaller portions, restaurants succeed by giving customers what they want and, at least for now, big portions fit that bill. What, then, to make of a report that means well, but is fraught with stumbling blocks for implementation?

For input on this, we called nutritionist and obesity researcher, Kathleen Keller, PhD, at the New York Obesity Research Center at Columbia University in New York City. The problem, she says, has so many layers that it is unfair to target restaurants alone and to ask them to change practices that have helped create their success. The food industry in general is part of the problem. Everything about food is getting bigger as packaged foods—already filled with calorically dense additives—are sold in larger sizes, increasing profits for manufacturers and boosting sales by value-driven customers.

HOW TO DOWNSIZE

Many American adults have lost the ability to gauge how much food their bodies need, eating big at home as well as when out. Combine that with the fact that they're not burning off enough calories. Excuses run the gamut from no time...too tired...or simply that there are no local sidewalks on which to safely walk. There are many issues at work here, including a reluctance to take personal responsibility for changing one's eating habits.

With all of this in mind, Dr. Keller makes the following recommendations...

•**Restaurants should consider adding healthier, less fattening sections to their menus.** Applebee's has done this with its Weight Watchers section, which lists the point value of foods as well as calories, fats and fiber.

•**The food industry should find ways to market smaller portion packages** that are as economical for consumers to purchase as the large ones. (In the meantime, she says, consumers should avoid preparing whole packages, but rather split and store contents of large packaged foods into smaller portions to assure appropriately sized servings.)

•**Communities must provide space and opportunity for all residents to walk regularly** and places for children to be physically active each day.

•**Education about health and food should begin early and become much more widespread.** Through education people can begin to learn or relearn to provide their bodies with what they really need, in terms of quantities as well as nutrition. But Dr. Keller cautions that this process has a long learning curve and takes commitment and discipline. It doesn't happen overnight, she adds, but eventually it is possible for people to learn how to listen to their body's signals...and eat when, what and how much their body actually needs.

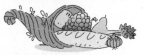

Healthier, Protein-Rich Vegetarian Diets

Sonja Pettersen, NMD, naturopathic medical doctor. She is licensed to practice primary care medicine specializing in natural therapeutics in Arizona and is based in Scottsdale.

Andrew L. Rubman, ND, consulting medical editor for *Bottom Line's Daily Health News* and director of the Southbury Clinic for Traditional Medicines in Southbury, Connecticut.

What's the secret to being a successful vegetarian? Can a vegetarian get enough protein without relying on dairy or soy, given that both are controversial with regard to their healthful benefits?

The short answer is yes, but it's a complicated question for two reasons. All protein is not created equal. Protein varies in "biological value" based in part on its amino acid content. Despite whatever other shortcomings they may have, meat, dairy and even some soy products tend to score high in the amino acid ratings. Vegetable protein (beans, nuts, whole grains) do not score as well as meat or dairy protein. The subject is further complicated by the fact that health experts—particularly those who are partial to vegetarianism—disagree about how much protein is really needed for optimal health.

T. Colin Campbell, PhD, whose China Project study—which is among the longest running epidemiological studies of dietary habits and health, investigated 65 counties and 6,500 adults—found a relationship between reduced rates of chronic degenerative disease and reduced animal protein intake. The generally accepted "recommended" amount of protein for an average adult—not too high, not too low—is 1 gram (g) per kilogram (kg) of body weight. This translates to a little less than half a g of protein per pound. For an "average" 140-pound person, that's about 63 g a day.

PROTEIN SOURCES

Assuming you're not a vegan, eggs—which are considered a complete protein—can be a great help here. But you'll need more than eggs or you'll need to eat a lot of them. One large egg has about 6 grams of protein. Nuts and seeds and most legumes are also decent sources, each with their own unique amino acid composition (amino acids are the building blocks of protein, and you need to take in at least nine essential ones through diet since the body can't make them on its own). That's why careful planning and combining is so important in a vegetarian diet.

Sonja Pettersen, NMD, is a naturopathic physician—and mother—in Scottsdale, Arizona, who maintains a vegetarian lifestyle and home. "Can you get enough protein?" she asked rhetorically. "Absolutely. But only if you pay attention." Dr. Pettersen is most concerned about people who simply eliminate meat and fish and consider themselves vegetarian. "A bag of chips and cola doesn't have meat in it, but it's not a healthy vegetarian meal," she says.

Dr. Pettersen says that it is critically important for vegetarians to know where their protein is coming from. "You need to learn the numbers." In her own practice, Dr. Pettersen recommends that her vegetarian patients write down what they're eating in order to be able to monitor their protein intake.

Dr. Pettersen suggests some tricks for upping the amount of high-quality protein in the diet without using soy or dairy...

• **Use whole grains whenever possible.** Two of Dr. Pettersen's favorites are amaranth and quinoa, both high in protein.

• **Combine grains** (barley, bulgur, cornmeal, oats, rice, etc.) with legumes (beans, lentils, peas)...or nuts/seeds (such as sesame seeds, sunflower seeds or walnuts) with legumes.

Examples: Peanut butter on whole wheat bread...rice and black beans...salad with beans, chick peas (legumes) and various nuts.

A note about whey: While many people recommend whey as a good source of protein, especially for vegetarians, *Bottom Line's Daily Health News* consulting medical editor Andrew L. Rubman, ND, points out that whey comes from cow's milk and contains two of the main allergenic proteins found in cow's milk—*alpha lactalbumin* and *beta-lactoglobulin*. So those avoiding the allergenic properties of cow's milk need to stay away from it.

IS VEGETARIANISM HEALTHIER?

"It's definitely healthier than the standard American diet," Dr. Pettersen says. "Vegetarians and vegans have less inflammation, and, if they're following a healthy vegetarian diet, they take in more fiber and antioxidants, all of which have protective benefits. And with plant foods you are also taking in enzymes that are helpful for your digestion."

But, she concludes, it may be easier "for most to just reduce the amount of meat in their diet as opposed to eliminate it."

Is Your Diet Making You Crazy?

Carol Simontacchi, MS, CCN, and author of *The Crazy Makers: How the Food Industry Is Destroying Our Brains and Harming Our Children*, Tarcher, as well as several other best-selling books on nutrition and health. She can be found at *www.flywithwings. com*.

In the early 1960s, Rachel Carson wrote the classic *Silent Spring* (Houghton Mifflin) in which she called for accountability from industrial polluters. Many have since been forced to clean up and undo the damage they've done. Similarly, there are those who believe that the food industry is polluting our bodies and needs to be held accountable.

Carol Simontacchi, MS, CCN (Certified Clinical Nutritionist), author of *The Crazy Makers* (Tarcher), says it isn't just a coincidence that use of medications for attention deficit hyperactivity disorder (ADHD) are on the rise as the quality of the American diet has declined.

YOU ARE WHAT YOU EAT

We've heard it before. You are what you eat. And, in particular, Simontacchi is concerned that not enough attention is being paid to the connection between our diets and our brains. The implications are enormous, influencing everything from behavior disturbances in childhood to memory loss and cognitive decline in old age. "The food industry has altered our consumption of basic nutrients so our brains are deprived of the essential building blocks required for them to function optimally," she explained. "Our food is literally making us crazy."

RESEARCH FOR THE CRAZY MAKERS

As part of the research for her book, *The Crazy Makers*, Simontacchi conducted a study on the influence of diet on cognition and mood. She gave a test group of typical high school students—who had been either skipping breakfast or grabbing a donut or some other carbohydrate-filled nutritionally devoid food—a breakfast shake of protein, carbohydrates, vitamins, minerals and omega-3 fatty acids. She did a before-and-after comparison of their results on a standardized mood test (Profile of Mood States, or POMS), which measures, among other things, tension, anger, depression, hostility, fatigue and confusion. "The results were so good, we had to rerun the statistics to verify the findings," Simontacchi told me. "The drink made a significant difference in how these teenagers felt emotionally. Since low levels of certain amino acids and essential fats have been frequently shown in both animal and human studies to be

173

associated with aggression, hostility and other behavior problems, the results were not surprising to her.

THE BIG 3

According to Simontacchi, there are three culprits that create the problem. They are sugar, sodium and food additives.

•**Sugar.** "The typical American consumes 200 pounds of sugar and artificial sweeteners a year," she says. "Sugar is an anti-nutrient. That means your body has to use up precious resources just to handle it. For someone deficient in zinc, or in the B vitamins, that's a huge problem. And when you sit down and have a breakfast cereal that has more sugar in it than cola, your blood sugar goes through the roof. Ultimately that leads to high insulin—a risk factor for diabetes and metabolic syndrome—and then to high cortisol, a hormone that has been shown to shrink the hippocampus in the brain."

•**Sodium.** "We don't commonly think about sodium," Simontacchi explains, "but kids typically consume huge amounts. Nearly all processed foods and snack foods have high sodium content and little potassium. Salty foods make you want more of them and set up a cycle of cravings." According to Simontacchi, sodium is our new "drug of choice." "When you have a steady intake of a lot of sodium and very little potassium for balance, as is typical in the American diet, it can cause anxiety, confusion, irritability and crankiness.

•**Aspartame and other food additives.** Finally, there are food additives. Asked to name a particularly bad one, she quickly named aspartame, the artificial sweetener known as NutraSweet. "There's not a lot of science to back this up," she points out carefully, "but here's what we do know. Aspartame is an *excitotoxin*—that means it works on the brain. There are more complaints to the US Food and Drug Administration (FDA) about aspartame than any other substance on the American market. Many of those complaints involve headaches, and some involve epilepsy.

I think the neurological effects of these chemicals is a whole area that needs to be explored in much greater depth."

"As far as the other chemical food additives, such as flavorings, colorings and preservatives, for example, no one is really studying them for their effects on behavior," she adds. "Sure, they've been 'found to be safe' in that they do not directly cause cancer—but what about the brain? It just makes sense that there might be neurological effects of using food additives, especially in the quantities in which we typically consume them."

WHAT TO TEST

Although testing of the effects of food additives on the liver, brain, kidneys, blood-forming organs and reproductive system is required under the Color Additive Amendment of 1960, it is impossible to test every additive, every pesticide, every herbicide and every other chemical in the environment. And some chemicals—such as pesticides used on agricultural products—are excluded from the definition of an additive. "Pesticides disrupt the endocrine and reproductive systems of insects," says Simontacchi. "It stands to reason that they could be having serious effects on our own systems, even if the science hasn't fully proved that yet."

The worst offenders in most American diets today, according to Simontacchi, are these...

1. Breakfast cereals (they have a high sugar content).

2. "Lunchables" (they contain 40 to 60 g of sugar and more than 750 mg of sodium).

3. Soft drinks (high sugar and chemicals).

4. Snack foods such as potato chips (high sodium).

5. Ice cream.

6. Juice drinks.

IS DEPRESSION FOOD RELATED?

"When an adolescent's nutritionally challenged diet has deprived his brain of the molecules needed to make calming, soothing neurotransmitters, and he feels overwhelmed with negative feelings, he lashes out in anger. He drinks more soft drinks and eats more junk food and this temporarily makes him feel better but escalates the bad mood. Some of the self-destructive behavior we see in teenagers may well be the result of depression they have no resources to resolve."

Adults pay the price for a diet heavy in processed foods as well. The cognitive decline often seen in aging—from "senior moments" to vascular dementia—is often accompanied by serious nutrient deficiencies. "Cognitive decline actually mimics deficiencies of folic acid and vitamin B-12," Simontacchi explains, "and B-12 is a particularly difficult nutrient for older people to absorb well."

WHAT YOU CAN DO

"It's really not complicated at all," Simontacchi says. "We need to go back to consuming real food."

"Older people are eating many more prepackaged entrees, and that's a big mistake." There's plenty of good-tasting and ready-to-eat food available at the supermarket. *Her favorites include…*

- **Roasted chickens**
- **Packaged salads**
- **Hummus**
- **Raw nuts and seeds**
- **Fresh, hearty soups** (*Note:* Watch the sodium levels.)

By eating more healthfully, you'll have more energy and brain cells available to be creative in your food preparation.

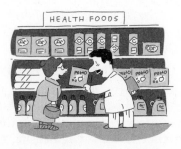

Shocking! New Rules Mean "Organic" Foods May Not Be Organic

Marion Nestle, PhD, professor of nutrition, New York University, New York City.

Many health-oriented consumers do not want their food tainted with synthetic chemicals, and they are willing to pay a premium for the "certified organic" label. However, the rules on what that label means have changed—along with the consumer's ability to trust what the label says.

Congress has recently loosened the definition of organic. According to Marion Nestle, PhD, professor of nutrition at New York University in New York City, organic standards have been put at grave risk, while potentially creating both confusion for consumers and the opportunity for food producers and manufacturers to mislead the public about the quality and healthfulness of their produce.

DILUTING THE MEANING OF ORGANIC

While organic produce account for only a tiny portion of food sales overall, it is one of the fastest growing segments of the agricultural industry, generating billions of dollars annually.

Food giants including Kraft and General Mills have jumped on the organic bandwagon, with just one caveat: Their goal has been to dilute organic standards…meaning foods could contain more synthetic chemicals but still carry the "organic" label.

Under federal organic standards previously adopted…

- **If an organic ingredient for a processed food** such as a granola bar or organic frozen pizza was not commercially available, one of 38 synthetic substances could be used instead. "Made with organic" means it must have 70% or more organic ingredients.

•**It was not necessary to inform consumers of this substitution** by listing the chemicals on a product's ingredient list.

While only time will tell what comes to pass under more recent legislation, here's what we know so far...

•**The number of synthetic substances permitted for use as an ingredient could skyrocket,** and consumers will still have no way of knowing what synthetic ingredients are in their "organic" foods.

•**In the past, the synthetic ingredients were closely overseen by the National Organic Standards Board.** The board could be stripped of this power. Theoretically at least, new synthetic substances could be approved as ingredients in organic foods on an emergency basis by the agricultural secretary, bypassing the National Organic Standards Board.

WHAT THIS MEANS FOR YOU

The meaning of organic standards depends on trust, explains Dr. Nestle. When the standards weaken, they lose their integrity and, therefore, trustworthiness. While food producers will be able to meet the labeling requirements to claim "Certified Organic," these newer rules frustrate consumer desires for pure, all-natural products, free from synthetic anything.

Dr. Nestle recommends writing your congressional representatives, and urging them to undo this new legislation. *Until or if that happens, your best bet is to look beyond the organic label...*

•**With meat, poultry, dairy products and eggs,** search for phrases on the labels such as hormone-free, antibiotic-free, free-range, cage-free and grass-fed.

•**When it comes to fruits and vegetables,** whenever possible shop at open-air green markets or local farm stands where you can purchase fresh produce straight from the farmers who grew them. Ask questions about any synthetic pesticide or fertilizer use.

•**Buy local fruits and vegetables in season,** and avoid purchasing produce grown internationally. Pesticides banned in the US are still used in other countries, and can find their way onto your plate.

•**When you find vendors or farmers you trust, patronize them on a regular basis.** Not only is this good for you personally, you will also be doing your part to encourage ecological, sustainable and humane agricultural practices. And that's good for everybody.

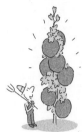

Tomatoes with Fish Genes and Other Scary Food Facts

Sheldon Krimsky, PhD, professor of Urban and Environmental Policy and Planning, Tufts University, Boston, and coeditor of *Rights and Liberties in the Biotech Age: Why We Need a Genetic Bill of Rights.* Rowman & Littlefield. Dr. Krimsky is on the board of directors of the Council for Responsible Genetics.

G enetically modified crops—sometimes known as *frankenfoods*—are foods that have been crossbred with other species of the same plant and sometimes with other organisms entirely in order to increase shelf life, reduce spoilage, etc. In so doing, food producers are looking at short-term profits rather than the long-term health implications.

Worse: This seismic sea change in the way we eat is taking place under the radar, with little attention to its impact on public health, notes Sheldon Krimsky, PhD, professor of Urban and Environmental Policy and Planning at Tufts University in Boston, and coeditor of *Rights and Liberties in the Biotech Age: Why We Need a Genetic Bill of Rights* (Rowman and Littlefield).

CROSSING THE SPECIES BARRIER

In genetically modified organisms (GMOs), genes from one organism (a plant, animal or microbe) are transferred into another. Genetic engineering permits scientists to cross the species barrier, most commonly for agricultural purposes (such as pest control or drought tolerance) and to a lesser extent to alter plants to produce pharmaceuticals (such as vaccines) and industrial substances (such as adhesive). As a result, you might find fish genes in tomatoes, viruses in fruit and human genes in tobacco. Thus far, at least 35 varieties of genetically engineered crops have been registered with the US Food and Drug Administration (FDA), the US Environmental Protection Agency (EPA) or the US Department of Agriculture (USDA).

A VAST, UNREGULATED EXPERIMENT

Although GMOs have only been around since the 1990s, they have already penetrated the food supply to a significant extent...as much as two-thirds to three-quarters of processed foods are thought to be manufactured with genetically engineered ingredients. The bowl of corn flakes you ate this morning probably contained corn that was genetically altered so that it would resist parasites in the field and spoilage in the box, while the salad dressing you use at dinner tonight may be made with oil from genetically modified canola or soybeans that allowed the oil to resist consumption by bacteria (and unfortunately, proper digestion by humans as well). Because there is no labeling required, there's no way to tell.

NOT JUST A FAT–TRANS FAT GAME— THE CONSEQUENCES OF GMOs

The long-term impact of this large-scale biotech transformation of the food supply is not yet known...and it's not just a game, cautions Dr. Krimsky. Genes interact with one another and the environment in ways that are impossible to predict. *Serious concerns include...*

•**Food allergies.** In one instance, genetically modified "StarLink" corn intended for animal consumption made its way into the human food supply through products such as Taco Bell's taco shells, causing allergic reactions in at least 44 people.

Another worry: Nut allergies. A study in *The New England Journal of Medicine* pointed out that people who were allergic to Brazil nuts were also allergic to genetically engineered soybeans that contained Brazil nut genes.

•**Nutritional quality.** Genetic engineering may render modified foods less nutritious than their natural counterparts. In one study, scientists found that genetically engineered soybeans contained fewer phytoestrogens than natural soybeans.

•**Unintended side effects.** According to the Council for Responsible Genetics, splicing a gene for human growth hormone into mice correctly produced larger mice, but splicing it into pigs resulted in skinny, arthritic pigs, and salmon reacted by growing too big, too fast...and turning green.

•**A scary new fairy tale.** In Ontario, scientists created the three little "Enviropigs"— named Wayne, Gordie and Jacques after three famous Canadian hockey players— who produce less smelly, environmentally damaging manure. In order to do this, they modified the pigs' digestion by splicing mouse genes and *E. coli* bacteria genes into pig genes. However, the long-term health consequences of ingesting mouse and *E. coli* genes with pork chops or ham remain unknown.

WHY THE SECRECY?

One of the most frustrating issues is the lack of labeling. This puts consumers at a distinct disadvantage. Without this basic information, there is simply no way to identify a genetically modified food as a potential concern—for example, for a person with nut allergies to know when a processed food has been genetically modified with nut genes.

Much criticism has centered on the cozy relationship between the giant agro-biotechnology industry and US regulatory agencies. Unlike genetically engineered drugs, the FDA does not require genetically engineered foods to be tested for safety. At the EPA, one of the agencies responsible for policing genetically modified plants (which are produced, by and large, by Monsanto), the second highest post used to be occupied by Monsanto's former top Washington lobbyist.

A SLOW BUT GROWING BACKLASH

While the federal government has been slow to intervene, several local governments have taken action. Genetically modified crops have been banned in Mendocino and Marin counties in California. In Vermont, the state senate unanimously passed the Farmer Protection Act to hold biotech companies legally responsible for contaminating other farmers' crops. In response to worldwide objections to tinkering with a key food crop, Monsanto was forced to abandon its plan to produce genetically engineered wheat.

Even the National Academy of Sciences (NAS), which originally gave genetically engineered foods a free pass, has voiced serious concern about traits of genetically modified organisms escaping into established ecosystems. The NAS has urged greater "bioconfinement" strategies to prevent genetically engineered plants and animals from breeding or competing with wild relatives, and to keep biological techniques such as induced sterility from invading the natural world.

Some in the business community are also beginning to respond to consumer concerns. Presumably in fear of a boycott, McDonald's squelched a plan to use genetically engineered potatoes in its french fries, while Anheuser-Busch objected to the cultivation of genetically modified pharmaceutical rice in the same state in which it grew rice to make beer.

WHAT YOU CAN DO

Genetically modified foods are the product of a "brave-new-world" technology that we still don't know enough about, and serious safety concerns remain largely unaddressed and unresolved. At a minimum, why not require labeling? Let consumers decide whether or not they're comfortable with genetically modified food on the dinner table.

In the meantime, if you're concerned about the risks, keep in mind that the usual healthful diet advice holds true here too—eat a variety of whole foods that are organically produced, and steer clear of processed and fast foods as much as possible. These include "precooked" or "heat-n-serve" products as well as items where you add water and then heat.

You also might want to drop a letter to Congress, encouraging your representatives to address food safety issues sooner rather than later.

10

Enjoying the Latest Healthy Foods

A "Berry Good" Fruit May Stop Cancer

A Brazilian berry known as acai (pronounced AH-sci-EE), is becoming the exotic new fruit juice of choice in health food stores. On the Internet, articles suggest that it can be used to fight cancer and boost cardiovascular health. Is there good science to back up these claims?

So far, the fact is that most of these healthful properties have yet to be tested scientifically. However, Stephen T. Talcott, PhD, assistant professor of food chemistry at Texas A&M University, has been studying acai berries and believes there is some basis for those claims. Acai berries are a rich source of disease-fighting antioxidants as well as health-promoting essential fatty acids, fiber and amino acids. Those attributes certainly make them a better-than-neutral choice, while we await the findings of research currently underway.

CANCER-FIGHTING POTENTIAL?

In his former post at the University of Florida, Dr. Talcott and his colleagues investigated the cancer-fighting potential of acai berries in the lab setting. They found that four out of six chemical extracts prepared from acai fruit pulp killed a significant number of leukemia cells in vitro. This was a lab study involving cells, not human beings, but the results are still encouraging. The next step at Texas A&M is to explore the impact acai has on healthy human subjects.

ALL BERRIES GOOD

Dr. Talcott said that products made with the processed berries have only been available here for a little over five years. The dark-purple acai berries, which are the size of blueberries, have a thin layer of

Stephen T. Talcott, PhD, assistant professor of food chemistry, Texas A&M University, Department of Nutrition and Food Science, College Station.

fruit surrounding a large seed. Dr. Talcott and other sources say they taste like a mix of red wine and chocolate. The berries grow on acai palms, which are abundant around the Amazon River. One reason the berries are relatively new to us here in the US is that they're highly perishable.

TRY SOME ACAI

An assortment of products made from acai is now available to consumers. If you want to try some acai, go right ahead—just don't forget to balance it with a variety of other health-promoting fruits and vegetables. For optimal health, make it a habit to enjoy fresh produce—familiar as well as exotic—nine times a day, every day.

Delicious Fruit with 10 Times More Antioxidant Power Than Broccoli

Jules Beekwilder, PhD, bioscience researcher, Plant Research International, Wageningen, the Netherlands.

For all you lovers of raspberries, there is more good news on the health front. According to recent research from The Netherlands, red raspberries rank just about at the top of antioxidant-loaded foods. In fact, the antioxidant activity in raspberries may be up to 10 times higher than that of tomatoes or broccoli and on a par with the "superloaded" blueberry. (Antioxidants, of course, are the soldiers that fight off damaging free radicals roaming the body and looking to cause trouble.)

A RASPBERRY BONUS

And there is yet another antioxidant bonus in red raspberries—*ellagitannins*, an important type antioxidant found in a short list of foods, make up about 50% of the antioxidant effect of raspberries. While ellagitannins belong to the tannin family (which are ubiquitous in fruits, notably in grapes, and thus red wine), this particular compound is found largely in a few fruits and nuts. Other food sources include strawberries, blackberries and walnuts. Seldom talked about due to their rarity, ellagitannins provide powerful protection in assorted ways.

THE POWER OF ELLAGITANNINS

Jules Beekwilder, PhD, led this research at Plant Research International in Wageningen, The Netherlands. We contacted him for more information about his findings. Dr. Beekwilder says that while raspberries have many other nutrients—vitamin C, folate, vitamins B-2 and B-3, magnesium and others and, of course, fiber—it is the ellagitannins that make the raspberry unique. In addition to being powerful antioxidants, these tannins are also antimicrobial and so inhibit the growth of bacteria such as *Salmonella*. Furthermore, the tannins, which are similar to those in red wine, act as relaxants for the blood circulatory system, a long-held tenet of traditional medicine that has held up in test tube studies. Indeed, people with circulation problems are often advised to drink raspberry-leaf tea, says Dr. Beekwilder. That said, people with diabetes and others with circulation problems should always check with a trained professional about their individual needs.

FRAGILE FEEDING

Unlike other power-packed foods such as broccoli, raspberries are among the most fragile of fruits. Purchase them fresh in season, during the summer, and refrigerate the berries—unwashed—immediately after purchase. Remove any that might be moldy or otherwise spoiled so that they do not damage the remaining healthy berries. Plan to enjoy the fruit within a day or so of purchase and wash just prior to serving. Dr. Beekwilder says, though, that you should make raspberries part of your diet year-round and thanks to flash freezing you can. While this process does destroy up to half of the vitamin C, it does not hurt the other antioxidants. Bags of flash-frozen berries are found in all supermarkets today.

"Concentrate" on Fruits for Health

Andrew L. Rubman, ND, consulting medical editor for *Bottom Line's Daily Health News* and director of the Southbury Clinic for Traditional Medicines in Southbury, Connecticut.

S cience has firmly established berries as a mother lode of antioxidants, compounds that battle harmful free radicals and are great for the body and the brain. In the summer, there is nothing more delicious or healthier than fresh, ripe berries. They're one of nature's true gems. Come winter, berries may still be available, but they're more expensive. So, here's a way to capture the summer and its goodness all year long—*berry juice concentrates*.

CONCENTRATEDLY GOOD

Not to be confused with juices, the concentrates are dense—it takes one cup of fresh blueberries, for example, to make one tablespoon of wild blueberry concentrate. Add a little of this to fruit juice or seltzer and you have a refreshing and very healthful drink.

We first learned about berry concentrates from *Bottom Line's Daily Health New's* consulting medical editor, Andrew L. Rubman, ND, as a way to ease some digestive inflammation. One of the best things about the juice concentrates is that the berries are picked just before they reach peak ripeness, which is when their nutritional benefits are highest. In addition, the berries and concentrates have what are called *cofactors*, or *pro-nutrients*—found in the fruit naturally but only when fruit is in its freshest state—that work in synergy and as facilitators with nutrients in foods

to maximize their absorption and utilization. It is such cofactors that make it best to get your vitamins from food rather than solely in supplement form.

TASTY VITAMIN TREATS

Concentrate flavors include blueberry, cherry and cranberry, among others, and are generally available in better health food stores—look for the concentrates that are syrup-like, without thickeners, additives and sugar. Dr. Rubman's favorite way to enjoy them is in a glass of sparkling mineral water with a slice of lime. Kids especially enjoy cherry concentrate; serve it in some seltzer or in a little juice. The cherry concentrate also makes an easy and healthy vinaigrette (olive oil, balsamic vinegar and cherry concentrate). It's a good way to sneak some extra vitamins into anyone's diet.

New Food Superstar— Pomegranate

Kelly Morrow, MS, RD, registered dietician and assistant professor, Bastyr Center for Natural Health and Bastyr University, Kenmore, Washington.

L ike other fruits and vegetables with vibrant, intense colors, pomegranates are antioxidant-packed superfoods. In fact, studies indicate that the juice contains even more disease-fighting antioxidants than green tea, blueberries or red wine. In addition to vitamins A, C and E—and potassium and iron—pomegranate juice is brimming with healthful components including *polyphenols, anthocyanins* and *tannins*.

Too many people make dull brown and white foods the centerpiece of their diets, observes Kelly Morrow, MS, RD, an assistant professor at Bastyr University in Kenmore, Washington. In her opinion, we would all be better off if we filled our plates with fewer empty carbohydrates and more richly pigmented produce such

181

as pomegranates, blueberries, kiwis, spinach and sweet potatoes.

HEART PROTECTION AND MORE

The pomegranate's abundant antioxidant and anti-inflammatory properties confer a wealth of health benefits. *Morrow describes some of the more well researched of these...*

•**Better cardiovascular health.** At the Technion-Israel Institute of Technology in Israel, researchers have found that drinking a glass of pomegranate juice a day slows cholesterol oxidation by nearly half, leading to less plaque in the arteries. In diabetic patients, who are at increased risk of cardiovascular disease, pomegranate juice successfully lowered blood lipids (fats) without affecting blood sugar. Morrow adds that preliminary evidence suggests that pomegranate may also modestly reduce blood pressure.

•**Potent cancer fighter.** Pomegranate also shows promise as a cancer fighter. At the University of Wisconsin in Madison, researchers demonstrated that pomegranate juice can stop the growth of prostate cancer in mice. In Israel, scientists discovered that pomegranate seed oil triggers *apoptosis*—a self-destruct mechanism—in breast cancer cells. They also found that the juice is toxic to estrogen-dependent breast cancer cells, while leaving normal breast cells intact.

•**Good news for expectant mothers.** Pregnant women at risk of giving birth prematurely may benefit from drinking pomegranate juice, according to an animal study at Washington University School of Medicine in St. Louis. Decreased oxygen and blood flow to a premature baby's brain can result in what is known as hypoxic ischemic brain injury. Researchers found that newborn mice whose mothers were given pomegranate juice were 60% less likely to experience this problem.

•**Skin support.** Pomegranate seed oil, readily available in health food stores or via the Internet, acts as a soothing moisturizer that protects the skin from ultraviolet radiation. While pomegranate seed oil can't replace conventional sunscreen, you can increase the effectiveness by applying the oil beneath the sunscreen. According to Morrow, vitamin C and polyphenols in pomegranate work together to support healthy collagen (the protein that makes up connective tissue) and prevent breakdown of the structural components of the skin. Naturally anti-inflammatory, the oil also can be used to relieve cracked, dry skin or a mild sunburn. In mouse studies, pomegranate resulted in a reduced incidence of skin cancer.

A POMEGRANATE A DAY

Most studies of pomegranate have focused on the juice, probably because the fruit is a bit messy and hard to get at.

Next time you're in the grocery store, think about giving pomegranate a try. Whether you sip a glass of juice, add it to your fruit smoothie or munch on the juicy red seeds, adding pomegranate to your diet is one simple yet positive step you can take toward good health.

Cloudy Juice The Clear Choice For Extra Nutrients

Sonja Pettersen, NMD, naturopathic medical doctor. She is licensed to practice primary care medicine specializing in natural therapeutics in Arizona and is based in Scottsdale.

Journal of the Science of Food and Agriculture, Jan Oszmianski, et al.

Many moms give their toddlers and young children apple juice boxes thinking it's a healthy choice. Truth be told, research indicates that the health risks of sugar-rich juice products can outweigh their benefits—especially in the quantities many children consume them in, and particularly in light of the national crisis of childhood obesity. Now some more research shows how processing in even the "all-natural" products affects the health value of apple juice.

THE CLOUDY AND THE CLEAR

To test the nutritive quality, Polish researchers made four batches of juice from two different varieties of apples (Champion and Ida Red). From each type, they produced one cloudy (like in apple cider) juice and one clear juice. Then they tested all four for antioxidants (those important compounds that can help fight cell damage). Regardless of which variety of apple was used, the cloudy version was better—in fact, antioxidant content of the cloudy juice was almost double that of the clear kind from the same variety of apple.

"The nutrient content of any juice depends on how it is processed and what's removed," explains Sonja Pettersen, NMD, an Arizona-based naturopathic physician we contacted in order to learn more about these findings. In their attempt to make clear juice, researchers in this study used an enzyme *pectinase*. The clear juice was then pasteurized in the same way as cloudy juice. The resulting clear, amber-colored juice looks appealing, and, not unimportantly, also has a longer shelf life—but a lot of what's good for you is lost in the processing, with the clarified product containing as little as one-quarter of the *polyphenol* content—and antioxidant power—of the unfiltered, unprocessed kind.

JUICE DRINKS vs. JUICE

And, notes Dr. Pettersen, this particular finding probably underestimates the variance between the juices, since many of the products available in supermarkets are even more processed than those the researchers produced for the study. "Many 'juices' given to children are actually 'fruit juice drinks,' which are primarily fruit-flavored sugar water," she says. Fruit juice drinks often contain as little as 10% juice, so consumers should look for labels that say 100% juice. "Even if it's

clear, a juice can be nutritious, depending on the fruit—it all depends on what they leave in, and what they take out." These researchers removed the pectin (an important fiber with cardiovascular benefits) and the pulp, the source of so many powerful plant compounds that make apples healthy.

MAKE YOUR OWN

Are any juices really good for you? Healthiest of all are those made at home. Two good juicer machine choices are Vita Mix (*www.vitamix.com*) or the Acme Juicerator (*www.healthnutalternatives.com*). These juicers range from approximately $160 to $700. At the supermarket, look for juices that are unfiltered and "cold-pressed" (meaning they are processed at very low heat if at all, preventing most of the enzymes from being killed).

But best of all, says Dr. Pettersen: "Eat an apple."

Amazing Way to Double the Nutrients In Watermelon

Penelope Perkins-Veazie, PhD, plant physiologist, US Department of Agriculture (USDA) Agricultural Research Service in Lane, Oklahoma.

Watermelon, like many fruits today, is in our supermarkets nearly year round, but it's still a hot summer afternoon that makes an ice-cold slice a real taste treat. Beyond being yummy, watermelon is full of healthful benefits—high in the antioxidant *lycopene*, a carotenoid pigment that produces the deep red color, and is fairly rich in vitamins C, B-6 and B-1 (thiamine), and beta-carotene. It also has magnesium and potassium—all for just 46 calories a cup. But now researchers at the USDA Agricultural Research Service in Lane, Oklahoma, have discovered a way to improve the melon's health benefits even more.

It's this simple: Just leave the melon out of the fridge for seven to 10 days if fresh-picked and a few days if store-bought before you open it. A watermelon kept at room temperature has double the level of beta-carotene and some 11% to 40% more lypocene.

MAXIMUM RIPENESS

Penelope Perkins-Veazie, PhD, was a lead researcher on this study. She says that allowing melons to be at room temperature for several days before eating gives them the chance to reach maximum ripeness. As the melon sits, the color of the red flesh inside becomes more intense and the rind thins, reflecting the fact that the fruit is continuing to ripen. For this study, watermelons were stored at 41° F, 55.4° F and 69.8° F, with 69.8° F representative of room temperature. If your room is warmer, keep in mind that increased heat will accelerate the process, she says. When you are preparing to serve the melon it is fine to chill it first, though this will slow any further increase in nutrients. How do you know when a melon is ripe? Completely ripened melon will sound almost hollow when tapped sharply.

EAT WHEN AT PEAK

Dr. Perkins-Veazie also cautions to refrigerate melon once cut or damaged because yeast organisms, bacteria and mold can easily invade it. But when you do open the fruit, you'll know that you have let the melon ripen too long if the rind is soft, pitted or has dark spots...or if the melon flesh has an orange tint and a pumpkin-type odor (which is not a surprise, since watermelons are in fact related to pumpkins).

While the study was performed on watermelons, tomatoes—another lycopene-rich food—as well as other fruits and vegetables are best eaten at their peak ripeness, and best bought when they have been harvested close to that peak ripeness to maximize their nutritional benefits.

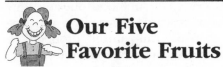

Our Five Favorite Fruits

Susan M. Kleiner, PhD, RD, CNS. Dr. Kleiner is owner of High Performance Nutrition, a consulting firm on Mercer Island, Washington, and author of several books, including *The Good Mood Diet: Feel Great While You Lose Weight* (Springboard), *Power Eating*, 3rd Edition (Human Kinetics) and *The Powerfood Nutrition Plan* (Rodale). Dr. Kleiner is cofounder of the International Society of Sports Nutrition.

Nutrition expert Susan M. Kleiner, author of *Power Eating* (Human Kinetics), from Mercer Island, Washington, shares her favorite healthful fruit choices, based on everything from antioxidant content to taste, accessibility and portability.

Dr. Kleiner generally recommends that her nutrition clients eat three pieces of fruit a day, including some type of berry (for the ***anthocyanins*** and vitamin C) and an orange-flesh fruit such as a peach, nectarine, cantaloupe, papaya or mango (for beta-carotene). Add frozen fruit to smoothies when fresh isn't available. You may be comforted to know that frozen is almost as good as fresh as long as it is completely ripe when frozen—which is generally the case.

See if any of Dr. Kleiner's top five fruits makes *your* list...

1. Dried plums (also known as prunes). Rich in fiber, especially pectin, a soluble fiber that may help decrease cholesterol. Packed with phenols that neutralize free radicals in the body and a good source of potassium and iron, too. "And because they're so portable, dried plums are on top of my list," says Dr. Kleiner.

2. Blueberries. These are full of super nutrients, including anthocyanins, *pterostilbene* and *ellagic acid*. They protect you from an assortment of health problems, including cancer, cardiovascular disease, vision loss and cognitive decline. And don't forget strawberries, blackberries or raspberries, says Dr. Kleiner, which are also rich in fiber and other health-protective nutrients.

3. Mangoes. Exotic and sweet, mangoes are rich in vitamin A, vitamin C and beta-carotene, plus potassium and fiber. The mango also has other nutrients that promote cardiovascular health and protect against colon cancer. Choose other beta-carotene-rich fruits, too, such as cantaloupes, peaches, nectarines and papaya.

4. Apples. Apples are antioxidant-rich and full of phytonutrients that may reduce your risk of cancer, heart disease, asthma and type 2 diabetes. Make sure you also eat the peel, which is rich in soluble and insoluble fiber (pectin)—great for gut health—plus compounds like *quercetin* and *proanthocyanidins*.

5. Bananas. Bananas are high in potassium, which may protect against high blood pressure, heart disease, stomach ulcers and bone loss. They are also surprisingly full of antioxidants.

EAT FRUITS IN SEASON

So should you eat brain-protective blueberries every day if dementia is in your family history? Dr. Kleiner thinks that's a miscalculation.

Better: Enjoy the wonderful fresh fruits of the season, which will give you a variety of delicious nutrients that help your body in assorted ways. You'll feel better and enjoy your food more.

Explained! How Food Keeps You Healthy

Boxin Ou, PhD, is president of Brunswick Laboratories, Norton, Massachusetts. Dr. Ou is a scientist who studies phytochemicals in plant foods, and his research has been widely published in peer-reviewed journals. He regularly collaborates with leading food companies and university research programs.

I f you are going to give thoughtful consideration to the healthful properties of the fruits and vegetables you eat, it's a good idea to get familiar with the appro-

priate terminology. One of those terms—ORAC—requires a little explaining.

ORAC BASICS

The letters ORAC stand for *oxygen radical absorbance capacity*, a reflection of the *antioxidant* ability of just about anything, including foods, to subdue the *peroxyl radical* (one of the harmful free radicals) in the test tube. Free radicals are highly reactive substances that can occur naturally in the body as a result of oxidation. When not being pressed into service by the immune system to attack pathogens, these free radicals might be considered the body's bad boys, having been shown to trigger much of the aging process and also to be involved in degenerative diseases. Antioxidants neutralize free radicals.

WHAT'S MAGICAL ABOUT ANTIOXIDANTS?

Studies at the Jean Mayer US Department of Agriculture (USDA) Human Nutrition Research Center on Aging at Tufts University in Boston suggest that consuming fruits and vegetables with a high ORAC value may help slow the aging process in both body and brain. Other research has shown that in middle-aged rats, foods with a high ORAC value can reduce loss of long-term memory and learning ability, maintain the ability of brain cells to respond to stimuli (thought to decrease with age) and protect blood vessels against oxygen damage. The assumption is that these high ORAC foods benefit people in much the same way. Most recently, Ronald Prior, PhD, and colleagues at the USDA reported on several small human clinical studies on high ORAC foods consumption with positive results.

WHICH FOOD IS BEST?

There isn't a simple way to measure antioxidant capacity or activity because different antioxidants respond to different pro-oxidants or radicals, much like different antibiotics kill different strains of bacteria. In fact, there are at least six kinds of potentially destructive free radicals... and when the original ORAC test was developed, it simply measured the ability of a food to fight *one* of these species specifically, the peroxyl radical, the one most abundant in the human body, says Boxin Ou, PhD, president of Brunswick Laboratories in Norton, Massachusetts, a leader in ORAC testing. Though the ORAC measure only relates to that, he explains that our bodies also have to defend against the other five. So Dr. Ou's team developed several other tests (with different designations, such as HORAC, NORAC, SORAC and SOAC) to describe how a food defends against the other types of potentially dangerous free radicals.

Carotenoids, primarily found in yellow and orange foods such as carrots, for example, score poorly on the standard ORAC test, Dr. Ou told us. Carotenoids do not defend well against the peroxyl radicals that are the basis of the ORAC test. But carotenoids defend brilliantly against a *different* type of free radical called *singlet oxygen*, measured by the SOAC assay. The antioxidant power rank assigned to them would depend on which test was used—but the only score you'd hear about would be the brilliant one.

MEANINGFUL OR NOT?

So should you pay attention to those claims about a product's ORAC value? The answer is, yes...but while it is true that a higher ORAC rating is better than a lower one, and any high rating is potentially good, just be sure that you realize the rating reported may be for an isolated and less prominent antioxidant action than the combined environmental assault you may be facing.

What are some high ORAC foods? See below...

ORAC values of common fruits and vegetables (per 100 grams—approximately 3½ ounces):

Spinach	1,515
Prunes	6,552
Raisins	3,037
Blueberries	6,552
Blackberries	5,347
Alfalfa sprouts	1,510
Broccoli	1,362
Beets	1,767
Red bell pepper	791
Strawberries	3,577
Onion	1,034
Raspberries	4,882

Source: United States Department of Agriculture, *www.usda.gov.*

"Grape" Way to Lower Cholesterol

Leo Galland, MD, director of the Foundation for Integrative Medicine in New York City. He is author of *The Fat Resistance Diet.* Broadway. *www.fatresistancediet.com.* Dr. Galland is a recipient of the Linus Pauling award.

Plant foods offer cornucopia of health benefits, and mounting evidence continues to reveal new plant chemicals that promote health. The latest darling is red grape juice. New studies are showing that compounds in the juice actually lower cholesterol and other cardiovascular risk factors.

GRAPE JUICE AND CHOLESTEROL

In one recent study in Spain, researchers took a group of 15 healthy subjects and 26 subjects who were receiving dialysis and gave all of them a total of 100 milliliters (ml) of red grape juice concentrate daily (100 ml is a little more than half a six-ounce can of the concentrate). Dialysis patients were chosen for the study because they're at a higher risk for developing cardiovascular disease.

After only two weeks of drinking the juice concentrate, all subjects had reductions in low-density lipoprotein (LDL) cholesterol (the "bad" kind), oxidized LDL cholesterol (the *really* bad kind) and total cholesterol. As a bonus, their high-density lipoprotein (HDL, or good) cholesterol went up. In addition, an important marker of inflammation, MCP-1, went down by half after three weeks.

**WHAT MAKES
GRAPE JUICE GO?**

Red grape juice is a rich source of *polyphenols*, potent antioxidants that "mop up" harmful free radicals, which are a big part of the aging process and are associated with degenerative diseases. The polyphenols (also known as *polyphenolics*) include all sorts of plant compounds such as *catechins* and *anthocyanins* that have been shown to be protective against various cancers and heart disease. "This is yet another piece of evidence for the importance of consuming fruits and vegetables that are rich in the polyphenolics," says Leo Galland, MD, an expert in nutritional and integrative medicine.

Dr. Galland explains that cholesterol metabolism in the body is influenced by a process known as oxidative stress—the damage that occurs when free radicals attack your cells and DNA, much the way oxygen attacks apple slices left out on your kitchen table and turns them brown. The phenolic compounds in red grape juice—and in other plant foods—work to disarm the free radicals. By preventing the oxidation of LDL cholesterol (which increases the risk for LDL to generate cardiovascular disease), the compounds have strong benefits on heart health.

GOOD RED FRUIT JUICES

The good news is that the phenolic compounds that lowered oxidation of LDL cholesterol, prevented oxidation and also lowered inflammation in the study are not specific to red grape juice. "You should be able to achieve similar results with other kinds of red fruit juice, like pomegranate, for example," Dr. Galland said.

Bottom line: Red grape juice contains antioxidant and anti-inflammatory compounds that rank high among the established benefits of other well-known antioxidants such as vitamin E, lycopene and vitamin C. And one of the benefits seems to be a significant improvement in cholesterol. Not only that…it tastes good, too.

Dig Into These Five Power Veggies

Susan M. Kleiner, PhD, RD, CNS. Dr. Kleiner is owner of High Performance Nutrition, a consulting firm on Mercer Island, Washington, and author of several books, including *The Good Mood Diet: Feel Great While You Lose Weight* (Springboard), *Power Eating*, 3rd Edition (Human Kinetics) and *The Powerfood Nutrition Plan* (Rodale). Dr. Kleiner is cofounder of the International Society of Sports Nutrition.

Carrots are an excellent source of nutrition. Of course, as healthful as carrots are, other veggies also pack a lot of disease-fighting power. What are the best? We called nutrition authority Susan M. Kleiner, PhD, RD—from Mercer Island, Washington, and author of *Power Eating*—to find out which five vegetables she considers the most healthful. A difficult task, since Dr. Kleiner says *variety* and what *looks good* to you as you shop should be your top priorities. There probably are thousands of health-promoting nutrients whose value is still unknown, so don't pass up the green beans you love because you think you should be eating broccoli every day, says Dr. Kleiner.

That said, here are Dr. Kleiner's top five vegetables…

•**Broccoli.** No surprise here, since *indoles* and *sulforaphanes* contained in broccoli are top cancer-fighters. Eat broccoli raw or lightly cooked. Or select other members of the crucifer family *Brassica* genus, such as kale, cauliflower, Brussels sprouts, kohlrabi and cabbage.

•**Garlic.** Along with onions and leeks, garlic is a member of the *Allium* group of vegetables, known for their cancer-fighting and immune-strengthening properties.

While the more pungent varieties of onions and garlic are richer in health-protective compounds, enjoy them all, including mild elephant garlic and sweet onions. No need to chew raw garlic cloves, says Dr. Kleiner. She uses lightly sautéed garlic liberally in her cooking.

•**Red chard.** This is a leafy green, like collard greens and mustard greens, but less bitter and simpler to prepare. Red chard is chock-full of vitamins and minerals, including high amounts of vitamin K, beta-carotene and potassium, plus cancer-fighting *anthocyanins* and fiber. Dr. Kleiner loves red chard stir fried with a bit of sweetened rice vinegar and soy sauce.

•**Carrots.** It's hard to beat carrots for their appealing taste, portability and nutrition. Carrots are rich in beta-carotene and vitamin K, plus carotenoids that protect against cancer, heart disease and vision loss. Also try other carotenoid-rich deep orange produce, such as sweet potatoes, apricots or cantaloupe.

•**Red peppers.** These are rich in beta-carotene and vitamin K, cardioprotective vitamin B-6 and folic acid, plus an excellent choice for *lycopene*, a carotenoid that can reduce your risk for certain cancers. Other good sources of lycopene are tomatoes, watermelon and pink grapefruit.

Select the freshest vegetables you can find, or buy quality frozen vegetables since they retain nutrients longer than veggies stored for a week at the bottom of your fridge, says Dr. Kleiner. Although cooking vegetables involves some degree of nutrient loss, don't be afraid to sauté them lightly, steam them or boil them briefly in water. Season vegetables with a little salt, pepper and grated lemon zest or healthful sauces—whatever it takes for you and your family to enjoy them regularly, says Dr. Kleiner.

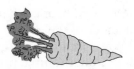

Eggs, Butter and More Secret Superfoods

Jonny Bowden, PhD, CNS, a board certified nutritionist, the "Weight Loss Coach" on iVillage.com and author of the best-selling *Living the Low Carb Life* (Sterling) as well as *The 150 Healthiest Foods on Earth* (Fair Winds). Find out more at *www.jonny bowden.com*.

Conventional wisdom on nutrition often shifts gears. Remember butter? And how about eggs? First they're evil, now they're our best friends. It is a good idea to periodically revisit some of our cherished beliefs about foods and health, so we spoke with nutritionist and weight-loss coach Jonny Bowden, whose book, *The 150 Healthiest Foods on Earth* (Fair Winds) has some surprising entries—and some surprising omissions.

FAT CAN BE YOUR FRIEND

"Many foods suffered from bad reputations in the past because of the deeply held belief that all saturated fat is bad for you," Dr. Bowden says. "Saturated fat is the general name for a collection of fatty acids—and some of these fatty acids are really good for you." For example, he says, "two of the healthiest foods on earth are whole eggs and coconut. Yet to this day people eat "Egg Beaters" and shun coconut oil because of the saturated fat."

EGGS—GREAT PROTEIN SOURCE

Dr. Bowden believes whole eggs are among the finest sources of protein on the planet. "On three of the four methods used by scientists for rating protein quality, eggs score better than milk, beef, whey and soy," he tells us. "Whole eggs contain all nine essential amino acids, plus they're loaded with vitamins and nutrients that are excellent for your eyes, brain and heart." Dr. Bowden explains that the fear of saturated fat causes people to shun one of the healthiest parts of the egg—the yolk. "The yolk contains *lutein* and *zeaxanthin*, two members of the carotenoid family that are emerging as superstars of eye nutrition. And the yolk is also one of the best sources of *choline*."

"Choline creates *betaine*, which helps lower *homocysteine*, a risk factor for heart disease. It's part of a compound called *phosphatidylcholine* that helps prevent the accumulation of fat and cholesterol in the liver. It's also needed to make *acetyl-choline*, which is critical for memory and thought," Dr. Bowden explains. Incidentally, he doesn't perceive the amount of cholesterol in whole eggs as a problem. "Virtually every study has shown absolutely no link between eating eggs and heart disease," he notes.

NUTS FOR COCONUTS

"In my view, coconut and coconut oil are superfoods," Dr. Bowden says. A half cup of shredded coconut has almost 4 grams (g) of fiber, 142 milligrams (mg) of potassium and almost no sugar. As for the saturated fat, he explains that in coconut, 50% of it comes from a fatty acid called *lauric acid*, which is antiviral and antimicrobial, and enhances the immune system. As for those saturated tropical fats that give coconuts a bad reputation…the saturated fat in coconut oil comes mostly from a family called MCTs or *medium-chain triglycerides*, making it particularly easy to metabolize. "The body likes to use it up as a source of energy, rather than turn it into a source of padding," says Dr. Bowden. "Long-term studies of people from the Pacific Islands who eat coconut and coconut oil regularly show that they have extremely low levels of heart disease."

BUTTER BARGAIN

Dr. Bowden has kind words to say about butter, too. "It's a rich source of vitamin A, needed both for maintaining good vision and the optimal functioning of the immune system. Butter also contains other fat-soluble vitamins, like vitamin K and vitamin D. And when it is made from the milk of healthy, grass-fed cows, butter contains CLA (*conjugated linolenic acid*), a kind of fat that has proven anticancer properties."

HEALTHY BREWS

Coffee's reputation has also been resurrected, says Dr. Bowden. Coffee is actually a major source of antioxidants in the American diet. "Caffeine is good for the brain," he explains, "and new studies show that it may be protective against type 2 diabetes and Parkinson's too. As long as you're not sensitive to the caffeine and you don't overdo it, coffee is fine for you." He also points out that black tea is nearly as good for you as green tea, because it, too, is loaded with *flavonoids* and *catechins* and antioxidants. But adding milk to your tea disables the antioxidants, so it's best to take it straight, with lemon or with your favorite sweetener.

NATURAL DISEASE FIGHTERS

Then there are the foods that are the unrecognized multitaskers in the health tool chest—like pumpkin. It has more potassium than a medium banana, is loaded with vitamin A, and has two carotenoids that are beneficial for the eyes—lutein and zeaxanthin. "Plus, pumpkin has less than 50 calories per cup, and you can season it with all kinds of great spices like cinnamon and nutmeg," adds Dr. Bowden. Another of his favorites is guava. "Guava has a whopping 9 g of fiber per cup. It's another potassium heavyweight, and it contains the cancer-fighting compound called *lycopene*," he said.

Cherries are another unappreciated fruit. These are loaded with *quercetin* and *ellagic acid*, two cancer-fighters. In addition, cherries have lots of natural anti-inflammatories, which is why they've traditionally been used to fight the pain of gout. And frozen cherries contain the same nutritional value as fresh, ripe fruit.

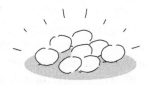

Go Nuts for Almonds!

Andrew L. Rubman, ND, consulting medical editor for *Bottom Line's Daily Health News* and director of the Southbury Clinic for Traditional Medicines in Southbury, Connecticut.

Nuts have gained popularity in recent years as an excellent source of protein and "good fats." One of the best nuts? Almonds. According to our consulting medical editor Andrew L. Rubman, ND, almonds are one of the most nutrient-dense, good-for-you foods there is.

ALMONDS BENEFITS

Although Dr. Rubman encourages eating a variety of nuts, just as you do fruits and vegetables, he particularly likes almonds because of their fatty acid content (almonds are high in monounsaturated fats). Furthermore, almonds have many health-promoting minerals, especially magnesium, but also potassium, which means the nuts help other dietary and supplemental sources protect cardiovascular health. Eating almonds with their skins provides significant amounts of vitamin E and flavonoids. Studies have shown that these two work synergistically to help boost low-density lipoprotein (LDL, or bad) cholesterol's resistance to oxidation by more than 50%, important because LDL cholesterol is not dangerous in and of itself. It is oxidation that makes LDL plaque-building and dangerous.

PROTEIN PROVIDER

Dr. Rubman adds that almonds are also a good source of protein (6 grams per ounce) nearly as much as one egg (6.3 grams of protein/egg)...and they have fiber and assorted vitamins and minerals. Visit *www.almondsarein.com* for more on their nutritional content.

DON'T ADD CALORIES

Still, some are concerned about the high calorie content of almonds and other nuts. Dr. Rubman has counseled many dieters about how to receive the health benefits of almonds without adding extra calories to their diet.

The solution: If you want to lose weight do not eat more than an ounce a day of unsalted almonds. That ounce would come to 23 nuts, he says, and the unsalted type is simpler because it is easier to stop at your limit with unsalted nuts than the salted, tastier form. Another good way to enjoy the health properties of almonds without toting up too many calories is to add them to other foods rather than eating them plain. Nuts toasted in a dry skillet are even more flavorful. Try chopping some into salads, sprinkling them over string beans or white fish. You can also coat fish or chicken with almond flour—make your own by grinding the nuts in a blender, food processor or even coffee grinder.

Latest News on Garlic

Matthew Budoff, MD, is associate professor of medicine at the David Geffen School of Medicine at UCLA and director of Cardiac CT at Harbor-UCLA Medical Center in Torrance, California. He has published more than 100 articles.

If there's ever been a spice or a food that just about everyone agrees is healthy, it's garlic. In his book, *The 150 Healthiest Foods on Earth* (Fair Winds), author Jonny Bowden calls garlic "a global remedy" and "one of the oldest medicinal foods on earth." More than 1,200 studies have been done on garlic, and even many conventional medical doctors agree that garlic helps lower cholesterol. In a meta-analysis published in the *Journal of the Royal College of Physicians*, garlic supplements lowered total serum cholesterol levels by 12% after only four weeks of treatment. Now a new study in the *Archives of Internal Medicine* throws some doubt on that, though there may be cause to be skeptical of the results. *Let's take a look...*

FAULTY RESEARCH

Researchers tested three forms of garlic (raw garlic, powdered garlic supplement and aged garlic extract supplement) on a population with elevated low-density lipoprotein (LDL) cholesterol and found disappointing results. They concluded that none of the garlic treatments had clinically or statistically significant effects. What gives? We went to Matthew Budoff, MD, a renowned researcher on the healing powers of garlic, to find out.

Acknowledging that the study was "a bit disappointing," Dr. Budoff stresses that it was not only "inconsistent with other studies," but that it also had more than a few problems in its design and methodology, including requiring participants to show up every day to receive both a sandwich (with garlic condiments or placebo condiments) and a pill (supplement containing garlic or a placebo) and then not checking to be sure they ate it.

Dr. Budoff also points out that this single study is hardly reason to question the many health benefits of garlic that have been documented in countless other studies. Put it in an overall context, he urges. The benefits of garlic are multifactorial, and not just about cholesterol. Garlic also lowers blood pressure and helps "regress" plaque—meaning the size of the blockage diminishes. Additionally, he notes that garlic decreases *homocysteine*, a dangerous inflammatory compound in the blood that has been linked to greater risk of heart disease and stroke.

WHAT'S IN A CLOVE

We also asked Dr. Budoff about another study, published in the *Journal of Agricultural and Food Chemistry*, reporting that crushing or chopping garlic before moderate cooking releases an enzyme that allows its active ingredients to work. (Dr. Bowden adds that chewing whole cloves may also be effective, though perhaps off-putting to friends and family.) "There are definitely challenges with studying garlic, and isolating its most active ingredients,"

he said. "When you take fresh garlic and process it differently, the benefits may be different. I think that's why there have been inconsistencies in the findings."

KEEP THE FAITH

In spite of this study, Dr. Budoff believes there's every reason to retain faith in the health properties of this food. "There is long-standing and consistent evidence that garlic consumption does improve your cardiovascular health," he says, adding that aged garlic extract (such as the widely available Kyolic brand) delivers similar benefits as well. It's just not quite so good in spaghetti sauce and soup.

Spice Up Your Health with Everyday Seasonings

Jonny Bowden, PhD, CNS, a board certified nutritionist, the "Weight Loss Coach" on iVillage.com and author of the best-selling *Living the Low Carb Life* (Sterling) as well as *The 150 Healthiest Foods on Earth* (Fair Winds). Find out more at *www.jonny bowden.com*.

It's exciting to see the increasing focus of research on the health benefits of everyday spices like chilies for prostate cancer...turmeric to reduce inflammation...ginger for nausea, to name just a few. Herbs and spices, derived from various plants, have a long history of medicinal use in Chinese medicine, Ayurveda and other traditional medical systems. What else is there in the spice rack that we can use to "healthify" our meals in a delicious way?

"Everyday spices are an amazing source of phytochemicals, which are plant compounds with extraordinary healing properties," explains nutritionist and weight-loss coach Jonny Bowden, author of *The 150 Healthiest Foods on Earth* (Fair Winds). "Many of these spices have been used in traditional medicine for hundreds of years, and Western medicine is just beginning to realize their potential." *Here are a few of Dr. Bowden's top picks for powering up your foods...*

CINNAMON

"There are anti-inflammatory compounds in cinnamon that can be helpful in alleviating pain, stiffness and even menstrual discomfort," says Dr. Bowden. "Additionally, compounds in cinnamon increase the ability of the cells to take in sugar, which is how it effectively lowers blood sugar and reduces the need for higher levels of insulin." A study published in *Diabetes Care* showed that cinnamon lowered not only blood sugar, but also triglycerides, total cholesterol and low-density lipoprotein (LDL), the "bad" cholesterol, in people with type 2 diabetes. Though it's not always the case with our other plant-based remedies, the inexpensive supermarket variety of cinnamon is basically as good as any of the pricier oils and extracts sold in specialty stores.

GINGER

Ginger, known as the "universal medicine" in Ayurvedic medicine, is often used to soothe an upset stomach and quell nausea. In fact, in one study on ginger root, it was shown to be as effective as Dramamine in holding seasickness at bay. Ginger also packs plenty of powerful antioxidants, Dr. Bowden says. "And animal studies show that ginger has antimicrobial effects and helps boost the immune system as well."

TURMERIC

Turmeric—the spice Dr. Bowden waxes most enthusiastic about—is a member of the ginger family, and also a heavy hitter in health benefits. "It's as close to a magical substance as you're likely to find in the kitchen cupboard," he points out. He attributes this spice's anti-inflammatory properties to *curcumin*, the substance responsible for making some Indian food and curry dishes yellow. In India, turmeric is used to treat arthritis precisely because of its ability to lower inflammation, Dr. Bowden says, noting that

research indicates that curcumin also may have an anti-tumor effect. If you're not an Indian food eater, you can try it in rice dishes or even on eggs. Do not use medicinal amounts of turmeric during pregnancy, though, because it stimulates contraction of the uterus.

OREGANO

Another spice touted for its health properties is oregano, which Dr. Bowden tells us "has been shown by research to have 42 times more antioxidant activity than apples and 12 times more than oranges." Oregano contains a powerful cancer-fighting compound called *rosmarinic acid* as well, and its anti-inflammatory properties make it useful in supporting joint function. Oregano is also a source of calcium, magnesium, zinc, iron and potassium.

GARLIC

Of course garlic is not always used as a spice, but it does have a well-deserved reputation for adding flavor and boosting health. One of the oldest medicinal foods we know of, it is recognized even by mainstream medical professionals as being helpful in reducing cholesterol. Dr. Bowden cites a study that found garlic reduces triglycerides by up to 17%. It has a small but notably positive effect on blood pressure. "In places where the consumption of garlic is high, there's a decreased risk of stomach and colon cancer," Dr. Bowden adds.

Some other spices that have health-promoting properties include...

• **Cardamom.** Another member of the ginger family, cardamom is found in spiced chai tea, used to flavor Turkish coffee, and is added to baked goods in Scandinavia. It stimulates digestion and flow of bile.

• **Mustard seeds.** These are a source of magnesium and selenium, and can be taken orally to stimulate appetite and circulation, and to help neutralize inflammatory materials in the GI tract.

• **Parsley.** A good source of vitamin K and potassium, parsley is also helpful for detoxification.

•**Rosemary.** Contains lots of antioxidants and anti-inflammatory compounds, plus substances that help prevent the premature breakdown of *acetylcholine*, a neurotransmitter that's vital for memory and healthy brain function.

•**Sage.** Contains rosmarinic acid (like oregano), which is both an antioxidant and an anti-inflammatory, along with *thujone*, which can be protective against *Salmonella* and *Candida*.

•**Thyme.** Helps relieve chest and respiratory problems, including coughs and bronchitis.

MORE THAN A PINCH?

How much of each seasoning is needed to make a difference? Dr. Bowden says it's usually more than is typically required for cooking to achieve a notable benefit —though it seems logical that adding a variety of spices, more often and in plentiful amounts, would have a cumulative positive effect. Though some of the dried spices retain their healthful properties, fresh herbs are usually nutritionally superior—not to mention delicious, and fun and easy to grow.

New Research Reveals Inside Story on Salt

Glenn Rothfeld, MD, clinical assistant professor, Tufts University School of Medicine, Boston. *www.wholehealthne.com.*

There is no question that salt is essential to life. It regulates numerous bodily functions. However, for some people, even a little salt is sometimes too much and can damage their health. Who are these salt-sensitive people? For details, we called Glenn Rothfeld, MD, clinical assistant professor at Tufts University School of Medicine in Boston, and a practitioner of integrative medicine who has long studied salt's role in health.

TWO TYPES OF HYPERTENSION

Salt sensitivity is when a person's blood pressure rises in response to salt intake. Although it's commonly assumed that anyone with high blood pressure (hypertension) is salt sensitive and so should greatly curtail salt intake, the data show this is not always the case. In fact, just over half of hypertensive people are salt sensitive. What about the others? Dr. Rothfeld explains that there are essentially two kinds of hypertension—one relates to volume, meaning an excess of fluid in the vessels, and the other to pressure, which reflects constriction of the blood vessels. For people who are volume sensitive, too much salt is a problem because salt can cause water retention and thus can *increase* the amount of fluid in the vessels. Those who have pressure-related hypertension are not as vulnerable to salt consumption problems.

OTHER PROBLEMS

But increased blood pressure alone is not the only indicator of salt sensitivity. About 26% of people with normal blood pressure are salt sensitive, making them vulnerable to possibly developing hypertension but also other health problems, as more research is showing. A National Institutes of Health (NIH) study revealed that salt sensitivity increases the risk of developing an enlargement of the heart's main pumping chamber, which compromises the chamber's proper functioning. Salt sensitivity also has been associated with kidney problems and now, says Dr. Rothfeld, it appears there is a relationship between salt sensitivity and insulin resistance as well. Our consulting medical editor Andrew L. Rubman, ND, says it is not surprising that researchers are finding a link between salt sensitivity and insulin resistance because both are regulated by hormones that are produced in the adrenal cortex.

It is important for anyone in the at-risk group to pay careful attention to salt sensitivity to protect his/her long-term health. *The following conditions, says Dr. Rothfeld, are indicators of being at risk...*

•**Having hypertension or a family history of it.**

•**Being obese.**

•**Having additional indicators of metabolic syndrome** (a cluster of findings that put people at elevated cardiovascular risk if they have three or more) such as high LDL cholesterol, an elevated C-reactive protein level, elevated triglycerides and insulin resistance.

•**Women with polycystic ovary disease** (ovarian cysts).

•**Being age 55 or older.**

•**Being African American.**

TESTING FOR SENSITIVITY

A definitive test for salt sensitivity, unfortunately, does not exist right now, although researchers at the University of Virginia are developing a genetic study for the condition that promises to have 94% accuracy. However, a simple blood test gives information about a person's *renin angiotensin-aldosterone system*, a hormone system that helps regulate blood pressure and blood volume, with results that suggest the type of hypertension the person has. The test is a good indicator of the presence of salt sensitivity as well, says Dr. Rothfeld.

It's also possible to do a two-week trial at home, although you will have to have a blood pressure measuring device. (Electronic ones are available at drugstores for about $70.) For two weeks, do not consume more than 2 grams (g) of salt a day (2,000 milligrams, or mg). Dr. Rothfeld says that some people notice a difference in just a few days because they lose puffiness, but the real measure is changes in blood pressure. If you have a five- to 10-point drop in the systolic reading (the higher one) at the end of the two-week period, it's highly likely you are salt sensitive.

SALT-REDUCTION STRATEGIES

Without question, our salt-saturated food culture leads people to consume far more salt than they need for health, even as much as 20,000 mg a day. If you are salt sensitive, restrict salt to 1,500 mg a day or less. This becomes much easier to accomplish by avoiding processed foods (including canned foods). Salt serves as a flavor enhancer and preservative in processed food, which in turn is the principal source of salt in the American diet. In fact, only about 10% of salt consumption comes from table salt.

Cheeses are often another culprit. Soft cheese in particular is high in sodium.

CALCIUM-MAGNESIUM-POTASSIUM BALANCERS

In addition to reducing salt, ensuring the adequate levels and balance of three minerals is crucial to addressing salt sensitivity, says Dr. Rothfeld. The three are potassium, calcium and magnesium. Imbalances in sodium can be caused by mineral deficiencies. Dr. Rothfeld recommends consuming 3,500 mg of potassium...800 mg to 1,000 mg of calcium—with 1,200 mg to 1,500 mg for post-menopausal women...and 500 mg to 800 mg of magnesium each day in addition to moderating salt intake.

Note: While it is safe to use supplements to ensure adequate levels of calcium and magnesium, it is not recommended to supplement potassium without a doctor's supervision. Excessive levels of potassium can be fatal. It is better to get your potassium through food. A list of potassium-rich foods can be found at: *www.vaughns-1-pagers.com/food/potassium-foods.htm.*

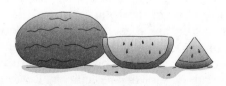

Uh-Oh! Milk Zaps the Healing Power of Tea

Verena Stangl, MD, professor, department of internal medicine, cardiology and angiology, Charité Hospital, University of Berlin, Germany.

Enjoying a cup of tea feels positively virtuous these days, given all we hear about the health-promoting antioxidants and flavonoids that researchers have discovered are in the brew. There's a surprising catch, however, for those who enjoy milk in their tea. According to a new study, tea with milk may do much less for your health.

TAKE TEA, THEN SEE

The study, from the Charité Hospital, University of Berlin, Germany, included 16 healthy postmenopausal women who, over the course of three clinical visits, drank half a liter of freshly brewed black tea alone...another time tea with 10% skim milk...another time just boiled water. Researchers measured the function of the endothelium (the cell lining) of the brachial artery before and for two hours after consumption of the beverage. The brachial artery was used since it is easy to access and measure and reacts quickly to inflammatory stimuli. Black tea alone, they found, improved the artery's ability to relax and expand, but adding milk to the tea inhibited this biological effect.

Further tests on rats measured the effect of both tea and tea with milk on the rodents' aortic tissue and endothelial cells produced similar results. This could explain why in some tea-drinking cultures, such as in Asia, the incidence of heart disease is lower than elsewhere, whereas in England, with its heavy consumption of tea with milk, it is not.

MORE RESEARCH COMING

Verena Stangl, MD, professor of cardiology and angiology at Charité, was the senior author of the study. She says that when combined with tea, the proteins in milk, called *caseins*, decrease the concentration of healthful flavonoids (*catechins*). Although only women were measured in this study, Dr. Stangl feels confident that the effect on men's endothelial function would be the same. She notes that other small studies have similarly shown that the antioxidant effects of tea are diminished when milk is added, but this hasn't been firmly established. Could a similar effect be noted in drinkers of coffee with milk? Does milk also diminish coffee's antioxidant effect? Dr. Stangl believes that theoretically this would be true, but says it hasn't been confirmed through research. She is now at work on another study to determine if there is any difference between the health benefits of green and black teas. Stay tuned for the results.

Bottled Teas Missing Healthy Ingredients

Marion Nestle, PhD, professor of nutrition, New York University, New York City.

It didn't take long for food manufacturers to jump on the news in recent years about the health benefits of assorted varieties of tea. Now consumers can find all sorts of exotic offerings, such as blueberry white tea and icy green tea spiked with ginseng. Indeed, sales of ready-to-drink teas have really grown. Tasty? Yes (to some). Healthful? No.

ALL TEAS ARE NOT CREATED EQUAL

The trouble is, all teas are not created equal. It's fairly well-established that freshly brewed teas of every stripe—white, green, oolong and black varieties from the *Camellia sinensis* plant—confer certain health benefits. Packed with high levels of antioxidants, *polyphenols* and other healthful compounds, drinking these hot teas on a regular basis may promote heart health and reduce the risk of health issues such as cancer, arthritis, osteoporosis, cataracts and dental cavities.

However, bottled teas contain considerably fewer of these beneficial components and, worse yet, many are essentially no more than diluted sugar water. At Oregon State University in Corvallis, researchers found that ready-to-drink teas typically had levels of polyphenols and antioxidant activity 10 to 100 times lower than those in conventionally brewed tea.

In addition, bottled teas are...

•**Usually made with low-grade commercial tea,** which means fewer antioxidants in the first place.

•**Packaged in glass bottles** that allow the photosensitive antioxidant compounds to degrade by exposure to ultraviolet light.

•**Packed with unnatural polyphenols** used as "natural" stabilizers and shelf-life extenders. These are added compounds that aren't naturally found in tea.

•**Packed with sugar or artificial sweeteners.**

FRESH BREWED IS BEST

Next time you think you're doing something good for your health by reaching for a bottle of iced tea instead of a soft drink, think again. It is hard to find a bottle of tea that does not contain sugars or artificial sweeteners, notes Marion Nestle, PhD, a professor of nutrition at New York University in New York City. If you want to include tea drinking as part of a healthful lifestyle, Dr. Nestle recommends that you stick with the freshly brewed variety either hot or on ice.

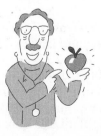

Health Food Phonies You Should Leave On the Shelf

Jonny Bowden, PhD, CNS, a board certified nutritionist, the "Weight Loss Coach" on iVillage.com and author of the best-selling Living the Low Carb Life *(Sterling) as well as* The 150 Healthiest Foods on Earth *(Fair Winds). Find out more at* www.jonny bowden.com.

Grocery store aisles abound with foods purported to be healthy. In fact, they are junk disguised in wholesome packaging.

A prime example of this is margarine. It was originally introduced as a healthy alternative to butter, but many margarines, loaded with trans fat, may be far worse for you than the butter it replaced. (It's possible that an exception is the plant sterol-enriched margarines recently brought to market, but we don't know enough about them yet, so the jury is still out on their health value.) And what about some of the other staples of the health-food industry? Are they really as "good" for us as we've been led to believe?

We spoke with board certified nutritionist and weight-loss coach Jonny Bowden, PhD, CNS, on that topic, and here's what we learned...

BREAKFAST CEREALS AND MEAL-REPLACEMENT BARS

The claim that many cereals are "whole grain" is wholly misleading. "The fact that something started as whole grain doesn't mean much if all the nutrition has been processed out of it," says Dr. Bowden. "Many cereal labels today say 'made from whole grains.' These 'whole grain' cereals have been processed to the point where they have around 2 grams (g) or less of fiber per serving, which is minimal." In Dr. Bowden's opinion, whole grain cereals with less than 5 g of fiber per serving are no better than the cereals they replaced.

"Additionally, many cereal- and grain-based breakfast products are loaded with sugar, some have trans fat, and most also have additives," says Dr. Bowden. He advises reading the labels carefully. Strive to find brands with about 10 g of protein (or close to that), no hydrogenated oils and no more than a couple of grams of sugar per serving. This doesn't mean you have to give up this convenient food category altogether. For example, the Atkins Advantage bars meet that criteria, as do a few—very few—others. "There are also good bars that have more sugar than three grams," he added, "but those are specialty whole-foods bars, such as Omega Smart... Bumble Bars...and LaraBars, made from nothing but real fruit, spices and nuts." All of these are healthy. Most other energy and meal replacement bars have very high sugar and belong in the candy aisle.

OY! SOY, TOO

Soy has been a health darling of recent years. It has become the primary source of protein in many protein-enriched products. Now, however, the bloom is off that rose. "I don't think soy is the worst thing in the world for you," Dr. Bowden says, "but I think it's been way oversold as a health food." The healthy kind of soy is that which is traditionally fermented, like miso and tempeh, or minimally processed, like edamame. Other soy products (such as those in some meal-replacement bars) should be enjoyed in moderation, according to Dr. Bowden.

CANOLA OIL: NO CAN DO

Neither is Dr. Bowden a fan of canola oil. "The presence of canola oil in the marketplace is a triumph of marketing over science," he says. "Canola oil is a highly processed oil that needs to be deodorized at high temperatures, which frequently creates trans fat," he notes. "In addition, the omega-3s in it are easily damaged by heating." If you want to use canola oil, stick to cold-pressed organic canola oil and use it for dressings, but not for cooking.

YOGURT

Yogurt—a major health craze a couple of decades ago—is not all that healthy in the drinkable and squeezable and high-sugar forms that are available today. What about frozen yogurt? "Its only resemblance to real yogurt is that they're both white," Dr. Bowden laughs. "Seriously, it can be a delicious dessert, but don't fool yourself that frozen yogurt is healthier than ice cream. In fact, the nonfat kind is often filled with aspartame, which can be a problem for many people," he says. Why not go ahead and eat the ice cream, and get the highest quality you can find? "Just eat it less often," he suggests.

FRUIT DRINKS

Another great pretender? Commercial fruit beverages, especially many of the kinds marketed and conveniently packaged for kids' lunches, are nothing but sugar water. "You are far better off drinking water and flavoring it with lemon or cherry or berry juice concentrate, which are high in antioxidants. Or, if you really want the juice, dilute it with water in a 1:4, solution so you take in less sugar," Dr. Bowden says. Healthy exceptions to the "no juice" rule are 100% juices made from cranberry and pomegranate, which do, in fact, contain plenty of important and desirable nutrients.

It's easy to be fooled by the advertising claims made for many products. Be skeptical, smart and look for foods that are minimally processed.

Start Your Day with a Super Breakfast

Jonny Bowden, PhD, CNS, a board certified nutritionist, the "Weight Loss Coach" on iVillage.com and author of the best-selling *Living the Low Carb Life* (Sterling) as well as *The 150 Healthiest Foods on Earth* (Fair Winds). Find out more at *www.jonny bowden.com.*

There's an old saying that goes 'Eat breakfast like a king, lunch like a prince and dinner like a pauper,'" says nutritionist and weight-loss coach

Jonny Bowden, PhD, CNS. "But most of us do the opposite." According to Dr. Bowden, this is exactly the wrong way to eat if we're trying to lose weight. It also works against us if we're trying to keep our energy up during the day and our performance level high. "Remember, you've just completed eight hours without food," he says. "You're literally breaking a fast. Your body is craving nourishment, and your brain needs glucose to function at its best. Skipping breakfast is one of the worst possible things you can do. You set yourself up for disaster in a number of different ways later in the day. People who skip breakfast are more than four times as likely to be obese than people who eat something in the morning."

EARLY EATER ADVANTAGES

Then there's performance. "Numerous studies over the years have shown that skipping breakfast impacts the behavior and mental performance of school kids," Dr. Bowden says. "Kids who eat breakfast have better memory, and higher math and reading scores. And kids who are hungry have a large number of behavior problems, including fighting, stealing, having difficulty with teachers and not acknowledging rules."

Additionally, people who eat breakfast are far more likely to get a healthy intake of vitamins and minerals than those who don't. In one study published in the *Journal of the American College of Nutrition*, researchers found that people who ate a hearty breakfast containing more than one-quarter of their daily calories had a higher intake of essential vitamins and minerals and lower serum cholesterol levels to boot.

THE BEST BREAKFAST

So what constitutes a good breakfast? "Higher protein breakfasts translate into a more sustained level of energy throughout the morning and possibly the day," Dr. Bowden says. "Protein fills you up longer, and you're less likely to have midmorning cravings. You're also less likely to overeat at lunch." And more protein at breakfast may increase metabolism, helping you to maintain a healthy weight. "In one study, a high-protein breakfast increased the metabolism of healthy young women by a shocking 100%," Dr. Bowden tells us.

"There are definite advantages to higher protein intakes in the morning," Dr. Bowden continues, "but that doesn't mean 10,000 calories of bacon." He recommends that at least one-third of your breakfast come from a lean protein source and the rest from healthy fats and fibrous carbs. "If you eat eggs, for goodness' sake, don't throw out the yolks," he urges. They're loaded with good nutrition, and may even lower your cholesterol levels, he added.

INSIDE THE BENTO BOX

"Moreover, don't be afraid to think outside the box," Dr. Bowden advises. He points out that in Asia, the traditional Japanese breakfast consists of a small piece of fish (like salmon), some light vegetables and a tiny portion of rice, accompanied by a small bowl of miso soup. "The health benefits of fish and vegetables in the morning are huge," Dr. Bowden reports. "And the omega-3s in salmon are terrific for your skin, plus they help regulate mood." *If salmon's a stretch for you, Dr. Bowden has his own list of favorite protein-packed breakfasts for more Western palates...*

•**Eggs.** "I think eggs are one of nature's perfect food sources," he opines. "They are loaded with protein and other nutrients such as *phosphatidylcholine* for the brain and heart."

A Bowden breakfast favorite: Scramble some eggs with spinach and sliced apples in some coconut oil, and season with turmeric and lemon pepper. "It's loaded with protein and nutrients for the eyes, like *lutein* and *zeaxanthin*," he explains. "Plus it includes turmeric, one of nature's great anti-inflammatories." (*Note:* Dr. Bowden strongly recommends free-range eggs—from hens that had access to the outdoors where they could run around and eat more natural food, which changes the fat and nutrition profile of their meat and eggs.)

• **Yogurt that contains active cultures.** "One of my favorite quick breakfasts is yogurt with nuts and red or purple grapes," Dr. Bowden says. "I always use goat's or sheep's milk yogurt because it's less likely to have added hormones in it and has a better nutrient balance. Then I sprinkle on some walnuts or almonds or pecans."

• **Peanut butter and banana sandwich.** "If you're someone who can tolerate grains," says Dr. Bowden, "buy a good whole-grain bread, preferably sprouted grain, take one slice and make a half sandwich using natural, unsweetened peanut or almond butter, a banana and, if you like, a dollop of yogurt on top."

• **Whey protein shake.** "Whey is my favorite protein powder," Dr. Bowden tells us, because it raises *glutathione*, the most important antioxidant in the body, and has shown in one study to lower blood pressure by about 5 millimeters of mercury (mmHg; a unit of pressure). "You can make a nutritious shake using water, whey protein and frozen berries, with a little cranberry or pomegranate juice. Or almond or rice milk. Throw in a handful of raw oats for texture—it tastes much better than it sounds. Adding a splash of olive oil to the shake will reduce the glycemic index and help the smoothie 'stick' with you a little longer. Experiment. Peanut butter is another great add-in."

• **Homemade muesli or granola.** According to Dr. Bowden, "Raw foods have a lot to offer. They contain enzymes, they haven't been processed, they tend to have fiber and they're loaded with nutrients."

Dr. Bowden's favorite: "Take some raw oats…soak in a little pomegranate juice…add nuts, berries or sliced apples, and flaked coconut. You can sweeten with *xylitol* if you need to (though it has been found to cause diarrhea in some), but it's delicious without it. You can also use raw cold-pressed honey or blackstrap molasses if you like."

Moove Over, Milk: Better Sources for Calcium

Mark A. Stengler, ND, naturopathic physician in private practice, La Jolla, California…adjunct associate clinical professor at the National College of Natural Medicine, Portland, Oregon…author of many books, including *The Natural Physician's Healing Therapies* and coauthor of *Prescription for Natural Cures* (both from Bottom Line Books)…and author of the *Bottom Line/Natural Healing* newsletter.

In spite of the US Department of Agriculture's (USDA's) latest dietary guidelines recommending milk as part of a balanced diet, evidence continues to mount that cow's milk is best left to the calves.

INTOLERANCE AND ABSORPTION ISSUES

Many Americans are lactose intolerant, meaning that they find it difficult to digest the milk sugar lactose, reacting with symptoms such as nausea, bloating, gas, cramps and diarrhea. Others have a milk allergy and cannot tolerate casein or whey proteins in milk. When they drink a glass, the uncomfortable consequences may include digestive disturbances, skin rash, vomiting, wheezing, immune system reactions and mucus build-up in the sinuses. Even Lactaid—a lactose-free milk made for lactose intolerant people—still contains casein. Organic milk poses other challenges of its own.

Not only is milk difficult to digest, it may also not be among the best forms of calcium for absorption, says Mark Stengler, ND, author of *Bottom Line Natural Healing* newsletter. He suggests that people who drink milk limit themselves to 24 ounces a week and bulk up on calcium-rich foods. This holds truer for children, due to the sensitivity of developing immune systems to milk's allergy-inducing properties, says Dr. Stengler. He notes that there is a possible association between cow's milk and recurring ear infections in children.

In other studies, cow's milk has been associated with cardiovascular disease and cancer. In the Harvard Nurses' Health Study (Boston), women with an increased intake of calcium from dairy products actually had a higher risk of bone fractures.

BETTER OPTIONS?

What *should* you put on your cereal and in your coffee?

Dr. Stengler points out that some people with an intolerance to milk seem to do better on goat's milk. However, those with allergies should use goat's milk with caution—it also contains casein-like proteins. Like cow's milk, goat's milk is packed with calcium. A cup of goat's milk supplies 327 milligrams (mg) of calcium along with 271 mg of phosphorus. In comparison, a cup of cow's milk provides 276 mg of calcium and 222 mg of phosphorus. Goat's—and sheep's—milk aren't adequate for babies under one year, since they don't contain the right amount of nutrients.

Other alternative sources of calcium include goat's and sheep's milk cheeses, as well as calcium-enriched plant-based milks such as almond, oat, hazelnut, rice and soy. Plant-based milks are good substitutes for people with milk allergies. While plant-based milks are not naturally rich in calcium, manufacturers fortify them. Dr. Stengler says that any of these enriched plant-based milks generally have just as much calcium per glass as cow's milk or more.

A WORD ABOUT SOY

Lately, there has been some controversy concerning soy products. Women with a history of, or existing, breast cancer should not consume soy milk, as it has an estrogenic effect on the body. In Dr. Stengler's opinion, children can have soy milk in moderation, but it is best to rotate with other plant milks.

Of course, if your goal is to find alternative sources of calcium rather than another kind of milk to drink, there are plenty of other food sources of calcium…

Food	Calcium (mg)
Broccoli, raw, ½ cup	21
Cereal, fortified, 1 cup	100 to 1,000
Chinese cabbage, raw, 1 cup	74
Kale, cooked, 1 cup	94
Orange juice, fortified, 6 oz.	200 to 260
Salmon, canned with bones, 3 oz.	181
Sardines, canned with bones, 3 oz.	324
Spinach, cooked, ½ cup	120
Turnip greens, cooked, ½ cup	99

Source: National Institutes of Health, Office of Dietary Supplements.

TOO MUCH OF A GOOD THING

We asked Dr. Stengler if he agrees with the standard government recommendations for calcium intake (1,000 mg/day for those age 19 to 50, and 1,200 mg/day for people age 51 and over). Because there are questions about a possible link between calcium and prostate cancer, until this issue is resolved, he recommends 500 mg daily for men.

A study published in the *Journal of the National Cancer Institute* reviewing 12 studies on this association concluded, "High intake of dairy products and calcium may be associated with an increased risk of prostate cancer, although the increase appears to be small." Another study found that calcium intake exceeding 1,500 mg a day might be associated with a higher risk of advanced and fatal prostate cancers.

Calcium is a vital nutrient for building and maintaining bone, but it is best to get it from a variety of sources, being especially careful to limit consumption from cow's milk and soy.

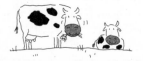

Incredible! Organic Milk May be Missing Nutrients

Ron Schmid, ND, naturopathic physician and director of the Alternative Medicine Center of Watertown, Connecticut. Dr. Schmid is author of *Traditional Foods Are Your Best Medicine* (Healing Arts) and *The Untold Story of Milk* (New Trends). He has prescribed raw milk for his patients for nearly 25 years.

As people become more health conscious and fearful of food products laden with growth hormones, antibiotics and pesticides, there is a growing market for organic foods. But there is an organic product that may not be as good as you would think—organic milk, now common in many grocery stores.

WHAT'S WRONG WITH ORGANIC MILK?

According to Ron Schmid, ND, a naturopathic physician at the Alternative Medicine Center in Watertown, Connecticut and author of *The Untold Story of Milk* (New Trends), organic milk—from cows who are raised antibiotic- and hormone-free—may in fact be less nutritious because it is frequently ultra-pasteurized to give it extra-long shelf life. "The ultra-pasteurization process is even worse than standard pasteurization since it kills not only the bacteria (both good and bad) but also many of the other beneficial properties in the milk, such as helpful enzymes and friendly bacteria," he explains. (Ultra-pasteurized milk is pasteurized at a higher temperature for a shorter period of time.)

"In fact," continues Dr. Schmid, "ultra-pasteurizing is so successful at killing things that the milk doesn't even have to be refrigerated afterward (if it's packaged in aseptic packaging). The only reason they do is because no one would buy milk if it was on the shelf next to cereal instead of in the cooler."

MILKING THE ORGANIC CONSUMER

To be labeled "organic," milk must meet criteria established by the US Department of Agriculture (USDA). It must come from cows that have not been treated with bovine growth hormone (BGH), which is done with cows that produce regular milk in order to increase production. Treatment with antibiotics is also not allowed in cows producing milk that will be sold as organic. Their feed must be grown without chemical pesticides—and the cows must have "access to pasture." (This final point has little meaning since the regulations don't stipulate how much time the cows spend in pasture.)

Though it is certainly true that the consumer has one layer of protection not found in "regular" milk—protection from the pesticides normally sprayed on cows' feed (grain)—organic milk producers have figured out how to bend the rules in other ways. "The natural diet of cows is grass, not grain," explains Dr. Schmid. "Most organic milk is produced in factory farms. Their cows start on pasture, but are then moved to outdoor feedlots full of grain. You still have all the same problems you have with regular milk—it is overly acidic (cows fed grains versus grass are more acidic and produce acid-resistant pathogens), the fat is lacking in omega-3s (grain affects omega-3 content adversely), and the real food value is destroyed during the processing."

GOT RAW MILK?

There is an alternative for people who believe in milk as a health food—but it's not always easy to get: "Raw" milk, which has not been pasteurized or homogenized. Literally coming right from the cow, with no processing whatsoever, the raw milk looks and tastes different—creamier, thicker, richer. Some people love it—and Dr. Schmid himself is a fan.

KNOW THE FARMER

However, primarily due to concerns about bacteria or pathogens not killed by the pasteurization process, raw milk is unlikely to be found in the dairy section of your local supermarket or food stores. In many states, it can't be sold legally at all, even on the dairy farm where the cows live. Further, states may impose heavier restrictions on suppliers of raw milk than on the suppliers of pasteurized, homogenized milk—organic or otherwise.

When it comes to any milk, as Dr. Schmid says, "ultimately, it is far more important to know your farm of origin than to rely on what the label says."

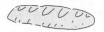

Is White Whole Wheat Bread a Half-Baked Idea?

Joy Bauer, MS, RD, nutritionist and coauthor of *Joy's LIFE Diet* (Collins) and *Joy Bauer's Food Cures* (St. Martin's). Bauer is a nutrition expert for the *Today* show.

Our health-care experts regularly urge a diet rich in whole foods (such as produce, lean proteins and whole grains) yet the food marketers seem focused on coming up with new ways to make their man-made versions of nature sound healthful.

Consumers who dislike the taste and texture of whole wheat bread will be happy to know that manufacturers have cooked up a new alternative—white whole wheat bread. The color of the bread is white or white-beige, but it is in fact made with whole wheat—albeit whole wheat made from a naturally white kernel. And, according to nutritionist Joy Bauer, MS, RD, coauthor of *Joy's LIFE Diet* (Collins) and nutrition expert for the *Today* show, white whole wheat bread, which can be found at most supermarkets, can be a good compromise for the many people—especially children—who are turned off by harsher whole grains.

LIGHTER, SOFTER AND SWEETER

White whole wheat bread is made with albino wheat, which is lighter in color, lighter in texture and sweeter in taste than regular whole wheat (which is more

correctly called "red" wheat). Regular whole wheat flour is dark in color and slightly bitter, due to the presence of phenolic compounds. The nutritional content of both these wheats is identical. Neither type of 100% whole wheat flour (red wheat or albino wheat) is refined, so in both cases you get the same vitamins, nutrients and fiber content. (To determine if bread is whole grain, check the label. The word "whole" should be listed as part of the first ingredient.) In contrast, regular white bread is made with refined grains, which are stripped of their vital nutrients.

BLOOD SUGAR IMPACT

One remaining issue regarding white whole wheat bread relates to its glycemic index, notes Bauer. The glycemic index is a ranking system for carbohydrates based on their effect on blood glucose levels. Eating low index carbs—such as fiber-rich veggies (broccoli, cabbage, peppers, etc.), which have a minimal impact on blood glucose—is healthier than eating foods with a higher glycemic index. Breads in general have a higher glycemic index than most vegetables. Generally speaking, the finer the flour, the quicker the rise in blood sugar, says Bauer. "Therefore, people with type 2 diabetes and blood sugar concerns need to make sure they moderate the amount of bread they eat—even the whole wheat varieties—and consume breads with lean protein to help minimize the sharp rise in blood sugar."

White whole wheat bread is nutritionally better than those refined white breads, and fresh-baked baguettes...but it may be healthier to view this product as a transition food. If you're not a fan of regular heartier whole wheat bread and other grains, consider using this new alternative to gradually retrain your taste buds away from the refined carbohydrates so common in the American diet and toward the heartier and healthier carbs, including whole barley, oats, brown rice, farro and quinoa.

The Latest Buzz on Honey

Rosa Ana Perez, PhD, researcher in the Department of Food Science and Technology in Madrid, Spain.

"Honeydew" honey (no relation to the melon of the same name) is superior to other honey, according to Spanish researchers, because it has a higher antioxidant capacity.

ABOUT HONEYDEW HONEY

Honey is actually a complex natural product produced (by honeybees, naturally) from one of two sources. The one most commonly available, produced by bees that feast on the nectar of flowers, is called, unsurprisingly, nectar honey. It comes in a variety of forms, some raw and some processed to the point where it could practically be called "liquid sugar."

In contrast, honeydew honey is an antioxidant-packed sweetener, with a rich, earthy, malty taste, made by bees that have relied on a different food source. These bees eat a kind of sap-like excretion (called honeydew) produced on trees and plants that have been attacked by insects.

A HONEY OF A STUDY

We contacted Rosa Ana Perez, PhD, a researcher in the Department of Food Science and Technology in Madrid to learn more about her study of honey. Her research group performed chemical analyses of 36 different Spanish honeys from a variety of origins. They found that the antioxidant properties of honeydew honeys were more potent and powerful than the conventional nectar honeys. The total *polyphenol* content is also higher in honeydew honeys, and their anti-browning properties (which, for example, can prevent apples from turning brown) further demonstrate antioxidant-capacity. It's possible that not everyone will like the different flavor of the honeydew honey, which has a darker, caramel color, a spicy, woody fresh odor and is not as sweet as traditional honey. However, it is quite common in other countries and is used the same way nectar honey is used. Given its health benefits, it may be worth a try.

Onions Reduce Cancer Risk Up to 88%

Carlotta Galeone, PhD, Istituto di Ricerche Farmacologiche "Mario Negri," Laboratorio di Epidemiologia Generale, Milan, Italy.

If you're a fan of TV chef Emeril, you know that he heaps on the onions and garlic when he cooks. Bam! The good news is that onions and garlic not only taste great, they are also very healthful. In a recent analysis of European studies, Italian and Swiss researchers discovered that the more onions and garlic people ate, the less likely they were to develop common cancers such as oral, colorectal and ovarian cancer.

For more information about the analysis, we consulted lead author Carlotta Galeone, PhD, of the Istituto di Ricerche Farmacologiche "Mario Negri" in Milan. According to Dr. Galeone, past research focused primarily on the protective role that onion and garlic played in the diet of Chinese, who have distinctive dietary habits. This study confirms that benefits also extend to Western populations, who consume considerably less garlic.

FLAVORFUL CANCER-FIGHTING COMPOUNDS

Onions and garlic are packed with natural cancer-fighting chemical compounds, notes Dr. Galeone. In particular, onions are rich in *flavonoids* (e.g., *quercetin*), disease-fighting antioxidants that prevent oxidative damage to body cells that can eventually lead to cancer. Garlic is packed with *organosulfur* compounds that inhibit tumor growth.

ONIONS, GARLIC AND CANCER

In the study, Dr. Galeone and her colleagues discovered that people who ate approximately one medium-sized onion a week reduced their colorectal cancer risk by 14%, in comparison with those who ate no onions. The protective benefits became more evident with higher intake. Eating at least two medium-sized onions per week reduced cancer risk at several other sites—larynx (56%), ovary (43%) and kidney (25%). Dr. Galeone found the results at even higher intakes even more interesting. People who consumed about one medium-sized onion a day reaped more protection in nearly all cancer sites studied (with the exceptions of prostate and breast cancer). The reduction in cancer risk for frequent consumers (seven or more medium-sized onions) varied from 56% for colorectal cancer to 88% for oral cancer. High intake of garlic was protective against all cancer in all sites studied (with the exception of breast cancer) in comparison with low intake. The reduction in risk ranged from 19% for prostate cancer to 57% for esophageal cancer.

AN OVERALL HEALTHFUL DIET

It is possible that combining onions and garlic with other healthful foods may have contributed to their protective effect, says Dr. Galeone. The researchers speculate that people who eat lots of onions and garlic are likely to follow a healthier, plant-based diet overall, which is known to be protective against cancer. In the Italian diet, for example, they are often eaten with tomatoes and olive oil in salads and pastas.

To help protect yourself and your loved ones, consider spicing up your dishes with plenty of garlic and onions. Simply toss into salads and stir-fries. And for even greater protection, don't forget to add a variety of other fresh, cancer-fighting veggies.

Note: Garlic also has blood-thinning properties. If you take blood-thinning drugs such as *warfarin* (Coumadin), or if you are about to undergo surgery, consult your physician before increasing your garlic intake.

 # Tomatoes' Latest Health Coup

Steven G. Pratt, MD, board-certified ophthalmologist. Dr. Pratt lectures nationally and internationally on the benefits of a diet based on whole foods and adopting healthy lifestyle choices to prevent diseases. He is author of *The New York Times* best-seller *Super-Foods Rx: Fourteen Foods That Will Change Your Life* (Harper), and *SuperFoods HealthStyle: Proven Strategies for Lifelong Health* (William Morrow). Dr. Pratt has appeared on various national TV shows including *Today, Oprah* and *The View.*

Not long ago the news media was abuzz with a new report about the connection between pizza and lower rates of prostate cancer. Everyone made a mad dash for the local pizzeria. The truth was a bit more nuanced—it turned out that men eating more than 10 servings per week of tomato-based products (including pizza) had lower rates of prostate cancer. The lowly tomato became reborn as a superstar of the produce section.

Now, tomatoes are back in the news. A recent report found that a tomato extract product actually lowered blood pressure in patients with stage 1 hypertension. The product—Lyc-O-Mato—is an extract of red, ripe tomatoes including *carotenoids* (especially *lycopene*), *polyphenols* and vitamin E, all known to have significant health benefits. To find out more about this latest news on tomatoes, we called Steven G. Pratt, MD, author of a number of books on "superfoods," and, as it turns out, he is a big fan of tomatoes.

"Tomatoes themselves have many bioactive compounds that are good for cardiovascular health," Dr. Pratt says. "In particular are polyphenols that can decrease blood pressure by causing vasodilation or widening of the blood vessels," Dr. Pratt explains. "Ninety percent of Americans are at risk for being diagnosed with high blood pressure at some point in their lives and reducing blood pressure by as little as a single digit produces a reduction in cardio risk factors."

THE GOOD TOMATO

Dr. Pratt explains that the benefits of tomatoes—and tomato extracts or tomato food products like tomato paste—go beyond just blood pressure and prostate cancer. "Two separate studies in the *American Journal of Clinical Nutrition* recently showed that tomato extracts have anti-platelet function, which means they help prevent your blood from clotting, reducing risk for stroke and heart attacks." This is precisely the benefit that many doctors want patients to get from taking aspirin. "The tomato extract does the same thing as aspirin and doesn't have any side effects except for those folks who are sensitive to nightshade alkaloids or allergic to tomatoes or other vegetables in the nightshade family, such as eggplant," says Dr. Pratt.

The tomato extract product, Lyc-O-Mato, is available in stores such as GNC and the Vitamin Shoppe. Dr. Pratt also sings the praises of other tomato products such as tomato paste. "I personally drink a daily tomato-based veggie cocktail, R.W. Knudsen Very Veggie Cocktail (Low Sodium). It has only 50 calories and 22 mg of lycopene per 8 ounces," he notes.

Great News! Chili Peppers Lower Insulin Levels

Madeleine J. Ball, MD, professor and head of the School of Human Life Sciences, University of Tasmania, Australia.

According to an important recent study from Australia, chili peppers may actually help improve health by affecting the hormone insulin that controls blood sugar.

Madeleine J. Ball, MD, one of the researchers from the study at the University of Tasmania, says that both some small animal and human studies have indicated that consumption of meals containing chili peppers or chili seasoning might increase both calorie burning and fat burning. What the researchers wanted to find out was whether the consumption of chili also affects insulin levels after a meal.

CHILI AND INSULIN

As it turns out, it does. "The subjects had similar blood sugar levels after eating the bland meals and the chili containing meals," Dr. Ball tells us, "but their insulin levels were different." Why does this matter? Because chronically high levels of insulin can be a risk factor for metabolic syndrome, heart disease, diabetes and obesity. "Chili is probably having some effect on the ability of the body to clear—or remove—insulin from the bloodstream," Dr. Ball says.

Though blood sugar went up about the same in all test subjects regardless of whether they were fed chili-containing meals or bland meals, those who ate the chili containing meals had less insulin in their bloodstream according to post-eating measures. The implication? The chili lowered the insulin-induced cortisol response to the meal, which promoted a more stable blood sugar level. Interestingly, the results were more pronounced in those with a higher BMI (body mass index).

CAPSAICIN'S HEAT

The chili preparation used in the study consisted of 30 grams a day of a chili blend that consisted of 55% cayenne chili plus a few other ingredients—such as water and sugar. Dr. Ball believes that *capsaicin* was responsible for the effect—the compound responsible for the heat or pungency in chili peppers. Capsaicin is also the active ingredient in pepper spray. While it's responsible for the burning heat you feel when you eat a really hot chili pepper, it also has significant health benefits. "We suspect it has significant antioxidant and anti-inflammatory properties," Dr. Ball says, which could also be important in reducing atherosclerosis.

More studies will no doubt come on capsaicin. In the meantime, the weather is getting cooler, so go ahead and enjoy that chili.

Take a Bite Out of Health Problems— Load Up on Sauerkraut

Thomas A. Kruzel, ND, naturopathic physician in private practice in Scottsdale, Arizona, past president of the American Association of Naturopathic Physicians and former vice president of clinical affairs and chief medical officer at the Southwest College of Naturopathic Medicine in Phoenix. Dr. Kruzel is author of *Homeopathic Emergency Guide: A Quick Reference Handbook to Effective Homeopathic Care.* North Atlantic.

Not only does sauerkraut (fermented cabbage) taste good—tart, tangy, sweet and sour all at the same time—it's also an extremely healthful food, good for the digestion and a potential weapon against a host of disease-causing microbes.

A JUICY GERM FIGHTER AND MORE

The digestive benefits of sauerkraut have been known for a long time, but recent interest in Korean fermented cabbage, kimchi, and its protective benefits in the fight against flu, indicate that it might be time to take an even closer look at this ballpark favorite. To learn more, we called Thomas A. Kruzel, ND, a naturopathic physician in private practice in Scottsdale, Arizona, and past president of the American Association of Naturopathic Physicians.

Dr. Kruzel confirmed our hypothesis— there are a wealth of benefits in eating sauerkraut, because it's...

•**A germ fighter.** Dr. Kruzel says that sauerkraut contains lactic acid, a natural by-product of the fermentation process that discourages invasive microorganisms such as disease-causing yeast, bacteria and viruses. This even includes the bird flu virus, according to Korean researchers at Seoul National University. (*Note:* The same benefits apply with kimchi and other fermented vegetable products, including pickles.)

•**A digestive aid.** In addition to fighting infectious germs, sauerkraut generates beneficial bacteria and healthy flora throughout the digestive tract. This helps support digestion, soothe stomach irritation, ward off food poisoning and boost immune function.

•**A weapon against cancer.** The fermentation of cabbage also produces *isothiocyanates*, a group of compounds that may help prevent breast, colon, liver and lung cancer. In addition, Dr. Kruzel points out that cabbage is a cruciferous vegetable, like brussels sprouts and cauliflower. According to the US Department of Health and Human Services, eating several servings weekly of cruciferous vegetables can reduce colon cancer risk.

•**A source of valuable nutrients.** Sauerkraut is rich in vitamins C and K, and also contains B-6, iron, folate, calcium, potassium and fiber. A one-cup serving has only 32 calories and no fat or cholesterol.

BUY FRESH OR MAKE YOUR OWN

Unfortunately, as with many foods, there's sauerkraut and there's sauerkraut. The stuff you buy in a can at your local supermarket does not provide the health benefits—not to mention the zippy flavor—of the fresh sauerkraut made at health food stores and old-fashioned delicatessens. The problem is that commercially processed sauerkraut no longer contains the live cultures that combat germs, as pasteurization kills off friendly, as well as unfriendly, bacteria. To get quality sauerkraut, Dr. Kruzel recommends that you buy the fresh variety, or if you're really ambitious make your own.

NOT FOR HOT DOGS ALONE

We're all familiar with sauerkraut as a topping for hot dogs, and after all, what's

206

a summer afternoon at the ballpark without a dog with the works? But sauerkraut is not for hot dogs alone. At juice bars, sauerkraut juice is increasingly popular. Sauerkraut is likewise a tasty accompaniment to meat dishes, a zesty addition to salads and soups, and an ingredient in ethnic favorites such as pierogies, knishes and strudels.

To learn more tasty ways to incorporate sauerkraut into your diet, visit one of the many Web sites that feature recipes (such as *www.sauerkrautrecipes.com*). Try hot potato salad with sauerkraut or Bloody Mary mix combined with sauerkraut juice instead of vodka.

Note: If you have high blood pressure or heart disease, watch out for the high salt content of some sauerkraut.

Unhealthy Elements in Your Healthy Produce

Devon Zagory, PhD, senior vice president, Food Safety and Postharvest Programs, Davis Fresh Technologies, LLC, Davis, California.

Americans may be gaining weight and exercising less, but they are at least taking their nutrition a bit more seriously these days. Consumption of fruits and vegetables is up, but produce-borne illness is also on the rise. In fact, produce has now surpassed meats, poultry and eggs as the cause of large-scale outbreaks of food-borne illnesses. Our editors called Devon Zagory, PhD, senior vice president, Food Safety and Postharvest Programs, at the consulting firm, Davis Fresh Technologies, LLC, in Davis, California, for his advice.

Dr. Zagory says that fruits and vegetables are always going to carry some degree of risk despite careful monitoring by the industry. Produce grows in nature where it could be exposed to bird and animal feces and sometimes polluted water.

Furthermore, much of the produce today undergoes additional steps on its journey from the field to the table. Heads of lettuce are wrapped, many are shredded and bagged, some are put out as part of a salad bar. Fruits get peeled, chunked and tucked into plastic containers. And unfortunately, the more food is handled, the more opportunities there are for contamination from nature or from human hands. *However, there are several key steps you can take as a consumer that will go far to ensure that the produce in your home is safe to eat...*

WORST OFFENDERS

Interestingly, cantaloupes and tomatoes have been particularly problematic. Pathogens can get inside produce, including tomatoes and cantaloupes, through cracks and fissures in the skin or even along the base of the stem. Dr. Zagory says to check produce carefully before you buy it and avoid any that is cracked. Wash all produce before you eat it by rinsing thoroughly under running water—this includes melons and bagged greens even if the label says they are prewashed.

SAY NO TO SOAKING

Some people prefer to soak produce, in particular leaves, but Dr. Zagory says soaking only makes the problem worse.

The reason: If a pathogen is on one leaf or spot on the produce, the water frees the pathogen and enables it to spread throughout the basin and onto the rest of the food. Should you have produce such as sandy spinach leaves that beg for a soak, you can eliminate any pathogens by adding a capful of *sodium hypochlorite bleach* (Clorox, or other household bleach, but be sure to check the label to be sure it is sodium hypochlorite) to a full basin of water.

CROSS OFF CROSS-CONTAMINATION

Cross-contamination is a major culprit in food safety, says Dr. Zagory, and careful hygiene is a must to avoid it. Wash hands carefully before and after handling produce. When slicing or peeling produce, always use a freshly washed knife and be sure the surface on which you are cutting is spotless. Cut out soft spots on fruits because that indicates the area has started to decay. Once produce is cut, refrigerate it—pathogens cannot thrive and multiply rapidly in cold temperatures. When sliced fruit or vegetables are allowed to sit out for any length of time, room temperature will liberate even a tiny speck of a pathogen that might have been on it and it will multiply. The same holds true of cooked produce. Refrigerate leftovers promptly.

But keep eating those fruits and vegetables. The benefits to health are countless.

Sweet News! Sugar Speeds Wound Healing

Thomas A. Kruzel, ND, naturopathic physician in private practice in Scottsdale, Arizona, past president of the American Association of Naturopathic Physicians and former vice president of clinical affairs and chief medical officer at the Southwest College of Naturopathic Medicine in Phoenix. Dr. Kruzel is author of *The Homeopathic Emergency Guide: A Quick Reference Handbook to Effective Homeopathic Care.* North Atlantic.

There may be a valuable and healthful use for sugar—wound healing. Research suggests that sugar is a natural disinfectant that helps destroy bacteria and speeds wound healing.

JUST A SPOONFUL OF SUGAR

According to Thomas A. Kruzel, ND, a naturopathic physician in private practice in Scottsdale, Arizona, and past president of the American Association of Naturopathic Physicians, sugar has been used in wound healing for eons. Its applications range from simple folk recipes that call for pouring granulated sugar on minor cuts and abrasions, to clinical treatments for more serious wounds using sugar mixed into a paste with adhesive hydrogel (gum). Since this combination of sugar and hydrogel also helps prevent or reduce skin contraction and scarring, it serves to amp up sugar's healing powers even more.

HOW SWEET IT IS

Sugar is a safe, nontoxic treatment for a variety of wounds. Dr. Kruzel has seen sugar used primarily in burn patients and in patients with minor wounds. Research indicates that sugar can also play an important role in treating diabetic ulcers. (*Note:* If you have diabetes, consult your health-care provider for the treatment of even minor wounds, especially those that occur on the arm and legs.)

In addition to its natural antimicrobial activity and the consequent infection reduction, this sweet remedy counters inflammation, pain and odor, and promotes easy removal of dead tissue. Moreover, sugar is inexpensive as well as easy and painless to apply. In clinical settings, sugar paste has proven particularly beneficial in the treatment of infected and malodorous wounds that fail to respond to antibiotics. It may well be that overwhelming microorganisms with pure sugar may not only put them off "attacking" the wound but actually may feed them to death, since pure sucrose, in the absence of other nutrients, can be quite deadly!

HOW TO USE SUGAR

Whenever you get a minor cut, scrape or other wound, the first thing to do is rinse it with cool, running water and soap to get the dirt out. Next, sprinkle sugar (powdered or granulated) on the wound and cover it with a sterile dressing. Other research demonstrates that sugar's close cousin, honey, has a similar healing influence on wounds and can be used in the same manner. So the next time your child scrapes his or her knee, consider opening the kitchen cupboard instead of the medicine cabinet.

Caution: Do not attempt to treat serious wounds yourself. If a wound is extensive or bleeding heavily, cover it with a sterile dressing and seek immediate medical attention.

A Drink a Day Keeps Kidney Problems Away

Tobias Kurth, MD, ScD, assistant professor of medicine, Harvard Medical School, Division of Aging, Brigham and Women's Hospital, Boston.

Evidence continues to mount that a little drink can go a long way toward boosting health. A recent study at Brigham and Women's Hospital in Boston in which researchers found that light to moderate consumption of alcohol may have a protective effect against kidney disease was particularly interesting.

According to study author Tobias Kurth, MD, ScD, assistant professor of medicine at Harvard Medical School, moderate alcohol consumption has long been identified as a factor with potential beneficial health effects on cardiovascular disease. Since traditional heart disease risk factors such as high cholesterol levels and smoking are also associated with kidney disease, it may not be surprising to learn that moderate alcohol consumption also can be beneficial for the kidneys.

ABOUT THE STUDY

Dr. Kurth and his colleagues examined data from 11,023 initially healthy men, ages 45 to 84, enrolled in the long-term Physicians' Health Study (Brigham and Women's Hospital, Boston). Over a period of 14 years, the participants reported their alcohol consumption and other behavioral and lifestyle factors and provided blood samples. Two of the most important measurements were creatinine levels and estimated glomerular filtration rate (both are indicators of kidney function). *Researchers found that compared with nondrinkers…*

•**Men who consumed seven or more drinks a week** experienced a 29% lower risk of developing kidney problems.

•**Lower alcohol consumption did not reduce risk.**

These results were published in the *Archives of Internal Medicine.* In the future, Dr. Kurth notes that further research

in broader segments of the population is needed. Because few participants reported heavy alcohol use, the effects of heavy drinking on the kidneys could not be measured in this study.

MODERATION IN ALL THINGS

Dr. Kurth is quick to point out that heavy alcohol consumption has many harmful effects, including damage to the liver, and this particular study does not suggest that, overall, drinking improves health. However, these data support that moderate alcohol consumption—generally considered to be up to one drink a day for women, and up to two for men—may have beneficial effects on some organ systems.

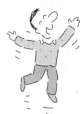

Seven Cheers for the Health Benefits of Beer!

Margo A. Denke, MD, associate professor of internal medicine, University of Texas Southwestern Medical Center, Dallas.

Meir J. Stampfer, MD, DrPH, chair, department of epidemiology, Harvard School of Public Health…professor of medicine, Harvard Medical School…physician, Brigham and Women's Hospital, Boston.

Good news, beer drinkers! Alcohol, it seems, is alcohol, and the health benefits we know to be found in wine are also found in alcoholic drinks like beer. The key word, of course, is "moderation"—most experts advise no more than two alcoholic beverages a day for men and more than one for women.

HERE'S TO YOUR HEALTH

An increasing body of serious research backs up beer's benefits…

•**Bone protection.** According to a medical team at Tufts University in Boston, beer may help prevent bone-thinning osteoporosis. Dietary silicon in grain products such as beer appears to reduce bone loss and promote bone formation. Beer contains silicate, a highly absorbable form of silicon that works by facilitating the deposit of calcium and other minerals in bone tissue. Margo A. Denke, MD, clinical professor of medicine at the University of Texas Southwestern Medical Center in Dallas, cautions that excessive alcohol intake is a risk factor for bad bones, perhaps because calories from nutrient sources are replaced with calories from alcohol.

•**Lower risk for cardiovascular disease.** Like wine, beer has well-documented heart benefits. Regular moderate drinking has a protective effect in both men and women against cardiovascular disease, confirms Meir J. Stampfer, MD, DrPH, chair of the department of epidemiology at the Harvard School of Public Health. He told us that moderate alcohol consumption in any form has an equivalent benefit—"Wine is not better than beer, red wine is not better than white and spirits (in moderation) are also associated with lower risk."

•**Better heart attack survival.** A study at Beth Israel Deaconess Medical Center in Boston concluded that moderate drinkers (who consumed more than seven alcoholic beverages a week) had a 32% lower risk of dying from a heart attack than those who drank no alcohol. Light drinkers (less than seven drinks weekly) had a 21% lower risk. Like other alcohol, beer acts as a blood thinner to help prevent clogged arteries. Other research links moderate alcohol consumption with improved blood circulation in the brain and lower risk for stroke.

•**Improved cholesterol levels.** In her research, Dr. Denke discovered that people who consumed one to three drinks daily had higher levels of high-density lipoprotein (HDL), the "good" cholesterol. She also found that regular moderate intake of alcohol resulted in lower blood insulin levels. In a related US Department of Agriculture (USDA) study, women who drank one alcoholic beverage daily lowered their low-density lipoprotein (LDL—"bad") cholesterol and levels of harmful blood lipids known as triglycerides.

•**Sharper brains.** In the long-term Nurses' Health Study (Harvard Medical School in Boston), Dr. Stampfer and his colleagues found that moderate consumption of alcohol seemed to preserve the mental abilities of older women. From 1995 to 1999, more than 9,000 women between ages 70 and 79 were interviewed regarding their alcohol use, and seven different tests of mental function were administered. Moderate drinkers scored better on five of seven tests, and on total overall scores.

•**Healthier kidneys.** Researchers found that men who consumed seven or more drinks a week experienced a 29% lower risk of developing kidney problems.

•**Antioxidant effect.** Japanese scientists have found that antioxidants such as *polyphenols* in beer may offer protection against cancer-causing chemicals. This repeats earlier research conducted in Portugal, which suggested that antioxidants slow the proliferation of breast cancer cells. According to Dr. Denke, *isoflavonoids* in beer are *phytoestrogens* that mimic the activity of the natural human hormone estrogen. In laboratory experiments, isoflavonoids have also been shown to inhibit the growth of cancers of the breast, prostate and colon.

PROCEED WITH CAUTION

Promising as all this research appears, talking about alcohol always requires special caution. It's all too easy to slip over the line from healthful consumption to overconsumption and physical damage, warns Dr. Denke. Yes, regular moderate consumption can benefit the heart, kidneys, bones and more. But drinking too much alcohol can seriously harm vital organs and processes in the body. As always, moderation in all things is the best path to follow.

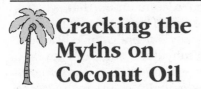

Cracking the Myths on Coconut Oil

Udo Erasmus, PhD, author of *Fats that Heal, Fats that Kill*. Alive. Learn more about Dr. Erasmus's work at his Web site, *www.udoerasmus.com*.

Is it a dangerous saturated fat or a tropical wonder that we should use in place of olive oil? Confusion and debate surround coconut oil. Mainstream organizations such as the American Heart Association and the National Cancer Institute recommend avoiding it because coconut oil is a saturated fat that, they say, raises blood cholesterol and cardiovascular risk. However, an increasing number of alternative voices are popping up on the Internet claiming that it was unfair to lump coconut oil in with unhealthful fats during the fanatical no-fat era, and this tropical oil is really a magic elixir, a virtual fountain of youth.

To learn more, we consulted Udo Erasmus, PhD, author of *Fats that Heal, Fats that Kill* (Alive). He says that it is difficult to determine where science ends and marketing begins, and both camps are misleading in their one-sided approaches. As usual, the truth lies somewhere in-between, he says. Coconut oil is neither as bad as traditionalists would have you believe, nor is it the miraculous cure-all hawked by aggressive Internet entrepreneurs.

NOT AS BAD AS TRADITIONAL CLAIMS

First, let's take a look at coconut oil as a saturated fat. Coconut oil and its tropical cousin palm oil are composed of medium-chain fatty acids that are relatively easy to digest, absorb and metabolize. In contrast, longer-chain fatty acids in beef and dairy fats (other than butter fats, which are short-chain) place a greater burden on the liver.

In other words, while it's not exactly a health food, coconut oil has nowhere near the artery-clogging impact of the saturated fats in hamburgers and milk shakes. Coconut oil is not an essential fat like the omega-3 fatty acids that we require for good health. However, Dr. Erasmus believes that it is a neutral fat that is safe to use in moderation, as long as you also make sure that you consume the right balance of essential fatty acids.

NOT AS GOOD AS INTERNET CLAIMS

And now for the health claims—you'll lose weight, have more energy, feel younger, and it will cure thyroid problems and banish wrinkles. *Dr. Erasmus responds...*

•**If you replace carbohydrates in your diet with fats such as coconut oil,** you will cut back on food cravings and turn on fat burning. True, and while essential fatty acids such as omega-3s are a better all-around choice in this regard, coconut oil will also help get the job done.

•**Coconut oil boosts metabolism and energy.** False. In fact, it appears to slow the metabolic rate. There is no evidence supporting coconut oil as a cure for thyroid disease.

•**Coconut contains good antioxidants,** and by thwarting free radical development you can, to some extent, counter the effects of aging. True, but you also can accomplish this in other ways by eating lots of fruits, veggies and cold-water fish.

•**Coconut oil can be a useful addition to skincare regimens.** True. For more youthful and supple skin, use moisturizing lotions, bath oils and cosmetics enriched with coconut oil.

MODERATION IN ALL THINGS

As always, there's some truth in marketing, but you have to take it with a grain (and sometimes a pillar) of salt. In the case of coconut oil's popularity, Dr. Erasmus believes that it is a fad riding on the coattails of essential fatty acid research. He points out that essential fatty acids are *essential* to good health and that coconut oil is not. That said, coconut is fine to use in moderation, and many people love its aroma. Always buy it in glass bottles (not plastic), and feel free to add a tasty tablespoon to smoothies or salad dressings.

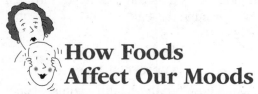

How Foods Affect Our Moods

Elizabeth Somer, MA, RD, author of *Food & Mood: The Complete Guide to Eating Well and Feeling Your Best.* Henry Holt.

Robert E. Thayer, PhD, professor of psychology, California State University, Long Beach, and author of *Calm Energy: How People Regulate Mood with Food and Exercise* and *The Origin of Everyday Moods* (both from Oxford University).

We often call it comfort food, but for millions of Americans, it is not comforting at all. Many people fail to make the connection, but how and what we eat has a direct affect on our moods. Not only is our consumption affecting us from moment to moment throughout the day, but bad eating habits can contribute to long-term mood troubles of all kinds, including depression.

Elizabeth Somer, MA, registered dietician (RD), and author of the book *Food & Mood: The Complete Guide to Eating Well and Feeling Your Best* (Henry Holt), says that it is not only what we eat but also our style of eating that contribute to our state of mind. The most important thing Somer recommends is that you actually eat. "Many people skip breakfast," she says, "and then wonder why they lack energy midmorning." Food is energy, and if we do not give our body fuel, it is going to run out of gas. Although we've all heard the advice about the importance of eating breakfast, it's astonishing how many people still start their day with a body that may not have eaten for more than 12 hours.

THE COMFORT OF CARBS

Somer also cautions against the "low-carb" craze that continues to sweep the nation, and recommends that we stop fighting our carb cravings. Our bodies, and specifically our brains, need carbohydrates. Carbohydrates raise our levels of *tryptophan*, which increases our *serotonin* levels. This actually calms us, increases our pain tolerance, improves our sleeping habits and reduces our cravings for more carbohydrates.

Somer's definition of carbs is not a double fudge sundae or chocolate chip cookies, however. She is talking about all-natural, low-glycemic index complex carbohydrates such as whole grains, fruits, vegetables, seeds, beans and nuts. Foods that are high in carbs, but also rich in nutrients, are the real comfort foods, with long-lasting effects.

CUT BACK ON SUGAR SHOCK

Somer recommends cutting back or eliminating refined and processed sugars and caffeine. For those people who are very sensitive to sugar, a sweet such as a single cookie can begin a vicious cycle of feeling bad, eating more sugar, crashing again and so on. If this sounds like you, eliminate all processed sugar from your diet. Look for the hidden sugars in condiments such as ketchup and salsa, canned fruits, juice drinks and other processed and prepared foods. If you are not as sensitive, Somer still recommends cutting back on concentrated sugars such as candy and pastries. In research studies, a significant decrease in sugar caused a direct decrease in feelings of sadness and anxiety.

CAFFEINE CAN SLOW YOU DOWN

Although caffeine may seem like a pick-me-up, studies show that it actually might add to depression. When tested on rats, researchers concluded that caffeine decreases the conversion of tryptophan to serotonin. For people who suffer from depression, caffeine can actually aggravate their symptoms.

BETTER PICK-ME-UPS

Robert E. Thayer, PhD, psychologist and author of *Calm Energy: How People*

Regulate Mood with Food and Exercise (Oxford University), says that most people make poor eating choices because they experience what he calls "tense tiredness." A lack of energy or increase in tension causes people to seek foods that will quickly raise their blood sugar. They often go for a sugar snack, which will temporarily "fix" the problem. Unfortunately, a snack high in refined, processed sugar will only relieve symptoms of tense tiredness for a short period of time, which is usually followed by a sugar crash.

A far better solution for tense tiredness is to release tension and/or increase energy. For people practiced in meditation or muscle relaxation techniques, taking a few minutes to relax will usually do the trick. For nonmeditators, Dr. Thayer recommends exercise. In most cases, a brisk, 10- minute walk increases energy for up to two hours, based on research findings.

Getting enough sleep and eating small meals throughout the day are also healthier ways to regulate your mood. If you have more energy, you are less vulnerable to tension, and you will be less likely to start the sugar binge cycle in the first place.

EVERYONE IS DIFFERENT

While Dr. Thayer has studied eating habits and their effect on mood, he is also a proponent of knowing your own body and habits. In his book *The Origin of Everyday Moods* (Oxford University), he suggests systematic self-observation. *Try this experiment...*

Notice the association between your thoughts, feelings and behavior before having a sugar snack. Rate your energy on a number scale. Are you a peppy 5? An exhausted 1? Then do the same after you eat your sugar snack. Note how long the energy lasts. Do this several times. Keep your findings in a notebook. Make a chart or a graph. Notice what the snack is doing to you. Then, try the same experiment before and after taking a walk or using relaxation techniques.

Knowing why you make food choices is the first step to lasting dietary changes and a healthier, happier state of mind.

11

Research Update on Vitamins, Herbs, and Supplements

Vitamin K—the Whole Body Vitamin

Some conventional doctors used to urge older patients who were on *warfarin* (Coumadin), to avoid vitamin K-containing foods and supplements. Why? Because vitamin K is essential for clotting...and it can interfere with the anticlotting effects of Coumadin, a blood-thinning (anticoagulant) medication.

But lately, there have been many reports of vitamin K's amazing powers. It plays a role in bone building. Some research shows that it may be involved in the prevention of atherosclerosis. Some forms of vitamin K are being used in current cancer research. Could the vitamin K story be more complex than was once thought?

BONE HEALTH

As it turns out, yes. Let's start with our bones. Vitamin K turns out to be the "Rodney Dangerfield" of bone health vitamins—"it don't get no respect" and no one talks about it. Instead, we talk about calcium and magnesium and vitamin D, which of course are all very important, but vitamin K is critically important for building strong bones as well. "Vitamin K actually activates a compound called *osteocalcin* that acts like studs inside the walls of a house. It's a structural framework that anchors calcium molecules inside the bone," explains Shari Lieberman, PhD, coauthor of *The Real Vitamin and Mineral Book* (Avery). So you can take all the calcium you want, but if it's not getting into the bones, it's not going to do

Shari Lieberman, PhD, CNS, author of several books including *The Real Vitamin and Mineral Book* (Avery) and *Glycemic Index Food Guide* (Square One). Dr. Lieberman is the founding dean, New York Chiropractic College's MS Degree program in Applied Clinical Nutrition, a member of the American Academy of Anti-Aging Medicine and board member of the Certification Board for Nutrition Specialists. She is also a past president of the American Association for Health Freedom.

you very much good and it actually can do you some harm by calcifying in other places in the body. "Vitamin K makes sure that you get that calcium into the bone where it belongs," she says.

HEART AND BONE PROTECTION

Vitamin K helps protect against heart attacks and osteoporosis. Dr. Lieberman explains that the very actions of vitamin K that protect the bones also help protect against *calcification* in the blood vessels, a prime risk factor for the artery-clogging disease called atherosclerosis. "Vitamin K produces opposite effects in bone and blood vessels. Proteins in bone *increase* mineralization when they're activated by vitamin K...but similar proteins in blood vessels *decrease* calcification in blood vessels." The end result? Vitamin K both helps build bones *and* protect against calcification in the blood vessels.

And, in the Nurses' Health Study (Harvard, Boston), of more than 72,000 women, those who got the most vitamin K were about one-third less likely to get a hip fracture. A double whammy—protection against atherosclerosis and osteoporosis.

VITAMIN K AND CLOTTING

Then there's clotting, vitamin K's original claim to fame. In fact, vitamin K got its name from the German *koagulation* when it was discovered that the vitamin was necessary in order to make the blood clot.

"The latest research shows that people on Coumadin can safely take 100 micrograms (mcg) of vitamin K a day," says Dr. Lieberman, "but they should certainly have their clotting levels monitored." *Bottom Line's Daily Health News* consulting medical editor, Andrew L. Rubman, ND, suggests, too, that taking vitamin E, ginko biloba and fish oil can also thin blood, so check with your doctor.

HOW TO GET VITAMIN K

Researchers now think that vitamin K is needed in larger quantities than what was once thought, particularly in aging adults. "According to the NIH (National Institutes of Health), the optimal daily intake (DV or daily value) for vitamin K is only 80 mcg," says Dr. Lieberman. "In my book I have a higher recommendation. Most multivitamins don't contain enough vitamin K for optimal health." Considering the importance of this vitamin, it's reasonable to ask yourself if you're getting enough. Fortunately, it can be found in assorted vegetables such as broccoli, turnip greens, green cabbage, spinach and tomatoes.

THREE FORMS OF VITAMIN K

Vitamin K actually has three forms—K1 is found primarily in foods and as *phylloquinone* or *phytonadione*...K2 is made in the body by intestinal bacteria and is found in some foods...and K3 is a synthetic form not generally available for humans. "Vitamin K2 appears to be the most active and biological form," said Dr. Lieberman. Since taking too much vitamin K can be problematic, it is best to get it from food. As much as 45 milligrams (mg) per day of supplemental vitamin K is being used for osteoporosis, cancer and heart disease—but under a doctor's supervision, says Dr. Lieberman. Recent research suggests that eating foods rich in vitamin K does not appear to interfere with anticoagulants (but don't make any drastic changes in your diet without consulting with your doctor). If you are taking additional vitamin K for health reasons and you are on an anticoagulant, check with your physician before supplementing with vitamin K.

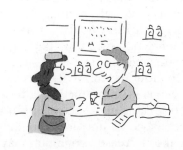

Common Vitamin Deficiencies and How to Fix Them

Andrew L. Rubman, ND, consulting medical editor for *Bottom Line's Daily Health News* and director of the Southbury Clinic for Traditional Medicines in Southbury, Connecticut.

Office of Dietary Supplements, National Institutes of Health, *http://ods.od.nih.gov*.

Even people with the most healthful diets can be deficient in a few key vitamins and minerals that are critical to vibrant health. According to our consulting medical editor Andrew L. Rubman, ND, diet alone is often insufficient to provide enough of these vitamins and minerals to meet a person's needs. That's when supplements come into play, but often at levels different than the government-recommended Daily Value (DV) or Recommended Dietary Allowance (RDA), which are not necessarily the levels for optimal health, says Dr. Rubman.

VITAMIN B-12: ESSENTIAL TO PROPER LIVER FUNCTION

One of the most common deficiencies of all is B-12, which the liver requires for optimal function in a myriad of roles including nutrient synthesis and transportation, and waste management and selective recycling, says Dr. Rubman. Older people, in particular, are very often deficient in B-12 for their needs. Normal government-recommended values are based on vulnerability to pernicious anemia (a type of anemia caused by extreme B-12 deficiency) rather than reflective of other needs. While most people don't develop this severe type of anemia, a significant percentage of the population has a functional deficiency such that they are unable to operate at an optimal level.

Given how essential B-12 is to brain and nervous system function, a functional deficiency can lead to neurological issues. Problems such as impaired memory, confusion and decreased cognition may seem subtle at first, but if the deficiency is not addressed, over time these problems may grow more pronounced. In older people, a B-12 deficiency is one contributing factor to dementia.

What you can do: Dr. Rubman encourages people to get a serum blood test to assess their level of B-12. If there is a functional deficiency, he recommends sublingual B-12 pills, either *hydroxocobalamin* or *methylcobalamin*, which are equally as effective as and less expensive than B-12 shots. (Avoid *cyanocobalamin*, which is poorly absorbed.) B-12 should be taken under a doctor's supervision. Because B-12 requires other B vitamins to function properly in the body, take a multi-B supplement twice daily (they do not last 24 hours in circulation).

Note: Take B-12 and a multi-B supplement under the supervision of your physician. You're taking in sufficient B if your urine remains yellow through the day.

CALCIUM AND MAGNESIUM: FOR BONE HEALTH AND MORE

Calcium is the most abundant mineral in the body, required for bone formation and for maintaining strong bones throughout life as well as for assisting in sleep and blood clotting. Insufficient calcium can lead to the bone-thinning disorders osteoporosis and osteopenia. While dairy products are the most popular sources of calcium, cow's milk is difficult to digest and may not be the best form of calcium for absorption. You may also try calcium-enriched plant milks (e.g., almond, oat, hazelnut, rice and soy) and leafy green vegetables such as spinach and kale.

Magnesium, the fourth most abundant mineral in the body, is required to ensure calcium absorption as well as proper muscle and nerve function, bone strength and to keep heart rhythm steady. Many people do not take in enough magnesium (through foods such as legumes, nuts, whole grains and vegetables), which is believed to offer protection against cardiovascular disease and immune dysfunction.

Gastrointestinal disorders such as insufficient stomach acid or Crohn's disease may impair the absorption of magnesium.

What you can do: Dr. Rubman often prescribes calcium and magnesium in the combination supplement Butyrex, made by T.E. Neesby. These capsules contain calcium/magnesium as *butyrates*, a form which makes them much easier for the body to absorb than that found in other commonly available supplements.

While the standard RDA for calcium is 800 to 1,200 milligrams/day along with magnesium in a 2:1 proportion, Butyrex's formulation is so well absorbed that the dosing is often lower. According to Dr. Rubman, patients often start feeling better within just a few days of taking Butyrex.

IRON: FOR OXYGEN
TRANSPORT AND ENERGY

According to the World Health Organization, iron deficiency is the most common nutritional deficiency in the world. On the other hand, too much iron can also cause problems, warns Dr. Rubman.

If you don't take in enough iron, oxygen is not transported efficiently to the body's cells. As a result, you're apt to feel tired and weak, and be more susceptible to infection. Women with heavy menstrual periods are at risk for iron deficiency anemia, as are pregnant women, children and teens, all of whom have a high need for iron. Gastrointestinal (GI) disorders such as Crohn's disease, celiac disease, ulcers and others, as well as the chronic use of antacids and acid suppressing medications, may impair the absorption of iron.

What you can do: Dietary sources of iron include animal proteins such as red meat, turkey, chicken and fish. Other sources include lentils, soybeans, kidney beans, spinach and enriched breads and cereals. If needed, it is fine to take iron as part of a multivitamin supplement, says Dr. Rubman. Otherwise, he recommends taking the iron supplement Proferrin, but only under medical supervision.

While you can pick up some of these supplements yourself at the local health food store, you should see a licensed physician. Remember that treating deficiencies is always a medical issue, no matter how readily available the pharmacy may be.

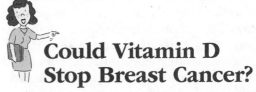

Could Vitamin D Stop Breast Cancer?

Carlo Palmieri, PhD, Cancer Research UK Laboratories and Imperial College, London.

Vitamin D, the "sunshine vitamin," has been the focus of intense study in recent years since researchers have found evidence it may help lower the risk of developing several types of cancers, including colon, prostate, pancreatic and breast cancer. A recent British study suggests that low vitamin D levels may play a role in the progression of breast cancer in women who already have it. The study involved 279 women...204 of them had early-stage breast cancer, while the rest were in advanced-stage cancer. While measuring the blood levels of vitamin D in all these women, the researchers discovered that those with early-stage cancer had significantly higher levels of D than the ones with advanced cancer.

D SPECIFICS STILL UNCLEAR

Carlo Palmieri, PhD, of Cancer Research UK Laboratories and Imperial College in London, was the lead author of the study. We asked whether he believes that vitamin D hinders the progression of breast cancer, or if the vitamin is depleted as a result of the disease. That's the big question, he acknowledges, and the answer is not yet evident. "What we do know is that lab tests have shown vitamin D inhibits the proliferation of breast cancer cell lines, somehow inducing them to die. We also know that in countries at higher latitudes, where there is less sunshine and people are more likely to be vitamin D deficient, there is a higher incidence of breast cancer." Yet more evidence—a case control study showed that women with no cancer had higher levels of vitamin D than women with breast cancer. (Results were only in Caucasian women.) We also know that vitamin D treatment boosts the activity of the p21 gene. This is important, says Dr. Palmieri, because the gene ensures that cells divide appropriately. "So, problems with adequate p21 activity could potentially lead to abnormal cell growth, and therefore, cancer."

MORE RESEARCH NEEDED

This is not a reason to rush out to get vitamin D supplements, however. According to Dr. Palmieri, his study adds to mounting evidence about the importance of vitamin D, but more research is needed to establish the case conclusively. For now, the best advice is to be sure you are getting a balanced diet full of all nutrients, and that you get regular, safe levels of sun exposure. And remember that vitamin D supplementation should only be done under the guidance of a knowledgeable professional, because too much can cause a medical emergency.

Take Two: The Healing Powers Of Vitamin C and E

Mark A. Stengler, ND, naturopathic physician in private practice, La Jolla, California...adjunct associate clinical professor at the National College of Natural Medicine, Portland, Oregon...author of many books, including *The Natural Physician's Healing Therapies* and coauthor of *Prescription for Natural Cures* (both from Bottom Line Books)...and author of the *Bottom Line/Natural Healing* newsletter.

Lately, some confusing and contradictory information has emerged concerning two popular vitamins—C and E. Some studies say they work, others say they don't. One recent analysis

suggests that high doses of vitamin E increase the risk of premature death. This was followed by a study reassuring consumers that both vitamins are safe in a broad range of doses.

What should we believe? For expert advice, we turned to Mark Stengler, ND, author of the newsletter *Bottom Line/Natural Healing* and the book *The Natural Physician's Healing Therapies* (Bottom Line Books). Dr. Stengler highly recommends vitamins C and E, and notes in particular that there were significant flaws in the vitamin E study.

VITAMIN C: AN IMMUNE-BOOSTING POWERHOUSE

A strong immune booster rich in antiviral and antibacterial properties, vitamin C acts as a powerful antioxidant to wipe out free radical molecules that are produced during—and may contribute to—inflammation. It is required for the synthesis of collagen (a vital connective tissue protein in skin, bones, arterial walls, etc.), and for the synthesis of the amino acid L-carnitine (which allows fat to be utilized for energy).

What it's for: Vitamin C can help enhance the immune system and reduce the duration and severity of colds. It is also beneficial to heart health, hypertension, high cholesterol, Alzheimer's disease, cataracts, glaucoma, easy bruising, allergies, asthma, diabetes, gingivitis, hepatitis, osteoporosis, infertility, preeclampsia, rheumatoid arthritis and cancer.

Dr. Stengler recommends that most people take 500 milligrams (mg) to 1,000 mg daily, though he considers doses up to 2,000 mg daily, which the Institute of Medicine (IOM) has set as a maximum, as a good general dosage. In some circumstances, he will recommend even higher doses. Dr. Stengler notes that these higher doses are a far cry from the US recommended daily allowance (RDA) of 75 mg for adult women and 90 mg for adult men. In Dr. Stengler's opinion, the RDA will keep you from dying from a deficiency but does not guarantee optimal health. Higher doses are needed to help counteract the effects of pollution and stress, he says.

Precautions: Check with your doctor before taking vitamin C if you have the genetic condition glucose-6-phosphate dehydrogenase deficiency, iron overload (such as hemochromatosis), a history of kidney stones or kidney failure. At doses of 2,000 mg or more a day, occasional gastrointestinal problems such as mild diarrhea may develop. According to Dr. Stengler, this is not a major concern. If you reduce the dose or stop taking vitamin C, the problem will go away. People who get stomach upset also may benefit from the use of a nonacidic C such as calcium ascorbate.

Vitamin C-rich food sources: Broccoli, red peppers, citrus fruits (oranges, grapefruit, etc.), currants, Brussels sprouts, parsley, potatoes, cantaloupe and strawberries. When possible, Dr. Stengler prefers the whole food (for example, oranges instead of orange juice).

About the controversy: Does vitamin C really help when you have a cold? Is this myth or reality? Modern research indicates that vitamin C cannot prevent or cure colds…but it can reduce their duration (by one day) and severity. Dr. Stengler often prescribes 3,000 mg to 5,000 mg daily for his patients who have colds.

VITAMIN E: A FREE RADICAL FIGHTER

Like vitamin C, vitamin E is a potent antioxidant that wards off free radical damage. It protects red blood cells and has an anticlotting effect. With some favorable studies and others not so favorable, Dr. Stengler weighs in on the pro side and continues to recommend vitamin E for the prevention of heart disease, Alzheimer's disease and prostate cancer.

Where E can help: Vitamin E can help lessen the symptoms and possibly prevent an array of debilitating diseases including heart disease, Alzheimer's disease, prostate cancer, AIDS, rheumatoid arthritis, diabetes, macular degeneration, hot flashes, premenstrual syndrome (PMS), fibrocystic breast disease, infertility, Parkinson's disease, epilepsy, carotid artery stenosis, intermittent claudication, angina and consequences of smoke exposure.

Dr. Stengler often prescribes 200 international units (IU) to 400 IU of vitamin E daily. He prefers a vitamin E blend that contains both tocopherols and tocotrienols, which work together synergistically for the best health effects. (Most multivitamins contain only alpha-tocopherol.) Natural vitamin E (d-tocopherol) is preferable to the synthetic form (dl-tocopherol), as it is better utilized by the body. In special circumstances—such as fibrocystic breast disease, hot flashes and eczema—Dr. Stengler recommends higher doses.

Precautions: People on blood-thinning medications such as *warfarin* (Coumadin) should check with their doctors before taking vitamin E. However, Dr. Stengler notes that doses of 200 IU and lower are generally safe for this group.

Vitamin E-rich food sources: Wheat germ oil, nuts and seeds, whole grains, egg yolks and leafy green vegetables.

About the controversy: A meta-analysis of 19 clinical trials reported that vitamin E supplements of 400 IU or more were associated with a 6% higher risk of premature death. However, Dr. Stengler says that the research was flawed in that it lumped together different types of vitamin E and different groups of patients (some of whom were already at higher risk due to heart disease or diabetes).

EVEN BETTER THAN ONE: TAKE TWO

Both powerful anti-inflammatory, disease-fighting antioxidants, vitamins C and E pack even more of a punch when taken together. This is because they protect different parts of cells—water-soluble C takes care of the watery components, while fat-soluble E stands guard on the fatty parts.

Herb That Boosts Energy and Eases Depression

Decker Weiss, NMD, an expert in integrative medicine and the first doctor to be recognized with the title Naturopathic Cardiologist. Dr. Weiss is the first naturopathic physician to have hospital privileges at a conventional hospital and the first naturopathic physician to be chosen as a Fellow of the American Society of Angiology. He is a consulting staff physician at the Arizona Heart Hospital in Phoenix, and is also in private practice in Scottsdale, Arizona.

Rhodiola rosea may be, as the famous Australian herbalist Kerry Bone describes it, "the new kid on the energy-boosting block," but this amazing herb isn't really new at all. It's actually been used since the times of the Vikings to boost endurance and treat fatigue and depression.

HORMONAL THERMOSTAT

"Rhodiola rosea is simply the best adaptogen plant I've ever seen or used," says Decker Weiss, NMD, a naturopathic cardiologist and consulting staff physician at the Arizona Heart Hospital in Phoenix. An adaptogen, Dr. Weiss explains, works like a thermostat. When a thermostat senses that the room temperature is too high it brings it down, but when it senses that temperature is too low it brings it up. An adaptogen does the same things with hormones. "All the good things you've ever heard about *Panax ginseng*, Rhodiola does," says Dr. Weiss.

"Cortisol is one of our main stress hormones," Dr. Weiss explains. "For example, if you drink coffee on an empty stomach, as many of us do, it's very hard to balance cortisol. Too much cortisol can lead to the feeling of being wired, yet tired. It contributes to weight gain, especially around the belly. And it can contribute to exhaustion, fatigue, depression and a whole host of ailments. By acting as an adaptogen—a kind of hormone thermostat—Rhodiola literally helps balance cortisol. If it's too high, it can bring it down. If it's too low, it can

bring it up." That's why, he says, Rhodiola is so useful for increasing energy while easing fatigue and depression.

PROOF OF PRODUCT

The research on Rhodiola is compelling. When Belgian researchers gave 24 people a placebo or Rhodiola (200 milligrams daily) the latter group experienced a noteworthy jump in stamina. According to a comprehensive review in *HerbalGram*, the journal of the American Botanical Council, the herb lessens the release of stress-related hormones and increases levels of feel-good compounds called *endorphins*.

"It's also great for time-zone changes because of its adaptogenic ability to modulate melatonin," Dr. Weiss says. "And it will help you sleep. It's one of the few herbs I won't travel without." Dr. Weiss recommends using Rhodiola manufactured by a reliable company to ensure product quality—he suggests Enzymatic Therapy, which makes it in pill form, or Herb Pharm, which makes it in a tincture. While generally thought of as safe, it is best to check with your trained practitioner before adding Rhodiola to your supplement mix. Rhodiola is a stimulant, so it is best taken early in the day on an empty stomach.

Peppermint: A Sweet Way to Relieve a Cold, Tame Your Tummy and More

David Winston, founding member of the American Herbalists Guild (AHG) and coauthor of *Herbal Therapy and Supplements: A Scientific and Traditional Approach* (Lippincott) and *Adaptogens: Herbs for Strength, Stamina and Stress Relief* (Healing Arts Press).

One of our favorite summer herbs is mint. It smells and tastes so fresh. It's delicious in salads and cool, refreshing drinks. Its stronger-flavored relative, peppermint, is especially soothing to the stomach.

David Winston, founding member of the American Herbalists Guild (AHG) and coauthor of *Herbal Therapy and Supplements: A Scientific and Traditional Approach* (Lippincott) and *Adaptogens: Herbs for Strength, Stamina and Stress Relief* (Healing Arts Press), highly recommends peppermint (mentha piperita) as a remedy for ailments ranging from gas and nausea to colds and fever. He notes that not only does mint taste good, it also has few significant adverse effects.

SOOTHING THE SAVAGE STOMACH

Peppermint possesses natural muscle-relaxing abilities that soothe the symptoms of digestive troubles such as stomachache, gas, nausea, vomiting, indigestion and irritable bowel syndrome (a common condition characterized by constipation and/or diarrhea). When the smooth muscles surrounding the intestine relax, spasms and accompanying indigestion are likewise calmed. Winston adds that he likes to combine peppermint with chamomile for treating digestive disturbances.

COLD, FLU AND FEVER RELIEF

Peppermint is also an excellent fever reducer and possesses antimicrobial qualities. Winston notes that mint's pleasing taste and aroma make it especially appealing to feverish children suffering from the cold or flu, who are likely to resist foul-tasting commercial syrups. For colds and flu accompanied by fever, Winston recommends a tea made with peppermint and elderflower (another herbal fever reducer). You can drink as much mint tea as you care to. Elderflower is also very safe, except those with strong pollen allergies should watch out for possible sensitivities.

CALM ITCHING AND INFLAMMATION

Applied topically, menthol, an active ingredient in peppermint, has a numbing and cooling effect. In your health food store, look for menthol-containing creams, ointments or gels to soothe skin irritations such as poison ivy, hives or contact dermatitis. These also may provide topical relief of joint and muscle pain.

According to *Bottom Line's Daily Health News* consulting medical editor Andrew L. Rubman, ND, in the past, people would simply chew a mouthful of mint leaves and then rub the resulting mush onto the irritated area. Supposedly the enzymes in saliva help the active ingredients to penetrate the skin.

REDUCE FRUSTRATION, FATIGUE AND HEADACHE PAIN

In a study at Wheeling Jesuit University in West Virginia, researchers found that the scent of peppermint in their cars decreased drivers' anxiety and fatigue. Adding cinnamon to the mix increased alertness. A whiff of the essential oil of peppermint also may help relieve headache pain.

MORE BENEFITS

Of course, that's not the end of mint's many benefits. We're all familiar with peppermint toothpastes and mouth rinses, which Winston points out not only freshen the breath but also kill bacteria and reduce plaque formation. Topical or inhaled menthol preparations can help open respiratory passages and ease stuffiness, and a cup of peppermint tea may be just what you need to soothe mild menstrual cramps.

HOW TO USE MINT

During the winter months, or for medicinal purposes, make a hot tea using a tea bag or one to two teaspoons of dried peppermint leaves per eight ounces of water. (Drink one to three cups daily.) In the summer, crush or tear a few fresh spearmint leaves and add them to iced tea, fruit salads or green salads. You also can use mint instead of parsley as a garnish on soups or casseroles. Or better yet, pick up a Middle Eastern cookbook and try out more exotic recipes using mint, such as tabbouleh (bulgur salad) or yogurt dressing.

Note: Although peppermint is generally a very safe remedy, it should not be used by those with gastroesophageal reflux disease (GERD), gallbladder inflammation or liver disease except under prescription. Also, the essential oil is for scent only and should never be taken internally.

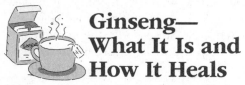

Ginseng— What It Is and How It Heals

Mark A. Stengler, ND, naturopathic physician in private practice, La Jolla, California…adjunct associate clinical professor at the National College of Natural Medicine, Portland, Oregon…author of many books, including *The Natural Physician's Healing Therapies* and coauthor of *Prescription for Natural Cures* (both from Bottom Line Books)…and author of the *Bottom Line/Natural Healing* newsletter.

Ginseng has been a mainstay in Chinese medicine for 2,000 years, but there is confusion about the different types of ginseng—there are three—and people worry that its stimulant properties may make it dangerous. Fortunately, explains Mark Stengler, ND, researchers have long studied all three types of ginseng and found many valid claims for their use.

BREAKING IT DOWN

Dr. Stengler says he often uses ginseng in his practice to address fatigue, low libido, weak immunity, type 2 diabetes and memory problems. But he adds that it is definitely important to know which type of ginseng to choose, depending on the desired result. Dr. Stengler cautions, however, that pregnant people should avoid ginseng…and those on blood-thinning medications should only take it under a doctor's supervision. Ginseng should also be avoided before surgery.

The three types of ginseng are *Panax schinseng-ginseng* (also called *Panax ginseng*, Chinese ginseng, Asian ginseng, Korean ginseng, Red ginseng and Ren-Shen)…Eleuthero (scientific name *Eleutherococcus senticosus*, also known as Siberian ginseng, though technically not

a true ginseng)…and American (scientific name *Panax quinquefolius L.*). Ginseng is also referred to as "hot" (yang) or "cool" (yin), depending on its particular effects, based on the Chinese medicine philosophy of yin and yang.

PANAX SCHINSENG-GINSENG (CHINESE GINSENG)

The oldest variety is Chinese ginseng, used in Chinese medicine to improve sexual function, energy and vitality…help recovery from illness…and slow the aging process. Another species, *Panax repens*, is occasionally found outside of China. Both the white and red forms of *Panax* are from the root, but red is heated through steaming and then dried and is, as the name implies, fierier and more potent (yang). Compounds thought to be responsible for many of the therapeutic effects of *Panax* are *ginsenosides*, the two most important being Rg1 and Rb1, which have been the focus of intense study. Rg1 has been shown to stimulate brain and central nervous system activity thereby increasing energy and intellectual performance. Rb1 has been shown to relax brain activity and lower blood pressure.

Today millions of people around the world use *Panax* for fatigue…immune enhancement, including during chemotherapy and radiation…mental alertness …cardiovascular disease…elevated cholesterol…type 2 diabetes…sexual function… athletic performance enhancement…stress …and anxiety.

Dosage: Dr. Stengler recommends using a product that is standardized between 4% to 7% ginsenosides. The standardized extract label will have the words *"Panax ginseng C.A. Meyer,"* referring to a specific type of ginseng and the one used in many studies.

Side effects: A high dosage can cause anxiety and insomnia. Do not use in combination with any kind of stimulant including caffeine or take before bedtime. People with high blood pressure and women who have a heavy menstrual flow or fibrocystic breast syndrome should use only under medical direction.

ELEUTHERO
(SIBERIAN GINSENG)

Eleuthero is not a member of Panax genus and so technically not a true ginseng, and its known active constituents are completely different from Chinese ginseng. The ones that have received the most study are a subgroup of saponins, plant chemicals called *eleutherosides*, some of which are thought to enhance energy. Siberian ginseng also contains polysaccharides believed to support immune function. Unlike white or red ginseng, Siberian ginseng has a neutral yin/yang compared with other ginsengs. Consequently, many people tolerate it well and can use it longer. Siberian ginseng seems to support adrenal gland function and helps cells better utilize oxygen, which promotes energy.

Dosage: Studies have used an alcohol extract at a dosage of 8 to 10 milliliters taken two or three times a day. Dr. Stengler has seen good results with a standardized capsule extract containing 0.4% eleutherosides.

Side effects: These are rare, though it may be too stimulating to take late in the day. Also, people with high blood pressure should take under medical supervision, as should those with heart disease.

AMERICAN GINSENG

Panax quinquefolius L. (meaning five-leafed *Panax*) is indigenous to North America. There are striking similarities between American and Chinese ginseng in their appearance and growth and in their active constituents—the ginsenosides, known to support adrenal gland function that helps the body better handle stress. However, researchers have found that American ginseng contains much more of the Rb1 group than the more stimulating Rg1 group found in Chinese ginseng and this is believed to give it properties that relax nerves, fatigue and fever and reduce blood pressure and pain. It also helps with digestion.

Dosage: American ginseng can be found in either tincture, extract or capsule form and varies as widely in potency as Chinese ginseng. Experts in botanical medicine consider powdered root (steeped in boiled water to make tea) the most superior form. American ginseng lowers blood sugar levels. It is best taken with meals, according to Dr. Stengler, and a doctor should monitor blood sugar levels.

Side effects: In healthy people, side effects are uncommon...though sensitive people may notice too much stimulation and may need to reduce dosage and avoid using before bedtime. People with high or low blood sugar should be monitored ...and, those pregnant or breastfeeding should avoid ginseng.

A QUICK GUIDE

Ginseng is a very powerful herb and can be helpful for some very challenging conditions. However, because it is so powerful, it is best to use under supervision of a trained professional, especially if you are taking other medications or remedies at the same time. *Dr. Stengler outlines the type of ginseng that is most appropriate to specific conditions...*

- **Asthma**—American ginseng
- **Athletic performance**—Eleuthero or Chinese ginseng
- **Diabetes**—American is best, Chinese ginseng is second
- **Fatigue**—all three are good though Chinese ginseng is strongest
- **Congestive heart disease**—Chinese ginseng
- **Low sex drive**—Chinese ginseng
- **Menopause symptoms, such as hot flashes**—American is best, Chinese ginseng is second
- **Poor memory**—Chinese ginseng and Eleuthero
- **Immune support**—all three, though Chinese ginseng is more specific to cancer

Think Ginkgo for Better Memory And More

Mark A. Stengler, ND, naturopathic physician in private practice, La Jolla, California...adjunct associate clinical professor at the National College of Natural Medicine, Portland, Oregon...author of many books, including *The Natural Physician's Healing Therapies* and coauthor of *Prescription for Natural Cures* (both from Bottom Line Books)...and author of the *Bottom Line/Natural Healing* newsletter.

If longevity of use is any indicator of effectiveness, ginkgo biloba (ginkgo) surely tops the list of natural remedies. The tree itself is one of the oldest around—fossils of the ginkgo leaf exist from prehistoric times some 200 million years ago—and the Chinese have made medicinal use of its leaves and seeds for thousands of years.

GINKGO'S POPULARITY

Today ginkgo extract, which comes from the tree's uniquely fan-shaped leaves, is one of the biggest selling herbal medicines in Europe and is growing in popularity in this country thanks to its anti-inflammatory powers and high-grade antioxidants. Controversies about ginkgo pop up occasionally, but none of them thus far have turned out to be serious...at the same time, studies that substantiate ginkgo's traditional medicinal claims continue to accumulate. We spoke with Mark Stengler, ND, author of *Bottom Line's Natural Healing* newsletter, about ginkgo's powerful place in the naturopathic physician's pharmacy.

OVERVIEW OF GINKGO

The ginkgo extract, explains Dr. Stengler, contains *flavonoids* and *terpene lactones*, two chemicals that are apparently responsible for its many healthful properties, including its well known anti-inflammatory performance and its powerful antioxidants that mop up disease-causing free radicals. Additionally, it can dilate blood vessels, thereby improving blood circulation throughout the body including to the brain, which is why, says Dr. Stengler, some of the most popular uses of ginkgo have been to treat circulatory disorders and improve memory. The extract also reduces the stickiness of blood platelets, which means that it is useful to prevent blood clotting. *Dr. Stengler often prescribes it for the following conditions...*

•**Alzheimer's disease (AD) and other dementias.** Some of the most exciting current research involves ginkgo's impact on early-stage dementia. Studies have shown that it increases cognitive function in elderly people with mild to moderate age-related memory impairment as well as improves some cognitive and social functioning—seeming to effect about a six-month delay in disease progression, according to some researchers' observations. (Unfortunately, Dr. Stengler says that recent research has shown that ginkgo does not improve normal age-related short-term memory lapses after people reach age 60, although it does seem to enhance memory and cognitive functioning in younger healthy people.)

•**Vision impairment.** Ginkgo has been shown to improve several aspects of vision, including early diabetic retinopathy and glaucoma. Diabetic retinopathy can develop in people who have had diabetes for many years as blood flow to the eyes becomes impaired, resulting in blurry vision and other problems. Dr. Stengler says that taking ginkgo for six months can significantly improve color vision in these patients. For those who have glaucoma of the normal tension type, ginkgo seems to improve previous damage to the visual field.

•**Intermittent claudication.** This symptom of peripheral artery disease (PAD) causes leg pain when PAD patients walk because of decreased blood flow to the legs during exercise. Patients taking ginkgo were able to walk considerably further pain free than those taking a placebo, says Dr. Stengler, though he cautions that gingko should *supplement* walking therapy exercise—not replace it.

•**Premenstrual syndrome.** When women took ginkgo starting on the sixteenth day of their cycle and extended it five days into the next cycle, Dr. Stengler says they reported significant relief in breast tenderness and PMS-associated psychological symptoms.

Other uses: Because of improvements in blood circulation, ginkgo helps reduce the number of attacks of Raynaud's syndrome, erectile dysfunction and eases high blood pressure. Ginkgo has also been helpful for altitude sickness and mild depression.

A general ginkgo dosage can be from 180 milligrams (mg) to 240 mg daily, says Dr. Stengler. People who weigh less than 150 pounds are often started on the lower dosage, but if after six or eight weeks they don't show clinical improvement, the physician may often increase the dosage at that point. Ginkgo is usually given continuously for a period of time. There are several different types of ginkgo on the market, but the one that Dr. Stengler recommends is a product standardized to 24% flavone glycosides and 6% terpene lactones. This information will be clearly marked on the label.

SOME PRECAUTIONS

You may experience side effects from ginkgo, on occasion. Watch to see if any of these develop, says Dr. Stengler—gastrointestinal upset, headaches, dizziness, palpitations, constipation or allergic skin reactions. He adds that side effects are generally mild and dosage can be reduced somewhat to see if the side effects fade, as is usually the case. If they do not go away, however, your physician should discontinue the supplement. Also, although the research at this time is still inconclusive, people who are taking blood-thinning medications such as *warfarin* (Coumadin) or aspirin for blood-thinning purposes… people who take a *thiazide*-type diuretic for high blood pressure…or people who will be having surgery may need to avoid ginkgo. Check with your doctor if you are taking any drugs or supplements before taking ginkgo.

New for You— Natural Blood Thinners

Ralph E. Holsworth, Jr., DO, cofounder and director of clinical and scientific research, NZymeCeuticals, Inc.
Clinical Hemorheology and Microcirculation.

Millions of Americans take blood thinners each day to avoid dangerous clots that could cause heart attacks, strokes or deep vein thrombosis, among other major conditions. But blood thinners (also called anticoagulants) are serious and tricky drugs. They are pharmaceutical "big guns," and include such medications as *warfarin* (Coumadin) or *heparin*. Anticoagulants lengthen the time it takes for the blood to clot, rather than "thin the blood," despite being called blood thinners. These are difficult to manage and can cause bleeding, as well as other side effects.

SOME NATURAL CHOICES

The good news is that there are quite a few natural supplements which also reduce clotting due to their antiplatelet activity—in particular garlic, ginger, ginkgo, fish oil and vitamin E. The bad news is that these vary considerably in efficacy from product to product, so it's hard to know how well any one in particular is working. And, there's little quantitative research that has been done on their efficacy. (*Note:* These natural herbs and supplements can also increase or decrease the effects of anticoagulants or antiplatelet drugs. So be sure to notify your doctor if you take any of them.)

NEW KID ON THE NATURAL BLOCK

Because of these complex challenges, a relative newcomer to the field, an enzyme called *nattokinase* (NK), is getting a lot of attention. It closely resembles *plasmin*, the human enzyme responsible for breaking down and dissolving blood clots. NK is extracted from natto, which is made by fermenting boiled soybeans. Natto has been a staple in the Japanese diet for centuries because of its healthful properties.

NK IN US

The clinical use of NK in supplement form was introduced to the medical community in the US just a few years ago by Ralph E. Holsworth, Jr., DO, a leading nattokinase researcher. In a recent conversation, Dr. Holsworth says that as we age, our production of plasmin begins to decline, sometimes making us vulnerable to potentially lethal clots. NK acts in assorted ways to protect us from clots. Specifically it prevents the formation of blood clots by decreasing Plasminogen Activator Inhibitor-1 (PAI-1), and increasing tissue plasminogen activator (tPA) and plasmin. Plasmin is the body's major enzyme to combat the onset of an inadvertent blood clot. NK also prevents platelets from sticking and it dissolves insoluble fibrin proteins—literally thinning the blood or reducing viscosity.

NK vs. ASPIRIN

Blood viscosity is a strong predictor of cardiovascular disease—making NK helpful for lowering cardiovascular risk, including high blood pressure. It also mitigates inflammation responses in the body, by keeping blood platelets from sticking and excess blood plasma proteins called fibrin from forming clots. Because it decreases the thickness of blood in general as well, Dr. Holsworth says that he sees no reason people can't take NK rather than a daily aspirin as a preventive measure against heart attack.

IS IT SAFE?

Tampering with the blood is never to be undertaken lightly, without physician direction. Some physicians use NK in combination with medication (only use the type of NK without vitamin K), adjusting dosages based on the patient's response. For instance, when people on warfarin also go on NK, they often are able to reduce their dosage of the prescription drug, says Dr. Holsworth. However, there is not sufficient research at this point to support going off warfarin altogether to take NK alone. Those who try NK (or for that matter any

other antithrombotics, including natural blood thinning products) must do so with medical supervision and monitoring.

Note: Natto naturally contains vitamin K, which affects blood coagulation. If you take an NK supplement, look for supplements that are formulated in a way so that vitamin K is removed.

The only side effect Dr. Holsworth has seen so far with NK is the occasional nosebleed in users who are also taking gingko, garlic, vitamin E and/or other supplements.

WHERE CAN YOU GET NK?

NK has been on the market as a supplement for some time, though some brands are better than others. To check for quality, look for the letters "NSK-SD," the trademark for a product from Japan Bioscience Laboratory Co., Ltd., which Dr. Holsworth says is of reputable purity...and the term "fibrin degradation units" (FUs) on the label, specifying fibrin degradation activity level. Dr. Holsworth generally recommends 2,000 FU per day for preventive use, but stresses that anyone considering use of NK or any natto product should only do so under the supervision of a trained professional who will monitor its use.

Supplement Combo That Reduces Pain by 79%

Mark A. Stengler, ND, naturopathic physician in private practice, La Jolla, California...adjunct associate clinical professor at the National College of Natural Medicine, Portland, Oregon...author of many books, including *The Natural Physician's Healing Therapies* and coauthor of *Prescription for Natural Cures* (both from Bottom Line Books)...and author of the *Bottom Line/Natural Healing* newsletter.

One of the most widely used natural remedies is a combination of glucosamine and chondroitin to ease the pain of aching joints for arthritis sufferers. But a major study investigating the supplements' effectiveness reported little impact. While previous small studies had shown positive results, this study was big—1,583 patients in a double-blind, multi-center investigation that included both a placebo control group and a prescription painkiller to measure against. The researchers' conclusions and the resulting negative headlines have served up confusion instead of clarity. We asked Mark Stengler, ND, editor of *Bottom Line's Natural Healing* for his opinion of the results. *This is what he had to say...*

STUDY RECAP

Here is a quick recap of the study, managed by the University of Utah. *It included five groups of people who had symptomatic knee osteoarthritis and took pills over the six-month study period in the following way...*

- **Group one**—1,500 milligrams (mg) of glucosamine daily
- **Group two**—1,200 mg of chondroitin sulfate daily
- **Group three**—a combination of glucosamine (1,500 mg daily) and chondroitin (1,200 mg daily)
- **Group four**—200 mg of *celecoxib* (Celebrex) daily
- **Group five**—a placebo pill daily.

The participants were also categorized into two groups determined by level of pain, mild or moderate to severe. All were allowed to take up to 4,000 mg of acetaminophen daily as "rescue" analgesia.

The results: Overall, glucosamine reduced knee pain by 3.9 percentage points over placebo...chondroitin sulfate by 5 percentage points...and Celebrex by 10 percentage points.

For patients whose pain was moderate to severe and who took the combined therapy of glucosamine and chondroitin sulfate, the results were impressive—79.2% pain reduction versus 54.3% for those taking placebo. The study's other good news

was that adverse side effects were mild and evenly distributed over all groups.

SOMETHING TO TALK ABOUT

One would think a 79.2% reduction in pain for people with moderate to severe knee pain would be something to trumpet, but that's not what happened. The report concluded that the two supplements alone or in combination "did not reduce pain effectively in the overall group of patients"...although it did add that "exploratory analyses suggest" the combination might help the subgroup.

WHY THE NEGATIVE PRESS?

Dr. Stengler's analysis: He says this study is interesting and that it would be a mistake to be misled by the negativity surrounding it. He points first of all to the fact that it confirms findings from 50 previous studies that showed glucosamine by itself or combined with chondroitin sulfate is effective when taken for osteoarthritis. The announced "ineffectiveness" of the supplements in this study reflected the larger numbers of participants in the mild-pain group. Even the study authors admit that the relatively low level of pain these volunteers experienced may have limited the effect of the supplements. In other words, it's hard to notice relief of pain when there isn't much pain to address in the first place.

NEGLECTED FINDINGS

Further evidence for the effectiveness of the combined supplements was a study result the media, oddly enough, did not report. The pharmaceutical drug Celebrex was not as effective for treating moderate-to-severe pain as was the combination of glucosamine and chondroitin sulfate.

Yet another overlooked and important finding: Chondroitin sulfate treatment was associated with a significant decrease of joint swelling, effusion (fluid seeping from inflammation) or both.

OTHER OBSERVATIONS

Dr. Stengler makes several other observations having to do with the supplements used in the study. Patients took glucosamine hydrochloride rather than glucosamine sulfate, the form that has been most widely studied and found to be effective. Glucosamine sulfate might have been more helpful in this study as well had it been used. Often people do better on the combination of glucosamine and chondroitin, which, of course, only one group was on in this study. Finally, there is that nagging issue of conflict of interest. Some of the study authors have had ties with pharmaceutical houses that sell arthritis drugs.

ADVICE

Given that this study in fact underscores the usefulness of these supplements, Dr. Stengler continues to recommend 1,500 milligrams (mg) of glucosamine sulfate and 1,200 mg of chondroitin daily for his patients with osteoarthritis. People who weigh more than 200 pounds are often advised to take a dosage of up to 2,000 mg of glucosamine sulfate. A small percentage of his patients found that the supplements caused them some digestive upset, and in that case they stopped taking it. Also, patients who are allergic to shellfish are advised to be cautious about taking them. *Other recommendations and reminders given to people with osteoarthritis...*

• **Methylsulfonylmethane (MSM)** is a natural anti-inflammatory.

Typical dose: 2,000 to 5,000 mg daily.

• **Fish oil,** frequently 1,000 to 2,000 mg daily, that combines EPA and DHA, helps reduce inflammation and lubricate joints.

• **Maintain a normal weight.**

• **Eat few simple sugars** because they can aggravate pain.

• **Acupuncture,** for pain relief

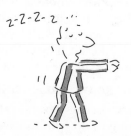

Good News for Sleep-Deprived Folks

Terry McMorris, PhD, professor, Centre for Sports Science and Medicine, University of Chichester, College Lane, Chichester, West Sussex, UK.

Recent findings from a British study about how the naturally occurring amino acid *creatine* can help those who don't get enough sleep caught our attention. To learn more about it, we consulted lead researcher Terry McMorris, PhD, a professor at the University of Chichester in England.

LACK OF SLEEP EXACTS A TOLL

Creatine acts as an energy source fueling muscular and nervous system activity. Our bodies naturally manufacture and pack it away in order to store energy. Insufficient rest puts demands on these energy reserves, while at the same time our activity level is drawing upon them. While the deficit created by the extra demand is small, it is significant enough to cause problems, especially with complex tasks such as problem-solving and decision-making, explains Dr. McMorris.

ABOUT THE STUDY

In the study, before undergoing a series of tests, 10 participants took five grams of creatine monohydrate four times a day for seven days, while nine took a placebo. The study was a double-blind trial, meaning that neither researchers nor participants knew who took creatine and who got the placebo. Next, participants were tested in areas such as movement, balance and mood after being deprived of sleep for six, 12 and 24 hours and performing moderate, intermittent exercise. They were tested at baseline and after each interval.

Researchers found that participants who took creatine were considerably sharper the day following sleep deprivation than those who took the placebo. According to Dr. McMorris, the creatine group not only maintained their baseline performance level on most tests, which researchers expected, they actually improved on some. Researchers concluded that creatine boosts mood and task performance after sleep deprivation places stress on the brain. Researchers found that recall was not affected as much as the ability to perform complex tasks. This study did not look at age as a variable. In another study, which was specifically conducted in the elderly, Dr. McMorris and his colleagues found that recall was significantly improved with creatine supplementation. According to Dr. McMorris, there may be differences in the ways in which the young and the elderly (age 70 and older) benefit from creatine supplementation.

REVERSING THE IMPACT OF SLEEP DEPRIVATION

Creatine is safe if taken in moderation, says Dr. McMorris. However excess creatine can cause problems with the kidneys (kidney stones, and over prolonged periods, kidney failure) and liver disease, so moderation is key, as with any nutrient, and your use should be supervised by your doctor.

Meet the Amazing Medicinal Mushroom

Mark Blumenthal, founder and executive director, American Botanical Council, Austin, Texas, and editor, *HerbalGram* and *HerbClip. www.herbalgram.org.*

Many mushrooms have strong healing powers. Compounds in various mushrooms have been shown to enhance immunity, fight off infections and cancer, and lower blood sugar and blood pressure. Among the most popular "medicinal mushrooms" is the maitake (*Grifola frondosa*), which is not only tasty but prized—particularly in Asian cultures—for its healing abilities.

To learn more about this versatile fungus, we consulted Mark Blumenthal, founder and executive director of the American Botanical Council in Austin, Texas. He tells us that maitake can be used by healthy people as well as those with health issues such as a compromised immune system, with no significant risk of adverse side effects. While incorporating mushrooms into the diet is always a good idea, maitake in the form of dietary supplements packs considerably more punch.

IMMUNE ENHANCEMENT AND MORE

The number-one use for maitake lies in boosting immune system function, though it has also been used for certain specific ailments. According to Blumenthal, some cancer patients use maitake-based preparations as part of their natural treatment regimens in order to reduce the adverse effects of chemotherapy drugs. Additionally, maitake has demonstrated the ability to increase *apoptosis*, the natural programmed death of old, worn-out cells that acts as a check against their becoming cancerous. (Cancer cells proliferate instead of undergoing apoptosis.) Maitake also has been shown to improve cardiovascular-related parameters such as blood pressure, cholesterol and glucose (blood sugar) levels.

HOW TO TAKE MAITAKE MUSHROOMS

Maitake preparations can be taken with vitamins and certain other dietary supplements, usually in the morning and evening or with meals. They are typically sold as liquid extracts, capsules or tablets containing dried maitake extract powder, says Blumenthal. Blumenthal recommends taking the "D-fraction standardized maitake," so indicated on the packaging, because it has the most powerful immune-stimulating activity, according to much of the published research.

Dosage depends on the intended use and the form of the product, notes Blumenthal. Given the power of maitake and the potentially severe conditions that it can be used for, it is best to work with a holistic physician, herbalist or other trained professional when starting a supplementation regimen. *Blumenthal notes that research shows that maitake can be used as an adjunct therapy for...*

•**High blood pressure and/or cholesterol levels.**

•**High blood sugar levels** associated with diabetes or metabolic syndrome.

•**Increased immune function** to help prevent colds and flu.

•**Supplementation to chemotherapy.**

NO SIDE EFFECTS BUT...

To Blumenthal's knowledge, there are no significant adverse side effects or drug interactions associated with the use of maitake mushroom preparations when used as directed. Still, as noted above, with serious diseases such as diabetes or cancer or high blood pressure, it is always best to add a trained alternative or conventional physician to your treatment team before taking dietary supplements. This is especially important if you are taking prescription medications for any of the above conditions.

Superstar of Antiaging Nutrients?

Mark A. Stengler, ND, naturopathic physician in private practice, La Jolla, California...adjunct associate clinical professor at the National College of Natural Medicine, Portland, Oregon...author of many books, including *The Natural Physician's Healing Therapies* and coauthor of *Prescription for Natural Cures* (both from Bottom Line Books)...and author of the *Bottom Line/Natural Healing* newsletter.

Recently, carnosine has been touted as the newest miracle "antiaging nutrient." Lots of people are selling it on the Internet. What's the real scoop? To find out, we went to frequent *Daily Health News* contributor Mark Stengler, ND, editor of *Bottom Line's Natural Healing* newsletter.

COUNTERACT SIDE EFFECT OF THE AGING

"I wouldn't say it's a super antiaging nutrient," says Dr. Stengler, "but I would say it can play an important role in protecting against cell damage related to the normal process of aging." The key to its effectiveness seems to be in its ability to fight the damaging effects of a process called *glycation*, in which proteins in the body interact with sugar. To get a picture of what glycation looks like, think of caramelization. Glycation is a reaction between protein and sugar that irreversibly alters the configuration of the proteins, making them sticky and jamming up the works. "The end result of this interaction is something called advanced glycation end products, or the aptly named AGEs for short," says Dr. Stengler.

AGEs AND AGING

However, there can be a dietary source of AGEs as well. Foods rich in protein and fat cooked at high heat tend to be the richest dietary sources of AGEs. High AGEs consumption triggers inflammation.

"These AGEs probably play a significant role in the aging process." Carnosine's claim to fame is that it helps prevent glycation from creating an inappropriately large accumulation of AGEs.

AGEs are known to have negative effects on the properties of proteins and on the tissues in which these proteins reside. Plus, they interact with free radicals, causing oxidation and even more damage in the body. "Carnosine, along with other antioxidants, may help protect against the damage from free radicals," Dr. Stengler tells us.

Since one of the main culprits in forming these AGEs is high levels of serum glucose, we wondered if carnosine might be especially helpful for people with diabetes. Dr. Stengler says that carnosine may protect against some of the degenerative changes suffered by people with diabetes like neuropathy, cataracts and circulatory difficulties, and so he recommends it highly for those with diabetes.

The bottom line? Dr. Stengler thinks carnosine is a safe supplement that is worth taking, especially for those with diabetes. Dosing runs from 500 milligrams (mg) to 1,000 mg per day—though it is best to talk to your own practitioner to determine what level, if any, is best for you.

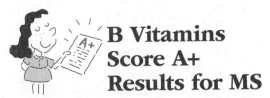

B Vitamins Score A+ Results for MS

Shinjiro Kaneko, MD, PhD, research fellow at Children's Hospital, Boston.

Allen C. Bowling, MD, PhD, consulting advisor at the Rocky Mountain Multiple Sclerosis Center, Englewood, Colorado.

There are 400,000 Americans with multiple sclerosis (MS). MS generally strikes people between the ages of 20 and 50, and two-thirds of them are women. Most MS patients are Caucasian of northern European descent, and having a sibling with MS makes the risk of developing it several times greater.

There isn't much conventional doctors can offer for treatment to ease symptoms and stall the disease, and what drugs are available come with difficult side effects, such as fever, chills, muscle aches and fatigue. But new hope—in the form of an everyday vitamin—may be in the offing for the many who have MS.

WHAT IS MS?

The complexity of MS has puzzled scientists for decades. Given that mostly women are affected, do hormones play a role? There is surely a genetic connection, but what? Scientists concur that MS is an inflammatory disease of the central nervous system (brain and spinal cord). It causes lesions to develop, apparently at random, on various spots on the nerve fibers (called axons). These lesions degenerate the myelin—material that coats and insulates nerves—damaging the ability of the axons to do their job, which is to transmit communication signals to and from the brain to nerves in the spinal column and elsewhere.

MANY SYMPTOMS

Because lesions can develop on axons anywhere in the central nervous system, they can affect a variety of signals…consequently MS has a wide and lengthy list of possible symptoms. These include fatigue, visual impairment, difficulty walking, spasticity, emotional and cognitive changes, pain and digestive problems. For most patients with MS, disease progression is slow, and their symptoms come and go, but about one-third of patients eventually need a wheelchair.

THE PROBLEM WITH DRUGS

Until the early 1990s there was no treatment for MS, but now there are several drugs that help reduce inflammation or preserve myelin in the early phase of the disease. However, these come with serious side effects and none have been successful in stopping the degeneration of axons that occurs in the later disease phase, which causes the greatest disability. Adding to everyone's frustration—especially people who have MS—there have been several promising medications that ultimately failed to deliver. All this makes a recent study on a common and inexpensive substance (that's unlikely to cause side effects) particularly exciting. Scientists at Children's Hospital Boston, affiliated with Harvard Medical School, have been working with a form of vitamin B-3 (commonly known as niacin) that seems to not only fight inflammation and stop myelin loss, but also appears to halt axon degeneration.

B-3 LOOKS GOOD BUT THERE'S MORE TO LEARN

To explain the study, it's useful to have a brief background about a coenzyme named *nicotinamide adenine dinucleotide*

(NAD). Coenzymes are organic chemicals that help enzymes do their jobs, and this coenzyme in particular is present in every cell. It is used by the body to produce energy. The precursor of NAD is nicotinamide, which is a form of vitamin B-3 closely related to niacin.

For these studies, the scientists bred mice to have an MS-like disease. When the researchers administered nicotinamide to the mice, it increased NAD levels in their nervous systems, and the increased NAD delayed the onset of neurological disability. The more NAD the mice had when symptoms developed, the less neurological damage they suffered...conversely, the mice with the least NAD had the most neurological damage. Furthermore, the scientists found strong evidence that administering nicotinamide protected against damage to the axons in the later chronic disease stage as well.

FURTHER STUDIES NEEDED

Shinjiro Kaneko, MD, PhD, a research fellow at Children's Hospital, Boston, was the lead author of the study. He says that the mouse studies were an extension of some they had done in the lab in vitro with the same results. Although B-3 (niacin) is often used by people who are trying to reduce high cholesterol levels, Dr. Kaneko says that this is the first study that researches how B-3 might be used in treating MS. The obvious question is whether B-3 should now be taken by all MS patients, but Dr. Kaneko says that it is too early to make that suggestion. He explains that the doses they administered to the mice in their studies were substantially higher than people normally take, and until clinical trials have been done to investigate further, he is concerned about safety issues.

We also checked in with Allen C. Bowling, MD, PhD, medical director at the Rocky Mountain Multiple Sclerosis Center in Englewood, Colorado, and author of *Complementary and Alternative Medicine and Multiple Sclerosis* (Demos Medical Publishing). Dr. Bowling agrees with Dr.

Kaneko that, based on these studies, it is too early to recommend B-3 to MS patients. He adds that other substances have seemed promising in studies, and then turned out to disappoint. We need to wait and see about B-3.

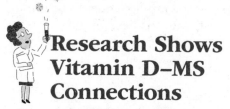

Research Shows Vitamin D–MS Connections

Kassandra Munger, MSc, research assistant, department of nutrition, at the Harvard School of Public Health, Boston.

Michael Holick, MD, PhD, program director of the General Clinical Research Center at Boston University School of Medicine.

Get out in the sun! This advice comes after a study involving data from Army and Navy personnel that revealed that those with the highest blood levels of vitamin D, the "sunshine vitamin," were 62% less likely to develop multiple sclerosis (MS). The results may help to shed light (no pun intended!) on why MS is more common in people living far from the equator, where exposure to year-round sunlight is less intense.

STUDY FINDINGS

Working with a military database, study researchers sorted through more than seven million Army and Navy personnel records and identified 257 cases of MS. Each MS case eligible for the study was assigned two matching controls (same age, gender, ethnicity and dates of blood collection). Vitamin D levels were obtained by blood samples taken before the onset of MS symptoms.

Decreased MS risk was very strong in people younger than 20 years old, suggesting that vitamin D exposure before adulthood could be particularly important. Interestingly, these findings were true for white study participants, but not for black or Hispanic ones, for whom no significant association between vitamin D and MS was found. According to Kassandra Munger, MSc, researcher at the Harvard School of Public Health in Boston, and lead author of this study, people with darker skin have lower vitamin D levels overall, because their pigmentation "blocks" UV light.

WHAT IT MEANS TO YOU

According to Michael Holick, MD, PhD, author of several papers on vitamin D, and program director of the General Clinical Research Center at Boston University School of Medicine, the findings do not change advice on tanning. During the summer months, 10 to 15 minutes a day (20 minutes or more for dark-skinned individuals), two to three days a week without sunscreen during the peak hours of 10 am to 3 pm, is plenty of exposure for a light-skinned person to produce adequate vitamin D levels.

SUN SUBSTITUTES

During winter in the northern latitudes, the strength of the sun's rays reaching the Earth are inadequate to produce beneficial amounts of vitamin D.

Dr. Holick says sunlamps that transmit UVB radiation can help the body produce amounts of vitamin D. However, he recommends that users limit "sunbathing" to 50% of the manufacturers' product guidelines in order to prevent skin damage that could increase cancer risk.

HOW ABOUT PILLS?

Should we now be taking vitamin D supplements to prevent MS? Munger is quick to point out that the study does not prove that increasing vitamin D levels will prevent MS, or that a lack of vitamin D causes MS. Future research is necessary to further illuminate the relationship. However, she reminds us that there is a growing body of evidence supporting vitamin D in overall health maintenance, including bone health. For this reason, individuals should ensure that their vitamin D levels are adequate—at 1,000 IU (international units)/day (and if you take the supplement form, look for the "natural" D-3, derived mostly from fish oil). People with chronic granulomatous diseases such as sarcoidosis should avoid high levels of vitamin D supplementation.

Omega-3s— Good for Your Heart and Bones!

Bruce A. Watkins, PhD, professor of food science, Purdue University, director of the Center for Enhancing Foods to Protect Health, West Lafayette, Indiana.

It is well known that omega-3 essential fatty acids are crucial for cardiovascular health, but now scientists have discovered that they also slow osteoporosis—the thinning of bones in older people, women in particular. Researchers at Purdue University's Center for Enhancing Foods to Protect Health conducted a rat study in which they removed the ovaries in two groups of rats, making them instantly estrogen deprived and therefore vulnerable to osteoporosis. They then fed one group a diet high in omega-6s (a ratio of 10:1) and the other a diet high in omega-3s (a ratio of 5:1). At the end of three months, the researchers evaluated the rats' bones and discovered that the 5:1 group preserved significantly more bone mineral than the other group.

TIME TO REMODEL

We spoke with Bruce A. Watkins, PhD, professor of nutrition at Purdue and the study's coauthor about the importance of the omega-3s to bone health. He explains that bone building takes place throughout life in a cycle called remodeling. Certain cells break down bone and remove the particles and other cells come in to rebuild. (Exercise enhances remodeling because, he says, the muscles surrounding the bones being used message these cells to build more "here.") Dr. Watkins says that estrogen deprivation seems to elevate the activity of bone removal relative to the rate of bone formation, and the omega-3s—with their anti-inflammatory properties—slow that escalation down again. Omega-3s might also help bones by setting the stage for proper mineralization and use of calcium, another nutrient needed to build bone mass.

HOW TO GET YOUR 3s

Because of the way food is processed today, few people are getting the health benefits of omega-3s. Omega-6s, found primarily in vegetable oils, have deluged 3s in the modern diet. The ratio of 6s to 3s is now 10:1 or higher, the optimal ratio is 5:1 or lower. Because omega-6s are ubiquitous—in the corn-based vegetable oils that fill processed baked and fried foods as well as in animal feed and thus in meats—it's crucial to increase omega-3s in the diet to establish a good ratio.

COLD-WATER FISH x THREE

The American Heart Association recommends three meals a week featuring cold-water fish such as salmon, herring, mackerel, sardines or tuna (packed in water, *not* soy oil, which is filled with omega-6s, Dr. Watkins says). Omega-3s are also found in leafy green vegetables, walnuts and flaxseed and its oil. The drawback of flaxseed, however, is that the only omega-3 it contains is *alpha-linolenic acid* (ALA), which the body must convert to the two most important omega-3s, *eicosapentaenoic acid* (EPA) and *docosahexaenoic acid* (DHA). To be sure you are getting enough EPA and DHA, our consulting medical editor Andrew L. Rubman, ND, advises taking 1,000 milligrams (mg) a day of a combination of both.

Best sources: Good-tasting fish oil products from Pharmax and Nordic Naturals.

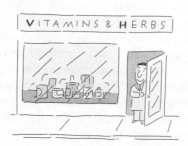

Supplement Conquers the Food–Depression Cycle

John P. Docherty, MD, CEO of Comprehensive NeuroScience Inc., adjunct professor of psychiatry, Weill Cornell Medical College, Cornell University, New York City.

All too often, depression can feed on itself. Such is the case for the approximately eight million Americans who suffer from *atypical depression*, a variety of depression in which sufferers have an increased appetite leading to weight gain, sleeping too much, excessive lethargy and hypersensitivity to interpersonal rejection. Although atypical depression symptoms are quite apparent and they account for about 42% of the 19 million Americans who suffer from clinical depression, the problem frequently goes undiagnosed.

RECENT RESEARCH CAN HELP

The good news for these people is that a recent study looked at the role of chromium salts in helping to control blood sugar, and in turn, cravings. For more on the subject, we spoke with John P. Docherty, MD, CEO of Comprehensive NeuroScience Inc., and adjunct professor of psychiatry at Weill Cornell Medical College, Cornell University in New York City, who says that the carbohydrates that patients overindulge in the most are not surprising—baked goods and pasta, both ranking high as comfort foods. The result is weight gain, which adds to patients' depression. Unfortunately, a common side effect of selective serotonin reuptake inhibitors (SSRIs)—antidepressant medications, such as *fluoxetine* (Prozac) and *sertraline* (Zoloft)—is weight gain, as well.

CHROMIUM PICOLINATE

The 113 participants in the eight-week study, all people with atypical depression and a mean body mass index (BMI) that was borderline obese, were randomized into a group taking up to 600 microgram (mcg) of *chromium picolinate* a day or a placebo. The findings showed that the chromium picolinate group had a significant improvement—65% versus 33% in the placebo group—in terms of decreased appetite and lowered carbohydrate craving.

Dr. Docherty says we don't know exactly why chromium picolinate works to decrease carb cravings, but it probably has to do with the fact that it seems to enhance insulin regulation. (Many people with type 2 diabetes take it for this reason.) The picolinate form of chromium was used in the study not because it's the most effective form to use, but because it is the most widely available

form. Chromium is abundantly available in whole grains, seafood, green beans and broccoli, among other foods, though it can be safely supplemented with physician oversight. People with diabetes especially should never start chromium supplements without medical supervision.

WEIGHT GAIN AND LETHARGY

Dr. Docherty stresses that it is important for all family members, friends and doctors to pay close attention when an individual starts to gain weight and seems unusually lethargic. These may well be signs that the person is suffering from depression or another physical illness such as sleep apnea disorder and should be evaluated.

12

Breakthroughs in Natural Healing

How Water Cures What Ails You

Hydrotherapy—the use of water in the treatment of medical conditions such as sore throat and fever—has been used effectively for centuries. We called on hydrotherapy expert Thomas A. Kruzel, ND, a naturopathic physician in private practice in Scottsdale, Arizona, and author of the *Homeopathic Emergency Guide: A Quick Reference Handbook to Effective Homeopathic Care* (North Atlantic) to find out the applications of hydrotherapy today. Dr. Kruzel says that this modality is being rediscovered and practiced by more and more health-care professionals, especially NDs who include hydrotherapy as a core discipline. It can help with everything from easing the symptoms of arthritis to providing relief from the side

effects of chemotherapy. These treatments are best performed under the watchful eye of an expert. However, individuals can use hydrotherapy to help with fevers, stress relief and detoxification.

HOW IT WORKS

Sometimes warm or hot water is used in hydrotherapy, other times cold...while alternating hot and cold has an especially intense impact on the body internally.

Heat calms and soothes, quieting the body, explains Dr. Kruzel. When you are anxious and your muscles are tense and tight, or after active sports, a hot shower or bath (Epsom salts and lavender are good to add) is just what the doctor ordered. In contrast, cold energizes and stimulates.

Thomas A. Kruzel, ND, naturopathic physician in private practice in Scottsdale, Arizona, past president of The American Association of Naturopathic Physicians and former vice president of clinical affairs and chief medical officer at the Southwest College of Naturopathic Medicine in Phoenix. Dr. Kruzel is author of *Homeopathic Emergency Guide: A Quick Reference Handbook to Effective Homeopathic Care*. North Atlantic.

When you are overtired and dragging, try a warm shower or bath followed by a short, cold rinse for a quick burst of energy.

According to Dr. Kruzel, hydrotherapy has a number of specific physiological effects on the body, depending on the type of therapy. *It can...*

• **Stimulate circulation, ease problems with digestion and thyroid function.**

• **Increase blood and oxygen flow.**

• **Boost white blood cell count and enhance immunity.**

• **Calm the central nervous system, easing anxiety, tension and insomnia.**

• **Loosen tight muscles.**

• **Kick body temperature up a half degree or more.**

HOW IT'S USED

Hydrotherapy comes in many forms. We're all familiar with hot baths and cold showers, but there are also sitz baths (baths taken in a sitting position that cover the hips and buttocks), foot baths, hot and cold compresses, steam inhalation, whirlpools, saunas and more. *Here are Dr. Kruzel's favorite do-it-yourself techniques...*

• **Reduce congestion associated with colds and flu.** Try a home steam treatment. Inhaling steam helps loosen secretions, thus reducing congestion. Simply fill a third of a bowl with boiling water, pull a towel over your head and inhale the steam for several minutes. (Some people like to add a drop or two of an essential oil such as eucalyptus to the water.) Warm compresses with Epsom salts can also help sinuses drain.

• **Melt away stress.** Soak in a hot bath, or better yet a whirlpool, which has a massage-like effect. You might want to add soothing herbs to your bath, including lavender and chamomile.

• **Reduce pain and swelling of hemorrhoids.** Dr. Kruzel suggests alternating hot and cold sitz baths. Women who have received episiotomies during childbirth may also want to ask their obstetricians or midwives for medical clearance to seek naturopathic advice about sitz baths to speed healing.

• **Treat vaginal infections of all types, including yeast.** Dr. Kruzel recommends that you alternate hot and cold compresses to your upper inner thighs and pubic area which improves lymphatic drainage in the specific nodes that often are involved with these infections. (To make a compress, simply wet a clean washcloth with hot or cold water and wring it out.) A compress with witch hazel also helps relieve symptoms like itching.

• **Sooth sore feet.** Add a tablespoon of Epsom salts and three to five drops of your favorite essential oil to a bowl of hot water. Soak feet for five to 15 minutes.

• **Sweat out metabolic wastes.** After your workout at the gym, visit the sauna or steam room for 15 to 20 minutes. To prevent overheating, wipe your face and neck frequently with a cold, wet washcloth.

Also: See precautions below.

For upper respiratory infections (URIs) and fever: Wet a T-shirt and socks with cold water, and wring as much water out of them as possible. Next take a warm shower, and afterward don the T-shirt and socks. Cover with a dry, warm sweat shirt and a dry pair of sweat socks, and climb into bed. Sounds uncomfortable, but Dr. Kruzel assures us that it calms the nervous system, and causes the fever to spike and then break.

Note: This treatment should be supervised initially by a health-care professional.

More fever relief: Wet a towel with cold water, and wring it out. Wrap the towel around the base of the skull and neck. This cools blood going to the brain. Try dunking your feet in ice water for only a minute and toweling dry. This can draw circulation down away from the head. Alternatively, just take a cool bath.

A FEW SIMPLE PRECAUTIONS

If you want to utilize hydrotherapy as part of a regular treatment plan and want specific guidance, Dr. Kruzel recommends that you seek the care of a naturopathic doctor (ND). *Other simple precautions to follow are...*

•**If you are pregnant or have abnormal blood pressure or heart disease**, do not use saunas or steam baths.

•**If you have diabetes,** do not apply hot applications to the legs or feet as you may not be able to have accurate temperature sensation in the limbs.

•**Do not use cold applications if you suffer from Raynaud's syndrome** (a condition that causes parts of the body—such as the fingers and toes—to feel numb in response to cool temperatures or stress).

•**The very young and the very old should avoid extended hot treatments.** And—those with heart problems, multiple sclerosis and pregnant people should follow these treatments while under the care of a physician.

There are many other hydrotherapy techniques that can help more challenging conditions—just speak with your naturopathic physician.

Expert Reveals Five New and Natural Sleep Aids

Chris D. Meletis, ND, executive director, the Institute for Healthy Aging, Reno, Nevada.

Oh, for a sweet sleep—and how Americans are clamoring to get one. For ways to foster sleep naturally, we called on naturopathic physician Chris D. Meletis, ND, executive director of education for the Institute for Healthy Aging located in Reno, Nevada.

IDENTIFY THE CAUSE OF INSOMNIA

Dr. Meletis says that if insomnia is a new situation, first consider what may be causing it. Is there something in your life that has increased stress—perhaps conflicts at work or a problem with your child—anything, in fact, causing anxiety that might interfere with sleep? Maybe the problem is something less apparent, for instance, your sleep environment. A mattress that has become uncomfortable or a pillow that is too hard or soft can be just enough of an irritant to intrude on good sleep. Is the bedroom dark enough and the temperature just right for you? Also consider whether you've started any new medications (or changed dosages) that might impact the quality of your sleep.

FOOD, DRINK AND SLEEP

Dr. Meletis also reminds people that what they eat and drink can impact sleep. Caffeine, of course, is often a culprit. Some people must avoid having caffeine after 2 pm, but super-sensitive types should stay away from caffeine completely. Only by eliminating, or vastly reducing, it for a few weeks will you know if you are in that group. Remember, too, that caffeine lurks in chocolate, colas and tea, as well as coffee. As for food, Dr. Meletis recommends having the last meal of the day provide a balance of protein and complex carbs—like vegetables (except tomatoes and peppers) and whole grains. This will fill you enough that hunger won't wake you up. Avoid spicy, fried and fatty foods and mint, all of which may increase acid reflux, and don't eat or drink liquids for two or three hours before bed to avoid middle-of-the-night treks to the bathroom. The ban includes alcohol, which also interferes with the quality of sleep.

SLEEPING PILLS, B VITAMINS

Anyone who is taking sleeping pills may need to be careful when weaning off of them, he says.

The reason: You can become dependent on the drug and need time to recover. Under supervision of the prescriber, gradually decrease dosage until you are off the medication completely. This process often takes several weeks. Dr. Meletis says that drinking green tea (during the day, since it also has caffeine) will help in this process because it has L-theanine, an amino acid that can help induce relaxation. He adds that B-complex vitamins also combat stress and, as a bonus, often make dreams more vivid. (Although necessary to take at least twice daily, unduly high B vitamin supplementations can contribute to sleeplessness because they can be energizing.)

HERBAL HELPERS

Certain herbs are also calming and can help produce a more restful sleep, including valerian, passion flower and chamomile tea.

Dr. Meletis says there are also herbal formulas that some people find helpful for occasional sleeplessness. He likes Herbal Sleep by Vitamin Research Products (*www. vrp.com*) that contains the following:

•**L-theanine (150 milligrams—mg)**

•**Hops (133 mg)**—*Humulus lupulus* extract, (strobiles)

•**Lemon Balm (133 mg)**—(*Melissa officinalis* extract, leaf)

•**Valerian (100 mg)**—(*Valeriana officinalis* extract, root with 0.8% valerianic acid)

•**Passion flower (133 mg)**—(*Passiflora incarnata*, aerial)

Consult a knowledgeable physician before you take any of the herbs or supplements above, as all botanicals can have side effects or interact with pharmaceuticals or other supplements.

OTHER IDEAS

Some nights, though, you may need other ways to quiet a mind that continues to churn. Dr. Meletis suggests keeping a note pad and pen next to your bed so that you can jot down whatever comes to mind. He also suggests the following self-healing techniques, based in part on existing sleep-inducing methods.

Try this for a brief mid-day meditation: Sitting up, close your eyes and observe your breathing without changing the way you breathe in any way. How much time do you spend breathing in and how much time breathing out? Pay attention to where the breath goes inside of you and what parts of you don't participate in the breathing process. Again, don't change the way you breathe, merely observe it until you feel completely relaxed.

For soothing yourself into sleep, try these techniques, both of which you should do slowly, gently and in bed.

•**On your back, rest your palms** on either side of your belly. As you breathe in, notice how your fingers go along for the ride as your belly gently swells on breathing in and recedes as you exhale. After many breaths, begin to gently, minimally lift one set of fingers, such as your thumbs, then switch to index fingers, just slightly so that ultimately the tips are barely off your skin as you finish breathing in. Allow them to return to the belly as you exhale and your belly recedes. The idea is not to breathe bigger or differently in any way, which is enough to induce stress. Instead simply observe what you do and repeat as necessary.

•**On your back, rest your arms** at your sides and bend your elbows so that one forearm is now perpendicular to the bed with your hands in a soft-fist position. Keeping your forearms upright, gently bend your wrists so that the palms face the bed. Do this slowly enough that you can feel that pull of gravity on your hands. (Your forearm position does not change.) You will see that your fists gradually and naturally unfold as you do this. Gently, slowly, return each hand to its original position where it will return to a soft fist, again, naturally. Repeat as necessary.

The Safest, Cheapest Sleeping "Pill"

Andrew L. Rubman, ND, consulting medical editor for *Bottom Line's Daily Health News* and director of the Southbury Clinic for Traditional Medicines in Southbury, Connecticut.

We've all lain awake at night on occasion, thanks to an upset stomach or over-indulgence during dinner. But, did you know that *what* you eat can also make you sleep *better*? In a country rife with sleep challenges, using healthful nutritional choices is a far safer and cheaper solution to getting a good night's sleep than whatever sleeping pill is being promoted on television. We spoke with *Bottom Line's Daily Health News* consulting medical editor Andrew L. Rubman, ND, about how normal digestive function is the key to getting a good night's sleep.

THE "GOOD NIGHT MOON" HORMONE

To begin with, we need to understand that the key ingredient to sleeping safe and sound is the chemical *serotonin*, which Dr. Rubman refers to as "the good night moon hormone." Increasing serotonin drops the "voltage" to the parts of the brain controlling creative thought and wakefulness, decreasing stress and anxiety levels and introducing a sense of calm and relaxation. Just the state you want to be in to gently drop off to sleep.

However, the body requires both sufficient levels of serotonin and the means to make efficient use of it in order to fall asleep successfully. Dr. Rubman notes that we take in plenty of *tryptophan*—the raw material for serotonin—through foods such as animal protein (especially turkey), eggs and fish. The trick is to optimize tryptophan's conversion into serotonin, a process you can contribute to by optimizing your digestion.

DR. RUBMAN'S PATH TO A GOOD NIGHT'S SLEEP

Dr. Rubman's path to a good night's sleep consists of the following…

• **Check your B-12 level.** If you have inadequate levels of B-12 your body cannot make the best possible use of tryptophan. The brain needs B-12 for most neurological processes and the liver requires it to break down metabolites (chemicals from digested food). With high-action, high-stress lives many Americans are quick to use up the B-12 they have…and so are running at a functional B-12 deficit. Dr. Rubman advises that you have your health-care professional assess your blood level of B-12. Your requirement for optimal function may be significantly higher than the reference lab values, so underline that point. If you suffer from this very common functional deficiency and display any of the symptoms associated with B-12 functional deficiency, you may be prescribed sublingual B-12 pills, which are equally as effective as (and less costly than) B-12 shots. One hour before bedtime, take 1 milligram (mg) of B-12 in the form of *hydroxocobalamin* or *methylcobalamin*. (Avoid *cyanocobalamin*, which may be more poorly absorbed.) B-12 should be taken under a doctor's supervision.

• **Take B vitamins.** For B-12 to function properly in the body, you must also have adequate levels of the other B vitamins, explains Dr. Rubman. He often prescribes a multi-B vitamin supplement (usually labeled as B-complex 50) twice daily, since B vitamins do not last 24 hours in circulation.

A marker of adequate additional Bs: If your urine is bright yellow, you're probably in good shape.

• **Consider calcium and magnesium supplementation.** Besides building strong bones, these nutrients are essential to a good night's sleep. Calcium and magnesium decrease irritability of the digestive tract and relax muscle tone throughout the body. The form of calcium you take is very important, notes Dr. Rubman. In particular, he most often prescribes Butyrex from T.E. Neesby in Fresno, California, which contains calcium in the form of a butterfat salt, resembling that provided in mother's milk. Most adults require 800 to 1,200 mg of calcium and 300 to 400 mg of magnesium daily. However, due to the high efficiency of its absorption, less may be required.

•**Avoid digestive stressors.** When the liver and intestine become overwhelmed, it can interfere with sleep. To give these organs a break, it's helpful to avoid alcohol, sugary foods, white flour and other refined carbohydrates (white bread, white rice, pasta, etc.), processed foods (especially those that contain trans fats or high-fructose corn syrup), fried foods and fast foods. Also, go easy on the red meat and fish. Large ocean fish such as tuna and swordfish are likely to contain mercury, and should be eaten no more than once or twice a week ...choose wild salmon, anchovies or sardines instead.

•**Bulk up on fiber.** Sufficient fiber—from oats, whole wheat bread, brown rice, steamed vegetables, ripe fruits, nuts, seeds, etc.—is yet another key to good digestion. If you don't take in enough, constipation, irritability and insomnia may result, warns Dr. Rubman.

His recommendation: Follow a diet that is composed of at least half unprocessed foods. Fiber stimulates the production of healthy flora in the gut, moves food efficiently through the digestive tract, and binds and transports excess cholesterol out of the system so it is not reabsorbed. To help ensure adequate fiber intake, Dr. Rubman may prescribe a soluble fiber supplement called glucomannan. Often a patient will take one capsule 30 minutes before lunch and dinner and again before bedtime with a large glass of water.

•**Eat three square meals a day.** Contrary to some popular thinking, snacking and grazing is not the best recipe for efficient digestion. Dr. Rubman recommends three square meals a day, in between

which you let your digestive system rest and regenerate. This also contributes to regular elimination.

More tips for better digestion: Limit beverages with meals, chew food thoroughly and avoid drugs that reduce stomach acid. Many people have trouble digesting cow's milk, adds Dr. Rubman, which in any case is not the best source of calcium nor a good food choice for humans. He believes that we're better off with goat or sheep's milk, as well as taking in calcium by eating plenty of leafy green vegetables.

FINISHING THE TRYPTOPHAN TALE

With improved digestion, people can fully digest the proteins that contain tryptophan. And, with adequate levels of B vitamins, tryptophan can be broken down into serotonin, which in turn allows people to relax.

Today's Best Sore Throat Soothers

Francis Brinker, ND, clinical assistant professor, College of Medicine, University of Arizona, Tucson. Dr. Brinker is author of *Herb Contraindications and Drug Interactions* and *Complex Herbs—Complete Medicines* (both from Eclectic Medical).

A scratchy, raw sore throat is often the harbinger of a cold, the flu or other illness. Or, it can be the result of breathing polluted air, smoking and allergies. Treatment options depend on the cause, though no matter what it is, there is no need to suffer undue pain.

Francis Brinker, ND, from Tucson, Arizona, and the author of *Herb Contraindications and Drug Interactions* (Eclectic Medical) and *Complex Herbs—Complete Medicines* (Eclectic Medical) shares some of his favorite sore throat treatments. Sometimes all that is needed is symptomatic relief. In other cases (as with strep throat), a more specific treatment is required. Additionally, resolving sore throats that are harbingers of colds can sometimes prevent the onset of the actual cold, Dr. Brinker, believes.

GARGLE YOUR SORE THROAT AWAY— FOR VIRUSES AND BACTERIA

For relief of sore throats caused by viruses or bacteria, Dr. Brinker highly recommends gargling with *Echinacea angustifolia* (or *Echinacea purpurea*) root liquid extract. Every two to three hours, mix one teaspoon in a small amount of water, gargle and swallow. Besides local and systemic immune enhancement, the *isobutylamides* from the echinacea root give good local pain relief for the throat.

Alternating echinacea and warm salt water gargles—or using salt water alone—can also bring relief, but do not swallow the salt water. In Dr. Brinker's opinion, antiseptic gargles such as Listerine are often not effective for bacterial sore throats.

USE LOZENGES AND COUGH DROPS

Zinc gluconate lozenges are another effective remedy for throat discomfort due to viruses, notes Dr. Brinker. He adds that to be effective, they must be kept intact in the mouth for a prolonged time—so, you should suck on them. Unfortunately, some people do not like the metallic taste associated with many zinc lozenges.

As an alternative, lozenges with slippery elm powder are soothing for sore throats of all kinds, whether caused by sickness or lifestyle.

Commercially available menthol-containing lozenges or cough drops help relieve discomfort, but Dr. Brinker warns that they are usually not good for throat infections because of their high sugar content—bacteria thrive on simple sugars.

MORE HERBAL REMEDIES

Another beneficial herbal remedy is "Throat Coat" from Traditional Medicinals (800-543-4372 or *www.traditional medicinals.com*), available at health food stores and some drug stores. According to Dr. Brinker, this combination herbal tea brings symptomatic relief for sore throats. It contains slippery elm bark, marshmallow root and licorice root extract, along with a few other herbs for flavor. Slippery elm bark or marshmallow root teas can be used alone for their soothing, coating action, but licorice adds antiviral activity and a nice flavor. Always consult your doctor before trying an herbal remedy.

CONSIDER COMPRESSES

Dr. Brinker also recommends compresses. To reduce local congestion in the throat, he advises a cold double throat compress. Just wrap a cold wet cotton or linen cloth snugly (but not tightly) around the neck, and cover it with a larger dry cloth. This will heat and relax the area, because the increase in blood flow to the area in response to the cold will warm the compress and dry it out overnight. Or, try the "wet sock compress."

Dr. Brinker's formula: Dip clean cotton socks in cold water, and thoroughly wring them out. Put the socks on and pull above the ankle, then cover the wet areas completely with long, dry wool socks. This helps all types of head congestion and promotes sleep, says Dr. Brinker.

WHEN THE DIAGNOSIS IS STREP

Strep throat (caused by *streptococcus* bacteria) is painful and can lead to potentially serious complications. It is diagnosed with a throat swab and treated with antibiotics. Usually accompanied by fever and frequently having a red appearance and white pustules in the throat, strep throat typically is associated with swollen, tender lymph glands in the neck beneath one or both ears, behind the angle of the jaw, explains Dr. Brinker.

He recommends that you enhance lymphatic drainage for throat congestion by doing a simple massage, moving the fingers, flat and open, down the neck, beginning below the ear and moving slowly down toward the breastbone. Repeat this three to four times on each side.

What to Do When Your Cough Won't Quit

Mark A. Stengler, ND, naturopathic physician in private practice, La Jolla, California...adjunct associate clinical professor at the National College of Natural Medicine, Portland, Oregon...author of many books, including *The Natural Physician's Healing Therapies* and coauthor of *Prescription for Natural Cures* (both from Bottom Line Books)...and author of the *Bottom Line/Natural Healing* newsletter.

Many people seeking medical care during the winter and early spring months do so because of the common cough. But according to the American College of Chest Physicians, cough syrups are not an effective treatment for cough.

We called Mark A. Stengler, ND, adjunct associate clinical professor at the National College of Natural Medicine in Portland, Oregon, to find out about natural cough treatment alternatives.

START WITH DIET

First, said Dr. Stengler, eliminate foods that encourage mucus production. These are dairy products...chocolate...bananas ...processed and refined foods...fried foods...and junk foods. Simple sugars should be avoided as well because they suppress immune function.

To thin mucus secretions, drink as much as a glass of water every two waking hours. And yes, your mother was right—homemade chicken broth does help clear mucus. Dr. Stengler suggests adding some garlic or ginger to your chicken soup for immune support (and a nice flavor kick, besides). Hot barley soup made with any kind of stock is another good choice to reduce phlegm.

HERBAL HELP

Dr. Stengler recommends several herbs for cough. For optimum effect, he suggests using more than one. *Many are readily available at your local health food store, but it is best to speak with a trained professional before using more than one of these...*

• **Echinacea and goldenseal.** For acute bronchitis with a wet, mucous cough, take both together in a dosage of 500 milligrams (mg) of each herb in capsule form four times daily...or 30 drops of tincture of each (total of 60 drops), four times daily. If it is a dry cough, then just take the echinacea at 500 mg four times daily...or 30 drops of tincture four times daily. Both herbs enhance immune function, and goldenseal works especially well in drying up mucus.

Side effects: None for short-term use.

• **Astragalus** (also known as *huang qi* in Chinese medicine). This herb is an excellent treatment for acute as well as chronic bronchitis. Astragalus strengthens weak lungs and increases the body's general resistance to infection. Dosage typically is 300 mg to 500 mg in capsule form, three times daily...or 2 milliliters (ml) of tincture three times daily.

Side effects: Astragalus is generally considered safe.

• **Licorice.** It reduces coughing, enhances immune function and soothes an inflamed respiratory tract. Licorice is effective with both wet, mucous coughs and dry, hacking coughs.

One cautionary note: Licorice is contraindicated if you have high blood pressure, though deglycyrrhizinated licorice (DGL) is generally considered safe for those with high blood pressure.

Dose: 30 drops of tincture four times daily...or one cup of licorice tea three times daily.

• **Cherry bark.** For short-term easing of dry, hacking cough, take 500 mg of the capsule daily...or 2 ml of the tincture four times daily.

Side effects: None for short-term use.

Finally, there's N-acetyl cysteine (NAC), which is not an herb but an amino-acid derivative. NAC reduces the viscosity or thickness of phlegm so that it is easier to expectorate. NAC is especially useful in reducing postnasal drip, which is a common cause of cough. NAC is also helpful for acute and chronic bronchitis, especially in smokers and in people with asthma or emphysema. Dosage is often 500 mg, in capsule form, twice daily.

Side effects: None, for short-term use.

Dr. Stengler prescribes more than one of these remedies at a time for his patients. It's best to check with a trained professional before you take these remedies on your own.

HOMEOPATHIC COUGH REMEDIES

As an alternative to over-the-counter cough syrups, Dr. Stengler recommends those homeopathic remedies specifically indicated for cough. For those who are not familiar with homeopathic remedies, they are *incredibly* specific with regard to the symptoms they impact. For example, the homeopathic products company Boiron produces a product called *Spongia Tosta*, whose label indicates it is effective for "croupy cough"...and another of its products, *Antimonium Tartaricum*, is indicated for "wet cough due to colds." Find the product that best addresses your symptoms.

Products by Boiron and another homeopathic medicine producer, Hyland's, are available in most health food stores. Hyland's products are sold at the national chains CVS and Walgreens pharmacies. Both companies have Web sites as well (*www.boiron.com* and *www.hylands.com*). That said, a holistic physician or other trained professional can best guide you to the product that fits your symptoms.

Remember that a lingering cough is a signal that something is wrong. If the above remedies don't work and the cough persists for more than a few days, see your doctor.

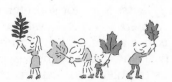

Airborne—
Help or Hype?

Mark A. Stengler, ND, naturopathic physician in private practice, La Jolla, California...adjunct associate clinical professor at the National College of Natural Medicine, Portland, Oregon...author of many books, including *The Natural Physician's Healing Therapies* and coauthor of *Prescription for Natural Cures* (both from Bottom Line Books)...and author of the *Bottom Line/Natural Healing* newsletter.

Some people swear by it, others say it's a lot of malarkey. Airborne is an extraordinarily popular new cold-fighting supplement. As anyone who has seen one of its many commercials knows, Airborne was created by a former elementary school teacher who was sick of coming down with cold after cold. Packed with germ-fighting vitamins, minerals, herbs, antioxidants, amino acids and electrolytes, Airborne is sold as tablets that you drop into water to create fizzy drinks. Its manufacturer recommends using Airborne as a preventative when frequenting airplanes, restaurants, offices, schools, health clubs—anywhere you are likely to be exposed to nasty germs...or, as many people do, at the very first sign of a cold.

To get the lowdown on Airborne, we consulted Mark Stengler, ND, author of *Bottom Line's Natural Healing* newsletter and author of *The Natural Physician's Healing Therapies* (Bottom Line Books). Dr. Stengler says that many of his own patients take Airborne to prevent colds, and he does indeed recommend using it if you feel as if you're coming down with a cold, are around people with colds or are planning to fly.

A GERM-FIGHTING POTPOURRI

Considering its mix of immune-enhancing ingredients, it makes sense that Airborne works. While you can also take these remedies independently, having them in a simple, all-in-one package just makes it a little easier. *Airborne contains...*

•**Vitamin C.** While some controversy always swirls around vitamin C and colds, several studies confirm that this powerful nutrient can reduce the length and severity of cold symptoms.

•**Vitamin A.** Dr. Stengler has found that vitamin A can be very useful in fighting and/or preventing upper respiratory infections. (*Note:* Vitamin A—and thus Airborne—should not be taken by pregnant women without a physician's approval.)

•**Herbs.** Airborne contains infection-fighting herbs such as echinacea. While some studies have panned echinacea, it is possible the methodology in some negative studies was flawed. Other reliable research supports this herb's usefulness.

•**Minerals.** The most useful mineral in Airborne is zinc, says Dr. Stengler. Zinc supports immune function.

Note: Since other supplements may have high doses of these ingredients, be sure to check with a physician before taking other supplements with Airborne.

With three flavors including lemon-lime, orange and grapefruit, Airborne is tasty as well as healthful. At the next sign of a cold, you might want to give it a try. However, be sure to take it at the first sign of a cold for maximum effectiveness. If you wait even a day or two, the "bug" may have time to take hold and results may not be as good.

Halt a Headache— Without Drugs!

Mark A. Stengler, ND, naturopathic physician in private practice, La Jolla, California...adjunct associate clinical professor at the National College of Natural Medicine, Portland, Oregon...author of many books, including *The Natural Physician's Healing Therapies* and coauthor of *Prescription for Natural Cures* (both from Bottom Line Books)...and author of the *Bottom Line/Natural Healing* newsletter.

When headache strikes, many people simply pop a pill. It's quick, easy and often effective. But, given increasing news about the dangers of nonsteroidal anti-inflammatory drugs (NSAIDs), which many take for headaches, there's good reason to consider nonpharmaceutical options. Mild dehydration is often the underlying problem, and drinking a glass or two of water helps. In other cases, the root cause is low blood sugar, and eating food sends headache pain packing.

Mark Stengler, ND, author of *The Natural Physician's Healing Therapies* (Bottom Line Books), shares some of his favorite healing therapies.

WATCH YOUR DIET

Diet can go a long way toward preventing and managing headaches, observes Dr. Stengler. *His suggestions include...*

•**To avoid headaches caused by food additives,** eat meals prepared from whole (not processed) foods.

•**To keep your blood sugar stable,** have five small meals throughout the day instead of three large meals. The meals should consist of a combination of protein...fruits and veggies...and complex carbohydrates—but watch it on the simple carbs, such as pasta or sweets.

Note: Bottom Line's Daily Health News consulting medical editor Andrew L. Rubman, ND, has found that for some patients, five small meals can sometimes aggravate gastric challenges. For these patients, not drinking beverages with meals and chewing more thoroughly will usually allow for the thorough and proper digestion of three large meals, keeping sugar stable. *Further suggestions include...*

•**Get enough fiber to reduce the chance of headaches due to constipation.** Dr. Stengler advises starting the day with one to two tablespoons of ground flaxseed with 10 ounces of water.

•**Drink a glass of filtered water every two waking hours.** The fluid will keep the muscles in your head and neck supple and will also flush out normal and environmental toxins.

•**Common triggers of headache include foods that contain the chemicals *tyramine* or *phenylalanine.*** Tyramine is found in cheese, chocolate, citrus fruits, coffee, cold cuts, herring, smoked fish, wine, alcohol, sausage, sour cream and vinegar. Sources of phenylalanine include monosodium glutamate (MSG), the artificial sweetener aspartame and nitrates (which are found in processed meats, especially hot dogs). If you have an allergy or sensitivity to such foods, eliminate them from your diet.

•**Avoid caffeine, alcohol and sugar products** as well as artificial sweeteners.

CONSIDER SUPPLEMENTS

Research also supports the use of supplements for coping with headache pain. *Dr. Stengler recommends...*

•**Magnesium and calcium.** Take 200 milligrams (mg) of magnesium and 500 mg of calcium twice daily to help prevent headaches. Reduce dosage if diarrhea develops. In a double-blind trial, magnesium successfully reduced the frequency of migraines. Headaches often are due to muscle tension, and calcium helps by relaxing muscles.

•**5-Hydroxytryptophan** (5-HTP). For headache prevention, take 50 mg to 100 mg three times daily. 5-HTP has a direct effect on serotonin levels, which affects circulation in the brain's blood vessels, and it increases the body's level of endorphins (natural painkillers).

Caution: Do not take non-prescribed 5-HTP if you are taking an antidepressant or antianxiety medication. The supplement increases serotonin levels, as do these pharmaceuticals, so the combination may theoretically produce too much serotonin and cause side effects.

If you develop a problem with recurring headaches, don't rely on supplements or over-the-counter medications alone. See your physician to get to the bottom of the problem.

HOMEOPATHIC OPTIONS

Another option is choosing the homeopathic remedy that best matches your symptoms. For acute headaches, Dr. Stengler recommends taking a 30C potency four times daily. For chronic headaches, take a 6X, 12X, 6C, 12C or 30C potency twice daily for two weeks. As soon as you notice improvement, stop taking the remedy (unless symptoms return). As with all treatments, it is best to start homeopathic treatments with the lowest potency (6X or 12X). According to Dr. Stengler, although it's fine to self-treat occasional headaches, it's always best to consult with a homeopathic practitioner or naturopathic physician.

Homeopathic options include...

•*Belladonna.* For headaches that begin in the back of the head on the right side and extend to the right eye or forehead. Pain is throbbing, face is flushed and the person feels better lying down in a dark, quiet room.

•*Bryonia.* For pain in the left eye or forehead that extends to the whole head. Symptoms are worse with movement, and there may be constipation, nausea and extreme thirst.

•*Cimicifuga.* For headaches accompanied by severe neck stiffness and pain, that often occur with the menstrual cycle or hormonal changes during menopause.

•*Gelsemium.* For a dull, heavy pain that begins at the back of the neck and spreads like a tight band around the head. The person feels tired, dizzy and may have blurred vision.

•*Ignatia.* For headaches associated with neck or back spasms. The pain may feel as if a nail was driven into the head, and may begin after experiencing emotional grief or trauma.

•*Nux vomica.* For headaches from stress, overwork and bad reactions to food or alcohol. Headache may be accompanied by stomachache and nausea, and feels better with cold compress applications.

•*Pulsatilla.* For headaches that occur around the menstrual cycle. Location of the pain changes rapidly. Symptoms worsen with heat or in stuffy rooms, and improve in the open air.

MORE NATURAL REMEDIES

Of course, these are not the only natural remedies for everyday headaches. One of the simplest things you can do is to massage the neck and temple areas to help relieve muscle tension. If that doesn't help, Dr. Stengler also likes stress-reduction strategies, such as biofeedback (using a simple electronic device to learn how to control your vital functions). He finds that many people with tension headaches unconsciously clench their head and neck muscles throughout the day—biofeedback can teach you how to spot this clenching reflex and stop it. Another helpful option is acupuncture. And in some cases, all you need to do is step out of your stuffy office and take a deep breath of fresh air.

WHEN TO GET HELP

Sometimes a headache signals a medical emergency. Seek medical help at once if you have a headache that is much more severe than any you've felt before, or if you experience a headache accompanied by alarming symptoms (such as double vision, confusion or disorientation, stiff neck, projectile vomiting, paralysis, vertigo, fever, deafness in one ear or extreme fatigue or weakness).

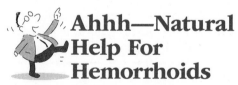

Ahhh—Natural Help For Hemorrhoids

Deborah Nagle, MD, chief of colon and rectal surgery in the Roberta and Stephen R. Weiner Department of Surgery and member of Harvard Medical Fauclty Physicians, both at Beth Israel Deaconess Medical Center.

Hemorrhoids are very common, but nobody wants to talk about them. That's fine, but all those suffering people could use some help. The truth is, over half the adult population in America will experience this "pain in the tush" some time by age 50. Hemorrhoids aren't usually life-threatening, but they sure aren't life-enhancing either. They can play havoc with your daily life if they are symptomatic and you get them frequently—but the good news is that they can often be treated with easy natural remedies.

WHAT ARE HEMORRHOIDS?

The term "hemorrhoids" (also called piles) describes a general condition in which veins in the area of the anus bulge. They swell, and if you have external hemorrhoids they can be seen (and felt) as bumps or lumps which may itch terribly and also hurt.

"Internal" hemorrhoids are less likely to hurt since there are no pain-sensitive nerve fibers in the area where they tend to occur, but they may be more frightening, since often the only symptom is rectal bleeding, typically from passing a bowel movement.

Internal hemorrhoids can also be more bothersome. Untreated, an internal hemorrhoid can become so swollen that it's pushed outside by straining. This is called a *prolapsed hemorrhoid*. (They can be felt with a probing finger.) Internal hemorrhoids that prolapse can become squeezed when the sphincter muscle contracts. If the prolapsed hemorrhoid stays outside the anal opening and its supply of blood gets cut off, it becomes a *strangulated hemorrhoid*, an uncommon, but much more painful affair that can make it particularly painful to have a bowel movement. It requires medical treatment.

THE COMMON CAUSES

There are several different causes of hemorrhoids—and anyone who has ever suffered with them will likely agree that preventing them is the best strategy. Constipation is a very common cause, due to the straining that usually accompanies it. (In fact, sitting on the toilet for longer than is necessary can encourage development of hemorrhoids.) Other risk factors include chronic diarrhea, obesity, a sedentary lifestyle (exercise stimulates peristalsis, the movement required for food to work its way through the intestine), lifting heavy weights and pregnancy and childbirth. If you're engaged in heavy work such as construction or if you regularly work out with heavy weights, make sure not to hold your breath and strain as you lift. Exhale!

FEW GET ENOUGH FIBER

For advice, we called Deborah Nagle, MD, chief of colon and rectal surgery at Beth Israel Deaconess Medical Center in Boston. She told us she can quickly help most people who come to her complaining of hemorrhoids. "The first thing I do is quiz them on their fiber intake," she said, noting that lack of fiber is the single most common reason for both hemorrhoids and constipation. Most people don't get anywhere near what she recommends as a daily intake—25 to 35 grams (g) (or approximately six to eight servings of whole grains, fruits and vegetables).

"Lack of fiber almost always translates to straining," Dr. Nagle says. "That, coupled with standing, puts increased pressure in the columns of veins around the anus that causes the hemorrhoids."

Fiber comes in two forms—soluble and insoluble. The latter is more important for digestion, Dr. Nagle explains, "since it passes through the colon undigested, and absorbs water to keep the stool formed and soft." Sources of soluble fiber include oat bran, dried beans and peas, nuts, oranges, apples and psyllium seed husks. Sources of insoluble fiber are many fresh vegetables and fruits, including green beans and dark green leafy vegetables, fruit skins and root vegetable skins, plus oat and corn bran, seeds and nuts.

HIGH IN FIBER

For the record, two widely available cereals that are high in fiber are Kellogg's All-Bran (10 g per ½ cup) and General Mills' Fiber One (14 g per ½ cup). Other whole grains can also be a good fiber source, especially old-fashioned oatmeal (but not the quick kind) with 2 g per ½ cup dry. High-fiber vegetables include spinach (5.8 g per cup), turnip greens, summer squash and cauliflower (2.5 to 5 g per cup each), cooked Swiss chard (3.7 g per cup), broccoli (3.9 g per stalk) and canned pumpkin (7.1 g per cup). Prunes are also a good source, containing 3 g per five consumed.

Also important, says Dr. Nagle, is water, especially when adding additional fiber to the diet—otherwise you're likely to suffer discomfort from bloating. Stool softeners can be effective for patients who do not tolerate fiber.

TO SOOTHE WHAT AILS YOU

Many people find that gentle creams like those containing aloe vera provide relief. Also helpful is witch hazel applied directly to the affected area. Warm baths (sitz baths) are soothing and healing too, and natural herbal suppositories can be a blessing.

Meanwhile, over-the-counter hemorrhoid remedies continue to be among the best-selling nonprescription medications. Popular brands include Preparation H and Tucks. Many remedies mostly contain a combination of emollient barrier-type creams and mild steroids, Dr. Nagle tells us, which are safe to use…though she cautions that symptoms—most especially rectal bleeding which can be a sign of something serious, like colon cancer—should be evaluated by your doctor. Note that some hemorrhoid relief ointments contain mercury and therefore should be used as sparingly as possible, says Dr. Nagle. (To view brands with mercury, go to *www.fda. gov/cder/fdama/mercury300.htm*.)

Astounding Relief at Your Fingertips

Joan-Ellen Macredis, ND, LAc, MAc, uses acupressure in her practice in Stamford, Connecticut.

Press on your hand and relieve a headache? Touch between your eyes and reduce anxiety? Sounds like a game you might play with children, but in fact it is part of the Chinese medicine technique of acupressure. Research studies have centered on the health benefits of acupuncture, in which fine needles are inserted into "acupoints"—specific places along the body's energy pathways called meridians.

BLOCKED ENERGY

Chinese medicine teaches that when energy gets blocked along meridians in one area, it can cause pain or discomfort in other, related places in the body. The idea is to stimulate the affected meridians to unblock the energy and restore its normal flow, which relieves the problem.

This can be done with acupuncture, which requires a professional trained in the use of fine needles to stimulate the meridians, or it can be done with acupressure, which actually predates acupuncture, and simply involves applying pressure on the correct acupoints. While acupressure also requires extensive training, there are a few simple strategies that anyone, with the proper instruction, can use to address some common discomforts in themselves or others. For information on how people can use this technique, we spoke with naturopathic physician and licensed acupuncturist Joan-Ellen Macredis, ND, LAc, MAc, who also uses acupressure in her practice in Stamford, Connecticut. *There are some differences in how various practitioners teach self-strategies, but Dr. Macredis says that the following general guidelines are what she has found to be best...*

•**To apply pressure to a point, use your thumb and press straight down to the stage of mild discomfort but not pain.** Less is often more in this case, she says. Some people find that rubbing clockwise on the point works well for them, but she prefers to start people with finger pressure and if results are good, stay with it.

•**Hold pressure for 10 seconds, release and reapply for sessions of up to five minutes.** Pressing longer than five minutes per session can create light-headedness, she cautions.

•**Never press off and on**—this can aggravate pain or create a general feeling of malaise, says Dr. Macredis.

•**Start with just one session a day.** You may not feel results until the next day and should too much energy be released, it may end up increasing discomfort. If that happens, adjust by shortening the amount of time you apply pressure or decrease pressure. Conversely, if you want more stimulation, add one or at most two five-minute sessions per day.

•**Drink a full glass of water before or after you start** and avoid practicing when you are hungry. Wait 20 minutes after eating, bathing or exercising.

TOP ACUPOINTS

With this in mind, following are the areas where energy commonly gets stuck, says Dr. Macredis...

•**Hand point.** This addresses any kind of problem in the area of the head including headaches, sinus pain, colds, etc. Close the space between your thumb and index finger to make a mound appear. Go to the top of the mound at the juncture between the thumb and index finger and press with your thumb. Try clockwise rotation rubbing if pressure alone doesn't work.

•**Toe point.** This is good for relieving muscular or skeletal pain, premenstrual symptoms, headaches or general irritability. Find the space where the first and second toes meet. Your finger will fall into a groove. It will feel as if your thumb has fallen into a small hole, she says, and is the correct point to apply pressure. To obtain greater relief, Dr. Macredis advises a pressure session for both the hand site and the toe site. Start with pressure on the same-side body points. If you want more relief, switch to doing it on opposite hand and foot sides instead. However, never apply pressure at all four points—in other words, don't apply on both hands and both feet. That would release too much energy in general, she says.

•**Wrist point.** Try this for nausea. Bend the inside of your hand toward you to form a crease at the wrist. Move your thumb the width of two thumbs toward the body and press.

•**Shin point.** This is the place where you can ease indigestion woes. Locate the shin bone (tibia) just below the knee cap. Place your thumb at the highest point and measure one thumb width to the outside of the bone, the right of the tibia, and slide your finger down the bone to locate any sensitive area to touch. This is your pressure point.

•**Ankle point.** If toe point pressure doesn't relieve menstrual cramps sufficiently, add this. Find the indentation on your inside leg between the ankle bone and the Achilles tendon. Go up about three thumb widths above the anklebone and apply pressure.

•**The third eye point.** This point is called the Yintang point and provides a handy way to soothe a headache or sinus pain, to calm a bad mood or anxiety and it serves as a general pick-me-up. Find the middle point between your eyebrows and press with your middle finger. Do not apply pressure for more than 30 to 60 seconds and do this only one time.

There are many more points and many other problems acupressure can address. More than this, though, requires hands that are properly trained in the art of energy release.

Duke University Uncovers Natural Health Breakthrough

Mitchell W. Krucoff, MD, director, Ischemia Monitoring Lab and Intervention Devices Clinical Trails, Duke University Medical Center, Durham, North Carolina.

Virtually every culture other than those in the Western world embraces the concept of *chi* (also known as *prana*, *qi* and others) as an internal energy that has an important role in mental and physical well-being. Western medicine, of course, has been far removed from acknowledging chi, given that it isn't visible...and evidence of its presence and effectiveness is anecdotal.

ENHANCING HEALING

But recently, in what may be the beginning of a breakthrough on this stance, researchers at Duke University Medical Center and at eight other prominent medical centers around the country, conducted a clinical trial to determine if employing internal energy forces and several other practices, including prayer, might have a measurable effect in enhancing healing. The paper was recently published in the prestigious medical journal, *The Lancet*.

STUDY STRUCTURE

The study participants, 748 patients undergoing possibly life-threatening cardiac procedures, were put into one of four groups—one received off-site prayer by congregations of various religions...one received MIT therapy (stands for soothing **m**usic, guided **i**magery and **t**ouch therapy—more on that in a minute)...one group received both prayer and MIT...and one group received nothing. While neither patients nor staff knew who was in the prayer group, obviously the MIT patients knew that they were receiving the therapy because it was a bedside activity. The nurses administering MIT worked with the patients before the procedure to teach them abdominal breathing rather than shallow chest breathing, and they had them select from among three types of music (easy listening, soft country or classical) to listen to. They then chose from three selections of imagery that represented the most beautiful place they had been or could imagine. Finally, the specially trained nurses conducted a 20-minute session on touch therapy, which is a hands-on method for moving energy through the body to help patients relax and perhaps enhance healing.

LOOKING AT THE RESULTS

Mitchell W. Krucoff, MD, the lead author of the study, says the study results showed that patients having off-site prayer, bed-side MIT or both prayer and MIT had comparable primary outcomes with regard to death, new signs of heart attack, rehospitalization and several other cardiac disease indicators. There was no difference between the control group versus MIT and prayer. But now it gets really interesting. Both groups of MIT patients, he says, did experience relief of preprocedural distress and at the secondary endpoint—mortality at six months after procedure—MIT patients were 65% less likely to die than those who did not receive it.

Dr. Krucoff stresses that in the statistical setting of multiple comparisons, these numbers are very interesting but also warrant cautious interpretation. Even so, he says that there are more analyses of long-term results to come. This study is just the beginning of further research to find whether such practices have a place for "promoting patient health in the modern medical setting."

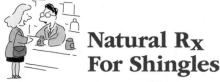

Natural Rx For Shingles

Chris Meletis, ND, executive director, the Institute for Healthy Aging in Reno, Nevada.

Approximately one million—mostly older—Americans get shingles (*herpes zoster*) each year as the virus reactivates from a childhood chickenpox (*varicella-zoster*) infection.

PAINFUL RASH

The virus typically travels along one nerve to the skin's surface where it eventually erupts into another rash with blisters. Before that happens, though, other symptoms may appear, including tingling, itching and sometimes pain or a burning sensation that can be so intense it has been confused with that of kidney stones, appendicitis or even a heart attack, depending on the location of the affected nerve. Once the rash does appear, typically on one side of the torso or face, it brings fresh misery with more pain and blisters. Patients are warned not to scratch because that might increase the potential for a secondary bacterial infection.

POSSIBILITY OF PHN

In most people, shingles resolves itself by five or six very uncomfortable weeks... although, for a few patients, a painful and debilitating complication called *postherpetic neuralgia* (PHN) can linger for many more months and even years. In fact, the recent development of a vaccine for shingles was partly to shield people from the possibility of PHN. While the vaccination is now a reality and is available to people ages 60 and over, we wondered about natural treatments that might both ease the discomfort of shingles and possibly reduce the amount of time it normally takes to run its course, as well as reduce the likelihood that it will develop into PHN. Naturopathic physician Chris Meletis, ND, executive director of education for the Institute for Healthy Aging in Reno, Nevada, often treats patients with shingles.

NATURAL Rx FOR SHINGLES

Dr. Meletis says that his first recommendation for shingles patients is to supplement with vitamin B-12. The reason, most importantly, is that B-12 has been shown to help prevent PHN. He says that it also helps bolster energy levels and eases the discomfort of the outbreak. Dr. Meletis often prescribes 1 milligram (mg) of B-12 in the form of *methylcobalamin* twice a day, preferably under the tongue (sublingually). Continue this for the duration of the outbreak and for two to three months after the resolution of the rash and other symptoms. Another useful vitamin for combating shingles is vitamin C. A potent antioxidant, vitamin C bolsters the immune system and helps patients cope with the stress of the disease. Some people find that vitamin C helps dry blisters as well and reduces pain to some degree, it may also hinder development of PHN. The dosage for many of Dr. Meletis' patients is 1,000 mg two to three times a day with meals. Vitamin C can cause diarrhea, in which case patients are directed to ease up slightly on dosage until they find the maximum level that is tolerated. If nerve pain does remain after the lesions have resolved, alpha-lipoic acid at a dose of 300 mg two to three times a day can be helpful.

One amino acid plays a particularly interesting role in shingles. L-lysine has been shown to be helpful in combating viruses, including another type of herpes virus called herpes simplex-1 that typically causes so-called fever blisters on the lips and herpes-simplex 2, which typically causes outbreaks of lesions on the genitalia. Use of L-lysine, however, must be prescribed and monitored carefully by a trained professional. L-lysine is contraindicated in pregnant women and those with elevated cholesterol or triglyceride levels.

TOPICAL RELIEF

Of course, it is important to have topical balms and creams to soothe the itching and pain of the rash. There are several available that Dr. Meletis has found to be helpful. Lysine cream is one (but do not put on open sores) and lemon balm is another. After the sores heal, a variety of capsaicin-containing creams on the market may provide pain relief. Capsaicin, the substance that adds heat to hot peppers, is said to inhibit nerve cells from sending pain messages to the brain. Capsaicin creams come in a variety of strengths. Whichever one you select, start small by using just a dab and apply four times a day. It will sting when you first put it on, but stick with it. It *will* help. After applying, wash hands with soap and water to avoid irritation on other parts of your skin.

Finally, Dr. Meletis reminds all shingles patients that your body needs time to restore itself. Use the time to take it easy and get lots of rest.

Six Essential Oils That Help Heal Cancer Patients

Cherie Perez, RN, quality assurance specialist in the department of GU Medical Oncology at M.D. Anderson Cancer Center in Houston.

Like so many New Age practices and beliefs, aromatherapy has ancient roots. The use of essential oils to affect mood and well-being can be found far back in Egyptian, Greek and Roman history. While scientific evidence about aromatherapy is scant, its long-standing role in spirituality and healing, along with anecdotal support of its benefits, gives essential oils an important role as a complementary alternative medicine therapy.

BOOSTING IMMUNE FUNCTION

Cherie Perez, RN, quality assurance specialist in the department of GU (genitourinary) Medical Oncology at M.D. Anderson Cancer Center in Houston, is a strong proponent of aromatherapy, including as an adjunct for cancer treatment. She teaches monthly classes for patients on the topic. We asked Perez about how aromatherapy can be useful for people who are healthy, as well as those with chronic illnesses. Used properly, Perez says essential oils can indirectly help bolster immune function in cancer patients, strengthening their ability to fight back against the disease by helping to ease pain, depression, sleeplessness and stress. The oils can also help relieve anxiety and improve memory, both frequent problems for people in cancer treatment.

ESSENTIALS ABOUT ESSENTIAL OILS

These essential oils have various scents such as floral, minty, citrus and masculine—and Perez advises using the ones you like best among the choices indicated for a specific treatment, since more than one oil may address the same problem. She explains that the limbic system, which is triggered by the sense of smell, is the emotional seat of the brain. It's the reason why people often respond strongly to certain scents—positively or negatively. Lavender, for example, might bring back warm memories of a trip to Provence, or sour thoughts about a dour relative who wore it as a fragrance.

DILUTION REQUIRED

All oils are highly concentrated distillations of plant parts, including the flowers, leaves, branches and roots. Because they are so potent (hundreds of times more concentrated than the culinary fresh or dried herb or herbal teas, and therefore easy to overdose on) they should be used only under the supervision of a knowledgeable practitioner, such as a naturopathic physician, registered nurse, massage therapist, clinical herbalist or aromatherapist. Some of the most popular oils include rosemary, eucalyptus, lavender and chamomile. Essential oils can be inhaled (safest with a simple diffuser), enjoyed in your bath or massaged onto your skin (but never directly in their undiluted form…because they can cause a rash or burning sensation).

Oils may come already diluted, and will say so on the ingredient label, but you can also dilute a pure oil yourself, with advice from your practitioner. Add three drops of an essential oil to a half tablespoon of scentless organic vegetable oil (such as sunflower or safflower) or to an unscented body lotion. People with sensitive skin should do a skin test before topical use. How much to dilute an oil depends on the type of oil and your skin's sensitivity. Thyme, for example, is quite irritating to some people, so it should be used more sparingly and with caution, whereas lavender is nonirritating to nearly everyone, says Perez. Citrus oils may cause sensitivity to sunlight, so avoid skin application if you are going to be in the sun. Because they're so pretty and fragrant yet highly toxic if ingested, they should be kept where children cannot reach them.

MENU OF OPTIONS

Here's a list of popular oils that address some common problems, as well as those common among people in treatment for cancer…

•**Lavender.** Great as a general relaxant, it also treats migraines and relieves stress. It is excellent for insomnia resulting from cancer treatment.

•**Rosemary.** For muscle pain, low blood pressure (do not use if you have high blood pressure) and cold feet and hands. Rosemary stimulates appetite.

•**Spearmint.** Used to ease nausea and to help digestion. Can help ease gas and other treatment-related digestive problems.

•**Eucalyptus or peppermint.** For rubbing on sore muscles. Eucalyptus may also help joints, including arthritic ones. Eucalyptus may increase the absorption of certain cancer drugs that are applied topically, so use caution and try a patch test first, avoiding application to the same area as the cancer drug.

•**Pink grapefruit or juniper berry.** Used with massage to encourage lymphatic drainage of toxins and waste. Pink grapefruit is one of Perez's favorites for cancer patients, as she believes it helps energize them and raise their spirits. This and all citrus-type oils should be avoided during chemo and radiation—and should not be used until you've spoken with your doctor.

•**Lemongrass, tea tree and orange.** Mix together into two cups of Epsom salts. Use five drops of each oil—a total of 15 drops—to make soothing bath salts (use one-half cup per bath).

WHAT TO LOOK FOR

Aromatherapy has become so popular that essential oils are now widely available, including in health food stores and supermarkets. However, Perez says that it is far better to purchase them from a shop with a staff knowledgeable in aromatherapy. Oils should come in dark blue or brown glass containers, which prevent light or heat damage. Avoid bottles with rubber droppers—the rubber breaks down and contaminates the oil. Finally, the label should feature both the common and the botanical name of the oil (for example, peppermint/*Mentha piperita*).

HOW TO TRY IT

If you would like to learn more about how to incorporate aromatherapy in your life, Perez recommends *The Complete Book of Essential Oils & Aromatherapy,* by Valerie Ann Worwood (New World Library), which she says is both thorough and easily understood. Again, as in the case with skin sensitivities, people with asthma or allergies need to avoid things that might trigger an attack—for example, chamomile, which is in the ragweed family.

People who want to try inhalation aromatherapy should use only two or three drops of essential oils in a basin of water or diffuser, or on a napkin. And—always consult with your doctor before using aromatherapy or any complementary therapy.

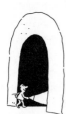

Hidden Causes of Chronic Insomnia

Mark A. Stengler, ND, naturopathic physician in private practice, La Jolla, California...adjunct associate clinical professor at the National College of Natural Medicine, Portland, Oregon...author of many books, including *The Natural Physician's Healing Therapies* and coauthor of *Prescription for Natural Cures* (both from Bottom Line Books)...and author of the *Bottom Line/Natural Healing* newsletter.

Rob, a teacher in his mid-sixties, generally stumbled along on just a few hours of sleep each night. Typically, he would fall asleep normally, then awaken three or four hours later and be unable to return to sleep. His chronic insomnia (six years' worth) was taking a toll physically and psychologically. His work was suffering, as he was having trouble maintaining focus on his lessons and students. He was also irritable and chronically tired, as his wife frequently reminded him.

ON THE RIGHT PATH

Finally, at his wife's urging, Rob called Mark A. Stengler, ND, for a consultation about his insomnia. Rob told Dr. Stengler that he had not sought advice from a medical doctor because he didn't want to take pharmaceutical medications, and he knew that the doctor would likely prescribe sleeping drugs and send him on his way. Rob had attempted self-treatment, trying several supplements known to be or associated with better sleep—these included a calcium supplement, as well as 5-HTP (Hydroxytryptophant) and melatonin. He had used each for a while, with so-so results, and then, seeing no significant improvement would move on to another, finding no lasting solution.

HORMONE DEFICIENCY

During the consultation Dr. Stengler discovered that Rob was not suffering from high stress other than his frustration about lack of sleep, he ate well and he exercised regularly. Given his general good health and moderate lifestyle, Dr. Stengler suspected Rob might be suffering from something more subtle and often overlooked—a hormone deficiency. He proceeded to give Rob a blood test to determine his level of testosterone and discovered it was not only low but in fact 80% lower than it should have been for a man his age. Other physical symptoms included low libido. His thyroid function was also low, which contributed to Rob's lethargy, although his growth hormone (IGF-1) was normal. (Low growth hormone can also cause insomnia.)

THE ROOT OF THE PROBLEM

Hormone deficiencies are often at the root of chronic insomnia in men and women 45 and older, but many medical doctors don't evaluate hormone levels as a possible cause, says Dr. Stengler. The fact that Rob's problems began in his early-sixties provided an important clue. A particular enzyme, lyase, a precursor of both testosterone and the estrogens, which may effect thyroid function, was likely responsible, since it is sensitive to both aging and stress. Without this perspective, doctors consequently end up treating insomnia with sleeping medications (hypnotics)—but Dr. Stengler says these drugs fail to address the underlying problem.

BIOIDENTICAL TESTOSTERONE

In Rob's case it was clear to Dr. Stengler that he needed a "bioidentical" testosterone—meaning it has the same structure and function as found in the human body. A substance derived from wild yam and soy is bioidentical to the testosterone normally made in both men and women and therefore potentially much safer than synthetics, says Dr. Stengler. He prescribed testosterone cream for Rob to apply to the inside of his arm each day. To address the slowed thyroid function he also prescribed a thyroid product called Armour Thyroid for Rob.

SWEET DREAMS ARE MADE OF THIS

Rob felt better almost immediately. Within just a few days his three to four hours of sleep had been transformed to a peaceful eight hours each night. Naturally his energy and mood greatly improved, and his memory improved as well. When Dr. Stengler met with him two months later, Rob reported with great relief that he now slept long and deeply every night.

But even bioidentical hormone replacement carries some risk if not carefully monitored, warns Dr. Stengler. For example, testosterone use has been associated with prostate cancer risk and so Dr. Stengler checked Rob's PSA levels and examined his prostate after one month, and again after the second to be sure that testosterone supplementation was not creating any problems for his prostate.

Medical Mystery Cured with Detox

Mark A. Stengler, ND, naturopathic physician in private practice, La Jolla, California…adjunct associate clinical professor at the National College of Natural Medicine, Portland, Oregon…author of many books, including *The Natural Physician's Healing Therapies* and coauthor of *Prescription for Natural Cures* (both from Bottom Line Books)…and author of the *Bottom Line/Natural Healing* newsletter.

The word "detox" often bears negative connotations, either because it's associated with drug addictions, or because practitioners who practice "detox" are often thought of as "wacky" by those who are not familiar with the practice. But detox does have its place. Mark Stengler, ND, makes this clear when he shares the details of a recent case, in which one patient's "mystery symptoms" were resolved with detoxification.

A 41-year-old airline pilot had the unpredictable schedule that is typical of airline crews. He was suffering from acne rosacea…on-again, off-again outbreaks of another type of rash…trouble getting to sleep and staying there…and even tinnitus, a nearly constant ringing in his ears. So those where the symptoms…what was the diagnosis?

TRACKING THE CLUES

Dr. Stengler says he suspected there were a number of reasons the pilot had developed a constellation of toxic challenges and needed to detox. The fact that his skin rashes came and went and that the pilot ate most of his meals in fast-food places and hotel coffee shops indicated this need…and the fact that his patient's bowel movements were irregular and sluggish confirmed the working diagnosis for Dr. Stengler. He chose to supervise his patient on a diet that featured much more healthful, natural and nutritious foods and give him special supplements that would cleanse his liver and kidneys.

The regimen was as follows…

• **Large amounts of produce**—with a produce ratio of 80% vegetables and 20% fruits. Although this man had a difficult schedule, he was easily able to greatly increase the number of fruits and vegetables he ate daily, in part by taking them with him and snacking on them as he worked and traveled.

• **Organic eggs and poultry, brown rice and small amounts of whole grains.**

• **No alcohol, sugar or coffee.**

• **A greens supplement** (six capsules daily of one called Deeper Greens, which is manufactured by Ortho Molecular Products, Inc. and available only through health-care professionals) that contains wheatgrass, chlorella, spirulina, barley grass and other greens. This helps the liver and kidneys to detox.

• **A second detoxification powder,** containing vitamins and minerals that support liver detoxification including vitamins E and C, carotenoids, selenium, magnesium, potassium, molybdenum, calcium, chromium, B vitamins and glutathione.

• **A combination liver support supplement** of milk thistle, dandelion root and burdock.

• **Saunas** (preferably a dry sauna) every other day. Fortunately, the patient belonged to a gym with a sauna and the hotels he stayed in on layovers generally had them. Sweating in saunas is an excellent way to pull toxins out of fat tissue.

• **Exercise.** A moderately intense cardio workout—at least 25 minutes a day—that made the patient break a sweat.

NATURE OF THE FAST

The cleansing regimen used for this patient lasted a few weeks. It is not unusual for people to feel somewhat worse before they feel better, primarily due to the increased movement of wastes out of the liver and into the intestinal tract. During the first two days, it is common for people to experience headaches and fatigue, and sometimes have skin breakouts, especially if their previous diet was particularly poor.

For most, though, the unpleasant side effects don't last longer than that. Within a reasonably short time, in fact, most people find they feel more energetic and they think more clearly. Their bowels move regularly, their skin begins to look better, and their mood improves.

The pilot noticed these kinds of changes, too. In fact, even his tinnitus improved, something that Dr. Stengler says is plausible but uncommon.

CLOGGED UP SYSTEMS

People who feel sluggish and have low energy or frequent low-grade depression often have poor eating habits (as did this patient), which challenges the body's functioning. Many times people turn to pharmaceutical or recreational drugs, alcohol or excessive amounts of sugar in attempts to pick themselves up. Unfortunately, those actions never help. In fact, they often make the situation much worse. A proper medically supervised detoxification protocol can help nearly all of these symptoms as well as chronic fatigue, allergies, headaches and digestive problems, including stomachaches and constipation. Dr. Stengler advises many of his patients to consider a detox of this nature every fall and spring to help them counteract the effect of the rich and fatty foods so common in our culture.

It is important not to try this detoxification on one's own, as blood pressure, blood sugar levels, heart and kidney function can be stressed from a radical detox.

Naturopaths—Today's Healing Experts

Jane Guiltinan, ND, immediate past president of the American Association of Naturopathic Physicians. She is a clinical professor at the Bastyr Center for Natural Health, Seattle, Washington.

I n North America, there are five naturopathic medicine programs currently accredited by The Council on

Naturopathic Medical Education (CNME), and one naturopathic program that is a candidate for accreditation by the CNME. Candidates for admission to these programs must earn a baccalaureate degree (or equivalent) prior to admission, including standard premed training. The naturopathic doctor (ND) degree is a doctoral degree and typically takes four years to complete, just like an MD.

There are many similarities between the naturopathic and conventional medical school curriculum. The first two years of both curricula involve basic science courses—anatomy, pathology, physiology, biochemistry, and other Western medical sciences. In addition, naturopathic philosophy courses expose students to the concepts and principles and practices of natural medicine, says Jane Guiltinan, ND, immediate past president of the American Association of Naturopathic Physicians. These include nutrition, homeopathy, botanical medicine, acupuncture and a variety of mind-body approaches.

During the third and fourth years, there's a mix of classroom courses such as gynecology, pediatrics and rheumatology, plus 1,200 hours or so of clinical training under the supervision of licensed naturopathic physicians. In this phase of training, naturopathy students observe and help manage patients in an outpatient setting.

THE NATUROPATH'S ROLE

Think of the ND as the equivalent of a family practice physician, said Dr. Guiltinan. Naturopaths provide excellent primary health care for individuals and families. Like the conventional general practitioner with an MD, an ND will assess your health and direct your treatment, either by treating you directly or by referral to mainstream or other natural care specialists such as chiropractors, acupuncturists, nutritionists or specialists in homeopathy, to name a few.

In Dr. Guiltinan's view, conventional physicians and naturopaths are most effective at different points in the spectrum of the health-care system. "At one end of the spectrum is crisis medicine," she says "and it's here where I think conventional medicine is excellent. Emergency care intervention, trauma care, serious infections—this is where conventional medicine excels."

OUTSIDE THE BOX

"Where I think conventional medicine has not done its most effective work is in chronic disease management and in conditions that don't really fit into a clear medical box—chronic fatigue syndrome, for example, fibromyalgia or depression," says Dr. Guiltinan. With these types of conditions, the conventional, technological or pharmaceutical approach is not always effective as it focuses on symptom suppression, rather than finding the underlying causes and addressing these to support healing and the creation of health and wellness. This is where naturopathic physicians can play an important role."

THE ND OFFICE VISIT: WHAT TO EXPECT

What is different about a visit to an ND? At your initial visit you'll be asked about your health history and receive a physical exam that is similar to the physical at a conventional medical office. And like a conventional MD, an ND may order lab tests or diagnostic imaging tests. So, what's different?

"You'll find much more in-depth questioning about your current lifestyle," says Dr. Guiltinan. Naturopaths ask about your diet—at minimum they will ask you to describe it but more likely you'll be asked to complete a diet diary, detailing your food intake for a week or so. "We're also very interested in finding out if you exercise or not, and what your mental and emotional state is," she adds.

PHILOSOPHY AND TREATMENT

Dr. Guiltinan says that extensive questioning is necessary to get to the underlying issues around a health problem and address them, rather than just addressing the presenting symptoms of a problem.

Because naturopaths believe that the human body has an incredibly powerful ability to heal itself if given the chance, she says, one principle is to take a look at what the "obstacles to cure" are in an individual patients' life. What are obstacles to cure?

Sometimes it's genetics, which we can do little about, but some obstacles can be removed (for example, eating poorly, being too stressed out with work, exposure to environmental toxins, lack of exercise). If you can add support in the form of a good diet, proper exercise and stress reduction to promote the healing responses of the body, then you can further capitalize on the body's ability to heal.

WHAT TO EXPECT

In naturopathic medicine, most treatment plans, regardless of the condition, begin with diet modifications. In addition, supplements (vitamins and minerals) may be prescribed. In some cases, NDs will do the nutritional counseling themselves. In others, patients may be referred on to a nutrition specialist.

Other common treatment modalities are homeopathy, botanical medicine, physical medicine and acupuncture and mind/body therapies. Again, depending on the patient's needs, the ND may provide treatment or refer the patient on to a specialist. Dr. Guiltinan says a big part of her naturopathic practice is preparing patients to make the little and big lifestyle changes that will impact their health.

HOW CAN I FIND A NATUROPATH IN MY AREA?

To find a qualified, licensed ND in your area, visit the American Association of Naturopathic Physicians Web site, *www.natu ropathic.org* and click "Find an ND."

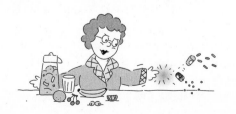

Is Your Doctor Prescribing Drugs When A Vitamin Will Do?

Andrew L. Rubman, ND, consulting medical editor for *Bottom Line's Daily Health News* and director of the Southbury Clinic for Traditional Medicines in Southbury, Connecticut.

There are many people these days who take the increasingly popular catchall prescription drug for nerve pain, *gabapentin* (Neurontin). According to *Bottom Line's Daily Health News* consulting medical editor Andrew L. Rubman, ND, Neurontin (which has been approved by the US Food and Drug Administration for epileptic seizures) is routinely prescribed off-label for neuropathy. In fact, Dr. Rubman notes, it has become one of the most popular off-label prescription drugs. How many people are taking Neurontin and putting themselves at risk for side effects that include dizziness, fatigue, poor coordination and worse—even suicide—when all they may need is a little more B-12?

A B-12 DEFICIENCY

Dr. Rubman says that many Americans are deficient in B-12, a vital nutrient that the liver and brain requires for optimal function. The deficiency can be caused by poor nutrition, an unbalanced diet or alcoholism, among other things. A lack of B-12 damages the myelin sheath that surrounds and protects nerves, which can lead to various types of neuropathy (in the extremities, from the hands and feet to the tip of the nose and the edges of the ears).

Some options…

•**Sublingual B-12 pills (either hydroxocobalamin or methylcobalamin)**, which are equally as effective as and less expensive than B-12 shots. Avoid cyanocobalamin, which is poorly absorbed.

•**Multi-B vitamins** (i.e., B-50) twice daily, as B-12 requires them to function properly in the body. The "twice daily" part is essential, since B vitamins don't last 24 hours in circulation, explains Dr. Rubman.

Vitamin B-12 should be taken under a doctor's supervision. To determine if you're taking in sufficient B vitamins, keep an eye on the color of your urine. If it's bright yellow, you're in good shape, says Dr. Rubman.

A NEURONTIN EXCESS

Several years ago, mega-drug manufacturer Warner-Lambert was fined $430 million for illegally promoting Neurontin for off-label use with neuropathy, bipolar disorder, drug and alcohol withdrawal and attention deficit disorder.

Unfortunately, Neurontin is but one example of the power that big drug companies and the medical industry structure has over our lives. On the one hand the pharmaceutical companies are wining and dining the doctors to encourage them to prescribe their medications. On the other hand, the doctors are prescribing based on the information they received from the pharmaceutical salespeople. Doctors have little time to keep up in detail with all of the new medical information (nor do most of them have nutritional training), so they rely on the information provided by the drug companies.

COLLABORATIVE MEDICINE IS BEST

To avoid getting a prescription for a drug instead of a recommendation for a vitamin, Dr. Rubman recommends that you add a trained, licensed naturopathic physician to your health-care team. To locate a naturopathic physician in your area, visit the Web site of The American Association of Naturopathic Physicians at *www.naturo pathic.org*.

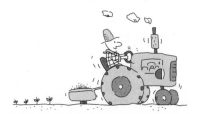

MS—Best Ways to Get And Stay Symptom Free

Thomas A. Kruzel, ND, naturopathic physician in private practice in Scottsdale, Arizona, past president of The American Association of Naturopathic Physicians and former vice president of clinical affairs and chief medical officer at the Southwest College of Naturopathic Medicine in Phoenix. Dr. Kruzel is author of *Homeopathic Emergency Guide: A Quick Reference Handbook to Effective Homeopathic Care*. North Atlantic.

National Institute of Neurological Disorders and Stroke, *www.ninds.nih.gov*.

Swank MS Foundation, *www.swankmsdiet.org*.

Conventional medicine generally looks at multiple sclerosis (MS) as an incurable disease typically marked by sporadic flare-ups and remissions. In contrast, naturopathic physicians generally do not view MS as incurable, and some have had great success in treating this unpredictable disease of the central nervous system to keep symptoms at bay. According to Thomas A. Kruzel, ND, a naturopathic physician in private practice in Scottsdale, Arizona, and past president of The American Association of Naturopathic Physicians, people who closely follow dietary, homeopathic and other naturopathic recommendations have the best odds of becoming and remaining symptom-free.

MS—A PRIMER

MS is believed to be an autoimmune disease in which the immune system mistakenly attacks the nervous system. This results in inflammation and damage to healthy myelin sheath tissue that insulates nerve cells. *Inflammation and demyelination of nerve cells disrupt the normal transmission of neural signals, which can lead to symptoms that include...*

- **Numbness**
- **A sensation of pins and needles**
- **Muscle weakness and spasms**
- **Tremors**
- **Impaired balance and coordination**
- **Paralysis**

- **Extreme fatigue**
- **Blurred or double vision**
- **Blindness**
- **Diminished bowel and/or bladder function**
- **Difficulties with memory and/or cognitive function**

Typically, the disease strikes adults between the ages of 20 and 40, with symptoms ranging from mild to debilitating. In people with a vulnerability toward MS, the disease can be precipitated by a physical or psychological trauma—for example, a death or divorce, a virus, or the body succumbing to some kind of long-term stress, illness, exposure to environmental toxins, poor diet, etc.

Conventional medications for MS, such as beta-interferon and steroids, are used to attempt to control recurrence and severity of the symptoms. They have serious side effects and varied success. In contrast, NDs use a mixture of less invasive modalities—from diet and nutrition to homeopathy to counseling and more —to address MS. *Here are some of the options that have been most successful for Dr. Kruzel's patients...*

THE SWANK LOW-FAT DIET

Most modern-day chronic, degenerative diseases are related to or worsened by a poor diet, and MS is no exception, observes Dr. Kruzel. He believes that it's no coincidence that the incidence of MS— along with the incidence of heart disease, obesity, diabetes and arthritis—rose as Americans increasingly adopted a pro-inflammatory diet high in saturated fat. There is also evidence suggesting that the more red meat a society consumes, the higher the incidence of MS.

Named for its creator, the late Roy Swank, MD, PhD, the Swank Low-Fat Diet is a strict, low-saturated fat program that has been demonstrated to ease the symptoms of MS, and possibly even cause the disease to go into remission.

While Dr. Swank recommended limiting the saturated fat in your diet, he also advised a teaspoon of fish oil daily. You are encouraged to eat more white fish and a specific amount of fatty fish such as wild salmon, tuna, and sardines, which count toward your daily allowance of oil. Fatty fish are also a good source of healthful essential fatty acids. Flaxseed oil is also rich in EFAs.

People who follow the Swank Low-Fat Diet can expect to start feeling better within four to six weeks, says Dr. Kruzel. The longer they follow it and the more strictly they adhere to it, the more they will improve. *The basic elements of the Swank Low-Fat Diet are...*

- **No red meat for the first year,** and only 3 ounces per week after that.
- **No more than 15 grams of saturated fat daily.**
- **No more than 50 grams of unsaturated fat per day.**
- **No processed foods that contain saturated fat.**
- **Any dairy product must have 1% or less butterfat.**
- **Take 1 teaspoon (or equivalent in capsule form) of cod liver oil daily.** A daily multi-vitamin and mineral supplement is also required.

HOMEOPATHY

Dr. Kruzel views homeopathy—treatments that stimulates the body's healing responses—as a cornerstone of his MS treatment approach. He points out that certain personality types tend to develop MS—most often serious or sensitive people who hold in their emotions and are reluctant to express them, possibly increasing stress. This makes homeopathy an especially appropriate treatment, since these remedies are intended to fit not only a person's symptoms, but also his/her personality, temperament and lifestyle. An ND is apt to prescribe homeopathic remedies such as *Natrum muriaticum, phosphorus* or *sepia*. It is important to work with a professional trained in homeopathy to ensure that you use the best remedy for your symptoms and persona.

BEE VENOM THERAPY

It may sound unorthodox, but Dr. Kruzel has seen many MS patients benefit from diluted bee venom injections, or apitherapy. Bee venom contains a variety of compounds—such as anti-inflammatory *mellitin* plus anti-inflammatory and pain-blocking *adolapin*—that work together to invoke the body's own natural immune reaction. Dr. Kruzel generally administers 20 sessions of bee venom therapy, one week apart. Unfortunately, the injections are painful, and some people cannot tolerate them. If they can, however, there is usually an improvement in symptoms.

Caution: Because a small percentage of the population is allergic to bee venom, this therapy should be closely supervised by your ND. There should be a bee sting kit available to treat any allergic reactions.

COUNSELING

Dr. Kruzel says he sees a huge mental and emotional component to MS. In his first lengthy consultation with each MS patient, he discusses not only physical symptoms but also core psychological issues and memories that may be an underlying cause of stress, thus aggravating the disease. Dr. Kruzel has found that once a person deals with these important emotional issues they begin to feel better. Once the emotional issues are dealt with, symptoms may abate. If the mental/emotional symptoms are not dealt with, or return, the MS may come back. That is why counseling in addition to homeopathic treatment is essential.

STRESS MANAGEMENT

Stress—whether due to a sudden shock such as an illness or loss, or a long-term battle with an unhappy marriage or legal troubles—is suspected to be a major contributing factor to worsening MS symptoms. To cope effectively with stress, Dr. Kruzel recommends modalities such as meditation, yoga and deep breathing.

EXERCISE

Exercise and physical therapy can keep neurological pathways functioning properly, says Dr. Kruzel. He adds that many people with MS unwisely give up on exercise. This is a big mistake which can lead to further muscle weakness and loss of muscle mass. When you work out, just be careful about heat, which can aggravate symptoms. Although there are people with MS who run marathons, most prefer less intense (and less heat-producing) forms of exercise such as swimming or yoga.

Reason: Becoming overheated aggravates symptoms of MS, so exercises that generate lower amounts of body heat are tolerated better.

NATURAL WAYS TO TREAT MS

While no two people with MS are alike and different individuals have different needs, certain supplements can benefit most people with this disease…

•**Essential fatty acids.** People with MS may be typically short on essential fatty acids, which are necessary for brain and nervous system health. Cod liver oil and other fish oils are good sources of essential fatty acids.

•**Antioxidants.** People with MS are apt to have higher levels of molecules called free radicals, which contribute to inflammation and demyelination. To control them, Dr. Kruzel recommends antioxidants such as alpha lipoic acid and vitamins C and E.

Other possible supplements: B vitamins (to support brain and nervous system function), vitamin D (to give the immune system a boost) and magnesium (to relieve stiffness and cramping).

HYDROTHERAPY

The alternate use of brief hot and longer cold applications—a short, hot bath followed by a long cool shower, alternating hot and cold compresses, etc.—is beneficial in a number of ways. According to Dr. Kruzel, this type of hydrotherapy increases circulation…delivers more oxygen to the blood…increases the white blood cell count…and promotes tissue rebuilding. Hydrotherapy treatments need to be

261

directly supervised by a caregiver and the benefits and risks should be reviewed by a physician in each individual case.

POSITIVE ATTITUDE AND COMMITMENT ARE ESSENTIAL

Dr. Kruzel finds that the people who are most successful in getting their symptoms under control have a commitment to getting well, follow naturopathic recommendations closely, live a "squeaky clean" life (no alcohol or smoking, little saturated fat or processed foods, regular exercise, etc.) and maintain a positive attitude.

To locate a naturopathic physician in your area, visit the Web site of The American Association of Naturopathic Physicians at *www.naturopathic.org*. To learn more about MS, visit Web sites such as the National Institute of Neurological Disorders and Stroke (*www.ninds.nih.gov*), the Multiple Sclerosis Foundation (*www.msfocus.org*), the National Multiple Sclerosis Society (*www.nationalmssociety.org*) and the Swank MS Foundation (*www.swankmsdiet.org*).

Natural Way to Quit Smoking Strengthens Lungs, Too

Jianhua Tsoi, OMD, LAc, Greenwich & Wilton Acupuncture and Herb Center, Greenwich, Connecticut.

Do your clothes smell at the end of the day? Are you bothered by the stains on your fingertips and nails, or the fact that you dread the thought of a flight of stairs? You probably know this already, but it is time to quit smoking. Maybe you have the will but think you need some added support. Acupuncture may be for you.

Jianhua Tsoi, OMD, LAc, licensed acupuncture practitioner, of the Greenwich & Wilton Acupuncture and Herb Center in Greenwich, Connecticut, says that acupuncture is a good way to quit. Using a five-session treatment plan, he treats approximately 20 smoking patients a month. People already suffering from a serious illness from smoking, such as emphysema or asthma, may require more than the usual five sessions.

HOW IT WORKS

Unlike many smoking cessation treatments that focus on the influence of nicotine on the body, Eastern theory maintains that acupuncture works by healing and strengthening the body, especially the lungs, by eliminating blockages of energy flow through the body. Clearing the energy pathways rejuvenates the lungs and increases their strength, which in turn reduces symptoms of withdrawal. The desire for a cigarette decreases with each session, until finally, all physical cravings are eliminated.

Dr. Tsoi says that sometimes patients who smoke but are not trying to quit come in to have their lungs worked on. These people will often unintentionally lose the enjoyment of smoking. He says the wife of one of his patients called to say that her husband had complained to her, "This acupuncture is no good. It makes my cigarettes taste bad."

Acupuncture can also be helpful for those who have already quit on their own. Even after quitting the body has remnant damage. Acupuncture helps by promoting healing and regeneration of the affected areas.

Although acupuncture can be effective in helping people quit smoking, Dr. Tsoi is quick to point out that it takes the will and desire of the patient to quit. Acupuncture is a physical treatment, not a psychological one, and it's not a miracle cure. You still have to make a conscious choice to put down the cigarettes.

13

Best Ever Secrets for Staying in Shape

Get More from Your Walking Workout

The popular 10,000-steps-a-day goal for physical fitness has been hugely successful since it has been promoted by the President's Council on Physical Fitness and Sports, and health organizations such as HealthPartners. The goal of taking 10,000 daily steps is a worthy one—it adds up to about five miles or an increase of about two-and-a-half to three-and-a-half miles a day over what most folks generally do. Everyone knows walking is good for you. So, a recent study about the effectiveness of the program was disheartening when it revealed that all that walking, while certainly better than nothing, may not be enough.

UNDERSTAND THE INTENSITY

To better understand the study, you need to know how scientists gauge intensity of exercise. Mild is defined as strolling (one to two miles per hour), a pace that allows for an easy conversation…at a moderate pace (three to four miles per hour) you become somewhat out of breath but can complete one or two sentences with ease…a vigorous level limits your ability to say anything more than one or two words. In this study, from the University of Alberta, Canada, researchers investigated how a low- to moderate-level (typical of 10,000-steps participants who choose their own pace) would compare with one done at a mostly vigorous level, in terms of health outcome measures. For the study, 128 men and women were randomly assigned to one of three groups for six months. One group followed the 10,000-steps program…the second group exercised in a traditional fitness program, gradually building to a vigorous level for 39 minutes, four times a week. The third group served as a control

Vicki Harber, PhD, University of Alberta, Physical Education and Recreation, in Edmonton, Canada.

263

group and did not add an exercise program. At the conclusion, researchers found that even though both exercise groups burned the same number of calories, the 10,000-steps program people improved oxygen uptake by 4%. But the traditional fitness program exercisers increased their oxygen uptake by an impressive 10%. The change in blood glucose was not different for participants in both groups—it didn't matter if they completed the walking program or the traditional program, they all improved fasting blood glucose. Systolic blood pressure was reduced significantly (10%) in the traditional group, but only reduced by 4% in the walking group.

HEALTH VERSUS FITNESS

We contacted Vicki Harber, PhD, who led the study. She stresses that in no way should this discourage people from taking on the challenge of 10,000 steps a day and walking for their health. However, she says that the study demonstrates that while walking is good, just a little more effort can make walking "great." Interestingly, Dr. Harber's definition of "great" is not "fitness," per se, but rather to create general health and wellness. What's the difference? To Dr. Harber, fitness aims at peak muscle and aerobic performance, whereas being healthy aims at sustaining healthy levels of calorie burning, oxygen levels and blood glucose regulation.

Dr. Harber says that the older exercise guidelines that scientists put out were strenuous and designed to make people fit, but these backfired when many people became discouraged and gave up. Consequently, scientists have rethought their guidelines to make them more approachable and still improve health measures. This is where the 10,000-steps-a-day goal comes in. Dr. Harber says it's time to raise the ante by adding a bit of huff and puff that will lead to more meaningful health gains and enhance quality of life.

TAILOR THE PROGRAM

The beauty of a 10,000-steps program, says Dr. Harber, is that it is so easy to in-

dividualize according to each person's current level and goal. *Here are her guidelines for how to tailor the program and take it to the next level...*

• **The truly sedentary should plan to build up to 10,000 steps per day** over a period of 12 to 16 weeks. You'll need a pedometer to keep track of your steps... using one will help inspire you to push a little harder as well as provide a feeling of accomplishment as you see your steps accumulate.

• **Once you have reached 6,000 steps daily,** gradually start to introduce a new pattern into your walking. About 10% of the time, speed up the pace for about 10 minutes. Do this several times each day.

• **When you have reached 10,000 steps**, add in three to five spurts of 800 to 1,000 steps at a moderate or even slightly vigorous level every day.

• **To determine how quickly you should increase intensity depends entirely on how your body feels.** If you feel great after an initial increase, stay at that level until your body becomes accustomed to it and then move on. If your body is sore, back off for a while.

ENTERTAIN YOURSELF

Pleasure, of course, should also be part of it. If you enjoy your exercise you'll increase the likelihood that you'll stick with it. Look for areas that you like to walk in, such as malls that are fun and easy to get to. Walking groups are a social way to exercise that many people enjoy. You can also build in private challenges that are entertaining and encouraging, says Dr. Harber. For example, once you know a walking route well, take one section and determine how long you need to complete it. Then challenge yourself to shave your time. Say it normally requires 10 minutes for you to get from point A to point B. Try to do it in nine and one-half minutes and once you are comfortable in that range, try to cut it back just slightly again. This will get you nicely to the moderate level and give you a sense of victory as well.

A New Way Of Walking

Wayne Westcott, PhD, fitness research director, South Shore YMCA, Quincy, Massachusetts. Dr. Westcott is author or coauthor of 20 books, including *Strength Training Past 50*. Human Kinetics. He is a consultant to many national groups, including the American Senior Fitness Association.

In the '90s, mall walking was the way to fitness. Now, Nordic walking, popular in Finland, is coming into fashion in the US. The secret to its success is the rubber-tipped poles that work the upper body and core to burn more calories during a revved-up form of fitness walking. Also known as pole walking, this technique was first used for summer training by cross country skiers, but soon became popular with the Finnish public.

For an inside look at this innovative sport, we checked in with Wayne Westcott, PhD, fitness research director at the South Shore YMCA, Quincy, Massachusetts, and the author of *Strength Training Past 50* (Human Kinetics). He says that Nordic walking supplies a better workout overall than normal walking, and many people enjoy this form of vigorous outdoor exercise that enables them to breathe in fresh air as they trek over varied terrain.

MORE BANG FOR THE BUCK

In Nordic walking, you use two lightweight aluminum or fiberglass poles to push off each step, as if you were a cross-country skier. This technique reduces wear and tear on the knees and ankles, since you are requiring your triceps, pecs and forearm muscles to take some of the weight off your joints. As for energy consumption or weight loss, Nordic walking provides more bang for the buck, too. Most Nordic walkers report not feeling like they have to work harder, yet they burn an additional 20% to 40% more calories compared with normal walking —primarily because the upper body is more involved.

IMPORTANT DETAILS

As with many forms of exercise, Dr. Westcott stresses that the right technique is essential. Nordic walking can be done on neighborhood streets (flat or hilly), or a more challenging hiking trail. The more challenging the terrain, the better the workout. The correct equipment is also important. Poles must be the proper length for your height or you risk back strain and diminished benefits. Most poles come with instructions, so read them carefully. You can learn more about Nordic walking at the Web site *www.nordic walking.com.*

FREQUENCY, INTENSITY AND CONSISTENCY

To keep energy and interest levels high, many people like to vary their exercises, choosing Nordic walking one day, biking or fitness walking the next. *Whatever exercise regimen you choose, Dr. Westcott points out that it must meet three important criteria...*

•**Frequency.** Try to get out there three or four days a week.

•**Intensity.** Activity should be vigorous enough to raise the heart rate 60% to 85% of maximum heart rate.

•**Consistency.** For your body to reap real benefits, workouts must be a minimum of 15 to 20 minutes long.

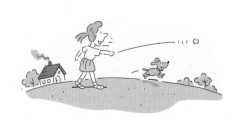

Think Outside the Gym For a Great Workout

Liz Neporent, MA, CSCS, coauthor of *Fitness for Dummies* and *Weight Training for Dummies* (both from For Dummies) and *The Fat-Free Truth* (Mariner). Ms. Neporent is an exercise physiologist and writer whose work has been featured in *The New York Times, Shape* magazine, the *New York Daily News* and *Fitness* magazine. She is president of Wellness 360, a corporate wellness consulting company. *www. w360.com.*

People feel great when they exercise outside. Whether it's a planned workout like a run, or simply a vacation activity such as kayaking or riding bicycles—activities that aren't mentally categorized as a "workout"—one can feel invigorated and energized in a very different way than from the usual indoor routines.

"There are some significant differences when you exercise outside," explains exercise authority Liz Neporent, MA, CSCS, and cofounder of Wellness 360, "though they have very little to do with calorie burning. Exercising outside is just more exciting and interesting. A rowing machine is just not going to be the same as rowing on the river. The movement on a machine is relatively predictable, but outdoors you're actually dealing with the elements—with the sun on your face, with pretty landscape going by and with getting rocked by the water.

Navigating the outdoor elements actually causes extra movement, which also makes it more of a challenge." Plus you get your fill of vitamin D from the sun, which improves your energy, calcium management and mood.

INDOORS vs. OUTDOORS

Neporent says that people believe that they burn more calories running outdoors than on a treadmill but that this really isn't true. "There's a slight difference between running up a hill and running on a treadmill," she explains. "You will burn slightly more calories on the real hill due to wind resistance and terrain changes. For the average person, it is hardly enough of a difference to matter, but physiologically speaking the difference is there," Neporent says. Other than that, she says, running/walking outdoors versus the treadmill test out virtually the same in terms of calorie burn.

But Neporent points out that exercising indoors has many advantages—safety being one of them. "Running on a treadmill in a gym is a lot safer than running outside in some neighborhoods, particularly at night," Neporent notes. "And the great thing about cardio machines is that they give you feedback about your speed, distance, pace and calorie burn, which helps ensure you exercise at an adequate level. It is also motivating, especially if you're one of those people who likes facts about your workout."

EXERCISE, THY NAME IS VARIETY

Some people who regularly work out outdoors skip strength training exercises. "You don't have to limit your outdoor workout to cardio," notes Neporent. *Some suggested exercises to mix in with cardio for a terrific outdoor circuit workout…*

- **Find a bench and do step ups.**
- **Stop and do some push-ups.**
- **Do tricep dips off a bench.**
- **Do a set of squats or lunges.**

So what's best? Variety. A little bit of both. When time is tight, or the weather is bad, stay inside. But on a beautiful sunny day, get out and enjoy the rich experience of an outdoor workout.

Most critical: Keep moving every day.

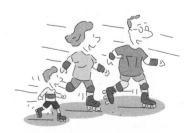

Improve Your Health By Sitting Still

Mark A. Stengler, ND, naturopathic physician in private practice, La Jolla, California...adjunct associate clinical professor at the National College of Natural Medicine, Portland, Oregon...author of many books, including *The Natural Physician's Healing Therapies* and coauthor of *Prescription for Natural Cures* (both from Bottom Line Books)...and author of the *Bottom Line/Natural Healing* newsletter.

Want to get healthier just by sitting? You can with what we can call "sweat therapy." Recently, we spoke with Mark Stengler, ND, author of *Bottom Line Natural Healing* newsletter (*www.drstengler.com*) and author of *The Natural Physician's Healing Therapies* (Bottom Line Books) about his use of detoxification strategies when treating patients. Sweating, in particular, is an easy and relatively risk-free method of reducing levels of toxins such as heavy metals (mercury, lead, aluminum, etc.), pesticides and other chemicals stored in fat tissue, Dr. Stengler says. This leads to a more efficient delivery of oxygen to cells and tissues, better circulation and immune system enhancement. *Here's how to sweat your way to a variety of health benefits...*

SWEAT YOUR WAY TO FITNESS

How you elect to go about sweating is an individual matter. According to Dr. Stengler, nothing fancy is required, and it's beneficial to simply work up a good sweat during exercise. The key here is intensity—it is regular, vigorous, sweat-inducing exercise (not just an occasional stroll through the park) that gets your heart pumping, stimulates perspiration, and keeps you leaner and fitter overall. Among your many options are power walking, jogging, bicycling, treadmill work and dancing. Almost any aerobic exercise will do it.

SOOTHING SAUNAS AND STEAM ROOMS

If you want to kick it up another notch and raise health benefits to the next level, visit the sauna or steam room following a workout at the local gym. The intense heat stimulates blood circulation near the skin, which triggers more intense sweating, and you may easily shed a pint or more of sweat—along with accompanying fats and toxins—even in a short stay. According to Dr. Stengler, saunas and steam rooms help wastes exit through sweat and sebaceous glands. In the end, which you choose is largely a matter of personal taste, though they tend to impact the body in slightly differing ways. *Here's what you can expect from the various options...*

- **Steam rooms** provide heated air that is moist.
- **Traditional European-style saunas** provide dry and then wet heat (when you splash water on hot rocks or a stove to generate steam).
- **Electric saunas** provide dry heat.

Benefits of intense heat and sweating in steam rooms and saunas include flushing of dirt and debris from the skin...general detoxification...pain relief from conditions such as arthritis, backaches and sports injuries by increasing blood circulation and removing accumulated pain-causing acidic metabolites...stress reduction, and an overall sense of relaxation and well-being.

NEW KID ON THE BLOCK: FAR INFRARED SAUNAS

Dr. Stengler also mentions a relatively new alternative—far infrared saunas. These special saunas harness infrared radiation to heat the skin without warming the air. An infrared sauna usually consists of a wooden box with several infrared heaters, with the box offering the atmosphere of the traditional sauna while heaters emit the actual radiation. People who are fans of infrared radiation point out that it offers the same health benefits as conventional alternatives, but with certain advantages. For example, traditional steam rooms and saunas may be more likely to spread germs because of the moist air, and some people have trouble breathing in air that is very warm. On the other hand, many people enjoy the sensations of relaxation and well-being they more typically associate with sweating out toxins in warm and/or moist air. Just be careful to avoid overcooking yourself with the penetrating radiant heat.

SAFE SWEATING IN THE SAUNA

Of course, there's a right way and a wrong way to go about using saunas and steam rooms. *To safely sweat your way to good health, Dr. Stengler recommends...*

•**If you are pregnant,** or if you suffer high blood pressure, heart disease, diabetes or other chronic health problems, check with your physician first. Intense heat makes your heart pump faster and raises your pulse rate by 30% to 50%.

•**Don't visit the steam room or sauna if you're not feeling well,** or if you've been drinking alcohol, and leave at once if you begin to feel nauseous, dizzy or otherwise unwell. Those on medications should check with their doctor before using a sauna or steam room. You should also avoid wearing jewelry when inside, so it does not get damaged.

•**Drink water before and afterward** —12 ounces for every 15 minutes in a sauna—and continue to sip water while inside. Dr. Stengler adds that an electrolyte solution would be even better, and that healthier versions than the usual Gatorade are available from health food stores. Also be sure to have plenty of salt in your system as well, especially if on medication or if you are prone to low blood sodium (a blood test can tell you if you are). Even a short session can result in significant fluid and salt loss, and you don't want to become dehydrated or sodium deficient.

•**Keep it short and sweet.** A general rule of thumb is 10 to 15 minutes in the steam room or 20 to 30 minutes in the dry sauna once or twice a week. Dr. Stengler adds that these numbers really depend on individual health, and healthy people can safely stretch their stays to 15 to 20 minutes in the steam room and as long as 60 to 90

minutes (with cooling off breaks every 15 minutes) in the dry sauna and 30 minutes (with a 15-minute break halfway through) in the infrared sauna. Conversely, people with conditions such as high blood pressure will need to keep sessions shorter. When in doubt, consult your physician for advice.

Fast Ways to Burn More Fat

Jason L. Talanian, exercise physiology researcher at the University of Guelph in Ontario, Canada. Talanian has coauthored several studies on exercise, training and adaptation, and was the recipient of a Gatorade Sports Science Institute grant for his proposal, "Effect of high intensity interval training on skeletal muscle metabolism."

There are two big challenges in sticking with an exercise regimen —keeping it interesting, since doing the same thing all the time gets so boring...and attaining the same level of health benefits from the same old workout, because your body gets more efficient as it gets increasingly fit. One method that meets both those challenges is what the Swedes call "*fartlek*," which means "speed play," a form of unstructured interval training popular with runners.

SPEED PLAY

This works by alternating intervals of high-intensity exercise with periods of what's called "active recovery," says Jason L. Talanian, an exercise physiologist at the University of Guelph in Ontario, Canada, and author of several studies on exercise performance. For example, if you're walking for an hour, try jogging for 30 seconds every few minutes. If you're already running, sprint for a half-minute. Talanian explains that these spurts of high-intensity exercise lead the body to physiological adaptations that help burn more fat, with the periods of rest making it possible for the body to meet escalating levels of challenge. One measure of aerobic fitness—maximum oxygen consumption (known as VO2max)—is also notably improved by interval training.

RESEARCH FINDINGS

In his most recent study, published in April in the *Journal of Applied Physiology*, Talanian asked eight college-age women to work out in his lab every other day for two weeks, for a total of seven interval sessions. During each workout, they performed 10 high-intensity intervals of four minutes each, following each with two minutes of rest time. The women were all over the map when it came to fitness levels—some had been fairly sedentary, but one was a triathlete and another played competitive soccer. About half were of average fitness and had been exercising in a conventional manner prior to the study (three times a week or so, at moderate intensity).

To track results of fat utilization, Talanian used a measure called *whole body indirect calorimetry*, which uses exhaled gases to calculate carbohydrates and fats burned.

BETTER FAT UTILIZATION

Talanian's study, which reinforces the benefits of interval training, was unusual in the duration of the higher intensity intervals (four minutes) and in measuring changes in fat utilization in the whole body. In previous studies, subjects ran all out for 30 seconds, followed by a lower intensity active rest period of two or three minutes, which he hypothesized was a key reason for the impressive results. The exact mechanism that resulted in improved fat utilization following interval training is not yet known, but Talanian says it may be the aerobic component…it may be that the fat is burned during recovery periods following exercise where the body replenishes its lost glycogen stores. "But at this time we really don't know why an exercise that requires primarily carbohydrate for energy results in improvements in fat burning," he told me.

SHORTER INTERVALS GOOD TOO

If four-minute intervals of high intensity seems daunting, you can get some of the benefits of interval training with much shorter intervals. An earlier study at McMaster University (in Hamilton, Ontario, Canada), found that between four and seven all-out bouts of 30 seconds each, alternating with a four-minute full-rest recovery period between intervals, still doubled the endurance capacity of the subjects in a mere two weeks of training.

GETTING STARTED

It's often helpful to work with a trainer for your first interval workout. If a trainer is not for you, Talanian suggests starting your interval training by computing your maximum heart rate (subtract your age from 220). Then you multiply by a percentage to get your range or goal. For example, a 40-year-old who wants to exercise between 60% and 80% of max would subtract 40 from 220—180. Then 60% of 180 is 108 (which stands for beats-per-minute), 80% of 180 is 144. His range is 108 to 144 beats-per-minute (in this case 80% is his high-intensity goal). You can, of course, work up to that, and you can also start with shorter intervals of low to moderate intensity and increase to longer ones as you improve.

Aerobics for Folks Who Have Trouble Moving

Karl Knopf, EdD, coordinator of the Adaptive Fitness Technician Program and Life Long Learning Institute at Foothill College, Los Altos, California, president of Keep Fit Over 50 and director of fitness for the physically limited at the International Sports Sciences Association. Dr. Knopf has authored numerous books and articles on older adult fitness and chronic conditions. For more information go to *www. keepfitover50com*.

Even people who are confined to a wheelchair or who don't have the ability to move around as freely as they used to can benefit from aerobic exercise. Fortunately, there are many practical options. *Here's what we learned when we went looking...*

IN THE SWIM

According to Karl Knopf, EdD, coordinator of the Adaptive Fitness Technician Program at Foothill College in Los Altos Hills, California, and president of Keep Fit Over 50, water can be a lifesaver—literally—for the person whose mobility is limited. Water presents a range of resistance to the muscles, he says. There are a variety of therapeutic pools designed exactly for this purpose—some where you can use a walker or wheelchair in the water, and also commercially available "swim spas" (also called "counter current" pools, which can often be found in physical therapy centers and are available for installation in private residences as well). In counter current pools, you can adjust the water flow so you can swim in place or walk with more of a challenge, he said.

WALKING IN WATER

Water walking can be another option. There are some people who use wheelchairs instead of walking because it's just simpler for them to get around and easier on their joints, but they actually have some ability to use their legs. By using a pool noodle (children use these brightly colored, foam tubes as pool toys) under their arms while in the water, a "mobile wheelchair user" can actually float in one place while moving his/her legs as though walking and get a lot of aerobic benefits, suggests Dr. Knopf.

Note: To avoid drowning, exercise caution and never go in the water unsupervised. You might even consider wearing a life jacket or an AquaJogger to make you feel safe in the water.

BICYCLES BUILT FOR YOU

Pedal exercisers (like bicycle pedals but without the bicycle) are easy to find, and easy to use for the mobility-challenged person who retains some (even if not much) ability to move the legs. This unobtrusive, relatively inexpensive (prices typically can range from $15 and up, depending on the materials with which they are made) device is widely available through medical supply stores. It consists of a small frame with pedals on which a "rider" can place his feet while sitting in a regular chair and pedal away, just like a regular bicycle.

ARM-ONLY AEROBICS

For people with absolutely no use of their legs, there are several ways to get aerobic exercise. Many gyms are equipped with a device called an *arm ergometer.* Almost like an inverted bicycle, according to Dr. Knopf, there is a seat on which the user sits while grasping a set of "handlebars" which rotate exactly like a bicycle pedaling device but powered by the arms. "This provides an excellent aerobic workout with no leg motion necessary whatsoever," says Dr. Knopf, with one warning. "Arm exercises generally elevate heart rate more than leg exercises, so if you're using one of these devices, don't rely on exercise heart rate to determine your intensity level." Instead, he recommends using the "*rate of perceived exertion.*" Ask yourself, "How hard is this on a level of one to 10, with one being the least possible effort (like sleeping) and 10 being the most effort you could possibly manage for a few seconds." Dr. Knopf suggests aiming for a workout that feels moderately challenging, like a 5 or a 6. Another option would be the talk test. If you can't carry on a conversation, you are training too intensely.

YOU CAN DO THIS AT HOME

There are video options, as well. Sit and Be Fit (*www.sitandbefit.org*) is a nonprofit organization that produces a television show for seniors and the mobility-challenged (it appears on PBS stations) and also sells a variety of video workouts for people facing physical challenges. With workout videos specifically for people with Parkinson's disease, arthritis, osteoporosis and MS, as well as for those who are mobility-impaired, the organization and its products come highly recommended by Dr. Knopf. The "Season 8 Workout" DVD, for example, has a warm-up, a seated circulation workout, seated towel exercises, seated weight workouts and optional leg strengthening and stretching exercises that require standing but not walking. While obviously not like running, these raise the heart rate enough to get substantial benefit.

JUST DO IT...WITH CAUTION

Of course, for people still able to walk even just a few steps, it's possible to get a workout the old-fashioned way, by just doing it. Dr. Knopf says people using walkers or even wheelchairs might still be able to exercise by walking, "albeit very slowly and carefully." For them, he recommends short exercise intervals. "They can stand behind the walker and walk five minutes then rest—and repeat for a few times, building up endurance." He points out that having a cell phone accessible helps people feel safer.

In all cases, it is important that people of limited mobility discuss their exercise strategies with their health-care professional, who can provide a recommendation to a physical therapist in your area. They are specially trained to provide exactly this sort of advice, and are quite often excellent motivators as well.

Easy Exercise Lowers Blood Pressure, Prevents Bone Loss And More

Wayne Westcott, PhD, fitness research director, South Shore YMCA, Quincy, Massachusetts. Dr. Westcott is author or coauthor of 20 books, including *Strength Training Past 50*. Human Kinetics.

It's well known that 30 minutes of aerobic exercise (walking, bicycling, etc.) three to five days a week helps prevent cardiovascular disease. What's less well known—or at least less practiced—is that strength training (e.g., lifting free weights or using weight machines) is equally important to good health, especially as we grow older. The American College of Sports Medicine (ACSM) recommends that adults perform two to three strength-training sessions each week.

A BOOST WHILE AGING

According to Wayne Westcott, PhD, fitness research director for the South Shore YMCA in Quincy, Massachusetts, strength training not only boosts metabolism and keeps blood pressure and glucose levels stable, it is also an excellent way to prevent the five-pound loss in muscle mass that people typically experience each decade as they age. *Dr. Westcott tells us more about the health benefits of strength training, and offers some useful tips on how to safely and effectively work out with weights...*

STRENGTH TRAINING: THE KEY TO SUCCESSFUL AGING

Lean muscle mass naturally decreases with age, but strength training (especially training with weights) can help reverse this trend. As you grow stronger and muscle mass increases, benefits multiply—you'll find that you are more energetic, have more stamina and feel better overall.

According to Dr. Westcott, strength training...

•**Lowers blood pressure,** which reduces the risk of cardiovascular disease. After two months, regular weight training can cause incremental drops in both systolic (top number) and diastolic (bottom number) blood pressure.

•**Encourages muscles to utilize glucose more efficiently.** This means less glucose circulating in the bloodstream, which lowers your risk of diabetes.

•**Stimulates the skeletal system,** which helps maintain bone density. This becomes increasingly important as we age, to prevent bone-thinning osteoporosis.

•**Enables you to manage weight more effectively.** Your best bet is to combine aerobic and strength-training exercise to raise your metabolism and burn off excess calories.

GETTING STARTED

Weight training with progressively heavier resistance is far and away the best way to build strength and muscle mass, notes Dr. Westcott. But if you're not familiar with free weights or weight machines, what's the best way to get started? Join a beginner's weight training class at the local gym, or schedule a session or two with a personal trainer who is knowledgeable in weight training. There are also helpful how-to books, such as Dr. Westcott's own *Strength Training Past 50* (Human Kinetics). If you're over 40 or have health issues, also see your health-care provider before taking on a new fitness program.

As for whether to choose free weights (barbells or dumbbells) or weight machines, such as Nautilus or Cybex, try both forms and see which you prefer. Free weights and machines work equally well, observes Dr. Westcott—though, of course, free weights can easily be done at home, without investing in expensive equipment or a health club membership. Muscles can't tell the difference.

GETTING THE MOST OUT OF YOUR WORKOUT

Once you learn how to work with weights, you'll want to focus on maximizing benefits of your workouts. An average strength-training regimen consists of two to three sessions a week, with one to three sets, using sets of resistance exercises to cover all the major muscle groups. *For optimal results, Dr. Westcott makes these recommendations...*

•**Begin with eight to 10 repetitions of a series of resistance exercises.** Consult a fitness trainer at the gym to determine appropriate starting weights, which should call on approximately 65% to 75% of your maximum resistance. At the gym, it's often not necessary to book a session with a personal trainer since many have "floor trainers" available to answer questions and offer advice on proper weight levels and lifting technique. At home, most women exercise with five- to 15-pound free weights, and most men lift 10 to 25 pounds.

•**Learn to lift weights properly, in a slow and controlled fashion.** It's not the amount of weight you lift, but how you lift it that counts. As a general rule of thumb, each repetition should last five to six seconds, and a series of 10 repetitions should take 50 to 60 seconds. When in doubt about technique, seek advice from a fitness professional.

•**Be sure sessions last 20 to 40 minutes.** Weight training should be performed three days a week, nonconsecutive days, at first. As time goes on and you grow more experienced, you can cut back to only two sessions a week, three days apart. This allows the muscles ample time to recover and prepare for the next workout.

•**Remember to breathe.** Holding your breath during weight training can lead to a dangerous elevation in blood pressure. Exhale when you lift, and inhale when you lower weights.

•**Vary your exercises.** For example, do one set of repetitions for the shoulders, move down to the abs, and then on to the legs. Don't overwork any one muscle group, as this can contribute to muscle fatigue and the risk of injury.

•**Increase weight when you successfully work your way up to performing 15 reps** with proper technique and without fatigue. However, to avoid strains and sprains, don't add more than 5%—of pound weight—at a time.

•**Stretch the muscles you just worked after each strength exercise**—or, if you prefer, following your entire workout.

MORE STRENGTH-TRAINING OPTIONS

Other forms of strength training also work well, if you don't enjoy weights or want to incorporate some variety into your fitness regimen. *Classes or activities you might consider include...*

• **Circuit training.** This handy, all-in-one exercise program combines strength training with aerobic activities such as the treadmill and stationary bike.

• **Pilates.** This approach emphasizes slow-moving stretches and resistance exercises (including using popular exercise resistance bands) to increase flexibility and strength.

• **Body sculpting.** While body sculpting—the modern day version of calisthenics with some light weights—does not pack the same oomph as other strength-training exercises, it will help slow muscle loss and moderately increase strength.

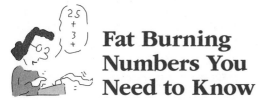

Fat Burning Numbers You Need to Know

Jonny Bowden, PhD, CNS, a board certified nutritionist, the "Weight Loss Coach" on iVillage.com and author of the best-selling *Living the Low Carb Life* (Sterling) as well as *The 150 Healthiest Foods on Earth* (Fair Winds). Find out more at *www.jonny bowden.com.*

The conventional advice about working at a lower heart rate to burn more fat is based on a complete misunderstanding of how the body works," says Jonny Bowden, PhD, CNS, nutritionist and fitness expert, and weight loss coach on iVillage. "Yet that information continues to get passed around in gyms and aerobics classes. It's even made its way into the computer programs on exercise machines."

FAT BURNING
TRUTH VS. MYTH

Dr. Bowden explains that at every level of activity—from sleep to running a marathon—you're always "burning" some mixture of fat and carbohydrates, with just the tiniest bit of protein thrown in for good measure. "There's always a mix of these two fuels," Dr. Bowden says. "The confusion about *fat* burning arose because many aerobics teachers don't understand the differences between percentages and absolute numbers."

FUELING YOUR SYSTEM

Here's how it works. You're always burning calories, even when you're sleeping. It "costs" calories to grow toenails, breathe and perform even the most basic metabolic activities. Those calories have to come from somewhere—and at rest, the highest percentage of them come from fat (or, more accurately, fatty acids, which circulate in the bloodstream and get stored in the hips, thighs and tummy). "But the total number of calories burned at rest—and at low levels of activity—is very small," Dr. Bowden explains. "The average person burns about a calorie a minute—or 60 calories an hour—sitting around watching television. Now the *percentage* of that 60 calories that comes from fat is pretty high—around 70%. But the *total* number of calories burned is very small. As you work harder, the *percentage* of fuel that comes from fat goes down somewhat, but the total number of calories burned goes way up." The result? You actually burn more *total* calories—and fat—when you're working harder even though the relative percentage of fat burning drops.

THE ARITHMETIC OF
FAT BURNING

"In seminars, I always ask the following question," says Dr. Bowden. "Would you rather have 90% percent of all the money I have in my pocket, or 10% of all the money Donald Trump has in the bank? Obviously, everyone chooses the Trump option, even though I'm offering a higher *percentage* of the money in my pocket. Why? Because clearly, the payoff in dollars for the person choosing a lower percent of a huge number is going to be way higher than the payoff for the person choosing a high percent of a low number! And it's the exact same thing with calories."

Dr. Bowden explains further: "At a high level of exertion, you might be

273

burning as many as 12 calories per minute, or 720 calories per hour. At that level of exertion, 30% of your calories are probably coming from fat. That sounds like a pretty low percentage, doesn't it? But the number of fat calories burned is actually 216 calories (30% of 720). Now at a very moderate rate of exertion, like they tell you to do on the "fat burning programs," you might burn only 5 calories per minute, or 300 calories per hour, and sure, a greater percentage—say 50% of those 300 calories—is coming from fat. But 50% of 300 calories is only 150 fat calories. Not bad, but you did better working harder!"

PAYING THE CALORIC DEBT

According to Dr. Bowden, the picture isn't as simple as how many calories you burn from fat during the exercise session. "People get very caught up in the concept of where their calories are coming from during the exercise session, but in the long run it doesn't much matter," he says. "Whether I pay a bill using nickels, dimes, dollar bills or savings bonds, in the long run I've still got to pay the debt. And it's the same thing with calories. Ultimately, to lose weight, you want to burn—or spend—more calories during the day than you take in. At some point in the day you may be using more fat calories, and at others you may be using more calories from carbs, but if you're in the red, calorically speaking, you're going to pay that debt from your savings account, which in this case is the fat around your waist, hips and thighs!"

"If you want to lose weight," Dr. Bowden says, "you want to work out as hard and as long and as frequently as you can." Of course, always check with your doctor before starting any exercise program.

So is there ever a reason to work out at lower levels of effort? "Absolutely," says Dr. Bowden. "It's always good to mix and match levels of intensity. Sometimes you go for a long slow run, other times you go for a series of sprints. Just burn the calories."

Better Way to Calculate Your Target Heart Rate

Liz Neporent, MA, CSCS, coauthor of *Fitness for Dummies* and *Weight Training for Dummies* (both from For Dummies) and *The Fat-Free Truth* (Mariner). Ms. Neporent is an exercise physiologist and writer whose work has been featured in *The New York Times, Shape* magazine, the *New York Daily News* and *Fitness* magazine. She is president of Wellness 360, a corporate wellness consulting company. *www. w360.com.*

Historically, exercisers have been told that the best way to estimate maximal heart rate—the maximum number of times your heart can beat each minute—is to subtract your age from the number 220. This formula, used for decades by many fitness professionals to design training routines, also forms the basis for the programs used on many aerobic exercise machines.

There's only one problem. The formula may not be accurate.

Previous research shows that this equation may *overestimate* maximal heart rate in younger people and *underestimate* it in older people, which in turn calls into question the validity of exercise routines using the traditional maximum heart rate calculation to determine how hard you should train.

Exercise physiologist Liz Neporent, MA, CSCS, president of Wellness 360 in New York City, explains it this way: "The standard heart rate formula is generally useful," she said, "but it can be off by 10 to 12 beats plus or minus." That would explain why a lot of older exercisers frequently complain that they barely break a sweat while staying in their recommended "target heart rate zone."

The research, funded by the National Institutes of Health and based on an analysis of 351 studies, proposes using a different equation that is claimed to be more accurate: maximal heart rate = 208 minus the figure you get from .7 times your age. This produces a slightly smaller age variance within the target area. Remember that training zones are found by calculating a percentage of the maximum heart rate figure. For example, a target zone of 70% to 85% of maximum heart rate is a vigorous-intensity aerobic training zone.

According to Neporent, the new formula is probably more accurate than the old one, but it is still not individualized. Neporent suggests that if you really want to know what *your* training range is, get it tested. "Any gym—or doctor—can do what's called a 'sub-max' test—where heart rate is measured and then through formulas or a chart it is equated to VO2 (a measure of oxygen consumption)—to give you a more individualized target range," she explains.

RATE OF PERCEIVED EXERTION

But Neporent has an even better, more user-friendly suggestion. "You could also abandon heart rate calculations altogether and use what's called the RPE scale—rate of perceived exertion," she told me. This is a very useful, subjective scale of how hard exercise feels to you. "It's a scale of 1 to 10," says Neporent, "with 1 being sitting in bed eating popcorn and watching a movie, and 10 being the last 30 seconds of a marathon running up a hill right before you just absolutely have to stop." Neporent suggests that the average person doing a workout keep his/her "perceived exertion" level at between 6 and 9, with perhaps 5 to 8 for beginners.

She also suggests doing "intervals," like periodic 20- to 30-second intervals at between levels 7 and 9 intensity alternating with a couple of minutes at level 6. "Unless you're an athlete fine-tuning your training, you're going to be just fine using the rate of perceived exertion scale of 1 to 10," said Neporent. "For a lot of people, all that heart rate calculation is just one more thing that's going to prevent them from exercising."

Why Muscles Ache— And How to Soothe Them

Stephen P. Sayers, PhD, assistant professor, department of physical therapy, School of Health Professions, University of Missouri-Columbia.

It's unlikely you know what "DOMS" stands for but very likely you know how it feels. DOMS is the acronym for "Delayed Onset Muscle Soreness"—the pain that peaks in overused muscles a day or two after you thought it would be a good idea to exercise really hard. Lactic acid buildup was thought to be the culprit behind DOMS, but scientists have since dispelled that notion. We wanted to find out what *does* cause the soreness and how to avoid it if possible. To get this information, we called Stephen P. Sayers, PhD, at the department of physical therapy, University of Missouri-Columbia, who has spent years researching exercise and its aftermath.

SURPRISING REASON WHY IT HURTS

Dr. Sayers first explained what's actually behind DOMS. When you exercise harder than usual or in a new way, the unusual strain creates tiny tears in the muscles, but that isn't what causes pain. (If it were, the pain would start immediately, not later.) Rather, the muscle damage puts in motion a delayed inflammatory response that releases chemicals that sensitize nerve endings. In time, these nerve endings send messages to the brain that say "ouch."

The cells that go into action to attend to the inflammation are white blood cells called *neutrophils*, but they generate free radicals that further damage the same muscles. That's when helpful cells called *macrophages* chomp away on the inflammatory debris and stimulate healing. The system might seem a bit odd, but that's how it works and it leaves you with muscles that hurt.

ECCENTRIC ACTIONS
AS TRIGGERS

The type of exercise that especially triggers DOMS is eccentric movement, which, curiously enough, feels the least stressful as you are doing it (running down a hill, lowering a weight, walking down stairs).

To explain: When you lift a weight, your biceps muscle brings it toward you and the muscle shortens—a contraction called concentric. But as you slowly lower it and lengthen the bicep, you are making an *eccentric* contraction. It's the same thing when you are using stairs or hiking—going up shortens muscles and is concentric, while going down lengthens muscles and is eccentric. Dr. Sayers says eccentric motions trigger more damage, which can lead to soreness because fewer muscle fibers are available to help eccentric actions...with fewer fibers pitching in to lighten the load, there is more stress on the muscles involved, therefore greater soreness.

DOES THIS HAVE TO HAPPEN?

Can one get fit without suffering DOMS? Some exercise professionals say no, DOMS is simply part of building strength. Dr. Sayers agrees, but says it does not have to be debilitating if you use caution. The key, he says, is to always start slowly and give your muscles time to gradually adjust.

Because strength training is the most frequent cause of DOMS, it is a good way to illustrate this approach. Using weights that are light enough not to overly stress your muscles, perform three sets of eight to 12 reps per exercise for your upper and lower body, three times a week on nonconsecutive days. (These rules change once you have reached a certain fitness level, as you will read in a moment.) As your muscles adjust to the weights you have been using, move up *gradually* to heavier weights. According to Dr. Sayers, "The greatest gains in strength seem to occur in the first eight to 12 weeks of resistance training. Gains can occur after that point of course, but they occur at a slower rate." Once you have achieved your goal, he says you can maintain it by using heavier weights and training just twice a week. Similarly when you're starting a new season's sport (skiing or tennis for example), if you haven't been working those muscles in the off season, then start gradually.

THE WARM-UP,
COOL-DOWN MYTH

The other area of chronic confusion concerns the need to warm up and cool down as a way to prevent injury to the muscles. Stretching is the usual approach to warming up, but, it does not prevent injury like people think it does, says Dr. Sayers. It does, however, enhance flexibility.

A warm-up is definitely required, though, because cold muscles are vulnerable to injury. Try with a brief cardio spurt at low resistance, such as on the bike or treadmill or walking briskly for a few minutes—anything that brings blood to your muscles, increases your body temperature and revs your metabolism slightly in preparation for the session to come.

A cool-down is to reverse the body changes you put into motion with your warm-up...just continue your exercise but slow the pace. Weekend warriors planning a hike or sports outing can reduce or prevent soreness by preparing with a few eccentric movements such as squats (for quads, using only your body weight) or sit-ups for several days beforehand. Stretching after exercise does not reduce DOMS.

ONCE DOMS SETS IN

Unfortunately, once DOMS sets in, there is little you can do to relieve it, though according to *Bottom Line's Daily Health News* consulting medical editor Andrew L. Rubman, ND, a hot bath with Epsom salts is somewhat helpful.

A recent study indicated that drinking tart cherry juice, with its ample antioxidants, might be useful, but the research is preliminary, says Dr. Sayers. Plenty of studies have focused on other sorts of treatments, including acupuncture, yoga, massage, icing, stretching and vitamin C, but to little effect. Nonsteroidal anti-inflammatory drugs (NSAIDs) have been the subject of multiple studies for DOMS relief, but Dr. Sayers notes that the results are split right down the middle as to whether or not they help. He wants us to remember, however, that our body's inflammation response is important to muscle repair and it probably isn't a good idea to routinely take NSAIDs before exercise, because they might slow the inflammation that is part of repairing muscle damage.

Dr. Sayers does offer one way to feel better, though. For a quick but short-acting fix, try this: Simulate the very exercise that caused your soreness, but do it lightly, just enough to get some blood flow to the muscles and release endorphins. The relief you get won't last long, but for a few minutes or hours, it may feel better.

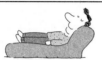

Surprising: Resting "Makes" You Sick

David Nieman, DrPH, director, human performance lab, Appalachian State University, Boone, North Carolina.

If you want to avoid a nasty cold this winter, go for a nice, brisk walk. Studies have shown that people who walk briskly for 45 minutes most days of the week have just half the number of sick days caused by colds or sore throats as nonexercisers. David Nieman, DrPH, director of the Appalachian State University Human Performance Lab in Boone, North Carolina, has researched the impact of exercise on human cells for more than 20 years. We called him to find out more about how exercise can maximize health in the cold, gray days of winter, the season of sniffles.

EXERCISE AND IMMUNE BOOSTING

Dr. Nieman says that moderate aerobic exercise creates favorable immune changes, including improvements in the killer T-cell function and improved immune system surveillance, which is the body's ability to detect and defend against pathogens. This improvement is triggered every time you exercise and lasts for one to three hours after the activity. The key, says Dr. Nieman, is frequency. Even though the change is just hours a day, over time it becomes protective. If you prefer, say, three 15-minute segments instead of 45 minutes, Dr. Nieman says it is probably equally effective as a cold fighter, but he can't confirm that until he completes more research.

TOO MUCH OF A GOOD THING

Dr. Nieman does have one important caveat about exercise, however—beware of the more-must-be-better trap. Over exercising, which is 90-plus minutes per day or running 60 or more miles a week, increases vulnerability to illness. Marathon runners, for example, are six times more likely to get ill in the one to two weeks following a race because excessive exercise suppresses the immune system. Dr. Nieman says that it pops back to normal quickly, but to get around the suppressed immunity period, superathletes need to be particularly careful to follow the rules of good health—avoid exposure to germs, eat healthfully and get enough sleep. In fact, studies have shown that lack of sleep as well as rapid weight loss and stress cause immune suppression.

IF YOU HAVE A COLD OR FLU

Should you continue exercising if you are getting or have a cold or the flu? Not if you have fever, aches and pains that are symptomatic of flu or other systemic illnesses. Heavy exercising will make symptoms worse and last longer, says Dr. Nieman. In the case of a simple cold, though, exercise is neutral—it will neither hurt nor help you.

As to the old saw that cold weather can increase vulnerability to colds and flu, Dr. Nieman says it's unlikely, assuming that your body is not cold. So dress warmly.

His advice: Get out and move, whatever the season. There is every reason to believe you are doing yourself a favor.

Surgery-Free Back Repair Works for 90% of Patients

Russell W. Nelson, MD, founder of the Nelson Spine Institute in Thousand Oaks, California.

Spinal discs are like small gel-filled balloons that rest between the vertebrae, sort of like little cushions separating the bones. But when something goes wrong with a disc—that is, it bulges or *herniates* (ruptures)—the pain can be terrible. A disc herniates when pressure on it causes a tear in the fibrous outer capsule and the soft inner part (the *nucleus pulposus*) protrudes, often pressing against a nerve.

A lumbar (lower back) herniated disc is a common cause of sciatic pain, which radiates down the buttocks and into the legs, typically to one side. But it can press on other nerves, as well. Occasionally, the disc presses on a nerve that controls the bowel or bladder, resulting in a loss of bladder or bowel control. This is *always* a medical emergency that calls for an immediate trip to the emergency room. But for all of the pain herniated discs might create, the patient is usually not in danger of long-term damage.

DISC DEGENERATION

A disc can herniate suddenly, as in the case of an accident or other trauma. Most of the time, though, it is the result of gradual degeneration. A portion of the disc deteriorates over time without symptoms until one day, the person bends over to tie his/her shoes and that small amount of pressure on the spine is just enough to make the disc herniate into the spinal nerves, sometimes resulting in excruciating pain. People most at risk include those who have a genetic predisposition to the problem. Smoking can cause spinal discs to degenerate as well. Disc degeneration can start early—MRIs indicate that about 30% of 30-year-olds already have signs of degeneration. Herniated discs are most common in people between the ages of 30 and 50. In older people, most spinal discs have flattened out too much to herniate, although the older spine is vulnerable to other problems.

FIRST AID FOR DISC DAMAGE

Many people assume that having a herniated disc means that they will eventually require surgery, but orthopedic surgeon Russell W. Nelson, MD, founder of the Nelson Spine Institute in Thousand Oaks, California (*www.nelsonspineinstitute.com*), says that is simply not true. Surprisingly, he says that up to 90% of people with herniated discs recover without surgical intervention. Dr. Nelson says that unless it's an emergency, he always starts conservative treatment for patients. The idea is to get the patient through the pain comfortably enough for healing to start. To reduce pain and inflammation, Dr. Nelson advises patients to take nonsteroidal anti-inflammatory drugs (NSAIDs) as the first line of treatment and ice the area in the immediate aftermath. (Wrapping a cloth around a bag of frozen peas to protect the skin works well.) Further treatment generally includes chiropractic adjustments or working with a physical therapist or both. Patients learn, among other things, to relieve their back pain by not doing the intuitive motion of bending forward, which actually adds to stress on the disc, but rather by arching the back as in a pelvic tilt.

Bottom Line's Daily Health News consulting medical editor Andrew L. Rubman, ND, adds that in addition to physical therapy, many patients have successfully alleviated the pain and suffering of herniated discs with interventions that include contrast therapy using cold and hot compresses as well as the use of anti-inflammatory natural remedies that often lie outside of the expertise of orthopedists.

EXTREME MEASURES

Often these efforts are sufficient, but if not, the patient can go to a specialist who assesses the disc and its location with an MRI. If the disc is taking up a large amount of space in the spinal canal, it may be necessary for the patient to have epidural corticosteroid shots around the spinal nerves. Within two to three days, they reduce inflammation and pain and that allows the patient to get back to other healing practices such as an exercise program. Dr. Nelson says that patients are allowed to have up to three steroid shots over a four- to six-week period and that for about 50% of patients, this course is successful.

SURGERY SECRETS

If the inflammation and pressure on the nerves cannot be relieved with non-invasive methods, the patient may opt for surgery. When the pain is so severe it interferes with daily life, many patients make that choice.

The classic procedure is discectomy (micro-surgery or endoscopic), which is still considered the gold standard. The surgeon makes a small incision over the area and removes the material that is causing pressure on the nerve tissue. Endoscopic discectomy involves a small scope inserted through small incision to view the area. Dr. Nelson says he prefers the microsurgery with a microscope because it allows the surgeon much better view of the affected tissue.

MORE RADICAL OPTIONS

Other, more radical procedures are disc replacement and spinal fusion, and there is much discussion and controversy in the world of spinal specialists concerning which is better. Replacement discs are made of hard plastic, metal or metal and plastic combinations, and doctors who prefer this method like it because of the motion the new disc preserves in the spine. However, there is also concern about the longevity of the disc prosthesis. If the disc fails in the future, how does the surgeon remove it without damaging the spine?

Fusion, in which two adjacent discs are fused together using bone grafts, does not present this problem, but there is a different risk. Eventually the pressure that caused the first herniated disc often simply

moves up another level, leading to another rupture and a second fusion. Dr. Nelson generally leans toward fusions, especially for people whose jobs require physical activity that puts constant pressure on the spine. He adds that for people who are active only in their leisure time, replacement surgery has worked well.

RECOVERY TIME

Recovery varies according to procedure. Replacement surgery requires two or three days in the hospital and no bending or exercise for three weeks. Fusion is also two or three days in the hospital, but patients are told to avoid bending for six to 12 weeks (and are often in a brace) to allow the bone the time it needs to heal. After that, patients of either sort can resume exercise and strengthening

Back surgery is far from a guaranteed fix, so it is far better to find nonsurgical options before taking such a drastic surgical measure.

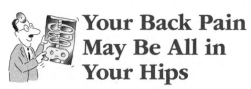

Your Back Pain May Be All in Your Hips

Andrew L. Rubman, ND, consulting medical editor for *Bottom Line's Daily Health News* and director of the Southbury Clinic for Traditional Medicines in Southbury, Connecticut.

Low back pain is a common reason why Americans see the doctor. Yet causes of back pain remain elusive, and more often than not, physicians can't clearly define the underlying reason. X-rays come back normal, MRIs come back normal, but still the pain persists. One common source of the problem, says *Bottom Line's Daily Health News* consulting medical editor Andrew L. Rubman, ND, is actually the misalignment of the hip and pelvic bones.

THE BACKBONE'S CONNECTED TO THE HIP BONE

One part of the body can profoundly affect another, says Dr. Rubman. In more than 25 years of clinical practice, it has been his experience that hip misalignment has caused or contributed to 75% of chronic back problems. The technical terms for the resulting spinal misalignments are *hypolordosis* and *hypokyphosis*.

The spine has a natural front to back curve (not side to side curve) explains Dr. Rubman. When this is disturbed for some reason—for instance, due to pregnancy and childbirth, an automobile collision or sports injury—the loss of curvature (or straightening of the spine) can throw the body's whole structure out of whack. A flattening of the thoracic spine, *hypokyphosis*, due to a misalignment of the pelvis and the sacrum, can cause a flattening of the lumbar curve, or *hypolordosis*, resulting in the compression of vertebral disks in the lower back. This can, in turn, compress nerves exiting from the spine, and muscles respond by trying to "lock down" to compensate, notes Dr. Rubman. The result is back pain—both chronic and acute due to spasms.

COPING WITH BACK PAIN

Proper diagnosis and treatment is required to restore the natural alignment of the hips, pelvis and spine. Unfortunately, conventional physicians are often quick to turn to drugs and surgery to remedy the problems…despite the fact that surgery has not been demonstrated to ease pain any better than less invasive techniques in many cases. To cure your aching back and get your hip bones and spine back into proper alignment, Dr. Rubman recommends that, after checking with your physician regarding safety, you try yoga, exercise and/or acupuncture, preferably with chiropractic or naturopathic oversight. Your physician may then prescribe specific manipulative, nutritional, dietary or physiotherapy interventions appropriate for your particular case.

It's generally safer to try the nonpharmaceutical and nonsurgical options in treating assorted medical conditions first. Lower back pain is no different. Of course, first check with your doctor to rule out any hidden medical condition.

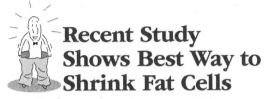

Recent Study Shows Best Way to Shrink Fat Cells

Barbara Nicklas, PhD, associate professor of internal medicine, Wake Forest University School of Medicine in Winston-Salem, North Carolina.

Metabolic syndrome, formerly called syndrome X, has become an important diagnostic tool for identifying people at risk for type 2 diabetes and cardiovascular disease, including heart attack and stroke. The World Health Organization came up with a definition of metabolic syndrome, and it has really taken off as a way of isolating specific conditions that predispose people to the above diseases. According to US guidelines, a person is classified as having metabolic syndrome if he/she has at least three of five symptoms in particular—elevated triglycerides…low HDL cholesterol…elevated blood pressure…elevated fasting blood sugar…and excess abdominal fat.

ABDOMINAL FAT

That last one is intriguing because it doesn't say generalized obesity, but specifically targets excess fat in the abdomen as presenting the greatest danger. Given that men nearly always put their excess weight on the belly, that definition covers just about all men who are heavy. But generally women become overweight in one of two different shapes—the apple shape with the large belly or the pear shape with wide hips and thighs. And clearly, while being overweight is never good because of a wide range of health-related reasons, being overweight with an apple-shaped body is even more troubling.

However, there is a secondary aspect to abdominal fat that also is an indicator of increased risk for heart disease and diabetes. According to Barbara Nicklas, PhD, associate professor of internal medicine at Wake Forest University School of Medicine in Winston-Salem, North Carolina, the size of abdominal fat cells themselves can also be considered a risk factor for these two diseases, independent of other conditions, including being overweight. Controversy has long swirled around whether the number of fat cells a person has can change, but Dr. Nicklas says it is well established that the size of fat cells can indeed change, describing them as similar to balloons that expand or deflate according to the amount of air they have.

HOW FAT IS FAT?

Dr. Nicklas and a team of fellow researchers at Wake Forest University recently published results of a study designed to evaluate the most effective way to shrink fat cell size. The study team set out to compare the impact of diet alone on abdominal fat cell size, the effect of diet plus low-intensity exercise or, finally, diet plus high-intensity exercise. Forty-five participants in the 20-week study were post-menopausal women with an average body mass index (BMI) of 31, which qualified them as officially obese.

The women were placed into one of the three groups. All groups were on a strictly controlled diet that created a deficit of 2,800 calories each week through diet or diet plus exercise. However, group one did not follow an exercise program while group two walked at a leisurely pace (about one to two miles an hour), for a maximum of 55 minutes three times each week. Members of group three walked at a higher intensity at 3.5 to four miles an hour but limited the time to just 30 minutes each session, also three times a week. Both exercise groups, however, burned the same amount of calories through walking at 400 calories per week.

BODY PROFILE CHANGES

At the end of the study, all of the women had changed their body profile to a similar degree regardless of the group they were in. The women had all lost between 19 to 23 pounds, lowered their fat mass, and reduced their waist girth by four inches and their hip girth by three to four inches. However, those who were in the diet-alone group, in spite of weight loss, did not have any significant change in the size of their abdominal fat cells. This compared with an impressive decrease of about 18% in the size of the fat cells that the women in both exercise groups achieved. How could they all lose the same, but have it be different? Not everyone lost fat cells deep in the abdominal section. Only the exercise groups did...the others lost weight in other parts of the body like the thigh.

REGULAR EXERCISE A MUST

Dr. Nicklas emphasizes the importance of understanding that weight loss through diet alone will not reduce fat cell size in the abdomen and it's the fat cell size in this location that is critical to reducing risk of heart disease and diabetes. In order to have healthy weight/fat loss, exercise of some kind must be added into the weight-loss program. Since both leisurely levels of exercise and more strenuous levels resulted in similar reduction in fat cell size, the key is to do it regularly and for sufficient amounts of time. Of course, more strenuous exercise is needed to build cardiovascular fitness via aerobic exercise.

Since even nonobese people can have oversized abdominal fat cells, the message once again to all is get off the couch and get moving. That doesn't change.

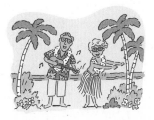

A Lot of Danger in a Little Extra Weight

Kenneth F. Adams, PhD, formerly at the National Cancer Institute, Nutritional Epidemiology Branch, Rockville, Maryland.

Even a few excess pounds can exacerbate gastroesophageal reflux disease (GERD) problems. This is well established. But a huge study conducted by the National Cancer Institute (NCI) indicates that the situation is far more serious. The study, of more than 500,000 men and women, confirmed that being obese increases mortality risk. But—and here's the surprise—it found that simply being overweight significantly increases risk as well.

SURPRISING STUDY RESULTS

Scientists analyzed the body-mass index (BMI) of study participants, ages 50 to 71 at the beginning of the study, and then followed these people for 10 years. At first glance, study results seemed to show that people who were either obese or underweight had an increased risk of death compared with people of normal weight. But then it got more interesting. The scientists removed data for all smokers and people with chronic diseases and did a follow-up analysis based on data from 186,000 people who had never smoked. After analyzing this information, scientists discovered that overweight people at age 50 were 20% to 40% more likely to die prematurely than people at the upper end of the normal-weight range (with a BMI from 23.5 to 24.9) and that obese people had a two to three times greater mortality risk than people at the upper end of the normal weight range (with a BMI from 23.5 to 24.9). Normal weight is defined as a BMI of 18.5 to 24.9.

MORE REASONS TO LOSE WEIGHT

Kenneth F. Adams, PhD, was the lead author of the NCI-led study. He explains that the study used the usual overweight criteria as a BMI from 25 to 29.9 and the obese one of a BMI of 30 or over. He says that they saw risk begin to increase in men at the BMI range of 26.5 to 27.9 and that for women, risk began at even a lower range, just 25 to 26.4. Dr. Adams adds that this study establishes that just being overweight directly increases risk of death and that when it comes to obesity, the risks are so high they are comparable to the risks from smoking.

These findings provide support to clear the confusion from a previous study that indicated people underweight were more at risk than those who were overweight. That particular study (from the Centers of Disease Control and Prevention) included data from smokers who have a higher mortality risk. Now that these people have been taken out of the mix, the data is definite that being pleasantly plump, as the old expression goes, can have unpleasant consequences.

The Deadly Dangers Of Desk Work

Harold Palevsky, MD, director of the Pulmonary Vascular Disease Program at the University of Pennsylvania Health System in Philadelphia.

Deep vein thrombosis (DVT) is quite literally what it says—a clot (*thrombus*) forming deep within a vein, generally in the leg or pelvis. Each year about two million Americans develop DVT and 60,000 to 200,000 of them die, often suddenly and without warning, because part of the clot has broken off and traveled into the lung (a pulmonary embolism) where it blocks blood flow to the lung's lobes. A known risk factor for DVT is being immobilized for any length of time as blood tends to pool in the legs. Although doctors worry especially about post-surgery patients, news in recent years has called attention to the potential risk of sitting still during long-range flights. And a recent study reveals a surprising new potential risk factor we need to be aware of—long hours at the desk.

A REVELATORY STUDY

The New Zealand study included 62 patients under age 65 who had been admitted to the hospital with blood clots. Researchers found that 34% of them had recently spent long periods of time seated at work. They either sat for eight or more hours a day with at least three or more consecutive hours spent without getting up...or 12 or more hours per day without getting up for one hour or more at a time. Does this mean that all of us desk-bound workers are in danger? To find out, we called Harold Palevsky, MD, director of the Pulmonary Vascular Disease Program at the University of Pennsylvania Health System in Philadelphia.

DESK ERGONOMICS

Dr. Palevsky explains that sitting at a desk involves bending the legs at the knees and the waist, thereby compressing or kinking the veins and impeding venous blood flow to some degree. Furthermore, when you sit still, your leg muscles are not engaging in the "squeeze and release" activity that ordinarily helps to pump blood against gravity back to the heart. He adds that in his own practice he has seen healthy people with no known risk factors develop DVT after periods of unusually long hours at their desks. This is because DVT is not a gradual process, he says, but rather can start from something as simple as sitting for hours at work with your leg folded under you.

FACTORS ADD TO RISK

Be aware that certain factors heighten risk, including smoking, obesity, having cancer, trauma to the vein from an accident or catheter, recent surgery, a family history of clotting, and synthetic estrogen (birth control pills and hormone therapy). Sometimes DVT develops without any symptoms, but be alert for swelling, pain and tenderness, and sometimes redness in a part of the leg, which may indicate DVT. The onset of unremitting or progressive symptoms in a leg is an emergency, requiring immediate medical evaluation.

TO REDUCE DVT RISK

Dr. Palevsky offers the following advice to reduce risk of DVT...

•**At work,** get up every one to two hours and walk around—and don't sit with your legs folded beneath you or crossed for long periods of time.

•**When driving,** stop and take a movement break every 90 to 120 minutes, and walk around.

•**On long flights stretch your legs and flex your ankles while seated at least every 30 minutes...**stand up frequently and roll from being flat on your feet to standing on your toes, or walk up and down the aisle a few times.

•**Eat fish at least once a week, and fruits and vegetables daily.** A recent study from the University of Minnesota adds to evidence that these foods lower DVT risk. It also found that the typical Western diet of red and processed meats, fast foods, refined grains, high-fat dairy products and a low intake of fish, fruits and vegetables increased risk by 60%.

Favorite Outdoor Workout

Liz Neporent, MA, CSCS, coauthor of *Fitness for Dummies* and *Weight Training for Dummies* (both from For Dummies) and *The Fat-Free Truth* (Mariner). Ms. Neporent is an exercise physiologist and writer whose work has been featured in *The New York Times, Shape* magazine, the *New York Daily News* and *Fitness* magazine. She is president of Wellness 360, a corporate wellness consulting company. *www.w360.com.*

When the weather turns nice, it's always fun to change things up a bit from your daily exercise routine at the gym, and take advantage of the healthful sunshine. What to do?

"Take it outside," says Liz Neporent, an exercise physiologist and coauthor of *Fitness for Dummies* (For Dummies), along with other titles. "Everything you've been doing on the machines can be done moving through space—instead of standing (or sitting) in one place. Biking, walking and jogging are great ways to exercise, and you can actually see the scenery, so you don't have to rely on bad movies on TV or headphones," she jokes. Neporent says that even the muscular workout from an elliptical machine can be replicated in a similar way outdoors. "Just find some hill courses for walking," she suggests.

FITNESS COURSES MAKE IT FUN

What about strength training? "Look for par courses, which are widely available in many cities, says Neporent "They are set up so you can do a full-body workout—plus they're fun."

A par course is basically a pre-designed fitness trail, with different exercise stations set up along the way. The starting point is clearly marked, so you usually begin there with a run (or walk or jog) to the first "station" (which usually takes two to five minutes, depending on what par course you are at or how fast you go). The stations typically have clear instructions and often pictures of the exercises to be done there, notes Neporent.

For example, first might be a place for you to do push-ups, with instructions to do as many as you can within one minute. Then you'd get up and continue your jog to the next station. Typically these courses include a station for squats, a place for a stretch and a chin-up bar.

THE DO-IT-YOURSELF VERSION

If you can't find a nearby par course, Neporent suggests designing your own. She advises basing it on the concept of circuit training, which many experts consider one of the most effective ways to get a full-body workout in a reasonable amount of time. "For example, you might run, walk or jog for five minutes, then stop by a park bench and do triceps dips for a set of 15. Then continue on your run for another five minutes and stop and do squats, standing in place. Five minutes more and you stop for push-ups."

Neporent explains that this kind of workout is infinitely flexible. "You can vary the intensity and duration." She suggests doing the first cardio exercise at a "warm-up" pace for five minutes, then the first "strength exercise" (push-ups, for example), followed by a "wind sprint" interval of 30 seconds to one minute before getting to the next "strength training" exercise. "You can carry a jump rope with you and skip rope for one of your cardio exercises," she suggests.

NO EQUIPMENT

One of the "no-equipment" strength exercises Neporent recommends is hopping on one leg. "This might be the best all-around calf shaper there is," she says. "Plus it allows you to work on balance and coordination." Since some body parts—like biceps and the back—are harder (but not impossible) to exercise without equipment, Neporent advises carrying one or two exercise bands with you. "They're lightweight and won't interfere with your run one bit," she says, "and they give you an infinite number of possibilities for every body part."

As for abs, one of her favorite exercises is the plank, easily done as one of the outdoor strength training exercises. "Balance on your forearms and toes, making your body straight, just like a plank," she says. "It makes your whole middle body work because you are supporting the position with 'core' muscles. At the end, you'll feel your whole abs work."

A TYPICAL WORKOUT PLAN

Following is one of Neporent's favorite "Take It Outdoors" workout circuits...

1. Walk (or jog) five minutes at a very moderate pace to warm up.

2. Stop at a park bench and do one set of triceps dips.*

*See How to do the Exercises section.

3. Do 30 seconds of jumping jacks.

4. Sprint for 30 seconds—full out. (Beginners, just walk faster, pushing your own "personal envelope.")

5. Jog for five minutes at moderate pace.

6. Stop and do a set of lunges*—10 reps per leg.

7. Jog for five minutes at moderate pace.

8. Stop and do a plank.* Beginners, hold for 10 seconds, working up to 60 seconds (advanced).

9. Jog for three minutes at a moderate pace.

10. Stop and do one set of push-ups. (Beginners, do as many as you can…advanced, go for as many as you can perform in one minute, even if you have to stop and pause every so often. It's okay to do the "assisted" version where your knees are on the ground.)

11. Sprint for 30 seconds—full out. (Beginners, just walk faster, again pushing your own "personal envelope.") Then jog at a moderate pace for three minutes as your heart rate comes back down a bit.

12. Stop and do a set of squats.*

13. Do 30 seconds of jumping jacks.

14. Jog at a moderate to slow pace as you cool down for five minutes.

15. Stretch.

The possible variations are endless, especially if you take the exercise bands with you, and mix it in with walking, jogging, kayaking, biking, swimming and all the other great outdoor activity options.

HOW TO DO THE EXERCISES

•**Triceps dips** (off a bench). Sit on the edge of a bench with hands firmly holding the edge of the bench, fingers facing out. Lift your butt up and away from the bench and lower it toward the floor by bending your arms at the elbows. Make sure your shoulders don't dip lower than

*See How to do the Exercises section.

the bench. Push back up. Repeat for 10 to 15 repetitions.

•**Lunges.** Stand straight and take a large step forward with your left foot, placing the left foot heel first on the ground. Then lower your hips down (bending the left knee) until the left knee almost touches the ground. Left knee should stay above left ankle. Come back up and repeat for 10 reps. Repeat on opposite side.

•**Squats.** Stand with feet shoulder width apart, toes pointing forward. Using the big muscles of your thighs, lower down until your thighs are parallel to the floor (resembling a sitting position). Keep knees above ankles. Repeat for 15 repetitions.

•**Plank.** Get on your hands and knees, then lower the top half of your body till you're resting on your forearms. Fully extend legs back (toes and forearms touching ground). Keep your back straight like a plank and hold the position (it's hard!). Beginners—10 seconds. Advanced—try for 60 seconds.

Workout for a Bigger, Better Brain

Arthur F. Kramer, PhD, professor of psychology, and director of the Biomedical Imaging Center at the University of Illinois at Urbana-Champaign. His research interests include cognitive neuroscience and brain plasticity.

S eems like there are new programs for brain health everywhere—new books, Web sites and board games focusing on "mental gymnastics" that are supposed to slow mental aging.

BRAIN BE NIMBLE

Recent research conducted in part by the National Institute on Aging showed that seniors who regularly practiced certain thinking skills maintained their ability to perform those skills better than those who didn't practice them. And a new study indicates that the right kind of physical exercise can actually build brain tissue, which may sharpen mental acuity.

The promise of a brain that's performance is nimble, sharp and quick well into our ninth and tenth decades grabs the attention of all of us. It's one thing to have the occasional "senior moment", as we all do, but quite another to experience the devastating affects of true cognitive decline—including dementia, from Alzheimer's disease or other causes. We've known for ages that exercise helps protect and strengthen the heart. Now we have evidence that it does the same thing for the brain.

BRAIN-BOOSTING AEROBICS

Many studies have already shown us that, with respect to cognitive performance, a brain with more associative pathways may offer an opportunity for better cognition. This latest research shows that regular aerobic exercise can not only enhance the ability of the brain to function, but can actually increase its size. Arthur F. Kramer, PhD, director of the Biomedical Imaging Center at the University of Illinois at Urbana-Champaign, recounts how he and his colleagues conducted the study using MRI technology on a group of 59 volunteers who did not exercise regularly. At the start of the study, the researchers took precise measures of brain volume to use as a baseline. "These folks were basically couch potatoes—healthy but sedentary, and ranging in age from 60 to 79," says Dr. Kramer. Half the group was enrolled in an aerobics program, starting at a moderate pace, but building up to a vigorous workout for one hour three times a week. The other group began a less strenuous "toning and stretching" program, using exercise bands at a pace slow enough that their heart rates were not significantly elevated. Both groups kept it up for six months. Diet was not studied or controlled in this research.

GRAY MATTER, WHITE MATTER

After the six months, all volunteers returned for follow-up MRI studies in which researchers measured the volume of both gray matter and white matter in their brains, comparing them with the initial exams. The gray matter of the brain is composed mostly of neurons or "computational units." Its purpose is to process inputs (electrochemical impulses) and create output, while the white matter consists of nerve fibers that carry information and are interconnections that act as conduits— "telephone wires between the neurons." In the group that had engaged in aerobic exercise, there was a notable increase in volume of both gray and white matter in several regions of the brain, compared with no change in gray or white matter in the "stretch and tone" group.

ANATOMICAL CHANGES

Prior to this study, there had been no known published research on whether exercise can bring about anatomical changes to gray or white matter in the human brain, Dr. Kramer says. He explains that plenty of studies had shown that exercise boosts the brain's functional capacities— such tasks as memory tests and the ability to count backward—but no one had investigated structural changes. So exercise actually increases the size of the brain? "That's exactly right," says Dr. Kramer. "And it doesn't take much. By walking 45 to 60 minutes, three times a week, people get measurable benefits."

Top Ways to Prevent Golf Injuries

David H. Janda, MD, director of the Institute for Preventative Sports Medicine, Ann Arbor, Michigan.

It's not exactly a dangerous game, but golf nonetheless puts many players at high risk for back trouble. Typically caused by an improper swing and/or inadequate conditioning, injury to the lower (or lumbar) back region, or the cervical spine (or neck), is common on the links. The good news, says orthopedic surgeon David H. Janda, MD, director of the Institute for Preventative Sports Medicine in Ann Arbor, Michigan, is that there are steps you can take to increase the odds you'll play through the season with nary a twinge. *Here's his advice on how to reduce the risk of a golf-related injury...*

GET CHECKED FIRST

Each year's first golf outing should be preceded by a pre-season check-up with your physician, says Dr. Janda. This is especially important if you have pre-existing health issues—including advancing age. Some older adults have an undiagnosed cardiac or lung issue that, left untreated, could make golf or any physical activity potentially risky. At this visit, it's wise to alert your doctor to muscle soreness or other sensitive areas. Do not play with injuries. Left untreated, minor soft tissue injuries can become major, possibly resulting in such problems as a herniated disc or torn muscles.

THE WARM-UP

Next, establish a conditioning program that includes stretching and strengthening in order to ease the stress golf's repetitive motions put on the lower back, upper back, and upper and lower extremities. Many fitness centers and YMCAs offer pre-season golf conditioning...or a trainer at the gym can put together a program you can do on your own. Once the season starts, make a habit of preparing for each outing with 10 to 15 minutes of simple stretches, followed by a 15- to 30-minute warm-up using your clubs. Most golfers do this by starting with long-arc strokes using a wood, but a more effective warm-up begins with small swings using a short iron, then medium strokes using a longer iron, and wrapping up with a wood to practice the big strokes. When playing, take a few minutes every half hour or so to gently twist and stretch your arms, legs and your back—tilting, bending and straightening.

DRINK UP

Dehydrated muscles are vulnerable to spasms and injury, so hydration is essential. While many choose sports drinks on the course, the best beverage for hydration is simply water (if you show no signs of dehydration) since it is free of excess sugar and other additives. On average, aim for approximately 16 ounces of water in the two-hour period before you start to play, and then sip regularly (about half a 16-ounce water bottle every 35 to 40 minutes) on the course. Though some people worry that drinking this much water will lead to lots of bathroom breaks, Dr. Janda points out that golfers lose so much water through sweat, they seldom need to go to the bathroom.

Note: Muscle spasms can be a sign of heat illness, caused by a loss of salt, electrolytes and dehydration. Stop playing and head for a clubhouse if this occurs.

A few caveats: If you take medication regularly, ask your doctor about hydration for golf. In most cases, the advice above is appropriate—but certain drugs and health conditions may require more or less fluids. In some cases, your doctor may also advise consumption of small amounts of salty snacks, to offset loss of sodium through sweating.

BAG IT

If you are strong and healthy, carrying your own clubs adds to your workout. Using a bag with wheels helps avoid back strain, while using a golf cart reduces risk of back injury even further (of course, then you'll get virtually no exercise).

Never play while in pain or injured, warns Dr. Janda. Toughing it out can make your back worse and ultimately prolong your time off the course. It's also a good idea to stretch again for another 15 minutes, after play.

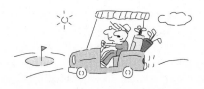

Innovative Treatment For Rotator Cuff Problems

Peter J. Millett, MD, director of shoulder surgery and partner, the Steadman-Hawkins Clinic, Vail, Colorado.

The shoulder is one of the most complicated and heavily worked joints in the body. It also has the greatest range of motion of any joint. As such, it is no surprise that it is also highly vulnerable to injury. The shoulder's rotator cuff is an important series of four muscle groups and associated tendons that connect the shoulder blade to the upper arm bone, or humerus. When the "cuff" is injured, it can become difficult, and even impossible, for a person to lift, throw, stretch or do any of the other chores assigned to the shoulder. Even getting dressed can be incredibly difficult.

COMMON ROTATOR CUFF PROBLEMS

Rotator cuff injuries are fairly common and quite painful. They can be caused by a traumatic accident such as a fall, or the repetitive-use stress that activities such as golf, tennis and other sports put on the shoulder. Job-related tasks that require reaching overhead, such as house painting, electrical work and carpentry, are other culprits. Age, too, can take a toll.

Our editors called orthopedic surgeon Peter J. Millett, MD, of the Steadman-Hawkins Clinic in Vail, Colorado, and formerly the codirector of Harvard Shoulder Service/Sports Medicine in Boston, for an update on rotator cuff injuries and treatment.

IDENTIFYING THE PAIN

Dr. Millett says that the most common rotator cuff injuries are to the tendons, both because of the stress they endure with activities that involve moving the arm, and because of the spontaneous degeneration that occurs with aging. Injuries to the rotator cuff range from inflammation and swelling of the tendon, to partial tearing, to "full-thickness" (complete) tears. The tendons can be injured in a variety of ways but one of the most common is when they become compressed between the humerus and the top part of the shoulder blade as the arm is raised overhead.

Pain at night is very common and is caused by inflammation in the area, particularly the bursa (bursitis), and by muscle spasm from the torn tendons. Another common complaint with rotator cuff injury is chronic pain that radiates down the side of the upper arm. Dr. Millett explains that this is actually called "referred pain" and comes from the nerves in the shoulder that course around the region of the tear.

DIAGNOSIS & TREATMENT

Trained orthopedists can often diagnose rotator cuff problems through physical examination and by observing the patient's mobility limitations. An MRI, which Dr. Millett says is the most accurate technology for imaging tendons, may be ordered to visualize the extent of the problem. When tears are only partial, first-line treatment may be anti-inflammatory medication (either over-the-counter such as Aleve or Advil or a prescription) along with physical therapy. Sometimes cortisone shots are used to decrease inflammation in the shoulder, but they are not a long-term fix. Unfortunately, there is little evidence that rotator cuff tears will heal spontaneously (without surgical intervention), and they certainly can progress in size over time, which leads to more functional limitations and disability. In severe cases, individuals may have severe pain and may not be able to raise their arms at all. In those whose symptoms persist, surgery is often advocated. With all such injuries, it is important to resist the temptation to return to previous activities before the recommended time, since the shoulder is particularly vulnerable to re-injury.

SURGICAL OPTIONS

While surgery for the rotator cuff is very inconvenient due to the lengthy recuperation process, in many cases it is the most predictable way to alleviate pain and restore function to the shoulder. "Rotator cuff tears do not heal spontaneously and thus require surgery to heal and to truly resolve the problem," says Dr. Millett. Rotator cuff tears have been repaired surgically for years, but the procedure used to require a large incision that was quite painful and necessitated a prolonged recovery. Now thanks to new technology, the surgery can be performed with less invasive methods.

Nationwide, many surgeries today are performed arthroscopically, with only small incisions for a tiny camera and surgical instruments. This technology has been applied to rotator cuff surgery as well. Over the last several years, Dr. Millett and others have developed innovative new surgical instruments and treatments for patients who have significant rotator cuff tears. These treatments are less painful and allow for a faster recovery. Dr. Millett performs essentially all of his surgeries this way, believing that arthroscopic repair is not only easier on the patient than traditional open surgery, but since less cutting is involved, there is also less damage to the overlying muscles with less scarring and less pain.

THE SURGERY PROCESS

Historically the best treatment for partial tears in the tendon or tendons with severe inflammation has been less clearly defined. Dr. Millett has developed a new innovative surgical treatment for these problems that is called a "marrow stimulation" or "healing response" technique, based on the fact that bone marrow contains both stem cells and growth factors. The idea is to get the stem cells and growth factors to the rotator cuff tendons to help them heal. Dr. Millett says this procedure can be performed entirely arthroscopically and as an outpatient procedure. To bring this about, Dr. Millett makes small perforations in the bone adjacent to the injured tendon, and then perforates the tendon as well. This allows the marrow, with its healing properties, to seep from the bone and stimulate repair of the tendon.

Essentially, this method triggers the body's physiological healing capabilities.

RECOVERY

Physical therapy (PT) following surgery is essential to restore full mobility and to protect the surgical repair. It's a commitment—three or four months of PT can be required to rehabilitate tendons. It's worth it, though, since it means the likelihood of complete recovery, whether from open or arthroscopic surgery, is excellent, says Dr. Millett.

To prevent rotator cuff problems initially, or to decrease the risk of a recurrent tear, Dr. Millett advises building strength through regular exercises designed for that purpose. Consult a physical therapist or trainer who is knowledgeable about the complexity of the shoulder, in order to learn specific exercises. Make sure to warm up properly and stretch before activities calling upon the shoulder joint, and don't overdo it. Avoid exercises that place the arm at extreme positions and abduction exercises with weights that require the arm to be fully extended, as these really stress the vulnerable rotator cuff tendons. Be especially careful early in the season when it comes to activities like golf or tennis. Have fun, enjoy your sport, but always use judgment and watch out for the "weekend warrior" syndrome.

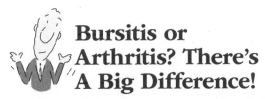

Bursitis or Arthritis? There's A Big Difference!

James V. Luck, Jr., MD, president, CEO and medical director, Orthopaedic Hospital, Los Angeles.

I t's not unusual for people to confuse bursitis and arthritis, says orthopedic surgeon James V. Luck, Jr., MD, medical director of Orthopaedic Hospital in Los Angeles. Both appear as pain in the joints and occur more frequently with age. But there's often not much you can do to cure arthritis, other than surgery, whereas bursitis can be treated and healed.

WHERE DOES BURSITIS COME FROM?

A bursa is a fluid-filled sac. These bursae or sacs are located throughout the body, wherever tendons or ligaments move across joints, to protect the bones, tendons and muscles surrounding joints from friction during movement. Sometimes, repeated pressure, overuse, acute physical stress or just age can cause bursae to become inflamed and secrete excess fluid, which pools inside. The affected area becomes painful and there may be swelling, heat or redness. While the body has more than 150 bursae, "bursitis" is most apt to develop in the elbows, hips, shoulders, knees, heels and toes.

WAYS TO IDENTIFY BURSITIS—HIP

Starting with bursitis of the hip (*trochanteric bursitis*), Dr. Luck says the easiest way to distinguish it from arthritis is usually by the location of the discomfort. Arthritic pain typically starts in the hip joint, which is found near the groin, at the midpoint on the crease between the thigh and the pelvic area. It may then move into the leg and sometimes even the knee, leading many patients to think the problem is there, says Dr. Luck. With hip bursitis, on the other hand, the pain is usually felt on the large bony protrusion of the upper outer thigh. It is sometimes referred to as the "hip bone," and more accurately called the greater *trochanter*. This is where the uppermost part of the thighbone juts out, along with muscles, tendons and, of course, bursae. Hip bursitis is most often triggered by long periods of sitting, standing or frequent bending from the hips. Most physicians feel physical deconditioning (loss of physical fitness) contributes as well.

ELBOW

Bursitis of the elbow (*olecranon bursitis*) develops in the back side of the elbow, where one often leans on things.

Inflammation of that bursal sac is tender to the touch, and creates a great deal of excess fluid and usually considerable swelling that feels like a balloon sitting under the skin. Infection occurs easily with elbow bursitis, says Dr. Luck. The inflammation is so near the surface of the skin that even a small cut can allow bacteria to enter and infect—making it very important to seek medical care for this bursitis. People most at risk are students (especially older ones) and those who bend their arm back and forth in work or for sports such as tennis and golf.

SHOULDER

Heavy use of the shoulder, for sports or work, puts people at risk for bursitis located there. This can be more complex, though, because it frequently appears in tandem with inflammation of the tendons—a combination referred to as impingement syndrome. The resulting pain radiates through the shoulder and is difficult to differentiate from arthritis, says Dr. Luck. One way to tell if pain is caused by bursitis is by raising the affected arm from the sides…if that causes pain, it is likely bursitis. (The converse is also true—pain moving the arm forward and back indicates the problem is more likely arthritis.) Complicating the picture further, there is often a concomitant rotator cuff tear (a tear in the shoulder's tendon and muscle group) since such tears, which are more common as people age, are often the trigger for bursitis. In contrast, arthritis of the shoulder would cause pain over a larger area and range of movement.

KNEE

Bursitis in the knee can flare in two different locations. *Prepatellar bursitis* is when the bursa overlying the kneecap can fill, feeling extremely swollen and spongy, says Dr. Luck. A bursa in the back of the knee (called a Baker's Cyst) can also fill with fluid, but in this case the fluid may be coming from the knee as well as the bursa itself. With this type of bursitis an MRI is needed to determine whether the knee is the real underlying source of the problem, in which case a different treatment plan is recommended.

TREATMENT FOR BURSITIS

Assuming there is no other injury that calls for medical attention (as may be the case in the shoulder or knee) most bursitis can be treated in the short term at home with R-I-C-E—that's Rest, Ice, Compression and Elevation. Consult your physician as to how to best use these strategies. Over-the-counter nonsteroidal anti-inflammatory drugs (NSAIDs) can help reduce both inflammation and pain. As always, you want to take the lowest dose possible and be alert to side effects.

For best healing, once the diagnosis of bursitis is confirmed, it is also crucial to build muscle strength with exercising. However, Dr. Luck advises patients to seek out a physical therapist or ask their physician about the correct exercises and ergonomic adjustments, since the wrong ones can do more harm than good. If these efforts fail to resolve the discomfort, your doctor may advise a corticosteroid shot to suppress the inflammation. If this doesn't work, excess fluid from the bursa can be drained with a syringe, which usually provides short-term relief and helps it heal. In extremely persistent cases, the inflamed bursa can be removed surgically, a short, relatively routine procedure, allowing the body to better heal the inflamed area.

PREVENTION IS THE BEST MEDICINE

Fortunately, there are things you can do to keep from getting bursitis. Keep your body strong with regular, low-impact aerobic exercise, but be careful—both at work and playing sports—to avoid overusing any joints. Stretching exercises are also important. Cushion joints that you lean or sit on, i.e., the elbows and buttocks, not only for comfort but to prevent irritation surrounding the bursae. In the event that you develop bursitis anyway, identify the activity that is the likely culprit and figure out what changes you can make to stay bursitis-free in the future.

Are Low-Cal Diets Bad for Your Bones?

Dennis T. Villareal, MD, associate professor of medicine at Washington University School of Medicine in St. Louis.

Here's a conundrum—we've long known that weight-bearing exercise is critical to maintaining bone mass, especially in post-menopausal women who no longer produce as much bone-protective estrogen. And of course, we know it's unhealthy to be overweight. Ironically, by carrying excess weight, overweight people perform "built-in" weight-bearing exercise in their daily activities, which in this case is actually beneficial to them. Does this mean that dieting—and having less weight for the bones to carry around all day—might reduce bone mass compared with weight loss from exercise?

STUDY SPECIFICS

This was the question Dennis T. Villareal, MD, associate professor of medicine at the Washington University School of Medicine in St. Louis, explored in a recent study of 30 women and 18 men, having a mean age of 57. Dr. Villareal assigned 19 participants to a diet that reduced calories by 16% for three months, and then reduced calories further to 20% for the following nine months...19 others had no dietary change but began an exercise program that expended 16% more calories for three months, and then escalated to 20% for the subsequent nine months. Ten participants did neither, but were offered general health information about the importance of eating right.

Results at the end of the year: Those in the calorie-restricted group lost an average of 18.1 pounds...while those in the exercise group lost on average 14.8 pounds. However, the calorie-restricted group also lost 2.2% bone density in the lower spine and hip and 2.1% at the very top end of the femur (the thigh bone), all high-risk fracture areas—while no one in the exercise group had any significant change in bone mineral density.

BONE TURNOVER

Dr. Villareal says that people in the exercise group did mostly aerobic exercise, including biking and walking and jogging. And they did a lot of it—six days a week for approximately an hour or a little over an hour each day. Interestingly, both weight-loss groups had an increased rate of bone turnover—usually an indicator of old bone being broken down and new bone developing. However, in the calorie restriction group, a marker indicating bone formation was lower, suggesting an imbalance in the bone turnover process after calorie restriction.

NEW BONE PRODUCTION

Dr. Villareal explains that bone turnover was actually more balanced among the exercisers, which means they had proper new bone creation. Regular exercise causes muscles to pull on bones, and it is believed that the strain stimulates new bone production. Consequently, bone turnover among exercisers is old bone being replaced by new, rather than simply lost mass.

Bottom line: To protect bone health during a weight-loss program, be sure exercise is on your daily menu.

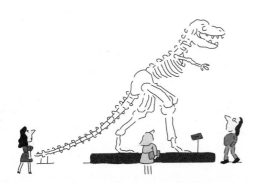

Speed Healing for Broken Bones

Susan E. Brown, PhD, certified nutrition specialist, director, the Osteoporosis Education Project, East Syracuse, New York.

Mark A. Stengler, ND, naturopathic physician in private practice, La Jolla, California…adjunct associate clinical professor at the National College of Natural Medicine, Portland, Oregon…author of many books, including *The Natural Physician's Healing Therapies* and coauthor of *Prescription for Natural Cures* (both from Bottom Line Books)…and author of the *Bottom Line/Natural Healing* newsletter.

Broken bones take many weeks, sometimes months, to heal. Is there anything people can do to mend broken bones faster?

REMODELING

The skeletal system has functions beyond serving as the frame upon which our bodies hang. Our bones are constantly busy with self-renewing cellular activity (a process called *remodeling*). Bones are hard, it seems, but that's actually only true of the outer shell, comprised mainly of calcium and phosphorous, and which serves as the body's storehouse for calcium, a mineral vital for regulating many body systems.

The spongy interior bone tissue, called the matrix, contains blood vessels, several types of cells and marrow, which produces both red and white blood cells.

FUEL FOR REPAIR

This complicated system uses energy, of course. We need the right fuel at all times, says Susan Brown, PhD, certified nutrition specialist, director of the Osteoporosis Education Project in East Syracuse, New York. But when our bones take on the added task of having to repair themselves, nutrition becomes even more important. Mending a fracture puts the metabolism into overdrive. Dr. Brown says that some experts suggest people with broken bones require as many as 6,000 calories a day for fracture mending. When endogenous stores of nutrients are scavenged, fluids collect as a replacement, often minimizing weight loss but compromising structure and function. You may not want or need to consume that many calories each day, but Dr. Brown stresses that this is definitely not the time for a weight-loss diet. She suggests boosting protein intake, which not only helps you feel better, but also promotes healing (fracture healing in the hip, for example, requires at least 20 grams of protein a day, she says).

IF IT'S A FRACTURE

If you feel sharp pain at the trauma site—especially when pressing upon or touching it—suspect fracture. If it is fractured, it should always be evaluated by your doctor, who will determine whether the fracture needs to be set, and if you should have any kind of cast or supportive garment. He/she will also give you instructions about activity restriction, and in many cases suggest physical therapy after the break has healed.

YOUR HIGH-POTENCY HEALING PROGRAM

In the meantime, kick off your own high-potency healing program. *How to supercharge your system with nutrients to maximize your healing power…*

•**Calcium,** of course, is a must, but absorption can be a challenge. Mark Stengler, ND, often prescribes 500 milligrams (mg) to 600 mg of calcium (look for formulations with citrate, citrate-malate, chelate or hydroxyapatite) twice daily, with meals, for best absorption. He counsels eating calcium-containing foods as well, including green leafy vegetables, nuts, molasses, salmon, oysters, sardines with the bones, broccoli and unsweetened yogurt with live, active cultures.

•**Vitamin D** is an important ingredient in maximizing calcium absorption. The usual prescription for vitamin D is 400 international units (IU) to 600 IU daily, but to boost bone healing, Dr. Stengler may prescribe a higher range of 1,000 IU to 2,000 IU per day.

•**Magnesium** is yet another nutrient that is always important, but it's especially critical for mending bone injuries. It's a requirement for proper calcium metabolism and bone formation, notes Dr. Stengler, adding that some experts consider magnesium as important as calcium. He prescribes 500 mg to 750 mg daily. Your physician will probably prescribe magnesium in conjunction with calcium.

OTHER NUTRIENTS

Two other important nutrients are phosphorous and vitamin K, but your decision to take these particular supplements, as with those above, should be discussed with your doctor. Phosphorous is generally adequate in our diet, says Dr. Brown…if you under-eat or are quite elderly, you may need to supplement. Recommended daily intake through diet is 700 mg. Vitamin K is important in forming a protein called *osteocalcin* that attracts calcium into the bone matrix, says Dr. Stengler. Foods that contain vitamin K include collard greens, kale and romaine lettuce. Though the standard vitamin K recommendation is 120 micrograms (mcg) for men and 90 mcg for women, the therapeutic dose prescribed for fracture patients is 500 mcg to 2 mg daily. Importantly, anyone taking a blood-thinning medication such as *warfarin* (Coumadin) must not take supplemental vitamin K (though dietary sources are okay under medical supervision).

ALSO HELPFUL

In addition to these macronutrients, your body continues to need vitamins C, B-6, B-12 and a number of micronutrients and trace minerals such as copper, manganese, boron, silica and zinc. Often a high-potency multivitamin may help to partially address your individual needs. At the table, fermented soy goods (such as miso, natto, tempeh and fermented tofu) are beneficial to bone health. Also, essential fatty acids found in walnuts, almonds, flaxseeds and fish are helpful.

Lastly, this is a time when cigarettes cause even more harm than usual—studies have shown that it takes smokers on average two months longer to heal a broken bone than those who do not smoke.

HANDS-ON HELP

Dr. Stengler reports that many of his patients find acupuncture helpful in promoting healing and reducing pain. But he has another technique—even easier and completely free—that you can do at home to help heal your fracture. This requires putting alternating hot and cold towels on the body part *opposite* the injury. (For example, the towels go on the left arm if the right arm is broken.) Start by applying the hot towel for two minutes, followed by the cold one for two more minutes. Repeat three times, twice daily. What this does, he explains, is trigger a reflex action that increases circulation in the opposite body part. That, in turn, directs all those excellent nutrients you are now getting into the broken bone, to maximize healing.

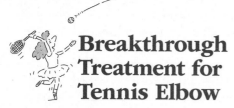

Breakthrough Treatment for Tennis Elbow

Allan Mishra, MD, of the Menlo Medical Clinic at Stanford University Medical Center, Menlo Park, California, *www.apexprp.com.*

Tennis elbow is an especially stubborn condition and an extremely painful one. Tennis elbow can go away after a few months (with or without treatment), but for some people the problem recurs and can become chronic. Treatment has traditionally consisted of rest, nonsteroidal anti-inflammatory drugs (NSAIDs) such as Advil or Motrin, wearing a brace, and physical therapy—with corticosteroid injections as a last nonsurgical resort. If all else fails, patients can have surgery to repair the damaged tendon, though surgery is not always successful. There may be new hope on the horizon, however, according to orthopedic surgeon Allan Mishra, MD, of the Menlo Medical Clinic at Stanford University Medical Center in Menlo Park, California. Dr. Mishra has successfully treated tennis elbow in some patients by injecting them with platelet-rich plasma, a component of their own blood.

WHAT PLATELET TREATMENT IS

If early success is confirmed, this remarkably simple approach may someday become the treatment of choice. Dr. Mishra says that platelet-rich plasma has been used to augment bone grafting during oral and maxillofacial surgery. His practice primarily treats soft tissue injuries such as ligament or tendon tears. He wondered if platelet-rich plasma could be useful for these types of problems. After considerable research, Dr. Mishra tested his theory by conducting a study with 20 patients with severe tennis elbow, none of whom had improved with extensive and prolonged nonsurgical treatment. These patients had suffered from tennis elbow for about 15 months and judged their pain as "severe" (a mean score of 82 on a scale of 100 as maximum pain).

For the study, Dr. Mishra took blood from each of the patients and sent each donation to a lab to isolate the platelets. Fifteen of the patients later received injections of a plasma suspension that contained their own platelets. The remaining five received an anesthetic injection.

To encourage absorption of the platelets, each tendon was injected six times with a total of one-half teaspoon of protein-rich plasma directly at that site, allowing the platelets to seep in. The entire procedure takes about half an hour. Afterward, patients were required to rest through the following day and then to start a stretching program. Two weeks later, they started a program to strengthen the arm. All patients were tested at four and eight weeks and again at six months.

IMPRESSIVE RESULTS

At eight weeks after the initial injection, the patients treated with the platelet preparation reported a 60% reduction in their pain compared with a 16% reduction in the control group. This reduction was statistically significant. Improvement continued in the platelet group. When these patients were evaluated at six months, they had approximately 81% less pain. Two years later, most of these patients reported complete satisfaction, all having returned to normal daily activities, with 94% once again active in work or sports.

WHY DOES IT WORK?

Dr. Mishra hypothesizes that the process works because growth factors in the platelets signal the need to bring new repair to the area. Observing that a few days following the platelet injection, patients reported that the surrounding area became warm and swollen, he postulates that the body may have circulated bone-marrow derived stem cells there, which would also facilitate ongoing repair. Since this procedure uses their own blood, rejection is not an issue and there have been no serious side effects reported.

MORE TRIALS NEEDED

But Dr. Mishra emphasizes that the procedure is still experimental. To confirm its long-term efficacy, national trials are under way to further evaluate this promising technique.

Bounce Back Faster After Joint Replacement

Daniel Rooks, PhD, assistant professor of medicine in the division of rheumatology, Beth Israel Deaconess Medical Center, a teaching hospital of Harvard Medical School in Boston.

Want to improve your joint replacement surgery experience and possibly get home sooner after surgery? Exercise regularly before surgery. That's the news from a recent study that found that contrary to what some osteoarthritis patients assume, an exercise program is not only possible, it may actually make a significant difference both before and after joint replacement surgery.

STUDY FORMAT

Daniel Rooks, PhD, assistant professor of medicine in the division of rheumatology at the Beth Israel Deaconess Medical Center in Boston, was the lead study author. He explains that they divided 108 patients with severe osteoarthritis—scheduled for either hip or knee joint replacement surgery—into one of two groups. Starting six weeks prior to surgery, one group of patients began to exercise three times a week, initially in the water and then switching to a land-based program. A research physical therapist tailored the exercise program to an individual's fitness and physical needs. The exercise program included strength training, aerobic and flexibility activities. The 54 members of the control group received the usual educational material but no physical training.

The results: Exercisers having hip replacement surgery improved their function and pain scores before surgery. Patients in the exercise group, both hip and knee replacement patients, increased leg strength by an average of 18% to 20% (leg-press scores) pre-surgery. Post-surgery, the exercise group reduced the odds of being discharged directly to a rehabilitation facility rather than going home by 73%. Similarly, 76% of the exercisers were able to walk 50 feet on the third day post-surgery compared with 61% of nonexercisers.

Another bonus: Dr. Rooks says that patients who exercised reported being well prepared mentally for their rehabilitation. This was in part because they were no longer afraid of exercise and they understood from first-hand experience how important it was.

TAILOR PROGRAM, GET STARTED

Dr. Rooks points out that this study demonstrates how even people with advanced osteoarthritis can benefit from an appropriate exercise program. However, with osteoarthritis you must have an exercise program tailored to your needs, he says. Ask your doctor for a referral to a physical therapist or specially trained fitness professional who can give you specific guidelines about what to do, how much and how often and how to determine progression. Your local Arthritis Foundation chapter is a good source for this information. It is also critical to find the types of exercise you most enjoy doing. That will help you keep up exercise as a life-long investment in health and better joints. Keep in mind that it takes time to build the kind of strength and flexibility that can be helpful. He urges everyone, whether with mild or more advanced osteoarthritis, to get started on it today.

Get Rid of Back Pain Without Surgery

Norman J. Marcus, MD, founder, Norman Marcus Pain Institute, New York City, past president, American Academy of Pain Medicine, and author of *Freedom From Pain*. Fireside. Dr. Marcus was voted one of New York City's Best Doctors for multiple years by *New York* magazine. You can visit his Web site at *www.backpainusa.com.*

Agency for Healthcare Research and Quality (AHRQ), *www.ahrq.gov.*

Andrew L. Rubman, ND, consulting medical editor for *Bottom Line's Daily Health News* and director of the Southbury Clinic for Traditional Medicines in Southbury, Connecticut

The conventional approach to treating some medical conditions is often more dependent on what's popular or traditional than what's based on evidence.

Case in point: Spinal fusion. Each year, about 325,000 of these back operations are carried out at an average cost of $50,000, when there is no significant evidence that they ease pain any more effectively than a combination of low-tech, low-cost and less risky approaches.

THE LOW-TECH APPROACH TO BACK PAIN

The spinal procedures themselves are risky. Some backfire and leave patients in even greater pain than before. Exercise, physical therapy and good ergonomics (designing your environment to protect the body from further injury) may be equally effective treatments, depending on the cause.

We asked New York City pain specialist Norman J. Marcus, MD how to address and prevent back pain. He says that in many cases, back pain is caused by improper body mechanics during heavy lifting, repetitive motion activities, awkward stances or sitting at poorly designed work stations (e.g., when you have to tilt your neck up to see your computer monitor, or rest your wrists against a hard desk).

WHAT YOU CAN DO

According to Dr. Marcus, simple, basic safety precautions will go a long way toward protecting your spine, back, neck and shoulders...

One of the best ways to protect your back is to maintain proper posture. Make sure that you stand so the spine's three natural C-shaped curves—inward cervical (neck) and lumbar (lower back) curves, and outward thoracic (mid-back) curves are maintained. *What to do...*

•**Keep your head up straight, chin in, shoulders back and chest forward.**

•**Avoid slouching, and do not lock or hyperextend** (straighten beyond normal range) your knees. In other words, if you do this, keep your knees slightly bent.

•**Distribute body weight evenly over both feet.**

At work or at the computer...

•**Use a proper chair with good lower back support.**

•**Make sure your work surface is at a comfortable height.** Dr. Marcus recommends that your desk chair be high enough so your arms at the elbow create a greater than 90 degree angle.

●**If you work at a computer,** you should be reaching down to the keyboard. The monitor should be straight ahead (never to the side) at eye level or slightly below.

●**When sitting for prolonged periods,** rest your feet comfortably on the floor or on a low stool.

●**Every half hour or so,** get up, stretch and walk around.

●**If you're on the phone a great deal,** use a headset. A wireless headset is even better, since it allows you to move around.

●**Avoid standing for long periods of time.** If you must do so, rest one foot on a low stool to keep the back from arching.

●**Wear comfortable, well-fitting, low-heeled shoes.**

On the road...

●**Move the seat close to the steering wheel** to support the curve of your back and allow your feet to easily reach the pedals.

●**When driving long distances,** put a pillow or rolled-up towel behind the small of your back.

●**Take periodic breaks** in which you get out of the car for a few minutes, stretch and walk around.

At night...

●**Choose a moderately firm mattress,** not too soft and not too firm.

●**Try sleeping on your back with a pillow under your knees,** or on your side with your knees bent and a pillow between your knees. (Sleeping on your stomach is often uncomfortable for many.)

●**Avoid reading or watching TV while lying in bed,** says Dr. Marcus. Sit up; it puts less strain on the neck muscles.

●**If you feel stiff when you get up in the morning,** Dr. Marcus notes that the sooner you start moving around, the better you will feel.

When you lift heavy objects...

●**Practice proper body mechanics.** When you lift heavy things, let the quadriceps muscles in the front of the thighs do the work, advises Dr. Marcus. Don't bend over and use your back muscles to carry or lift a load.

●**Before lifting,** face the object and bend your knees, keeping your back straight.

●**As you stand up and lift,** hold the object close to your body. Holding objects away from the body puts more load on the spine.

●**As you rise,** stand upright without twisting.

●**If the object is very heavy,** ask for help.

●**Use a backpack to tote your belongings.** Using a traditional one-shoulder bag places strain on your back. It's better to distribute the weight evenly across your back.

LOOK BEFORE YOU LEAP

Before you resort to drastic solutions such as surgery, be sure to thoroughly investigate less invasive approaches to back pain. In addition to ergonomic adjustments, consider the Kraus exercise program, designed by Hans Kraus, MD, the back doctor for President Kennedy. The exercises are designed to produce minimal strength and flexibility in the key postural muscles by sequentially teaching relaxation, limbering, stretching and only then strengthening. You can find these exercises on Dr. Marcus' Web site, *www.back painusa.com.* When in doubt (or in pain), a physical therapist can help you design a safe and effective program.

Bottom Line's Daily Health News consulting medical editor, Andrew L. Rubman, ND, adds that it is important to check if the source of your back pain might actually be in your hips or pelvis. In his over 25 years of practice, 75% of lower back problems that he has treated involved hip or pelvic bone misalignment.

Most important: Think twice before agreeing to back surgery. Odds are you may not need it.

Heal Headaches (Even Migraines) Without Drugs

Mark V. Wiley, OMD, PhD, editorial manager and health consultant, The Healthy Back Institute, Gaithersburg, Maryland, *www.losethebackpain.com*. Dr. Wiley is author of 10 books including *Outwitting Headaches*. Lyons.

Mark A. Stengler, ND, naturopathic physician in private practice, La Jolla, California...adjunct associate clinical professor at the National College of Natural Medicine, Portland, Oregon...author of many books, including *The Natural Physician's Healing Therapies* and coauthor of *Prescription for Natural Cures* (both from Bottom Line Books)...and author of the *Bottom Line/Natural Healing* newsletter.

National Institute of Neurological Disorders and Stroke, Headache Information page, *www.ninds.nih.gov/disorders/headache/headache.htm*.

Not all headaches are the same. Of the approximately 45 million Americans who suffer from chronic, recurring headaches, each have symptoms and headache triggers that differ. The most common are tension headaches, a catchall term for diffuse, mild to moderate pain over the head. Next come migraines, afflicting 13% of Americans with symptoms such as nausea, pain around the eye, aura and throbbing in the temple area. Makers of *ibuprofen* (Advil, Motrin), *naproxen* (Aleve), among others, love headaches, because these nonsteroidal anti-inflammatory drugs (NSAIDs) are generally the first-line defense in the multi-billion dollar headache market. However, as we all now know, NSAIDs come with significant risk when used regularly. What are better, safer options?

THE MIND/BODY APPROACH

To learn more about headaches and how to cope with them, we spoke with Mark V. Wiley, OMD, PhD, and author of *Outwitting Headaches* (Lyons). He says that it is not the particular label you put on a headache that is important. Taking a multi-pronged approach to returning your body to its natural, balanced state is preferable—the state in which headaches are less likely to occur. After suffering from painful migraines himself for 27 years, he developed the following integrated mind/body approach to preventing headaches of all kinds.

IDENTIFY AND AVOID HEADACHE TRIGGERS

It is not normal to have headache after headache. You need to take action to break this destructive pattern, Dr. Wiley stresses. In his view, the key to ending headache pain is proactive avoidance of its causes rather than reactive treatment of symptoms. Major headache triggers include chemicals in food and beverages and even toxins in the body and air, dehydration, lack of exercise, as well as the stress you harbor and the sleep you miss. In order to reestablish what he calls cellular balance, he says that one must remove the toxins and stressors that tax the body, or learn to deal with them in new ways. For most people, this means a major lifestyle change.

What you can do: Start by looking at your diet. Eat more fresh and fewer processed foods. Also, try eliminating suspected food triggers one by one from your diet for two to three weeks, and monitor what happens with your headaches. Common culprits include cheeses such as Brie, feta and Gorgonzola, pickles, chocolate, dairy products (from goats as well as cows), alcohol (beware the notorious "red wine headache"), processed meats (bologna, pepperoni, salami, hot dogs, etc.), onions, nuts, raisins and products that contain MSG, aspartame or tyramine.

DRINK PLENTY OF WATER

When we become dehydrated, the digestive system, lungs, liver and kidneys can no longer do their jobs as effectively, and this can lead to a headache.

What you can do: Drink plenty of water every day to help your body clear hazardous chemical residues and toxic buildup. Water cleanses the colon, flushes the liver and kidneys and empties the bowels. Dr. Wiley recommends two quarts of bottled or filtered water daily, and cautions that caffeinated coffees and teas, carbonated sodas and sugar-filled fruit drinks and diet drinks don't count toward that total.

HOW TO BREAK STRESS PATTERNS

Stress, in its many forms, is a leading cause of headaches, Dr. Wiley observes. So, to control headaches, you must break the pattern of stress. There are many ways to go about doing this.

To reduce tension and tightness in the shoulders, neck and back, which can lead to a headache, see a massage therapist or do daily gentle stretches. A chiropractor can work with misalignments which can occur as a result of constantly tensed muscles…and acupuncture does wonders for keeping energy levels balanced. Dr. Wiley also recommends meditation and deep breathing to quiet the mind and relax the body's nervous system. Others benefit from tai chi, yoga, qigong or other gentle exercises that stretch the body and soothe the soul. Taking a multiple B vitamin, at least twice daily, also helps fight the stress reflex. For many people, a magnesium supplement may be useful as well.

Dr. Wiley recommends an exercise for progressive relaxation.

What to do: Lie down comfortably with your arms at your sides, and inhale as you tense your toes. Hold for a moment, and then exhale as you consciously relax them. Gradually and slowly continue up the rest of the body, mindfully tensing and relaxing the feet, calves, thighs, etc., as you inhale and exhale.

TAKE A DEEP BREATH

In addition to stress relief, deep breathing ensures a continuous flow of fresh oxygen into the body. Many people breathe shallowly, which can limit the amount of oxygen that goes to tissue.

GET SUFFICIENT SLEEP

Some people get cranky and headachy when they don't get enough sleep. To prevent headaches, it's essential to establish deep and constant sleep patterns.

What you can do: Avoid caffeine and overly stimulating activities such as intense exercise six hours before bed. Stop working at the computer at least an hour or more before bed. Instead, establish a regular, soothing routine, such as a warm bath and a good book before retiring. (As long as it is not a thriller, which can overstimulate and cause sleeplessness.)

Side sleeping is the best sleeping position if done correctly. To begin, side posture should mimic the fetal position. That is, both knees bent, and hands held close to the body. This is a normal and inherent sleeping posture. A pillow should be placed under the head and pulled to the shoulder for optimal neck support. The hands should be parallel and below the eyes. To avoid hip pain while sleeping on your side, place a pillow between your knees to create proper distance between them, thus keeping the hips in proper balance. The legs must be parallel, so the hips remain square and there is no strain on the lower back. If you were not previously a side sleeper, you may be able to retrain your body by falling asleep in that position each night and then readjusting each time you wake up.

ENGAGE IN REGULAR EXERCISE

Exercise reduces stress, releases endorphins, improves blood flow, works through muscle tension and keeps the body firm and supple. Engaging in basic activities such as brisk walks and simple stretches will go a long way toward preventing headaches, as well as improving overall health.

What you can do: Exercise at the same time every day, buddy up with a friend or group for accountability and support, and consider a trainer (if only for a few sessions) to help you establish a safe, personalized program. Even very easy, do-it-yourself stretches are beneficial for headache prevention. For example, try the chin-to-chest stretch. To stretch and release tension in the shoulders and upper back, use your hands to gently push on the back of the head to press the chin toward the chest. Repeat several times daily.

WHEN HEADACHES STRIKE AND YOU NEED RELIEF

With lifestyle changes, you can hopefully reduce the frequency and severity of your headaches. Of course, on occasion a headache will arise and you may want immediate relief. Then what?

Mark Stengler, a naturopathic physician in La Jolla, California, and author of Bottom Line's print newsletter *Bottom Line Natural Healing*, suggests a number of options for immediate headache relief...

•**Mother Nature's aspirin.** Take 240 milligrams (mg) of *salicin*, the active component in white willow bark. This natural pain relieving component is the ingredient from which aspirin is derived. Do not take with NSAIDs.

•**Homeopathic medicines.** Options include *Gelsemium sempervirens* (yellow jessamine) for a dull, heavy pain at the back of the neck...*Nux Vomica* (Poison Nut) for headaches from stress...and *Pulsatilla pratensis* (pasque flower) for headaches around the menstrual cycle. For an acute headache, an average dosage consists of a 30C potency, four times daily.

•**A cup of tea.** Take a timeout with a soothing and relaxing cup of peppermint, chamomile or passion flower tea.

•**Herbal rub.** Gently massage peppermint or menthol cream into the temple area.

•**A compress.** Lie down in a darkened room and apply a compress to the painful area. Depending on the headache, some people prefer cold compresses, others warm ones.

•**Hydrotherapy.** Wrap a few ice cubes in a thin towel and apply to the back of the neck and upper back. At the same time, immerse your feet in a bucket of warm water for 10 minutes.

WHEN A HEADACHE MAY SPELL TROUBLE

While Dr. Wiley's strategy is effective for most headaches, there are times when the pain requires immediate medical attention.

According to the National Institute of Neurological Disorders and Stroke (NINDS), you should seek prompt medical care if you experience any of the following...

•**An abrupt, severe headache,** or a sudden headache associated with a stiff neck.

•**A headache associated with fever or convulsions,** or accompanied by confusion or loss of consciousness.

•**A headache following a blow to the head,** or associated with pain in the eye or ear.

•**Persistent headache in a person who was previously headache-free.**

•**Recurring headaches in children.**

New Research Proves NSAIDs Don't Help Tendinitis

Sabrina M. Strickland, MD, assistant attending orthopedic surgeon, Hospital for Special Surgery, New York City.

Tendinitis is frequently diagnosed among otherwise healthy people who play golf, tennis and other sports, or who participate in activities that require repetitive motion. Most people let the problem go for a time, even a period of many weeks, until pain becomes severe. Doctors typically then tell them they have tendinitis, an inflammation of a tendon, and to take NSAIDs (nonsteroidal anti-inflammatory drugs including *ibuprofen*, *naproxen* and others) to calm the inflammation. So it was a surprise to read an editorial from the *Clinical Journal of Sport Medicine* that reported there is seldom a reason to take NSAIDs for tendon issues.

The reason: most so-called tendinitis is actually an entirely different condition. Some experts are calling this situation "the tendinitis myth."

TENDON MYTHOLOGY

For more information, we called Sabrina M. Strickland, MD, assistant attending orthopedic surgeon at the Hospital for Special Surgery in New York City. Dr. Strickland explains that nearly all cases labeled tendinitis are in fact *tendinosis*, a condition that has nothing to do with inflammation. According to an article in the *British Medical Journal* (BMJ), animal studies show that within two to three weeks of an initial tendon injury, tendinosis is already present and inflammatory cells are absent. The problem is that many tendon injuries start out as tendinitis...however, the inflammation is not treated immediately. By waiting, the injury degrades into the damaged tissue of tendinosis. The ending "itis" refers to inflammation, but the "osis" ending means degeneration and that is what tendinosis is—degeneration of a tendon, most commonly in the elbow, knee, shoulder and/or ankle. Although some people associate age with degenerating tendons, in fact age affects only tendons in the shoulders.

MORE DIFFERENCES

In tendinitis there is redness and swelling. This is best seen in the hand or wrist, where there is little soft tissue to mask the telltale evidence. In tendinosis, which can been seen on an MRI scan, the affected area of the tendon is whitish and gray because it is dead tissue. Dr. Strickland agrees that there is no biological basis for taking NSAIDs to treat tendinosis since there is no inflammation present to reduce—although the drugs may help ease pain of tendinosis caused by the surrounding vital tissue becoming tender due to the proximal dead tissue. A better approach is to follow a plan to resolve tendinosis and its pain.

THE RIGHT WAY TO TREAT

So, if NSAIDs are the wrong way to treat tendinosis, what is the right way to treat?

According to Dr. Strickland, the first order of business when tendon pain develops is to quiet the affected area. Stop the particular activity, put ice on the joint (she recommends warmth only for muscle spasms and those are nearly always in the back) and wear a special cuff or band, found in sporting-goods stores or drug stores, just below the area. The band decreases stress on the tendon and is good for pain management as well.

Physical therapy: Interestingly, most tendon injuries are not from overusing a tendon, but from incorrect form, such as flexing the wrist incorrectly when gardening or playing tennis. Consequently, working with a coach or other expert or physical therapist on the proper physical motions to use for a given activity is crucial.

Therapists design individualized exercise programs to improve range of motion and strength. The exercise technique used recently to treat tendinosis is called *eccentric loading*, which involves stressing the muscles in the extended phase rather than the more usual contracted phase. For example, therapists may have a patient squat on the stronger leg and lift the weaker (eccentric) leg—the one being rehabilitated. Therapists also, and importantly, help refine proper techniques for patients to use in the sport or activity that caused the tendon injury in the first place.

Dr. Strickland also urges flexibility training. Interestingly, she says that if you stretch regularly, for example, with yoga, Pilates, stretch classes or others, there is no need to stretch before or after an activity. The key is to have and maintain ongoing flexibility.

Finally, strengthening exercises are good as well because building muscles around the joint will help protect it from additional stress. Again, work with a physical therapist on appropriate exercises to build the muscles around the tendons.

Dr. Strickland suggests that people follow this action plan for several weeks, but if the tendinosis hasn't resolved itself by then, check back with the doctor regarding additional steps.

Note: Doctors used to give corticosteroid shots for tendinosis, but, like with NSAIDs, these shots treat inflammation, so while they may relieve pain temporarily, they do not have any lasting affect on healing. One exception for using corticosteroid shots is in treating shoulder cuff tendinosis because bursa, fluid-filled sacs between tendons and bones that provide a slippery surface, sit atop the rotator cuff, and these often are inflamed and respond to anti-inflammation treatment—at least temporarily.

THE EUROPEAN WAY

A European technique for treating tendinosis and one that is making a few inroads in the US is *extracorporeal shock wave therapy* (ESWT), similar to what is used to break up kidney stones. In ESWT, scar tissue is broken down while creating inflammation in surrounding tissues, which in turn helps regenerate healthy tissue. Dr. Strickland says studies have shown ESWT to be effective in the elbows but not in the knees or shoulders. In any case, it is still unproven in the US and insurance companies do not pay for the procedure.

Surgery is a last-resort option for tendinosis...the doctor removes the dead part of the tissue and the body regenerates the tendon or other tendons compensate.

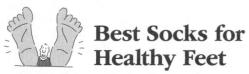

Best Socks for Healthy Feet

Howard J. Palamarchuk, DPM, assistant clinical professor, Temple University School of Podiatric Medicine, Philadelphia.

For those of you who play sports, jog or just go for walks, have you checked your socks lately? Choosing the right socks is critical—they protect your feet from blisters, infection and the like, as underscored by a recently released study.

COF AND BLISTERS

A group of biological engineering students at the University of Missouri-Columbia tested a variety of socks to determine at what point the material in each would start to slip—what's called the coefficient of friction (COF). The reason COF is important is that a high COF makes feet vulnerable to blistering, especially when moisture is present, which the students factored in by testing in a humidity chamber. The study showed that all-cotton socks, often favored as a natural product, were actually the worst.

The best: Socks that combined cotton and synthetic.

ALL-COTTON SOCKS vs. BLENDS

Howard J. Palamarchuk, DPM, assistant clinical professor at Temple University School of Podiatric Medicine in Philadelphia, has consulted for numerous marathons. He tells us that all-cotton performs poorly for two reasons. It tends to wear out and that makes it abrasive. Even more to the point, though, cotton doesn't wick moisture away from the skin and so, much like a wet cotton ball, it sits and sticks. Dr. Palamarchuk says this is why runners are most likely to blister on days that are rainy or hot and humid. The soggy sock can't slide over the skin and blisters result.

He agrees that blends of synthetic and cotton are best, though wool with synthetic is also good. The key is to have a combination of softness, good absorbency and glide. Premium socks are big business today with some costing $10 and up. Because many of them have cushioning for different parts of the foot, Dr. Palamarchuk says they are good for diabetics with circulatory problems or for marathoners. But for most people bargain socks with the proper material blend are perfectly fine.

HYGIENE HELP

Always wear clean socks. If you exercise on a hot day, wash your feet with soap and warm water and towel dry well afterward. Interestingly, do this even when you wear socks that wick. Check socks regularly and get rid of any that are starting to wear, whatever the blend.

A NOTE ON BLISTERS

Don't pop a blister yourself, but if one does burst, clean it with soap and water. Put Neosporin or Betadine ointment on it to prevent infection, and cover. If you should ever see red streaks around the blister, call the doctor immediately. Red streaks indicate the onset of an infection that can turn serious. For people who tend to blister, Blist-O-Ban (available at *www.sammedical. com*), a special type of protective bandage, can help, says Dr. Palamarchuk.

Fun Fitness For Seniors

Selene Yeager, fitness expert based in Emmaus, Pennsylvania, and author of *Selene Yeager's Perfectly Fit*. Rodale.

By now, every adult knows that exercise is a vital part of lifelong health—and that you don't get a pass because of age. But when many Americans think of exercise, they think of gyms, weights and boredom. We called Selene Yeager, author of *Selene Yeager's Perfectly Fit* (Rodale), based in Emmaus, Pennsylvania, to discuss the possibility that older adults might actually have fun while they are getting fit.

KAYAKING

Yeager's first suggestion is one that will get you to the water, but not in it—kayaking. Kayaking involves paddling a one- or two-person boat ("shell") in a continuous motion. It is becoming increasingly popular in both city and rural settings among older adults, she says, and with good reason. Kayaking is a low-impact sport so there are no injuries from pounding, and it can be done at a pace that suits the individual. It is particularly good for strengthening back and upper body muscles, making it easier to stand tall. One of the best aspects of kayaking is that since it's so much fun and generally done in scenic places, people don't realize they're getting a good workout at the same time. Yeager says some people are hesitant because the boats can roll over, but while learning to upright yourself is a necessary safety step (as is wearing a life jacket), in actuality, capsizing seldom happens. For greater comfort, select a boat that has some kind of back support and bring along small cloths, such as washcloths, to put between your knees and the boat's hard surface.

OTHER OUTDOOR OPTIONS

Some hobbies lend themselves to incorporating exercise, says Yeager. Birding, for instance, can become active if you pack your things into a backpack and walk the mile or two to various sites rather than driving.

Another popular hobby with surprising exercise rewards is gardening. Yeager says that in some studies, gardeners—because of their constant bending and lifting—had stronger bones than the runners in the same study. Gardening is also great for increased flexibility and stretching.

Hiking provides a little more adventure. It can range from scaling mountain peaks to taking a pleasant, vigorous walk. Yeager points out that there are trails of some kind in virtually every community, from local parks to wooded areas. All you need is a good pair of hiking shoes and information about where to go. Check with the Chamber of Commerce or at your town's Web site. Or go on a day's adventure to a hike in a nearby park or town.

Winter is no excuse to stay indoors. Snowshoeing is one of the best forms of exercise there is. Today's snowshoes are far removed from the tennis racquet-like footgear of old. There are a variety of types, and they all fit easily onto hiking boots. Yeager says the snow base should be at least four to six inches. As you walk along you will discover you hardly sink at all. Skating of course is another good cold-weather exercise, but Yeager doesn't advise it unless you're experienced, due to the risk of falling. This is especially important for people taking medications, such as some high blood pressure drugs, that can cause balance problems.

AND DON'T FORGET BIKING

One last outdoor activity Yeager is especially enthusiastic about for older adults is bicycling. She says that manufacturers are catering to this market because biking is easy on the joints, it is aerobic, strengthening and a whole lot of fun. A bike she particularly likes is by Electra called the Townie (*www.electrabike.com*). This model has a low seat that enables riders to put their feet easily on the ground and to sit upright, which allows them to comfortably look around. It is also a more relaxed position than the standard bending forward position of most bikes. Happily, this design does not intrude on the bike's pedaling mechanics. You may not win the Tour de France on the Townie, but you will have fun.

WHEN THE WEATHER TURNS SOUTH

What to do on those rainy days? Ballroom dancing is becoming a favorite with many older adults. Whether you decide to learn new steps—perhaps the salsa or merengue, or swing, foxtrot or quickstep—the activity is aerobic and weight bearing, so it's good for your bones. Most communities have a nearby dance school, or you can check with the YMCA, churches and senior and community centers for dance events.

Finally, Yeager says that any discussion of exercise for older adults cannot end without mention of weight work because it is absolutely crucial. Without strength training, muscle mass starts to diminish in your 30s, and after age 60, the loss escalates. But take heart, there are ways to make strength training more fun. Fitness clubs today offer a bevy of classes (and remember that Pilates and gentle yoga build strength as well as flexibility) including those that cater specifically to the older crowd.

Instead of meeting friends for lunch, Yeager suggests setting up a workout group. Hire a trainer at a club to supervise your group. This way you'll be socially active, more motivated and together you'll build the muscles you need for better living.

IF YOU'RE JUST STARTING

For those who are just getting started in the exercise world, Yeager suggests talking with your doctor to be sure you have a clean bill of health or to get information on how to accommodate any physical problems into your program. Your doctor's okay will give you peace of mind and the freedom to become more vigorous as you get stronger, more experienced and have more fun.

The Skinny on Weight-Loss Surgery

David S. Zingmond, MD, PhD, assistant professor of medicine, UCLA School of Medicine.

Nikhil V. Dhurandhar, PhD, associate professor, Pennington Biomedical Research Center, Louisiana State University System, Baton Rouge.

Weight-loss surgery may seem like a good way to help morbidly obese people who are unable to lose weight through conventional means to stay out of the hospital in the long run. But that assumption may not be true, it turns out. A study recently published in the *Journal of the American Medical Association* showed that California adults who underwent the *Roux-en-Y gastric bypass* (RYGB) surgery, the most common type of weight-loss surgery, had twice the rate of hospitalization in the year following surgery than they had in the year before surgery. What's more, RYGB patients who were followed for three years spent roughly $20,000 on post-surgical hospitalizations in addition to the surgery's $33,000 tab. That's sobering news—for both patients and insurers.

RECENT STATISTICS

Gastric bypass surgeries promote weight loss by restricting food intake and reducing the amounts of calories and nutrients the body absorbs. After RYGB surgery, patients can lose roughly 60% to 70% of their excess weight and enjoy improvements in chronic conditions such as diabetes, high cholesterol, high blood pressure and obstructive sleep apnea.

On the downside, patients may experience nutritional deficiencies and digestive problems, and, as the California study found, about 20% of patients go back into the hospital for surgery-related complications, such as ventral hernia repair or gastric revision.

To qualify for gastric bypass surgery, a person must have a body mass index (BMI) of 40 or more (about 100 pounds overweight for men and 80 pounds overweight for women) or a BMI between 35 and 39.9 and a serious obesity-related health problem, such as diabetes, heart disease or sleep apnea. Deciding whether the surgery's risks outweigh the potential health benefits gets a little more complicated when recognizing the potential for additional health problems and hospitalizations, not to mention the extra costs.

HEALTH BENEFITS
VERSUS SURGICAL RISKS

To get some background on the matter, we spoke with the study's lead author, David S. Zingmond, MD, PhD, of the University of California, Los Angeles, who with his colleagues examined data from about 60,000 patients who underwent RYGB surgery in California. The average age of the patients in the study was 42...84% were female. Of those patients followed either for one year or for three, about 20% were readmitted within a year of surgery. (About 8% of the patients in these two groups had been admitted in the year before surgery for obesity-related reasons.)

Should people take these findings to mean they shouldn't have the surgery? Dr. Zingmond says no. "The message isn't, 'Don't get the surgery. You're not going to derive health benefits.' It's, 'If you have the surgery, there's a good chance you will be rehospitalized after the procedure. Be ready for it.'"

Dr. Zingmond pointed out that weight-loss surgery, like any surgery, carries risks. So the question is, are the potential benefits of surgery worth those risks?

INCREASING CHANCES
FOR SUCCESS

It's obviously preferable if you can lose weight without surgery. But people who decide to undergo gastric bypass surgery can improve their chances for a better outcome by picking an experienced surgeon, Dr. Zingmond says. They can also maximize the effectiveness of the surgery by finding a surgical program that involves dietary changes and behavioral help in the year before surgery. Although these, he adds, won't decrease the risk for surgical complications, they will improve the patient's physical state in preparation for the surgery.

GO LAPAROSCOPIC?

Another option is laparoscopic bypass surgery, in which surgeons use smaller incisions. Laparoscopic procedures result in less tissue damage and blood loss, shorter hospitalization, a faster recovery and fewer complications than open surgery. But laparoscopic procedures aren't right for everyone. Once again, be sure you choose a doctor and hospital well-experienced in the procedure.

Dr. Zingmond says that we don't have many years of significant data with regard to the safety and effectiveness of weight-loss surgeries. "We don't know what's going to happen in another 15 years to people who undergo the surgery," he told me.

OBESITY IS NOT A SIMPLE ISSUE

Nikhil V. Dhurandhar, PhD, obesity researcher and associate professor at Pennington Biomedical Research Center at Louisiana State University wants people to understand that obesity is not simply a matter of willpower deficiency. "There are multiple causes for obesity—hormonal, genetic, viral and environmental. The problem is," he says, "conventional doctors treat all overweight and obese people the same way—with diet and exercise. These can be effective at getting weight off but they aren't effective enough at keeping it off. We need to determine the causes of obesity and offer treatment directed to each cause."

As evidence, Dr. Dhurandhar points to his own research, which showed that a person infected with the human adenovirus, AD-36, which increases the number of fat cells in people, is more likely to be overweight or obese. "There are people who gain weight easily and then some who don't," he says. Of course, these exceptions are not what is underlying the obesity epidemic in the US today, nor are the majority of people who are opting for gastric bypass surgery suffering from these unusual conditions.

TAKE A TEAM APPROACH

Dr. Dhurandar notes that people who take a team approach to weight loss are more successful at losing weight and keeping it off. Often, weight-loss clinics at universities, hospitals and wellness spas provide a team of experts—physicians (conventional and/or naturopathic), dietitians, nutritionists, exercise physiologists and psychologists—plus support groups.

But for people who aren't able to visit a clinic? Make your own team, Dr. Dhurandhar advises. Get help from a family doctor, who can refer you to other experts. Hire a personal trainer, even for a few sessions. Visit a registered dietitian or take a nutrition class (many hospitals and adult schools offer them). Join a gym or a Y, or find an exercise class. Join a weight-loss group. Buddy up with committed friends who have the same goals. Don't try to go it alone.

Done right, you won't need to weigh the risks versus the rewards of gastric bypass surgery.

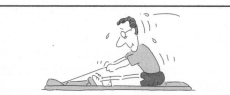

Can Sit-Ups Heal a Skinned Knee?

Charles F. Emery, PhD, professor of psychology, Ohio State University, Columbus.

Whether it is a cut from a kitchen knife or a surgical incision, the faster a wound heals, the better. But as people age, wound healing slows. Researchers at Ohio State University have identified a very unique source of healing help—exercise.

The study, led by Charles F. Emery, PhD, professor of psychology at Ohio State University in Columbus, included 28 healthy adults, average age 61, who had not exercised for at least the prior six months and who perceived themselves as not stressed. One half of the group started a workout program that consisted of 75 minutes of warm-up, cool-down, aerobic and strength exercises, three times a week, while the others continued to be sedentary. A month later, all participants received a tiny puncture wound in their upper arm that was then monitored for its rate of healing. The study also measured participants' levels of the stress hormone cortisol both before and after a stress test conducted prior to the study and again at the study's completion.

THE RESULTS

Exercisers healed faster, in 29 days versus 39 for the nonexercisers. Doctors were not surprised to see that exercise sped healing, given that it typically increases nutrients to and wastes from the site, but the second finding concerning changes in cortisol levels was quite another story. Exercise normally causes an immediate rise in cortisol levels, but after the initial stress test, neither groups' cortisol levels rose. This peculiar result indicates that age slows the body's ability to regulate cortisol. Such a dysregulation would indeed hinder healing because cortisol plays a role in increasing the efficiency of the immune system. After the post-study stress test, cortisol levels did increase in the exercise group. Dr. Emery says that this finding leads them to believe that exercise enhances cortisol regulation and seems to combat even the natural decline of regulation that comes with age. This also offers further evidence that exercise enhances wound healing.

Although the exercise group partook in vigorous activity, Dr. Emery says that doing less more often would likely be equally beneficial for healing. He advises the usual recommendation of 30 minutes a day, most days of the week.

An Exercise Program For Every Attitude

Wayne Westcott, PhD, fitness research director, South Shore YMCA, Quincy, Massachusetts. Dr. Westcott is author or coauthor of 20 books, including *Strength Training Past 50*. Human Kinetics. He is a consultant to many national groups, including the American Senior Fitness Association.

P ilates...yoga...aerobics...stairmaster...treadmill...jogging...water aerobics—the list of exercise options goes on and on. For people who are starting an exercise program, it is easy to get discouraged if they pick a program that doesn't work well for them. Once discouraged, it may be bye-bye exercise.

NO "ONE SIZE FITS ALL"

When it comes to weight loss, we all have different "diet and exercise personalities." And if there's one mantra that virtually every fitness professional has come to embrace, it's the one that says, "no one program works for everyone." One size simply doesn't fit all. What works for your neighbor may not work for you, and what your neighbor hates most may be number one on your own personal hit parade. So, how do we choose the right diet and exercise program for our own personal situation?

"There are a number of ways to accomplish weight loss," Wayne Westcott, PhD, a researcher in the field of exercise, explains. How you approach weight loss depends on your exercise attitude, of which there are several types.

•**Attitude Type One:** "I hate to exercise." *If this is your attitude, Dr. Westcott makes these recommendations...*

Diet: Reduced-calorie diet (typically 1,600 calories or less per day for women, 1,800 for men).

Strength training: Only two times per week, 15 minutes per session (see strength training circuit below for specifics).

Aerobic exercise: Only two times per week, 15 minutes per session (aerobics can be anything that gets the heart rate up to 50% to 75% of maximum heart rate for your age—running, jogging, walking, swimming, step class, etc.). Target heart rates can be found at the American Heart Association Web site at *www.americanheart. org/presenter.jhtml?identifier=4736*).

"That minimum amount of exercise—just one hour per week—will actually maintain muscle and cardio fitness," says Dr. Westcott.

•**Attitude Type Two:** *"I like exercise but don't like strength training much"...*

Diet: Less calorie restriction than Type One (1,700 to 1,750 for women...1,900 to 1,950 for men).

Strength training: Same as Type One above (two times per week, 15 minutes each circuit).

Aerobic exercise: Four times per week, 15 minutes per session (or twice a week, 30 minutes per session).

The extra aerobic exercise allows you to eat slightly more than Type One.

•**Attitude Type Three:** *"I like to exercise hard"...*

Diet: Continue what you normally eat.

Strength training: Two to three times a week, 30 minutes per session (circuits).

Aerobic exercise: Two to three times a week, 30 minutes per session.

"Those strength-training circuits burn a lot of calories," says Dr. Westcott. "Remember that the more vigorously you exercise, the more calories you need in your diet."

STRENGTH TRAINING: WHAT TO DO

Dr. Westcott recommends a "circuit" of exercises. A circuit is performed by doing an exercise and moving on to the next with minimum rest in between. When you've performed each exercise in the series, you've done "one circuit." You can repeat the circuit up to three times in a session. Studies have shown that unfit people performing just one hard circuit, twice a week with a one-minute or less rest between exercises will get measurable results from this routine. Those who are more fit and conditioned to begin with have to up the ante a bit in order to get serious improvement—either by performing more circuits or using heavier weights.

TWO ACTUAL CIRCUITS

Here are two of Dr. Westcott's recommended strength-training circuits. Weight for each exercise should be enough that you can complete eight to 12 repetitions. If 12 is too easy, and you feel you could continue, raise the weight. If you cannot complete eight, lower the weight until you can finish the set.

The first circuit is composed of exercises that use multiple muscles (called "compound exercises"). The second includes specific arm exercises. Either is effective, and you may alternate. They can be performed at home or at the gym. (Note: For an excellent illustrated explanation of how to perform these exercises with correct form, see *Weight Training for Dummies* (For Dummies) by Liz Neporent and Suzanne Schlosberg.)

STRENGTH TRAINING: CIRCUIT ONE

1. Leg press or squat
2. Dumbbell bench press (if at home) or chest press machine (if at the gym)
3. Bent-over row (home) or rowing machine (gym)
4. Dumbbell shoulder press (home) or shoulder press machine (gym)
5. Chin-up (home: have someone assist you) or assisted chin-up (gym)
6. Incline dumbbell bench press (home) or incline chest press machine (gym)
7. Crunches

STRENGTH TRAINING: CIRCUIT TWO

1. Leg press or squat
2. Chest press
3. Bent-over row (home) or seated row (gym)
4. Shoulder press
5. Lat pulldown (gym only)
6. Triceps press
7. Bicep curl
8. Crunches.

PICKING AEROBIC EXERCISES

As for the aerobic portion of your workout, the key is to make it enjoyable. Be sure to choose an activity that is fun for you—and remember that it doesn't have to be the same one every time. In fact, your muscles will respond better if you mix it up, so that you exercise slightly different muscle groups each time you work out. You can ride a bicycle one day...use a cross-country ski machine another...and swim on a third. Or take an aerobics or dance class. In good weather, kayaking will give you a good upper body workout, while cycling or a fast walk will exercise your lower body on alternating days.

If a certain exercise gives you pain, then don't continue. Pick a different one that doesn't strain your "trouble spot(s)."

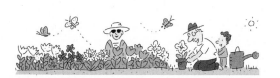

Will Quick Workouts Do the Trick?

Len Kravitz, PhD, exercise physiology, University of New Mexico, Albuquerque.

Americans looking for a quick fix were very excited recently by a report promising that six minutes of very vigorous exercise (per *week*) was just as good for getting fit as two hours of moderate exercise three times a week.

File this one in the "if it sounds too good to be true then it probably is..." bin. Sorry, folks.

REAL TIME INVOLVED

It *is* true that super-intense exercise can boost fitness fast. In the study, Canadian researchers found that men and women who cranked out four 30-second full-on (fast and as hard as possible) sprints (with four minutes of rest or easy pedaling between efforts) on exercise bikes, three times a week reaped identical fitness gains to those who pedaled two hours at a moderate pace three times a week. But it's a little misleading to say that you only need six minutes a week, because though the hard work only totaled two minutes per exercise session, if you include the four minutes of easy pedaling or rest, these cyclists were actually exercising for 14 minutes per bout.

NOT FOR BEGINNERS

What's more, this type of exercise is extremely challenging and *not* appropriate for beginner exercisers—the usual audience looking for quick exercise fixes. "Very intense exercise bouts are not for people just starting out," says exercise physiology expert Len Kravitz, PhD, of the University of New Mexico in Albuquerque. "You need to build a good foundation by exercising consistently for at least several months so your muscles, joints, connective tissues and heart are conditioned to withstand that level of work, impact and intensity." Otherwise, you're just asking for an injury or even a heart attack.

WORKOUT SUPPLEMENT

Instead of trying to cut corners and whip yourself into shape overnight, use high-intensity exercise bouts as a supplement to your regular workout to take your fitness to the next level. Short, vigorous sessions also can help you maintain fitness when you're going through a busy period at home or work and you're crunched for time. "Exercising 30 to 60 minutes most days is still your best bet for health, weight loss and fitness," says Dr. Kravitz.

What's Worse— Skipping Your Workout Or Blowing Your Diet?

Liz Neporent, MA, CSCS, coauthor of *Fitness for Dummies* and *Weight Training for Dummies* (both from For Dummies) and *The Fat-Free Truth* (Mariner). Ms. Neporent is an exercise physiologist and writer whose work has been featured in *The New York Times, Shape* magazine, the *New York Daily News* and *Fitness* magazine. She is president of Wellness 360, a corporate wellness consulting company. *www.w360.com.*

Every once in a while, you're so busy you might have to skip a workout. And sometimes when you're out to dinner you might have the key lime pie.

So if you have to cheat on either diet or exercise, which cheat does the least amount of damage?

"The research says that when you're trying to lose weight, you're probably going to get better results if you emphasize diet over exercise," says noted New York City fitness expert Liz Neporent, MA, MS, CSCS and coauthor of Fitness for Dummies (For Dummies). "But for *maintaining* weight loss, nothing supports success as well as exercise does."

In other words, if you're trying to lose weight, stick to the diet. If you're trying to maintain weight loss, don't skip the exercise regimen.

TO LOSE WEIGHT

When it comes to losing pounds, diet trumps exercise every time. "It's so easy to do damage with overeating," says Neporent, "because taking in calories is so much easier than burning them off." She points out that burning off the calories in one big doughnut—which you can eat in a minute—could easily take you more than one hour of exercise.

WEIGHT MAINTENANCE—
EXERCISE IS KEY

On the flip side, The National Weight Control Registry—which tracks the behavior of people who have lost at least 30 pounds and kept it off for at least a year—shows very clearly that incorporating a regular exercise program into your life is critical for success. "No matter how they lost the weight, Registry members who exercise regularly are the ones who wind up keeping it off successfully," Neporent says. She explains that exercising regularly for those weight-loss winners in the registry meant walking off about 1,000 calories a week (the equivalent of about five half-hour sessions) *plus* burning up another 1,800 calories in other exercise activities. "That other 1,800 calories a week can be from anything—though most people did a high-intensity activity such as an aerobics class, running or weight training."

"Of course, it isn't really an either/or choice," she adds. "To lose weight, you should be doing both—watching your diet and working out *regularly*." Neporent stresses that an occasional lapse on either diet or exercise is not particularly meaningful, so you probably shouldn't sweat it. "It's the consistent pattern that makes the difference, not the once-in-a-while slip."

14

The Latest on Drug Safety

The Dangers of New And Improved Drugs

In July 2005, the FDA halted the sale of a powerful new pain reliever called Palladone. After just five months on the market, they concluded that this new extended-release form of the narcotic *hydromorphone* could be dangerous—even fatal—if taken with alcohol. The problem is that alcohol speeds up its time release, and when the drug floods the body too quickly, depressed breathing and possibly death can follow.

Fortunately, for the 11,500 people who had already taken Palladone, no adverse reactions or deaths were reported. But the moral of the story is this: *New is not necessarily better when it comes to medications.*

NEWER IS NOT NECESSARILY BETTER

According to Jay S. Cohen, MD, from San Diego, California, and author of *What*

You Must Know About Statin Drugs and Their Natural Alternatives (Square One), newer or stronger drugs are not necessarily better than the drugs that came before them. This is a myth perpetuated by Big Pharma, which is almost invariably motivated by profit margins to sell the newest, most expensive drugs.

However, drugs with a long track record for safety that have been on the market for some time are nearly always preferable to new drugs...unless the new drugs *really* accomplish something new and exciting. And the truth is, most don't.

MOST NEW DRUGS ARE COPYCAT DRUGS

When older drugs go off patent and can be made more cheaply in generic versions, it

Jay S. Cohen, MD, adjunct (voluntary) professor of family and preventive medicine, University of California, San Diego. Dr. Cohen is author of *What You Must Know About Statin Drugs & Their Natural Alternatives* (Square One) and *Over Dose: The Case Against the Drug Companies* (Tarcher/Putnam). Visit his Web site at *www.medicationsense.com*.

311

is in the financial interest of pharmaceutical companies to come up with so-called new and improved versions. They slap a patent on these new drugs, aggressively market them directly to consumers via print ads and TV, and send thousands of drug reps out to doctors' offices and flood them with free samples for patients.

The problem is that the majority of these expensive, new drugs are copycat, me-too drugs, warns Dr. Cohen. Often they are modeled closely on the profile of older, equally effective, less expensive drugs. Take *rosuvastatin* (Crestor), for example, a relatively new and strong cholesterol-lowering statin drug. With greater strength comes a greater risk for side effects. According to Dr. Cohen, the majority of people would be better off with an older statin such as generic *lovastatin*, which is not as strong, causes fewer side effects and is less expensive.

WHAT YOU CAN DO

To exercise the utmost care with new drugs...

•**View them with a healthy dose of skepticism.** Don't get taken in by slick advertising campaigns. Just because a celebrity says one pill is better for you than another, doesn't mean that it really is.

•**Beware of free samples and copycat drugs.** If your physician hands you a free sample of a new drug, inquire whether it is different from the old drug you were taking, and if so, in what way.

•**Ask whether generic or over-the-counter alternatives are available.** Very often, older, safer, less-expensive drugs are equally effective.

•**Read the fine print.** Potentially serious side effects of new drugs are commonly glossed over. In addition to consulting your doctor and pharmacist, carefully read the package insert and closely follow the directions.

•**Make sure the drug prescribed for you is truly necessary.** Ask your healthcare provider whether it's safe to first try alternatives such as lifestyle changes before turning to drugs. For example, Dr. Cohen notes that mildly elevated cholesterol responds well to a healthful diet, regular exercise and weight management.

If the time comes when you must take a drug, tell your physician that whenever possible you prefer medication that has well-established effectiveness and a long track record for safety, and start with the lowest recommended dose.

FDA: Are They Watchdogs or "Lapdogs"?

Marcia Angell, MD, senior lecturer, department of social medicine, Harvard Medical School, Boston, Massachusetts, and author of *The Truth About the Drug Companies: How They Deceive Us and What to Do About It*. Random House. In 1997, *Time* magazine named Dr. Angell one of the 25 most influential Americans. She is former editor-in-chief of *The New England Journal of Medicine*.

Jay S. Cohen, MD, adjunct (voluntary) professor of family and preventive medicine, University of California, San Diego. Dr. Cohen is author of *What You Must Know About Statin Drugs & Their Natural Alternatives* (Square One) and *Over Dose: The Case Against the Drug Companies* (Tarcher/Putnam). Visit his Web site at *www.medicationsense.com*.

Given the blasting the US Food and Drug Administration (FDA) has lately taken for its failure to properly monitor and regulate drug safety, our editors thought it would be helpful to review some of the issues in question. As a starting point, it is fair to point out that the challenges this agency faces are daunting—keeping Americans safe while encouraging innovation from the profit-driven pharmaceutical industry—and its resources limited.

However, the FDA received a blistering report from the Institute of Medicine (IOM) that highlighted shortcomings of the agency and provided 25 recommendations on ways the FDA could better protect Americans and improve drug safety. Drug after drug has proven to have safety issues (not infrequently life-threatening) after being approved by the FDA, often even as they are aggressively marketed directly to the public. The recall of *rofecoxib* (Vioxx) after it was implicated in heart attacks and strokes is just one of the most publicized examples of late—but there are many others. The FDA and the Department of Health & Human Services requested the IOM to assess the US drug safety system and report back with recommendations. The Drug Safety Oversight Board was also created in February 2005.

HOW CAN THIS BE?

According to its own mission statement, the FDA is responsible "for protecting the public health by assuring the safety, efficacy and security of human and veterinary drugs" as well as biological products, medical devices, the nation's food supply, cosmetics and products that emit radiation…"for advancing the public health by helping to speed innovations that make medicines and foods more effective, safer and more affordable"…and for "helping the public to get accurate science-based information they need to use medicines and foods to improve their health."

Though initially funded with tax-payer money through Congressional budgets, as it should be, since 1992 the FDA has been authorized to collect fees from drug companies to help cover the cost of reviewing their products. Recently, the agency responded to criticism of its effectiveness in the review process by proposing a 22% jump in the yearly user fees to be paid by drug developers (an additional $87.4 million).

CONFLICTS OF INTEREST

In the opinion of Marcia Angell, MD, senior lecturer in the department of social medicine at Boston's Harvard Medical School and author of *The Truth About the Drug Companies: How They Deceive Us and What to Do About It* (Random House), this constitutes an obvious conflict of interest, in effect putting the FDA on the payroll of the drug companies it regulates. Jay S. Cohen, MD—(*www.medicationsense.*

com), and author of *Over Dose: The Case Against the Drug Companies* (Tarcher/Putnam)—believes the FDA devotes more of its resources, both in terms of staffing and financing, toward pushing drugs to market than to monitoring their risks and benefits, before and after they become available.

TOO LITTLE, TOO LATE

Given that user fees now pay more than half the costs of getting drugs through the approval process, the net effect is that instead of being the watchdog protecting the health and well-being of American consumers, "the FDA has become the lapdog of the drug companies," says Dr. Angell. With post-approval resources for follow-up study scarce, multiple drugs—e.g., Vioxx, *valdecoxib* (Bextra), *fenfluramine* and *dexfenfluramine* (the "Fen" in Fen-Phen) and *astemizole* (Hismanal), to name but a few—have been yanked from the market only after harming, sometimes even killing, consumers.

PHARMACEUTICAL PITCHING

Another critical safety issue is direct-to-consumer advertising—the promotion of prescription drugs through TV, newspaper, magazine and Internet ads. This, too, is in the FDA's domain. We are one of only two industrialized countries to permit this kind of advertising. Everyone should be aware of how aggressively the pharmaceutical companies are pursuing us. They spend billions of dollars annually pitching their products to vulnerable consumers, with advertising directed toward making an emotional connection (Wish you had a more fulfilling sex life? Are you allergic to your new puppy?) and barely mentioning risk factors. In fact, according to Dr. Cohen, new drugs (like Vioxx) become best sellers largely on the strength of TV, newspaper and magazine ads.

PROMISES, PROMISES

In addition to asking for higher user fees from drug companies, the FDA has responded to the IOM report by proposing changes, such as assessing the safety

313

of drugs longer after they are approved and marketed. It's a baby step in the right direction, say critics.

In Dr. Angell's opinion, more substantive changes are required. She believes that drug companies' user fees to the FDA should be terminated, and the US government should once again cover these substantial costs. Drug safety is, after all, frequently a matter of life and death.

BETTER SAFE THAN SORRY

Clearly, the FDA needs to take a stronger, more aggressive regulatory approach to being careful before a drug is approved—as well as more closely monitoring and responding to dangers and health risks that become evident once a drug (as well as the medical devices, cosmetics, foods and other products the agency oversees) has been approved. One step recommended by the Institute of Medicine is a moratorium (waiting period) on direct-to-consumer advertising for new drugs, until established usage reveals more certainty about their risk-benefit profiles.

Additional recommendations include mandatory registration of clinical trial results, a boost in staffing and funding, an increased role for the drug safety staff and more. The FDA itself and Congress are proposing changes as well, including public databases and stricter safety regulations. But consumer activists are unimpressed as these fall "dramatically short of the changes needed to overhaul the nation's drug safety system," according to the Consumers Union, a consumer watchdog group, in a *Wall Street Journal* piece on the subject.

IF DRUGS ARE REQUIRED

In the meantime, it's up to us as individuals to be vigilant. Drugs that are newer and "in the news" aren't necessarily safe and effective. Try to consider drugs a last-choice solution to other more healthful and natural treatment options when it is safe to do so. If drugs are required, ask your physician if it is possible to prescribe medications in the lowest appropriate doses that will still help your condition, and to prescribe drugs that

have a long track record for safety. Also, when available, request less expensive generic alternatives.

Ten Great Ways to Minimize Rx Side Effects

Jerry H. Gurwitz, MD, executive director, Meyers Primary Care Institute, University of Massachusetts Medical School, Worcester, Massachusetts. A specialist in geriatric medicine, Dr. Gurwitz has published numerous articles, commentaries and book chapters on the optimal use of drug therapy in seniors.

Andrew L. Rubman, ND, consulting medical editor for *Bottom Line's Daily Health News* and director of the Southbury Clinic for Traditional Medicines in Southbury, Connecticut.

There are pills to control high blood pressure, keep arteries clear, maintain normal blood sugar levels and build strong bones, as well as medicines to manage many other age-related ailments. We have become a pill-popping society, driven by doctors who are trained to provide medication to resolve symptoms and by patients in search of quick fixes for what ails them.

MANAGING DRUGS

Unfortunately, along with these benefits come serious concerns about overmedication or conflicting medication. Older people take an average of four drugs daily. Not surprisingly, they also face the greatest risk of side effects and drug interactions. And, unfortunately, the "solution" to the side effects is all too often yet another drug.

To learn more about wise drug management, we contacted Jerry H. Gurwitz, MD, the executive director of the Meyers Primary Care Institute at the University of Massachusetts Medical School in Worcester, who has written a number of articles regarding drug use and the elderly. He offers some essential advice about the safe use of medications, especially for older people.

THE MEDICATED GENERATION

There is a cycle of drugs, in which one drug creates side effects, so another drug is given to counteract it and another and another. For example, heart medications and sleeping pills can cause depression, that can lead to an antidepressant prescription, which can prompt sexual dysfunction and pills for erectile dysfunction, and so on. This drug cascade happens all too frequently in older people, who take multiple medications and may be more susceptible to side effects, observes Dr. Gurwitz. *To counter this, he recommends exercisizing the following precautions...*

•**Know the name of every medication you take and the reason you're taking it.** Most people—whatever their ages—don't have this information, says Dr. Gurwitz. Don't take a drug without understanding why it is necessary, he says. Do not leave the doctor's office without a full explanation for every prescription you are given.

•**Start all medications at the lowest dose appropriate for your specific condition and slowly increase as necessary.** Older people are often more susceptible to side effects because their liver and kidneys are slower to clear drugs, explains Dr. Gurwitz.

•**Consider any symptom in an older patient a side effect until proven otherwise.** Too often a change in energy, mood, concentration or memory is attributed to "old age," when it is actually a side effect of a medication, warns Dr. Gurwitz. Read the accompanying contraindications/warnings that come with all prescriptions so that you are familiar with potential side effects. If you suspect that a drug is causing side effects, notify your doctor and ask him/her if drug therapy is absolutely necessary. If not, ask about alternatives.

•**Schedule a brown bag checkup.** Often older people have a number of specialists, and take different medications prescribed by different doctors. As a safety precaution, once a year gather all your medicines—both prescription and over-the-counter (OTC), including vitamins and supplements—and bring them to your primary care provider's office. He/she can check for unnecessary overmedication, drug interactions and side effects.

•**Give each physician you visit a list of all medications you take, both prescription and OTC.** One doctor may not know what the others are prescribing. Let each doctor know what you are taking. (According to *Bottom Line's Daily Health News* consulting medical editor Andrew L. Rubman, if you are taking vitamins and other natural supplements it makes sense to have a naturopathic physician on your team, too.)

•**Fill all your prescriptions at the same pharmacy.** This is another safeguard against any unnecessary duplication of therapy. Additionally, Dr. Gurwitz points out that pharmacists are very knowledgeable, and may be more familiar with drug side effects than doctors.

•**Take all medicines exactly as prescribed by your physician.** According to Dr. Gurwitz, many people skip doses because they are wary of side effects or because they lose track or try to save on drug costs. There are many types of pill organizers available that can help you keep track of your medications and ensure proper dispensing.

Note: Again, if you notice side effects, contact your doctor immediately.

•**Put a support system in place.** According to the American Psychiatric Association, up to one-quarter of older people experience symptoms of mental illness, such as anxiety, depression or psychosis. If these symptoms result in skipping important medication—such as heart or diabetes drugs—a stroke, heart attack or diabetic coma may ensue. In such situations, a family member or home health aide is essential to ensure that older people take medications on schedule and refill prescriptions on a timely basis.

•**Whenever possible, take generic drugs, with your physician's consent.** Generics are usually lower-priced than brand-name products and are just as safe and effective, explains Dr. Gurwitz. Also, consider tried-and-true drugs instead of the newest brand-name drugs, since many newer drugs don't have the same track record for safety as do well-established drugs.

•**Avoid drug samples.** In the long run, samples will not serve an older person well, notes Dr. Gurwitz. You might get by for a few months on free samples, but then you are stuck with a higher-priced medication.

Drug Manufacturers— Are They Making You Sick?

Jay S. Cohen, MD, adjunct (voluntary) professor of family and preventive medicine, University of California, San Diego. Dr. Cohen is author of *What You Must Know About Statin Drugs & Their Natural Alternatives* (Square One) and *Over Dose: The Case Against the Drug Companies* (Tarcher/Putnam). Visit his Web site at *www.medicationsense.com*.

US Food and Drug Administration, *www.fda.gov.*

It's come to this—according to a recent front page article in *The New York Times*, pharmaceutical companies are now recruiting college cheerleaders to hawk their wares to doctors. After all, who has a bigger smile, a more enthusiastic disposition, a better ability to sell a product than an attractive young cheerleader?

Some experts fear that this is yet one more manifestation of a pharmaceutical culture run amok. Boundaries have been blurred, and it is increasingly difficult to determine where the science ends and the marketing and cheerleading begin.

DRUGS IN SEARCH OF DISEASES

Big Pharma has us trained to believe that there is a pill for every problem. And now, in search of ever broader markets

and more customers, drug companies are pushing the boundaries into grayer areas. Rambunctious child? Medication may be the answer. Getting older and less frisky? The TV commercials make tantalizing promises about intimacy drugs.

Increasingly, drug manufacturers are no longer marketing merely pills themselves, but the diseases they are intended to treat. According to Jay S. Cohen, MD, author of *What You Must Know About Statin Drugs and Their Natural Alternatives* (Square One), there is no doubt that some people truly suffer from conditions and diseases that drugs effectively address...but are these medications necessary on such a widespread basis? Not every boisterous child has attention deficit hyperactivity disorder (ADHD), nor does every man not batting 1,000 have erectile dysfunction.

SIDE EFFECTS ABOUND

All drugs have side effects, and Dr. Cohen points out that nonpharmaceutical approaches should be the first line of attack against most health-care concerns. However, this is not the message sent by the glitzy drug ads that are now ubiquitous on TV and in magazines and newspapers.

REPACKAGING DRUGS TO INCREASE SALES

Pharmaceutical companies routinely try to come up with new conditions or indications to broaden the use of individual drugs, observes Dr. Cohen. For example, Zyban—which is prescribed to help people quit smoking—is really the same drug as the antidepressant *bupropion* (Wellbutrin XL). Although Zyban's short-term effect on smoking cessation appears promising, the long-term outlook is less certain.

But no drug is without side effects, and bupropion—whatever its brand name or purpose—is a serious drug with serious side effects. Shortly after its introduction, Wellbutrin was withdrawn from the market because of an unacceptable incidence of seizures, involving convulsions and loss of consciousness. Although that withdrawal was brief and the drug returned to market, a *Journal of Emergency Medicine* article confirms that seizures continue to be a problem for takers of bupropion. In fact, the authors found it to be the third leading cause of drug-related seizures. (Cocaine is number one.)

SELLING BUPROPION

Bupropion may also cause side effects such as dry mouth, difficulty sleeping, agitation, skin rash and weight loss. Ironically, although there are far healthier ways to lose weight (think "eat less and exercise more," instead of taking a pill that can cause seizures), the manufacturer Glaxo-SmithKline commissioned a study from Slim-Fast on bupropion and weight loss. Their conclusion was that bupropion in combination with lifestyle changes could help sustain weight loss in obese people.

THE FEMINIZATION OF PROZAC

Everything old is new again when it comes to Serafem, the "new" pink-and-lavender capsule that was approved by the FDA to treat premenstrual dysphoric disorder (PMDD)—severe symptoms of PMS that affect about 5% of menstruating women. In reality, Serafem is *fluoxetine*, also known as Prozac. It's just been repackaged and renamed by manufacturer Eli Lilly. This clever marketing ploy gave Lilly additional patent protection for a major moneymaking drug. That is, when the patent on Prozac expired and the drug became available generically, Lilly could no longer charge top dollar for it. Brand name Serafem, however, could still command high prices.

Dr. Cohen notes that there is considerable controversy about PMDD. In the "bible" of psychiatry, the *Diagnostic and Statistical Manual of Mental Disorders* (DSM-IV), it is listed as a disorder still under evaluation. In a parallel instance, no one looked at menopause as a disorder or disease until Big Pharma spent millions promoting hormone therapies for it.

PROMOTING OFF-LABEL USE OF DRUGS

In the case of the anticonvulsant drug *gabapentin* (Neurontin), Warner-Lambert went too far in searching for ways to sell its wares. In fact, the company went so far that the FDA slapped it with $430 million in fines. Neurontin was approved as a supplemental treatment for epileptic seizures. But without getting further FDA approval, its drug reps/cheerleaders illegally promoted the off-label use of Neurontin for a veritable kitchen sink of ailments, including various pain disorders, amyotrophic lateral sclerosis (ALS), attention-deficit disorder, bipolar disorder, migraine, drug and alcohol withdrawal seizures and restless legs syndrome.

According to the FDA, Warner-Lambert paid physicians substantial fees to attend "consultants' meetings," which were essentially expensive dinners and junkets where doctors did little or no consulting. At supposedly independent educational events, the company planted people in the audience to ask questions highlighting Neurontin's benefits. Even worse, doctors were paid to allow sales representatives to see patients with them, and make recommendations about Neurontin.

THE LATEST AND POSSIBLY GREATEST: STATINS FOR ALL

Of course, recent controversies over the risk versus reward of statin drugs haven't stopped manufacturers from seeking new and creative ways to market them. First they were beating the drum of low cholesterol for all. Then it became statins for bird flu. Researchers studying data of both flu and pneumonia patients noted that the people taking statins actually had lower incidence of influenza and serious complications from the infection. Should further research bear this out, we may all be told to take statins every flu season in lieu of more healthful immune-boosting strategies.

PEEKING BEHIND THE CURTAIN

Remember that drug making is a for-profit business. Pharmaceutical giants aim to expand the uses of their drugs and hopefully obtain longer patent protection in order to make more money. The upshot of all this is that we now have a host of disease labels for what were formerly considered normal conditions. How can consumers avoid falling prey to such sophisticated marketing strategies?

•**When your doctor prescribes a new drug, ask what it is, what are its possible side effects and why he/she is prescribing it.** Drug representatives lure in doctors and patients with free samples of brand-name drugs, when more established generic drugs may be equally effective, less expensive and have a longer safety track record.

OTC Pain Killers Raise High Blood Pressure Up to 93%

John P. Forman, MD, hypertension researcher and associate physician, Brigham and Women's Hospital, Boston.

As if assorted types of painkillers (analgesics) haven't gotten enough bad press lately, researchers at Brigham and Women's Hospital in Boston decided to investigate what role if any the drugs might play in the development of high blood pressure (hypertension).

Result: Add another notch in the belt of dangers of these all-too-common drugs.

The study investigated two groups of women—an older (ages 51 to 77) group of 1,903 women from the long-term Nurses' Health Study I, and a younger (ages 34 to 53) group of 3,220 women from the Nurses' Health Study II. Participants recorded frequency of painkiller use in days per month and the number of tablets and dosage per day. The researchers considered high-dose usage as more than 500 milligrams (mg) per day of *acetaminophen* (Tylenol) or more than 400 mg per day for nonsteroidal anti-inflammatory drugs (NSAIDS)—the equivalent of one extra-strength acetaminophen tablet daily or two over-the-counter (OTC) *ibuprofen*

(e.g., Advil or Motrin) each day. The study also separated out women's use of analgesics to treat headaches because some people believe that headaches can be a symptom of hypertension.

WHAT THEY FOUND

Although aspirin use was not significantly associated with development of hypertension, the other results were indeed sobering...

•**Older high-users of acetaminophen other than for headache** had a 93% increased risk of developing high blood pressure.

•**Younger women in the high-usage group had an increased risk of 60%.**

•**Older high-users of NSAIDs other than for headache** had an increased risk of 78%.

•**Younger high-users of acetaminophen had twice the risk of nonusers.**

UNDERSTANDING THE RESULTS

John P. Forman, MD, who headed the study, suggests that there are several possible reasons for this increased risk. The drugs might harm endothelial function (cellular lining of blood vessels), and they may inhibit hormones that help keep vessels dilated. Dr. Forman also theorizes that the drugs may cause retention of sodium, which is known to potentially affect blood pressure.

OTHER CONCLUSIONS

We asked Dr. Forman if the OTC analgesics also might be a problem for people who are already hypertensive. Although this study didn't look at this, he says there is reason to assume that the drugs contribute to established hypertension as well. Prior studies have suggested that NSAIDs work against the action of antihypertensive medications. He also says that it is likely that men and women are equally affected by analgesic use in terms of the drugs' influence on hypertension because the hormones that control blood pressure are similar for both sexes.

WHAT ABOUT ASPIRIN?

So, should people stick with old-fashioned aspirin when they need a painkiller fix? Dr. Forman answers that his concern is not recommending one drug or another. The message about these drugs, he says, is that even though they are easily available, they are not completely safe and should be used as a last resort for most minor ailments, including basic tension headaches and minor aches and pains.

If you had to pick one of the bunch? Our consulting medical editor Andrew L. Rubman, ND, would go for aspirin for the occasional use, but be on the lookout for any stomach irritation.

The Dangers of Blood Thinners

Larry Sasich, PharmD, MPH, assistant professor, public policy expert and pharmaceutical research analyst, Lake Erie College of Osteopathic Medicine (LECOM) School of Pharmacy, Erie, Pennsylvania.

National Consumers League, *www.mybloodthinner.org*.

When you are taking a blood thinner like *warfarin* (Coumadin) to prevent blood clots, otherwise minor cuts can suddenly become major bleeds, especially if you and your doctor have not yet arrived at your proper dosing level. Blood thinner dosage levels can be difficult to fine tune.

SERIOUS HEALTH CHALLENGES

According to a recent survey by the National Consumers League (NCL), people who take prescription blood thinners typically face far more serious challenges than previously believed. These drugs—most commonly prescribed for individuals who are at risk of stroke, have mechanical heart valves, suffer from atrial fibrillation (a heart rhythm disturbance), or who have had recent knee or hip replacement surgery—may successfully prevent life-threatening blood clots. However, blood thinners are also especially difficult to manage in terms of balancing the dosage, the effectiveness and side effects, observes assistant professor and public policy expert Larry Sasich, PharmD, MPH, of the Lake Erie College of Osteopathic Medicine (LECOM) School of Pharmacy in Erie, Pennsylvania.

BAD REACTIONS

Blood thinners may cause adverse reactions such as bruising, bleeding and dizziness, and interact dangerously with other drugs, vitamins, supplements and foods.

MINIMIZE RISK

Even though the vast majority of participants in the NCL survey reported adverse reactions of one kind or another, more than half admitted that they had done nothing about them. The good news is that there are specific steps you can take to ensure that blood thinners function properly, thus minimizing your risk of dangerous adverse effects, says Dr. Sasich.

GET REGULAR BLOOD TESTS

Blood thinners are effective within a very narrow range, and even a slight variation outside this range can pose significant health risks. To stay safe, regular blood testing is critical, notes Dr. Sasich. These tests measure how fast your blood clots and is known as the international normalized ratio (INR), which should fall somewhere between 2 and 3. If the number is off, problems can develop and the physician will adjust your dosage accordingly. At the onset of treatment, testing is required on a weekly or sometimes even daily basis. As time goes on, you may only need monthly testing.

TELL YOUR DOCTOR ABOUT ALL DRUGS AND SUPPLEMENTS YOU TAKE

Other medicines, vitamins and herbal supplements can interact dangerously with blood thinners, changing the way they work in your body, warns Dr. Sasich. These substances can affect clotting in either direction, rendering it either too likely or not likely enough to occur. As a result, you must be sure to tell your doctor about all substances you take. Dr. Sasich cautions that you must pass on this information *before* you begin taking blood thinners. Also inform your pharmacist, who is better trained in possible interactions.

CONSISTENCY IN DIET IS KEY

Significant changes in diet also affect the way blood thinners work in the body. For example, if you start eating lots of foods rich in vitamin K (which is the vitamin that helps with blood clotting)—e.g., green vegetables such as spinach or broccoli—your INR number may drop below 2, at which point the blood may clot too quickly. On the other hand, suddenly cut back on leafy green veggies, and you can raise the INR over 3, which means the blood may clot too slowly and raise your risk of severe bleeding.

Note: People should consult with their doctor if they drink a lot of alcohol, as it may also have an effect.

This does not mean that veggie lovers should give up their greens if they already eat them on a regular basis, stresses Dr. Sasich. The watchword here is consistency. Do not make radical changes in your diet one way or the other without informing your physician.

PAY ATTENTION TO
WARNING SIGNS

When you are taking a blood thinner, it is normal to be more vulnerable to getting bruises. However, promptly report any large bright red or sudden or unusual forming bruises to your physician, advises Dr. Sasich. If you experience even a minor cut or nosebleed that won't stop bleeding, he recommends that you immediately check with your doctor or go to the emergency room.

It is also critical to suspend use of blood thinners before any medical procedure—including dental cleanings—that might cause bleeding. Check with your doctor for how and when to adjust your dosing for the procedure. If you have a hard fall,

check with your doctor, because it can cause internal bleeding.

DO YOUR HOMEWORK

Doctors and other caregivers need to make a more concerted effort to inform patients how to use blood thinners safely, emphasizes Dr. Sasich. In the meantime, however, ask questions of both your doctor and pharmacist, read the drug inserts and make it a habit to inform all health-care providers about all the products you take, whether prescription or over-the-counter. You can also learn more about blood thinners at the NCL Web site, *www.mybloodthinner.org.*

 # Eight Ways to Lower Cholesterol Without Drugs

Jay S. Cohen, MD, adjunct (voluntary) professor of family and preventive medicine, University of California, San Diego. Dr. Cohen is author of *What You Must Know About Statin Drugs & Their Natural Alternatives* (Square One) and *Over Dose: The Case Against the Drug Companies* (Tarcher/Putnam). Visit his Web site at *www.medicationsense.com.*

Even with all the controversy about cholesterol-lowering statin drugs, sales of them are still in the billions of dollars. There are indeed some people with extremely high cholesterol that can be helped by statins, but many users can be better served with any number of natural alternatives. To learn more about these, we spoke with Jay S. Cohen, MD, author of *What You Must Know About Statin Drugs and Their Natural Alternatives* (Square One).

THE PRECISION-PRESCRIBING
METHOD

In Dr. Cohen's view, most people are far too quick to turn to pharmaceuticals to cure every ill. He warns that all drugs have side effects, and the side effects of statins—the top-selling drug group in the US—are often underestimated. They range from muscle discomfort to gastrointestinal problems to fuzzy thinking and lack of concentration. Many people who begin taking statins are bothered by these side effects, which leads them to stop taking them…and this can lead to greater risk for heart attack or stroke (and perhaps heart failure).

Dr. Cohen's solution lies in what he calls the *precision-prescribing method.* This means that before taking any drug, first consider nutrition, then natural interventions and only then pharmaceuticals. *When considering natural interventions, Dr. Cohen's favorite cholesterol-reducing options include…*

GARLIC

Some experts swear by garlic for cholesterol control, while others believe that its claims are vastly overrated.

What it does: Garlic has a modest impact on lowering total cholesterol, LDL (the so-called "bad") cholesterol and harmful blood lipids called triglycerides.

Dr. Cohen says: Garlic is a nice adjunct to a cholesterol-lowering program. It is tasty, inexpensive and safe—so why not toss a fresh clove or two into your next dish? However, keep in mind that its benefits are not as dramatic as those of more aggressive cholesterol-lowering agents.

GUGGULIPID

This Ayurvedic remedy from the guggul tree has been used for centuries in India.

What it does: Guggulipid reduces cholesterol and inflammation, acts as an antioxidant and reduces platelet aggregation to make blood thinner. High doses also may reduce C-reactive protein (CRP), a marker of inflammation that increasingly appears to be as significant a risk factor as cholesterol.

Dr. Cohen says: Recent studies suggest that guggulipid may not be as reliable as was previously believed. Dr. Cohen recommends its use only under close medical supervision. Talk to your doctor about the best brand to use. A standard dose is 250 milligrams (mg) or 500 mg twice daily with meals, although doses of up to 500 mg three times a day also are used. Side effects include nausea, gas and bloating.

NIACIN

Physicians split ranks on the subject of niacin supplementation. Mainstream doctors for the most part prescribe US Food and Drug Administration (FDA)-approved Niaspan, and natural practitioners prefer niacin derivatives that are associated with fewer side effects.

What it does: Niacin, the first supplement therapy shown to improve cholesterol levels, reduces total cholesterol and low-density lipoprotein (LDL), and raises the level of "good" high-density lipoprotein (HDL) cholesterol.

Dr. Cohen says: Niaspan is associated with side effects such as flushing, nausea, vomiting and agitation. A possible side effect of Niaspan is hepatitis, so you should get regular blood tests to check liver enzyme levels while taking this drug. He prefers a niacin derivative known as *inositol hexaniacinate*. A typical dosage is 600 mg twice daily.

Note: A B-50 supplement needs to be taken twice a day in conjunction with the Niaspan in order to avoid an induced deficiency in other B vitamins.

OMEGA-3 FATTY ACIDS

Mainstream and natural physicians agree: Omega-3 fatty acids are good for your heart.

What they do: Omega-3 fatty acids in fish and fish oil supplements increase your good HDL cholesterol, lower levels of harmful triglycerides, help control inflammation and blood clotting and contribute to overall blood vessel health.

Dr. Cohen says: Take your fish oil capsules. An average dose consists of 2 grams (g) to 3 g daily.

Another option: Eat wild salmon (or other wild ocean fish such as sardines) once or twice a week. Dr. Cohen advises avoiding farmed fish, which tend to be high in mercury and other toxins.

Caution: Do not take fish oils with blood thinners or if you have a bleeding disorder without checking with your physician.

PLANT STEROLS

The American Heart Association and the National Cholesterol Education Program Expert Panel recommend plant sterols as adjunct therapy to reduce potentially harmful LDL cholesterol.

What they do: When you eat plant sterols, they impair the absorption of cholesterol from the intestines.

Dr. Cohen says: With plenty of research to back up their benefits, plant sterols are a good, safe way to reduce cholesterol. Small amounts are present in vegetable oils, seeds, nuts and some vegetables and fruits, or you can buy supplements in health-food stores. Studies show that 1.8 g a day reduces LDL by an average of 10%. Dr. Cohen does not recommend margarines enriched with plant sterols if they also contain harmful trans fats. (Check the labels.)

POLICOSANOL

Made from sugar cane in Cuba and commonly produced from citrus peels in this country, many experts believe that policosanol is a safe and natural substance that can be as or even more effective than statin drugs in lowering cholesterol (and without the side effects).

What it does: When you take policosanol, your liver produces less cholesterol overall and absorbs more LDL cholesterol. In addition, blood is thinner (which protects you from heart attack and stroke) and inflammation is reduced.

Dr. Cohen says: The jury is still out on policosanol, with mixed results from the various studies. However, the good news is that it's safe and inexpensive. If you want to give policosanol a try, Dr. Cohen recommends the sugar cane-based variety, which seems to be of higher purity. Check the labels. The usual starting dose is 5 mg or 10 mg a day taken with dinner.

RED YEAST RICE

It is this traditional element of Asian cuisine that imparts a rich red color to Peking duck.

What it does: Red yeast rice contains a natural form of *lovastatin*, the active ingredient in the statin drug Mevacor. Less expensive and with fewer side effects than statins, this supplement lowers total cholesterol, LDL and triglycerides. It also may reduce elevated CRP.

Dr. Cohen says: Red yeast rice is well researched, and its benefits have been clearly demonstrated. Dr. Cohen cautions that it may produce side effects similar to those of statins, and should be taken only under the supervision of your health-care provider.

SOY

According to the FDA, 25 g of soy protein a day, as part of a diet low in saturated fat and cholesterol, may reduce the risk for heart disease.

What it does: Soy reduces total cholesterol by as much as 9%, as well as lowering LDL and triglycerides. It also may have a beneficial impact on the smaller-particle LDL-cholesterol, a newly recognized risk factor for heart disease.

Dr. Cohen says: It's hard to take in 25 g of soy every day—the equivalent of about six ounces of tofu. Moreover, some controversy surrounds the intake of large doses of soy, which critics warn may have a negative impact on estrogen-sensitive tissues and the thyroid. That said, Dr. Cohen recommends including a moderate amount of soy in your diet as a useful adjunct to more aggressive cholesterol-lowering treatments.

DO NOT SELF-TREAT

Although you can purchase all of the dietary supplements listed above on-line or from quality health food stores, Dr. Cohen says that it is always best to consult first with your health-care provider. What works for one person may not work for another— recommended dosages and combinations can vary according to each person and his or her condition, and many dietary supplements must be used with caution (if at all) with prescription drugs. In addition, regular blood tests are required to determine whether supplements are successful in bringing risk factors within target range.

REDUCE INFLAMMATION

Additionally, reducing inflammation has been identified as being even more critical to lowering heart attack risk than reducing cholesterol levels. And, important lifestyle adjustments to benefit your heart include a healthy diet low in saturated fat and rich in veggies, fruits (especially berries), soy and wild ocean fish...regular exercise...maintaining a healthy weight...not smoking... and managing stress.

The ABCs of Beta-Blockers

Catherine Ulbricht, PharmD, senior attending pharmacist at Massachusetts General Hospital in Boston, assistant professor, Northeastern University and the University of Rhode Island, among others. She is a founder of Natural Standard Research Collaboration, which provides high-level complementary and alternative medicine information for clinicians, patients and health-care institutions. Dr. Ulbricht is also chief editor of the *Journal of Herbal Pharmacotherapy*.

Erica Seamon, PharmD, clinical research associate, Natural Standard Research Collaboration, author and editor of numerous publications, and a pharmacist in Florida.

Beta-blockers are considered quite versatile, and are prescribed for high blood pressure (hypertension), and a variety of other conditions. According to Catherine Ulbricht, PharmD, senior attending pharmacist at Massachusetts General Hospital in Boston, and Erica Seamon, PharmD, her colleague at Natural Standard Research Collaboration in Cambridge, beta-blockers are also used to relieve chest pain (angina)...prevent additional heart attacks in heart patients...correct abnormal heart rhythms (arrhythmias)...manage chronic heart failure...treat tremors... prevent migraines...and treat glaucoma.

BETA-BLOCKERS—A PRIMER

Beta-blockers work by blocking the effects of adrenaline on the body's beta receptors, explains Dr. Ulbricht. This action slows down nerve impulses through the heart, relaxes the heart and slows the heart rate. By reducing its workload, beta-blockers may successfully decrease the heart's need for blood and oxygen. Taken over the course of time, as these medications routinely are, beta-blockers can transiently improve the heart's pumping ability.

Dr. Seamon says that the body has two main beta-receptors...

- **Beta-1 receptors.** These are responsible for heart rate and the strength of your heartbeat.

- **Beta-2 receptors.** Beta-2 receptors are responsible for part of the function of smooth muscles.

She notes that some beta-blockers are selective, meaning that they block beta-1 receptors more than they block beta-2 receptors. Nonselective beta-blockers block both beta-1 and beta-2 receptors.

COPING WITH SIDE EFFECTS

Dr. Ulbricht says that fatigue is a very common side effect that has been reported with beta-blockers. Along with fatigue, there may be a reduced capacity to engage in strenuous physical activity.

Fortunately for most people, the fatigue diminishes over time, says Dr. Ulbricht. However, if you find that you are still feeling unusually tired and washed out after a couple of months of taking a beta-blocker, ask your physician and pharmacist about a change in medication or dosage. A different beta-blocker or a lower dose may be effective for you while causing fewer side effects. Taking beta-blockers with food may also prove beneficial, as slowing absorption of the medication can reduce side effects. You may want to work with a nutritionist or naturopathic physician to develop a food plan that ensures proper absorption of the medication.

Dizziness and lightheadedness are likewise common with beta-blockers, observes Dr. Seamon. These side effects are typically most intense when you first get out of bed in the morning or stand quickly after sitting for an extended time. Your best bet is to take your time and rise more slowly.

Other possible side effects include weakness, dry eyes and mouth, difficulty sleeping, nightmares, diarrhea, constipation, impotence and loss of sex drive. When these side effects are troublesome and interfere with your day-to-day life, talk to your doctor.

VULNERABILITY OF THE ELDERLY

Dr. Ulbricht and Dr. Seamon caution that older people may be more susceptible to the side effects of beta-blockers, notably dizziness and fatigue, making them especially vulnerable to accidental falls. Beta-blockers may also make elderly patients more sensitive to cold temperatures, especially if circulation problems already exist. When this is the case, lower doses may be required.

TALK TO THE DOCTOR

Always tell your physician and pharmacist about all other medicines you take, both prescription and over-the-counter (herbs, vitamins, nutrients, etc.), and about any other medical problems you have. With this information, he/she is more likely to shield you from both side effects and dangerous interactions, assuming he is familiar with all the products that you take. If you need more information about these therapies, encourage your physician to visit *www.naturalstandard.com*, which is a trustworthy resource.

Note: If you experience increased shortness of breath, difficulty breathing, wheezing, skin rash, weight gain, a slow, fast or irregular heartbeat, swelling of the ankles, feet or lower legs, or chest pain, contact your doctor and pharmacist at once. These are signs of serious potential problems or allergic reactions to the medication.

WHICH BETA-BLOCKER IS BEST?

According to Dr. Ulbricht, there are a number of different beta-blockers, and doctors tend to prescribe specific beta-blockers to prevent symptoms of specific conditions. For example, she points out that agents specifically indicated for arrhythmia include *esmolol* (Brevibloc) and *sotalol* (Betapace). Beta-blockers used to reduce pressure in the eye in cases of glaucoma include eyedrops containing *timolol* (Timoptic) and *betaxolol* (Betoptic).

People with asthma or other breathing problems may want to avoid nonselective beta-blockers, advises Dr. Seamon. Nonselective beta-blockers such as *propranolol* (Inderal) affect the beta-2 receptors located in the lungs and blood vessels and may precipitate breathing problems. In her opinion, this group is better off with beta-1 selective beta-blockers like *atenolol* (Tenormin) and *metoprolol* (Lopressor), which have fewer effects on the lungs. With all drugs, Dr. Seamon notes, individual responses may vary.

info To learn more, visit MedlinePlus, the National Library of Medicine and the National Institutes of Health's Web site at *www.nlm.nih.gov/medlineplus* and type in "beta-blockers."

Warning: The Side Effect of Medical "Cures"

Andrew T. Chan, MD, MPH, assistant professor of medicine, Harvard Medical School, staff physician, Massachusetts General Hospital, Boston.

Drugs can be a double-edged sword. At their best, medicines save lives. (Think of penicillin or insulin.) On the other hand, many drugs turn out to have such dangerous side effects that they are abruptly pulled from the market. (Remember Vioxx?)

A recent examination of data from the long-term Nurses' Health Study offers yet another example. Researchers found a correlation between high aspirin consumption and reduced risk for colon cancer...but the dose required is so high that it also increases the risk for intestinal bleeding.

ABOUT THE STUDY

At Massachusetts General Hospital in Boston, lead researcher Andrew T. Chan, MD, MPH, and his colleagues looked at data from 82,911 initially cancer-free women. The women provided information on their aspirin use from 1980 through 2000. During this period, there were 962 documented cases of colorectal cancer.

Researchers discovered a high correlation between high aspirin use and reduced incidence of colon cancer. However, the protective benefits were dose- and time-related. Compared with women who reported no use, the greatest reduction in colon cancer risk occurred in those who took more than 14 standard-dose 325 milligrams (mg) tablets per week for more than 10 years.

Of course, that's a lot of aspirin, and all drugs—especially in high doses—have side effects. For every one to two cases of colon cancer prevented, high doses of aspirin caused eight additional cases of serious intestinal bleeding. In contrast, an 81 mg baby aspirin taken daily for cardiovascular protection is less likely to cause bleeding, but does not prevent colon cancer.

These results were published in the *Journal of the American Medical Association*.

BEST PROTECTION— A HEALTHY LIFESTYLE

According to Dr. Chan, while the study implies a possible role for aspirin in cancer prevention, any substantial impact of aspirin on cancer was seen with early initiation and prolonged, consistent use of relatively high doses. He says that future studies will need to thoroughly consider the risk-benefit profile for aspirin among various risk groups, and compare such a strategy with other potential prevention efforts. At this point, for most people, the best way to prevent colorectal cancer continues to be regular screening, exercise and a diet that is high in fiber and low in saturated fat and other inflammatory foods.

Surprising Side Effects of Common Medicines

Alan Winter, DDS, periodontist in private practice and associate clinical professor of implant dentistry at the New York University College of Dentistry, both in New York City. Dr. Winter has published several medical journal articles on gum disease.

American Dental Association, *www.ada.org*.

Drugs can cause negative side effects in the mouth and affect oral health. Everyone is aware that medications can cause assorted and sometimes serious side effects in our bodies, but somehow mouth trouble isn't usually on the radar.

Alan Winter, DDS, a periodontist in private practice and associate clinical professor of implant dentistry at the New York University College of Dentistry, both in New York City, says that many medications affect the mouth and in a number of different ways.

DRY MOUTH

Hundreds of medicines can prevent the salivary glands from manufacturing enough saliva to keep the mouth moist, resulting in an uncomfortably dry mouth. The most common medications that cause dry mouth include blood pressure medications, antidepressants, anti-diarrhea drugs, antihistamines, antipsychotic drugs, decongestants, diuretics, muscle relaxants, oral inhalants for asthma and tranquilizers. The consequences of dry mouth range from simple discomfort to an abnormal taste in the mouth to an inability to generate enough saliva to soften and chew food and in turn properly digest it, to inflammation and dental decay.

What you can do...

•**Make it a habit to frequently sip water.**

•**Avoid sugar.** A dry mouth makes you more prone to decay, so sugar is a no-no.

•**Steer clear of caffeinated drinks, alcohol and tobacco.** These can dry out the mouth.

•**Suck on sugarless hard candy** or chew sugarless gum to stimulate saliva flow.

•**Use a humidifier.** If it's winter and you live in an airtight apartment or house, a humidifier will help keep the air moist.

•**Ask your doctor about a lower dosage** or alternate drug.

ALTERED TASTE

This is another common complaint that may be brought on by cardiovascular drugs, central nervous system stimulants, NSAIDs (nonsteroidal anti-inflammatory drugs), respiratory inhalants or nicotine patches. Often it is difficult to distinguish smell from taste disorders, and advancing age may play a role in impairment, says Dr. Winter. Fortunately, an altered sense of taste or a "bad," metallic taste in the mouth is often a temporary phenomenon.

What you can do...

•**Ask your doctor about changing to a different medication,** or decreasing or eliminating the drug. Perhaps a natural treatment with fewer side effects is an option.

•**Consult your physician about a B-12 test.** Impaired taste can be a sign of a vitamin B-12 deficiency.

SUGAR AND TOOTH DECAY

Although this is beginning to change, not so long ago nearly every children's cough and cold medication came in a sugary red, green or orange syrup. Obviously, the more sugar, the more tooth decay. Other potentially sugary meds or supplements include liquid medications in general, cough drops, vitamins, antacids and antifungal agents.

What you can do...

•**Whenever possible, opt for sugar-free alternatives.**

•**When these are not available, rinse your mouth (or your child's mouth) after taking a medication.** This will get rid of most of the sugary, syrupy residue. This is especially important for medications taken prior to bed.

GUM AND TISSUE REACTIONS

Other oral disturbances—inflammation, sores and tissue discoloration—may be related to blood pressure medications, immunosuppressive drugs, oral contraceptives or chemotherapy. Enlarged gum tissue or overgrowth can be caused by anti-seizure medications, calcium channel blockers or immunosuppressants. This is probably one of the more serious side effects of medications, since tissue overgrowth in the mouth could also signal effects in other areas of the body. The swelling of the tissues comes from the connective tissue...this is called *hypertrophy*, says Dr. Winter.

What you can do...

•**Ask your doctor about changing to a different medication** or whether non-pharmaceutical treatments exist.

•**Pay strict attention to oral hygiene.** Brush at least twice daily and floss once a day. If you neglect your teeth and gums, the problem will only grow worse.

•**If a red patch or white patch, sore or other lesion doesn't heal on its own in seven to 10 days, see your dentist.** While the vast majority of these are benign, only your dentist can determine whether this is a sign of a more serious underlying problem.

BLEEDING IN THE MOUTH

Some medications—such as *heparin*, *warfarin* (Coumadin) and even aspirin— reduce blood clotting, which can lead to bleeding. Dr. Winter adds that certain dietary supplements, notably vitamin E and garlic, are also anticoagulants. This is an important side effect to be aware.

What you can do...

•**Before undergoing any oral surgery or periodontal work,** consult with both your dentist and physician. To prevent excessive bleeding, it may be possible to temporarily adjust your medication or stop taking dietary supplements.

•**If unexpected or excessive bleeding occurs,** make an appointment for a dental checkup to address periodontal disease or an underlying problem. However, if you are taking Coumadin and get excessive bleeding from flossing that does not stop, you should see your physician if you have not had a recent INR (international normalized ratio) test (this checks clotting time). If a recent INR test was within normal limits in the previous three to four weeks, see your dentist for the bleeding.

Note: Not all drugs in all drug categories listed above will result in the specific side effect described. However, there are too many specific drugs to list them all. Read medication warning labels carefully for potential side effects, and be alert to changes in your oral health after you start taking the medication.

DON'T STOP TAKING
YOUR MEDICINE

If you experience uncomfortable side effects in your mouth and suspect they're due to medications, do not simply stop taking your medicine. Instead, consult your physician and dentist. Very often, your doctor can prescribe other treatment options that do not have the same side effects, and your dentist can offer helpful tips on how to cope with problems and keep your teeth and gums in tip-top shape.

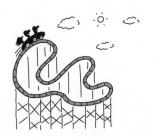

Boning Up on Antidepressants

David Goltzman, MD, director of the McGill Centre for Bone and Periodontal Research, McGill University, Montreal, Canada.

If you're one of the millions of Americans taking antidepressants, be careful, suggests results of a Canadian study.

Antidepressant medications called SSRIs (selective serotonin reuptake inhibitors), which include the well-known drugs *fluoxetine* (Prozac), *paroxetine* (Paxil), *sertraline* (Zoloft), *escitalopram* (Lexapro) and *citalopram* (Celexa), are huge sellers. Sales for SSRIs are already more than $10 billion in this country alone. Older adults are a significant slice of the SSRI market, given that an estimated seven million Americans age 65 and over suffer from depression.

Particularly worrisome for this group is a complicating factor revealed recently by a Canadian study: Use of these antidepressants by older adults substantially increases bone fracture risk. The study came out of the large Canadian Multicentre Osteoporosis Study, designed to research numerous factors of osteoporosis, such as risk factors and intervention success. Scientists followed 5,008 people (age 50 and over at the onset of the study) for five years, by collecting data via questionnaire each year and through intermittent X-rays of participants.

SSRI USE
BONES AND FRACTURES

One of the study authors, David Goltzman, MD, director of the McGill Centre for Bone and Periodontal Research at McGill University in Montreal, Canada, says that previous studies had already shown that SSRI use might predispose people to fractures, and that this particular study confirmed this connection. The study went beyond the previous association between depression meds and bone fracture, in order to look specifically at whether the drugs alone would impact fractures, independent of other conditions that might be present in older individuals taking SSRIs that could also affect bone strength. Study results confirmed that these drugs do appear to predispose users to an increased risk for fractures. Dr. Goltzman adds that some basic data from mice studies have suggested that the drugs' action on serotonin receptors in bone might decrease bone mass and strength.

The numbers weren't large—just 137 people in the total group were taking the drugs, and 18 in this subgroup experienced a bone fracture. But Dr. Goltzman says that the evidence appears to be sound and the researchers have statistical confidence in the study conclusions.

KEEP BONES HEALTHY

SSRIs can be very effective against depression and these findings should not preclude their use when necessary, says Dr. Goltzman. But doctors and older patients should be aware of this added risk when considering use of SSRIs. Dr. Goltzman advises older adults to have a bone mineral density test before starting SSRI treatment, then annually thereafter for as long as they continue the medication. It's also important to maintain a lifestyle that is bone-healthy, he adds—with physical exercise (especially weight-bearing exercise)…adequate intake of calcium, magnesium and vitamin D…a nutritious diet…and not smoking.

What's Unsaid About NSAIDs

Steven E. Nissen, MD, chairman, department of cardiovascular medicine, Cleveland Clinic, Cleveland, Ohio. Dr. Nissen is past president of the American College of Cardiology.

For people suffering from arthritis or headache pain, the solution used to seem relatively simple—take one or two aspirin, ibuprofen or other NSAID (nonsteroidal anti-inflammatory drug) as per label instructions and the pain will go away, or at least recede to a manageable level. However, that advice has become suspect in recent years. Ever since hidden cardiovascular risks forced the withdrawal of the NSAID *rofecoxib* (Vioxx) from the market because it was linked to increased risk of heart attack and stroke, all kinds of questions have arisen about the safety of NSAIDs.

UNDER A CLOUD

Recent criticism has been leveled at the popular over-the-counter pain reliever *naproxen* (brands such as Aleve and Naprosyn), which had been considered the safest cardiovascular choice among the NSAIDs. Steven E. Nissen, MD, chairman of the department of cardiovascular medicine at the Cleveland Clinic and past-president of the American College of Cardiology, says that, in his opinion, the study criticizing naproxen was flawed, in that it was terminated early—but he does concur that this entire class of drugs is under something of a cloud, and agrees that people with cardiovascular problems should be very careful about taking any NSAID (as should people with a long list of other health problems, too, including digestive, liver and kidney disorders).

A FLAWED STUDY

The ADAPT (Alzheimer's Disease Anti-Inflammatory Prevention Trial) research study was designed to compare naproxen and *celecoxib* (Celebrex) in the prevention of Alzheimer's disease. However, the National Institutes of Health (NIH), in response to concerns from the ADAPT Steering Committee, halted the study prematurely (before a reliable conclusion about its potential for Alzheimer's could be made from the data) after Merck withdrew Vioxx and a second study showed increased risks with Celebrex. According to Dr. Nissen, the decision to stop the naproxen trial was made "in a panic" after the publicity about the risks of Vioxx and Celebrex. The details of the study were published two years later.

According to Dr. Nissen, stopping the trial before its intended completion resulted in data that cannot be reliably interpreted—either relative to Alzheimer's disease or cardiac risks. He describes the warnings about naproxen as "the medical equivalent of yelling 'fire' in a crowded auditorium," and he believes the premature termination of the drug trial was not decided for scientific reasons.

TAKE ALL NSAIDs WITH CAUTION

It's important to understand that, to varying degrees, all NSAIDs have cardiovascular and gastrointestinal side effects. In various studies comparing naproxen with other NSAIDs, naproxen has often come out as least harmful to the heart—and one of the hardest on the stomach. Therefore, in the opinion of Dr. Nissen, naproxen is still the safest NSAID for a person with cardiovascular risk factors, although someone who has ulcers might be better off with other alternatives.

LOOK FOR ALTERNATIVES

That said, if you don't need a drug, don't take it, emphasizes Dr. Nissen. If you are experiencing such severe pain that you need to take something, take the lowest possible dose for the shortest possible period of time. For example, people with osteoarthritis have good days and bad days. They should take pain medication only when they are really suffering and need relief. If you have unrelenting chronic pain, such as from rheumatoid arthritis, and must take pain relievers every day, ask your health-care provider to weigh the risks and benefits of the drugs, and discuss if a drug or non-pharmaceutical option—such as meditation, massage, Reiki or music—is a possibility for you.

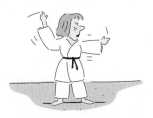

Accutane: Far From the "Clear" Choice for Acne

Peter Rost, MD, author of *The Whistleblower: Confessions of a Healthcare Hitman*. Soft Skull.
PDRHealth, *http://pdrhealth.com/drug_info/rx drugprofiles/drugs/acc1003.shtml.*

When teenage girls receive an Accutane (*isotretinoin*) prescription for acne, they have to register with a federally mandated iPLEDGE program (*www.ipledgeprogram. com*)...sign a consent form regarding the danger of birth defects...read a pamphlet ...watch a video...promise to use two forms of effective contraception simultaneously...have two negative pregnancy tests before beginning therapy...and take monthly pregnancy tests thereafter.

UNNECESSARY EXPOSURE

This elaborate process is the FDA's newest effort to rein in fetal exposure to isotretinoin, which is known to cause birth defects. In spite of this process, many experts feel that far more people are taking this drug than truly need it, unnecessarily exposing thousands to its serious risks.

DANGEROUS ADVERSE EFFECTS

As with too many drugs, overprescription is a major problem with isotretinoin. While the FDA has approved it for a particular form of acne (severe disfiguring cystic acne), it has been prescribed increasingly for milder forms of acne. One study in the *Journal of the American Academy of Dermatology* found that the percent of prescriptions for severe acne from 1993 to 2000 fell from 63% to 46% while isotretinoin treatment for mild and moderate acne increased from 31% to 49%. In addition, over this eight-year period, total prescriptions increased by 250%. Despite all the warnings, many of these women become pregnant.

To make matters even worse, this is far from the only problem with isotretinoin. There are also reports of depression and suicide in people taking it, and in a recent study at the University of California, San Francisco, researchers demonstrated that isotretinoin raises serum lipid levels and that of a liver enzyme, which experts suspect increases the risk for potential heart and liver problems. And still it continues to be prescribed.

IT'S ALL ABOUT MARKETING

You see this over and over again in the drug industry, observes Peter Rost, MD, a former vice-president of marketing at Pfizer and author of *The Whistleblower: Confessions of a Healthcare Hitman* (Soft Skull). He told us that this is a classic way of approaching a difficult drug. Big Pharma gets a narrow approval for limited use of a drug, but then doctors can prescribe it for whatever they want. And, according to Dr. Rost, around half of all prescriptions may be for off-label purposes. It's all about marketing, notes Dr. Rost. He points out that even when drug companies are fined millions of dollars by federal regulators for improperly marketing drugs, it's small change to them compared to the billions of dollars they rake in as profits. And, clearly, there's no one watching the doctors' use—or misuse—of certain drugs.

Your bottom line: The strongest drug is not always the best drug, and you need to think about safer alternatives—in this case, consider benzoyl peroxide or topical tea tree oil. Accutane and its lengthy list of serious risks is just one example of a drug that comes with a big cloud surrounding its silver lining.

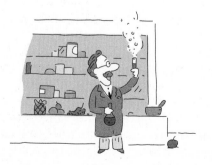

Weight Loss Drug Fills You Up with Side Effects

Larry Sasich, PharmD, MPH, assistant professor, public policy expert and pharmaceutical research analyst, Lake Erie College of Osteopathic Medicine (LECOM) School of Pharmacy, Erie, Pennsylvania.

Alli, the no-prescription-needed diet drug being stocked on drugstore shelves sounds friendly—but can this lower-dose, over-the-counter (OTC) version of the weight loss drug *orlistat* (Xenical) be trusted? At half the dose of Xenical (60 milligrams [mg] versus 120 mg), Alli is said to deliver 85% of its weight loss benefit. But there have been serious concerns about side effects of prescription Xenical, including digestion-related side effects such as flatulence, oily stools and occasional loss of bowel control. Can we expect this version of the drug to behave so differently? And, what are the risks associated with using it without a doctor's supervision?

FRIEND OR FOE?

We spoke with Larry Sasich, PharmD, MPH, assistant professor and public policy expert at the Lake Erie College of Osteopathic Medicine (LECOM) School of Pharmacy in Erie, Pennsylvania. According to Dr. Sasich, who argued before an FDA committee against Xenical's approval (granted in 1999), Alli has no significant health benefits, yet it does have significant side effects.

RISKS APLENTY

Like Xenical, Alli works by blocking the digestion and absorption of fat in the intestine, thereby blocking calories from that fat. Food that is not absorbed simply passes through the system, which can lead to digestion-related side effects such as flatulence, oily stools—and occasional loss of bowel control. In addition to preventing the absorption of fat, Alli also inhibits absorption of some fat-soluble vitamins in food. As though all that wasn't bad enough, the Public Citizen's Health Research Group protested against Xenical, pointing to studies that linked it with precancerous changes in the intestine. Dr. Sasich also cites more recent concerns about a possible link with gallstones.

SAFETY vs. BENEFITS

When it comes to any drug, safety is always weighed relative to benefits. In Dr. Sasich's opinion, the benefits of this drug are not significant. He equates its impact on weight loss efforts with substituting a hamburger for a cheeseburger. You may lose a few pounds, but in the long run this is more cosmetic than healthful. There is no compelling evidence that orlistat (in either the Xenical or Alli formulation) is linked with significant, long-term weight loss that leads to a successful battle against obesity or forestalls diabetes or heart disease, says Dr. Sasich.

NO SHORTCUTS

For most people, there is one simple formula for weight loss: Eat less and exercise more. There are no shortcuts, and even those who advocate for Alli say that it should be used along with a reduced-calorie diet and regular exercise.

How Antibiotics Can Make You Sick

David N. Juurlink, MD, PhD, assistant professor in the department of medicine at the University of Toronto, Canada.

John Mohr, PharmD, assistant professor of medicine-research at the University of Texas Health Science Center at Houston.

Infections are an ongoing risk for those with diabetes, bearing with it serious, even life-threatening complications. Antibiotics, of course, have been the standard pharmacologic treatment for infections. So it was disconcerting when a recent Canadian study showed that one antibiotic, *gatifloxacin* (Tequin), has significant risk of hypoglycemia (low blood sugar) and hyperglycemia (high blood sugar) in people, both those with and without diabetes.

Even before the study results were published in *The New England Journal of Medicine*, the Canadian government issued a warning to consumers that stated that people with diabetes should not use Tequin. Since then, the drug maker Bristol-Myers Squibb has returned the rights of the drug to a Japanese drug company, and Bristol-Myers Squibb has stopped selling and manufacturing Tequin.

WHAT ABOUT OTHER ANTIBIOTICS?

The good news is that very few antibiotics carry the same risk, due to differences in how they work, says David N. Juurlink, MD, PhD, one of the study's authors from the University of Toronto. His study did reveal that there was a slightly increased risk of hypoglycemia with *levofloxacin* (Levaquin), but no such risk was seen with *moxifloxacin* (Avelox), *ciprofloxacin* (Cipro) or certain *cephalosporin* antibiotics (such as *cefuroxime*).

Dr. Juurlink points out, though, that it's important to remember that infections themselves can cause swings in blood sugar, especially for people with diabetes. It's not always exclusively the drug.

John Mohr, PharmD, at the University of Texas Health Science Center at Houston Medical School, agrees. His own research suggests that the class of antibiotics known as *fluoroquinolones* (of which Tequin is one and Cipro, Levaquin and Avelox are others) have been more associated with glucose abnormalities than other classes of antibiotics.

DOSING AND KIDNEYS

Another aspect to be aware of in all of this, says Dr. Mohr, is the dosing issue as it relates to kidney function. For fluoroquinolones that are excreted through the kidneys, attention should be paid to the dose, especially for those patients that have impaired kidney function. Diabetics can have impaired kidney function…they may not be able to eliminate the drug properly…and they can be retaining too much of the drug, unless dosages are reduced, which can produce swings in blood sugar levels.

Diabetics are not the only ones who have impaired kidney function, Dr. Mohr points out. Renal function declines with age, so age is a risk factor for these events as well.

SAFETY STRATEGIES

Dr. Mohr suggests that diabetics taking antibiotics should monitor their blood sugar more frequently than usual and be especially aware of symptoms indicating *dysglycemia* (a blood sugar imbalance). Diabetics are well aware of these, but since sugar imbalance can affect nondiabetics as well, we asked him to enumerate the symptoms.

What to watch for: Increased perspiration…heart palpitations…increased hunger and/or thirst…confusion.

If you experience these symptoms while on a fluoroquinolone, whether you have diabetes or not, you should seek medical care. If you experience sudden changes in mental status or confusion, you should go to an emergency room. However, increased thirst or hunger may not necessarily be due to the fluoroquinolone, and a follow-up in your physician's office should suffice.

New and Risky Treatment for Weight Loss

Anton W. Steiner, MD, PhD, founder and medical director, TriStar Medical Clinic, Los Angeles. He is an active member of the American Society of Bariatric Physicians, an organization for physicians who specialize in the medical treatment of obesity. He can be reached at *www.tristarmedical.com*.

People are choosing to take prescription drugs for weight loss (and doctors are choosing to prescribe them)

that are known to cause weight loss as a "side effect." While prescribing off-label drugs—drugs for an ailment different than what it was originally tested and approved for—is commonplace, seeing the "drug cocktails" for weight loss (for example, an antidepressant and an antiseizure medication) raises all sorts of red flags.

Anton W. Steiner, MD, PhD, a Los Angeles bariatric physician (a doctor who specializes in the medical treatment of obesity), uses prescription medications in his practice, but he combines them with nutrition and exercise recommendations and supplements to design customized weight loss programs.

OFF-LABEL DRUGS

"The whole concept of using drugs 'off-label' has been around for a very long time in general medicine," Dr. Steiner says. "But it snowballed in the weight loss field after the 'fen-phen' experience." Fen-phen was a combination of two drugs—*phentermine* (used to decrease appetite) and *fenfluramine* (a serotonin enhancer)—that was used to produce weight-loss…but the combination was never approved as a weight loss drug, even though many doctors used it for just that purpose. Fenfluramine was taken off the market when it was found to have serious side effects, but phentermine remains the go-to warhorse among weight-loss drugs.

RAISING SEROTONIN

Phentermine (Fastin and Adipex-P) raises levels of two neurotransmitters, dopamine and norepinephrine, resulting in a decrease in appetite and an increase in energy for most people. The other half of the combination—the now off-the-market fenfluramine—worked by raising serotonin. "Our experience with 'fen-phen' back in the 90s taught us that there may be some value in raising serotonin for weight-loss clients even though fenfluramine wasn't the way to go," he says. "This knowledge has sent physicians to another class of drugs that can also raise levels of serotonin, the antidepressants known as selective serotonin reuptake inhibitors (SSRIs; e.g., *fluoxetine* [Prozac], *citalopram* [Celexa] and *escitalopram oxalate* [Lexapro]), as an adjunct in their weight loss protocols."

BESIDES SSRIs

In addition to testing the use of SSRIs, doctors are also prescribing other lesser-known drugs such as *bupropion* (Wellbutrin), an antidepressant that is believed to work by affecting dopamine and norepinephrine, and *topiramate* (Topamax), an antiseizure medication used for migraines, in addition to others. In Dr. Steiner's view, "Wellbutrin doesn't work through serotonin pathways like other antidepressants, but chemically it's very similar to a well-known weight loss drug called *diethylpropion* (Tenuate), so I'm not surprised that some doctors are using it. Topamax is an antiseizure medication and during studies, the observation was made that people lost weight on it. So, in spite of side effects that include skin problems, dizziness, memory loss and sleepiness, doctors are increasingly prescribing Topamax for a variety of off-label situations."

RISKS OF THE REWARD

Dr. Steiner has significant reservations about this "drug cocktail" approach. "As indicated above, each of these drugs has known adverse side effects. However, there are lesser known side effects that can be unpredictable," he says. "For example, high doses of Topamax can produce cognitive impairment. Lexapro can produce nausea. When you have a combination of four psychoactive drugs—that is, drugs that each work on brain chemistry—you may get effects that are totally unpredictable."

Besides the risk associated with the individual drugs, Dr. Steiner notes that "There are almost no studies on combinations of these drugs, and when you get into using three or four or more, what side effects are caused are anyone's guess."

LONG-TERM EFFECTIVENESS?

We asked Dr. Steiner about the long-term effectiveness of this treatment approach. Specifically, how long does he keep his patients on these cocktails? And, does the weight stay off once they are drug free? "If I prescribe a combination of drugs, I will typically use it for three to four months and monitor progress," he says. "If patients aren't making progress in regard to weight loss, we stop the combination." Dr. Steiner says that there are no good studies that indicate weight stays off after discontinuing the drug combination. "In our office, after stopping any drug combination therapy, we do continue with our other modalities such as behavioral and nutritional counseling."

While Dr. Steiner has had success with this therapy in very special cases, and he does not choose this course lightly, we think, there are far safer ways to lose weight especially when long-term results of this protocol are not proven.

New Study Shows COPD Drugs May Be Deadly

E. Neil Schachter, MD, medical director, respiratory care, Mount Sinai Medical Center, New York City, and author of *The Good Doctor's Guide to Colds and Flu*. HarperCollins.

US Food and Drug Administration, *www.fda.gov*.

Chronic obstructive pulmonary disease (COPD), an umbrella term for lung diseases including emphysema and chronic bronchitis (in combination or alone), affects more than 15 million Americans. Because COPD can only be managed—not cured through conventional means—medication is crucial to control symptoms.

TWO GROUPS OF MEDS

Medications for these conditions include bronchodilators—either anticholinergics such as *tiotropium* (Spiriva) and *ipratropium* (Atrovent) or beta-2 agonists. Beta-2 agonists are used singly or in combination with anticholinergics. Beta-2 agonists—with the drug names *metaproterenol* (Alupent), *formoterol* (Foradil), *salmeterol* (Serevent, Advair, Diskus) and *albuterol* (Proventil, Ventolin, Volmax and others)—are widely used, which makes a recent study from Stanford University particularly worrisome.

BETA-2 AGONISTS

The study was a statistical analysis of previous trials on the drugs as used by a total of 15,276 participants. It found that patients using anticholinergics reduced severe respiratory events by 33% and respiratory-related deaths by 73% compared with a placebo. Conversely, however, the use of beta-2 agonists showed an increased risk of respiratory death that was more than twice as high as that of a placebo. This alarming statistic prompted our editors to call pulmonologist E. Neil Schachter, MD, the medical director of respiratory care at the Mount Sinai Medical Center in New York City and author of *The Good Doctor's Guide to Colds and Flu* (HarperCollins).

STUDY LIMITATIONS

Dr. Schachter says that while this is a worthwhile study, even the authors point out its limitations. First, while the study reviewed results from 22 previous studies, the majority of patients were from a few larger trials. Second, it investigated patients only as an overall group without consideration of the impact of higher-risk subgroups. In fact, there are two subgroups of patients at greater risk when using beta-2 agonists—patients with underlying cardiovascular disease and those with a genetic variant that is particularly prevalent among African Americans. However, he says that these are generally considered to be good drugs used successfully by millions of patients for many years.

LABS ADVISORY

Still, the US Food and Drug Administration (FDA) notified drug manufacturers to update product labels with revised warnings on certain long-acting beta-2 agonists (LABAs) for use by asthmatics. *The FDA's advisory stated…*

•**LABAs should not be the first medicine used to treat asthma.** LABAs should be added to the treatment plan only if other medicines do not control asthma, including the use of low- or medium-dose corticosteroids.

•**Do not stop using your LABA or other asthma medicines that your health-care professional has prescribed for you** unless you have discussed with your health-care provider whether or not to continue treatment.

•**Do not use your LABA to treat wheezing that is getting worse.** Call your health-care professional right away if wheezing worsens while using a LABA.

•**LABAs do not relieve sudden wheezing.** Always have a short-acting bronchodilator medicine with you to treat sudden wheezing.

Thus far the FDA has not issued anything further on LABAs, even after the recent COPD study.

DISCUSSION WITH DOCTOR

Even so, while Dr. Schachter urges patients not to stop taking their medications, he says they should discuss their individual situation with their doctor. He especially cautions anyone who might have—or be at risk for—cardiovascular disease to immediately discuss these drugs with their doctor…and that African Americans should ask about having the test for the gene variant that puts people at risk. He adds that although the statistics of a bad outcome are low for beta-2 agonists, there is no need for anyone at risk to take them because alternative drugs are available.

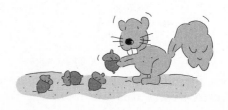

Research Update: Statin Drugs Don't Prevent Cancer

Michael White, PharmD, associate professor of pharmacy practice, University of Connecticut/Hartford Hospital, Hartford, Connecticut.

Statin medications were originally introduced for people at high risk of cardiovascular disease as drugs that would decrease their cholesterol levels. However, in the ensuing years, studies emerged that associated statin use with a number of other benefits as well. The studies that most excited people were those that showed a link between statins and decreased cancer risk, but we now have more recent information on the subject.

CANCER RATES

Researchers at the University of Connecticut/Hartford Hospital analyzed data from 26 controlled studies (studies on statins and cancer that went as far back as 1996 through July 2005) that involved about 87,000 people taking statins. Their finding was clear. Statins do not affect cancer rates, as much as the statin manufacturers would like us to believe otherwise.

DIFFERENT FINDINGS

This was surprising news in light of the reported findings of earlier studies. We called the study's lead author, C. Michael White, PharmD, to find out more about the situation and his findings. Dr. White explains that the reason for the different outcomes was the nature of the previous studies. The originally reported studies were case-controlled ones in which researchers looked back at databases of patients with or without cancer and then investigated which of these people were taking statins. Case-controlled studies do not investigate any other factors about the population—for example, age, education levels, lifestyles, gender, differences in levels of cholesterol—some of which would

have an important impact on outcomes. This can lead to false conclusions.

CONTROLLED STUDIES

Dr. White's research evaluated only randomized controlled studies, considered the gold standard in research. In these controlled studies, researchers split their test subjects evenly and start one group on the drug under investigation and a second group on a placebo. The groups are "blind," which is to say that they don't know if they are on the drug or the placebo. In evaluating the results at the end of the study, the researchers adjust for any factors other than drug use that would affect outcome so that findings will reflect the influence of the medication only.

NO CONNECTION

Dr. White's study went so far as to isolate individual statins as well as types of cancer and still found no relationship. His conclusion is that people who need the protection statins can provide against cardiovascular risk should take them. But no one should be taking statins in hopes of preventing cancer—or, for that matter, assume that because they are taking statins they don't need to follow other cancer-preventive measures.

Breakthrough Drugs Do More Than Just Treat Symptoms

Scott J. Zashin, MD, rheumatologist with practices in Dallas and Plano, Texas. Dr. Zashin is author of *Arthritis Without Pain*. Sarah Allison.

One of the biggest problems with many drugs is that they are non-specific. While they are "fixing" what ails you, they also are affecting other parts of your body, often with unpleasant or dangerous side effects. Enter *biological response modifiers* (biologics for short), a potentially exciting new class of drugs derived from living organisms that are designed to target specific components of the immune system with the goal of treating the underlying causes of serious disease rather than the symptoms. These drugs have been in use for some time in the treatment of rheumatoid arthritis (RA) and are starting to make their way into other areas.

HOW THEY WORK

An exciting difference in biologic drugs versus most current medications is that they offer more than symptomatic relief—they focus on underlying issues that cause symptoms. Scott J. Zashin, MD, Texas rheumatologist and author of *Arthritis Without Pain* (Sarah Allison), has been using biologics to treat patients with rheumatoid arthritis. He says that three biologic agents—*etanercept* (Enbrel), *adalimumab* (Humira) and *infliximab* (Remicade) are often effective in controlling RA in people who do not respond to conventional medications known as disease-modifying drugs (DMARDs).

BLOCKING TNF

Enbrel, Humira and Remicade work by blocking a substance manufactured by the immune system called tumor necrosis factor (TNF). People with RA and related inflammatory diseases—including juvenile rheumatoid arthritis, ankylosing spondylitis, psoriatic arthritis and psoriasis—have too much TNF in their bodies. This overwhelms the immune system's ability to control inflammation, resulting in painful, swollen joints or, in the case of psoriasis, redness, itching and thick, silvery scales on the skin.

Note: These medications are approved for RA and psoriatic arthritis...Humira and Remicade are also approved for ankylosing spondylitis...Remicade is approved for Crohn's disease and ulcerative colitis, etc. They are also used on an off-label basis for those inflammatory problems for which they are not approved.

TNF-blocking biologics are essentially man-made versions of proteins that the body produces naturally, whose job it is to bind to and deactivate TNF molecules before they can do their damage. This interrupts the chain of events that leads to some forms of inflammation, and much of its resulting pain and damage.

PROS AND CONS OF BIOLOGICS FOR RA

According to Dr. Zashin, each of the three primary biologic drugs for RA (which are essentially blocking agents) have their pluses and minuses. *One minus is that they can weaken the immune system...*

•**Enbrel.** Given by self-injection under the skin once or twice a week, Enbrel can provide rapid relief, often with the first shot. Dr. Zashin reports that relief tends to come faster with Enbrel than with Humira. With both Enbrel and Humira, injection site reactions that include pain, redness and infections are a concern, and, as mentioned above, all three biologics can weaken the immune system. Alert your physician at the first sign of any infection.

•**Humira.** This drug is also administered by injection, but a significant advantage is that shots are required on average only twice a month. In his practice, Dr. Zashin sees fewer upper respiratory infections caused primarily by the suppression of the immune system with Humira than with Enbrel. However, he adds that this is only his own experience, and research has yet to corroborate this effect.

•**Remicade.** Dr. Zashin recommends Remicade only when Enbrel and Humira prove ineffective. This drug must be given intravenously and administration takes about two hours. It is usually given three times during the first three weeks of treatment, and every eight weeks thereafter. Dr. Zashin cautions that with IV administration, there is a small but real risk of infusion reactions. Remicade is also considerably more expensive than the other biologics and brings with it similarly dangerous side effects. Remicade also has been approved for use in the treatment of Crohn's disease and ulcerative colitis.

OTHER BIOLOGICS

A fourth biologic, *anakinra* (Kineret), is also available, but in Dr. Zashin's opinion, it is less effective than the others. Newly approved *abatacept* (Orencia) is a second-generation biologic that works differently from the TNF-blockers because it targets a different element of the immune system. Only time will tell whether this new medication is "safe and effective." Keep in mind that "safe and effective" is a category description that the FDA uses, not a guarantee that the drugs will be safe for all—or safe in the long term.

A RISK FOR SERIOUS SIDE EFFECTS

As with any drugs that affect the immune system, Dr. Zashin warns that biologics have a serious downside. *Risks that he mentions include...*

•**Serious infections,** including tuberculosis and sepsis

•**Nervous system diseases,** such as multiple sclerosis

•**Blood problems**

•**Heart problems** (for example, congestive heart failure)

•**Allergic reactions**

•**Malignancies,** including lymphoma

Also, Dr. Zashin warns that the long-term effects of these drugs are simply not known. If you are taking a biologic, you must be very careful to meet regularly with your doctor to monitor your progress and any side effects.

TREATMENT MUST BE CAREFULLY INDIVIDUALIZED

RA can be a crippling disease, and some sufferers look on biologic medications as lifesavers. On the other hand, not everyone with RA needs to take biologics, warns Dr. Zashin. These are serious drugs that should be used only when they are absolutely necessary, and some people may be able to get by with nonsteroidal anti-inflammatory drugs (NSAIDs), such as ibuprofen, and more natural treatments.

The most important thing is to carefully individualize treatment, emphasizes Dr. Zashin. While one person with RA needs only NSAIDs, another might experience such rapidly developing damage that early and aggressive intervention with biologic medications is warranted.

Blood Pressure and Painkillers

Charles H. Hennekens, MD, DrPH, Sir Richard Doll research professor, Charles E. Schmidt College of biomedical science, Florida Atlantic University, Boca Raton, Florida.

Research has shown repeatedly that frequent use of nonaspirin pain relievers raises high blood pressure in women. Interestingly, research has not shown the same connection for men. This, however, does not give men a free pass, says Charles H. Hennekens, MD, DrPH, an architect of the Women's Health Study at Harvard and now research professor of biochemical science at Florida Atlantic University in Boca Raton.

THE LATEST RESEARCH

The latest research results regarding a connection between pain relievers and high blood pressure were reported in the *Archives of Internal Medicine*. At Brigham and Women's Hospital in Boston, researchers looked at data from more than 8,000 men, ages 53 to 97, enrolled in the long-term Physicians' Health Study. At the start of the trial, no participants had high blood pressure. Over a six-year period, the men recorded their use of NSAIDs (nonsteroidal anti-inflammatory drugs such as *ibuprofen* [Advil, Motrin, etc.]), aspirin and *acetaminophen* (Tylenol). Their blood pressure was also monitored during this time.

After six years, about one-quarter of the men developed high blood pressure. However, researchers found no clear link between the frequency of pain reliever use and the occurrence of hypertension. Sounds like a free pass, right?

HOLES IN THE LOGIC

According to Dr. Hennekens, by causing salt and fluid retention, all NSAIDs can contribute to high blood pressure in anyone, male or female. This study may have been skewed in that it researched only physicians, who may be more likely to take better care of themselves than the general public.

In Dr. Hennekens' opinion, we need large epidemiological studies that focus on direct, one-on-one comparisons of over-the-counter (OTC) pain relievers in different populations. Until that time comes, if you need to take a painkiller for any substantial length of time—for example, to cope with a chronic condition such as arthritis—he recommends that you proceed with caution. *Keep in mind...*

•**Are you prone to cardiovascular risk?** From a cardiovascular perspective, you are better off with aspirin.

•**Do you suffer from gastrointestinal (GI) discomfort?** Aspirin and NSAIDs can cause stomach ulcers that bleed as well as GI bleeding in most people. The longer you take an NSAID, the greater the risk. Do not take an NSAID for more than 10 days without consulting your physician. Do not take more than the dose listed on the package...and take less if possible.

•**Consider acetaminophen,** which is not associated with GI bleeding. However, if taken in higher doses than recommended, Tylenol can lead to liver and kidney problems, particularly when taken with alcohol or other medications that contain acetaminophen (such as OTC cold remedies, cough syrups and prescription pain medications). Often these problems are irreversible and life-threatening.

NO PERFECT PILL

The bottom line is that all drugs have side effects, and there is no easy answer, no one perfect pill to cure what ails you. The best you can do is carefully weigh the risks versus benefits, consider your medical history, talk to your doctor and come to a decision about which is best for you individually. Also, don't forget that there are many safer alternatives to pills. For example, nondrug approaches to arthritis management include diet, exercise, acupuncture and stress management.

15

Breakthrough Healing For Women

Ladies: Best Ways to Pump Up Your Heart

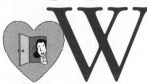omen truly have a lot of catching up to do when it comes to awareness and information about heart disease—even in light of the fact that heart disease is the number one killer of American women, claiming more lives each year than all cancers combined. Thankfully, that's changing, and attention is at last being paid, largely due to the efforts of the American Heart Association's (AHA) annual campaign for women's heart health. The AHA has released its guidelines for preventing cardiovascular disease in women to address and, it is hoped, change the fact that today nearly one in three women die of cardiovascular disease (CVD). The really good news about the recent guidelines is that they focus on prevention of heart disease

in women, not merely on the differences in how it manifests and should be treated.

SETTING THE BAR REALLY HIGH

While the guidelines are replete with good-health recommendations including don't smoke, exercise regularly and eat a heart-healthy diet, they are also complex, lengthy and ambitious, aimed at encouraging women to view lowering CVD risk as a lifelong pursuit. With this goal in mind, the guidelines urge women as young as 20 to make the effort to determine their personal risk and, if necessary, take action to lower it. They advise women to get at least 30 minutes of exercise most days of the week or every day. They also recommend 60 to 90 minutes of exercise most days or every day for those who need to lose or maintain weight loss (which is many women since two-thirds are overweight). Nutrition advice includes consuming fruits

Kelly Anne Spratt, DO, clinical associate professor of medicine, University of Pennsylvania Health System, Philadelphia.

and vegetables…whole-grain, high-fiber foods…and fish (especially oily fish) at least twice a week. Then it gets complicated, advising restriction of saturated fats to no more than 10% of daily caloric intake and limiting cholesterol to 300 milligrams (mg) a day, plus more.

There is general agreement that the AHA guidelines are a noble effort, but some fear their complexity and scope may overwhelm many women who will, as a result, give up entirely and return to the couch with their potato chips.

HERE'S HOW TO DO IT

Without question, simplifying and prioritizing the information would increase the odds that more women will incorporate enough of these guidelines to lower CVD risk and enhance their overall health. Cardiovascular specialist Kelly Anne Spratt, DO, clinical associate professor of medicine at the University of Pennsylvania Health System in Philadelphia, shares the concern that women will find the guidelines overwhelming, but she says they are nonetheless vital—if for no other reason than to reinforce the importance of building health-enhancing habits while you are still young.

START SLOWLY AND BUILD

Regarding nutrition and exercise, Dr. Spratt believes that everyone, whatever age, should start with the easiest possible improvements and make gradual positive changes. She suggests starting an exercise program by walking 10 minutes each day (even busy people can usually fit this in). Once that becomes a habit, increase your daily walking time by five minutes each week until you're up to at least 30 minutes per day.

Her nutrition advice is equally straightforward. Avoid high glycemic foods, she says: Just cut back on all white foods—white bread, white rice, pasta and sugar—and eat more whole grains and a variety of brightly colored fruits and vegetables. You'll be well on your way to improved heart health.

DOES YOUR DOCTOR DO THIS?

Many women, young and middle-aged, rely on their gynecologists for health exams. That's fine, as they are able to perform the routine screenings the AHA recommends. Just make sure they are being done. *In Dr. Spratt's opinion, here are the health screenings that even 20-year-olds should have at least annually…*

• **Blood pressure check,** along with a discussion about the reading.

• **Women should be weighed at regular exams and they should also get a height measurement,** so they can calculate their body mass index (BMI) and figure out if weight needs to be modified through diet and exercise. Though BMI is thought to be an imperfect measure of weight-related health risk, it's the best we have at present—and better than no measure at all. To calculate body mass index, go to the Centers for Disease Control and Prevention's Web site at *www.cdc.gov/nccdphp/dnpa/bmi/index.htm.*

• **Moving beyond basics,** Dr. Spratt suggests women in their 20s should also have lab tests for cholesterol and glucose levels—not because heart problems are apt to show up at this young age, but again, because this helps raise awareness of these health measures for heart disease risk factors (diabetes and high cholesterol) and build lifestyle habits that will protect them down the line.

JUST REMEMBER THIS…

Dr. Spratt has one final and important point: Women's symptoms of heart disease and heart attack are often more subtle than those of men, typically including shortness of breath (especially in association with exertion), persistent fatigue and a pain or dull ache in the arm, jaw and/or neck, shoulder or back (most especially if in more than one location, won't go away and can't be connected to any other obvious cause). Other symptoms include chest pain, nausea, indigestion and feeling faint. These may be signs of a serious problem, and should always be investigated by your doctor, she says. If you suspect a heart attack, call 911 immediately. Dr. Spratt says that women tend to call for help three hours later than men, losing priceless time that doctors could use to save heart muscle, and perhaps even your life.

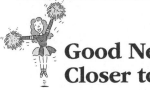

Good News!
Closer to the Cure

Stephanie Kaplan, ND, A Woman's Time, Portland, Oregon.
American Cancer Society, *www.cancer.org.*

For 20% to 30% of women with breast cancer, there's renewed hope with a drug called *trastuzumab* (Herceptin). This treatment represents a major breakthrough for those who produce too much of a breast cancer-related protein known as HER2. Not long ago, these women suffered from an aggressive and stubborn form of breast cancer with a poorer prognosis, greater chance of recurrence and lower likelihood of survival than women with HER2-negative breast cancer.

According to Stephanie Kaplan, ND, a naturopathic physician at the women's health-care clinic, A Woman's Time, in Portland, Oregon, Herceptin is one of a number of promising treatments that bring us closer to an actual *cure* for breast cancer.

CUTTING CANCER
RECURRENCE IN HALF

In 1998, Herceptin was approved for the treatment of metastatic breast cancer that had already spread through the body. However, in recent years researchers have begun to explore the drug's use in women with less advanced cancers.

In April 2005, the preliminary findings of two clinical trials of Herceptin were so promising that the National Cancer Institute halted them early to make the results public. In more than 3,300 women with early stage HER2-positive breast cancer, researchers found that those who combined Herceptin and chemotherapy experienced a 52% decrease in cancer recurrence, in comparison with women who had chemotherapy alone.

Unfortunately, this positive impact comes at a price beyond high cost. Herceptin must be administered intravenously, and common side effects during the treatment include fever, chills, weakness, nausea, vomiting, cough, diarrhea and headache. In addition, Herceptin may increase long-term risk for heart problems such as congestive heart failure, hypersensitivity reactions (including life-threatening anaphylaxis) and respiratory distress. In rare instances, these have been fatal.

ONE STEP CLOSER TO A CURE

Herceptin is currently FDA-approved for advanced metastatic breast cancer in HER2-positive women and, combined with other cancer drugs, for treatment of HER2-positive breast cancer after a mastectomy or lumpectomy. As with any medication, women who are candidates for Herceptin (especially those with early-stage cancer) should carefully discuss its risks versus benefits with their physicians, keeping in mind that the long-term impact of Herceptin is not yet known due to the newness of the drug.

It's not perfect and it's not for everyone, but for some HER2-positive women, Herceptin can literally be a lifesaver.

Closing In on a
Cure for Breast Cancer

Elizabeth M. Whelan, ScD, MPH, president, American Council on Science and Health, New York City.
National Cancer Institute, *www.cancer.gov.*
US Food and Drug Administration, *www.fda.gov.*

Is it possible that we are finally approaching a cure for breast cancer? According to Elizabeth M. Whelan, ScD, MPH, president of the American Council on Science and Health in New York City, the answer is yes—at least in the case of early-stage tumors. Although we are routinely bombarded with bad news on the cancer front, she points out that significant progress has been made in recent years, with deaths from breast cancer falling. The latest good news involves the new class of drugs called *aromatase inhibitors*.

THREE FACTORS BRING US NEARER TO A CURE

Dr. Whelan says it's important to understand that there are several factors that are increasing survival rates for breast cancer, some of which have nothing to do with medications...

•**Early detection through mammography.** As more women undergo screening for breast cancer, more tumors are being detected in early stages when there is a greater likelihood of a cure. Dr. Whelan notes that an increasingly large percentage of tumors are being found when they are at stage 0—technically a pre-cancer known as "breast cancer in situ"—or stage 1, when the cancer is less than ¾ inch in size and has not spread to the lymph nodes or elsewhere.

•**Effective treatment of early-stage breast cancer.** Dr. Whelan points out that the treatment of stage 1 cancer has become so effective that already it essentially amounts to a "cure." The current course of treatment typically consists of lumpectomy, followed by six weeks of radiation and then drug therapy. New research suggests that shorter courses of radiation may be just as effective as longer courses.

•**Hormone therapy.** Seven out of 10 women with breast cancer have tumors that are estrogen-sensitive, meaning that the hormone estrogen encourages their growth. By reducing estrogen levels, hormone therapies lower the risk of breast cancer recurrence. *Tamoxifen* (Nolvadex) has long been the standard hormone treatment for women with estrogen-receptive breast cancer as well as for women at higher risk than usual for the disease (for example,

if they have had breast cancer in situ or a close family member with the disease).

There is no doubt that tamoxifen has had a major impact, reducing the risk of recurrence by some 40% in clinical trials. However, recently, new hormone-therapy drugs known as aromatase inhibitors (AIs) have seized center stage, demonstrating great promise in reducing recurrence rates even further.

PROMISING AROMATASE INHIBITORS

While tamoxifen has saved many lives, its effectiveness has come at a cost. There is growing concern about the relatively uncommon but real and very serious risks associated with this drug, including uterine cancer, severe blood clots and stroke. Enter AIs, a newer class of hormone drugs with fewer (although still significant) side effects and potentially even greater effectiveness. So far, three AIs have been approved by the US Food and Drug Administration (FDA)—*anastrozole* (Arimidex), *exemestane* (Aromasin) and *letrozole* (Femara).

What the research tells us: There have been three recent randomized controlled trials of AIs in postmenopausal women with breast cancer. In all the trials, AIs significantly improved disease-free survival. This proved to be the case both when AIs were given as the initial hormone therapy compared with tamoxifen, and when they were given sequentially after tamoxifen therapy (for example, taking tamoxifen for two years and then switching to an AI).

How aromatase inhibitors work: AIs reduce estrogen by blocking the enzyme aromatase, which enables tissues other than the ovaries to make estrogen. Since this makes them effective in women whose ovaries no longer manufacture estrogen, these drugs are used mostly in postmenopausal women.

Possible side effects: While generally well tolerated, AIs are nevertheless powerful drugs with potentially powerful side effects. These include joint pain, pain in the muscles and bones, bone loss (osteoporosis) and increased fracture rates. To counter potential reduction in bone density, Dr. Whelan recommends calcium and vitamin D supplements, and osteoporosis drugs as necessary. Good news is that adverse events associated with tamoxifen—uterine cancer, severe blood clots and stroke—are significantly lower with AIs.

LOOKING TOWARD THE FUTURE

Not only can AIs effectively reduce breast cancer recurrence in postmenopausal women, research increasingly suggests that they may play a vital role in preventing it in the first place. Clinical trials to determine their effectiveness in this regard are currently underway in the US and Canada. Readers can learn more about the ExCel study at *www.excelstudy. com*. Studies comparing tamoxifen with AIs also continue, with the goal of determining whether AIs should ideally be given in place of tamoxifen or as part of a sequential treatment. In all cases, researchers are looking at ways to prevent or mitigate treatment-related side effects.

MORE GOOD NEWS

The sister drug to tamoxifen, *raloxifene* (Evista), is currently approved for osteoporosis and breast cancer prevention in certain postmenopausal women. *Trastuzumab* (Herceptin) is a drug that represents a major breakthrough for women who produce too much of a particular breast cancer-related protein (HER2).

Digital Mammograms— Better Detection

Etta D. Pisano, MD, Kenan professor of radiology and biomedical engineering, as well as vice-dean for academic affairs, University of North Carolina at Chapel Hill School of Medicine. She is also director of the UNC Biomedical Research Imaging Center.

Digital technology has won yet another battle over film. This most recent victory won't affect your point-and-shoot handheld camera, but it does prove that going digital could improve the effectiveness of your next mammogram. In some cases, it could even save your life.

Those are the implications of a study published recently in *The New England Journal of Medicine*. The study compared traditional film mammograms with digital mammograms in 42,760 women.

What the researchers found: The digital mammograms allowed for earlier detection of more cancers in women under 50, women with dense breasts, and pre- and perimenopausal women. Many of these cancers were early-stage invasive cancers— precisely the type that must be detected early in order for treatment to be effective.

DIGITAL POWERS THROUGH THE CLUTTER

What makes digital better? The answers are still being researched, but it likely has to do with being able to manipulate the image after the fact (much like removing red-eye from your home snapshots before printing them)—something that can't be done with film.

"We can play with the contrast of the image and make it clearer so you can see through the dense areas better," says the study's lead author, Etta D. Pisano, MD, Kenan professor of radiology and biomedical engineering at the University of North Carolina at Chapel Hill School of Medicine, and director of the UNC Biomedical Research Imaging Center. Improved viewing of dense breasts seems to be the key factor, and it also explains why there's no noticeable difference between film and digital in those who are over age 50 or postmenopausal, as well as in those with less dense breasts. Breast density changes over time—and breasts typically get less dense with age.

IT'S EXPENSIVE

Unfortunately, digital mammography isn't widespread—according to Dr. Pisano, only about 10% of mammography units in the US use digital systems. The changeover is happening slowly, mostly due to the price of the digital machines, which cost up to four times as much as film mammography units.

THE DIGITAL OPTION

So what's a patient to do? First, talk to your doctor to find out if digital mammograms are available in your area and if they would benefit you. (If digital is an option, contact your insurer to find out about coverage—at this point, it still varies, although the results of this study have had a positive impact.) If your doctor believes a digital mammogram is clinically important for you, ask him to contact your insurer. Often, when physicians cite strong clinical need to an insurer, a specific test that otherwise would not be covered, will be.

If digital is not yet available in your area, ask your doctor to be on the lookout for its availability—or if you are at high risk, if it is possible to travel to a facility where the procedure is performed.

In the end, though, remember this: Whether digital or film, what matters most is that you have your regularly scheduled mammogram. This screening is too important to skip.

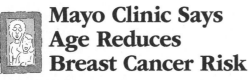

Mayo Clinic Says Age Reduces Breast Cancer Risk

Lynn C. Hartmann, MD, oncologist, Mayo Clinic, Rochester, Minnesota.

A long-held medical belief is that breast cancer risk increases as a woman ages. In fact, age alone is considered a risk factor. But a fascinating study from the Mayo Clinic has found that for many women, normal aging might actually *reduce* risk.

Reason: The breasts have numerous milk-producing glands called lobules and,

not surprisingly, as women age, these lobules shut down, a process called lobular regression or involution. The scientists at Mayo Clinic discovered that the fewer the remaining lobules women had—or, in other words, the greater the involution of the breast—the lower the woman's risk of breast cancer. This makes complete sense because the vast majority of breast cancers start in the lobules of the breast...so the fewer of them, the fewer places for these cancers to begin.

RESEARCH BACKGROUND

For the study, pathologists evaluated 8,736 tissue samples from breast biopsies (benign results) taken between 1967 and 1991 at the Mayo Clinic. They then used this large number of samples to evaluate what types of benign breast findings were associated with increased cancer risk. (These biopsies were done because of a lump or mammographic abnormality, for example.) Having such a vast number of tissue samples gave the researchers the opportunity to study how changes in breast tissue itself might provide risk clues.

THE INVOLUTION FACTOR

When they evaluated the degree of involution, they discovered that women with no involution had twice the risk of developing cancer than did women who had complete involution. They also found that 53% of the women age 70 and over had complete involution...women who had never used hormone replacement therapy (HRT) had slightly more involution as well. Others with increased involution were women who had never given birth and those who had had only one child. Interestingly, breast feeding history made no difference in the amount of later involution.

A COMPLEX PUZZLE

Mayo Clinic oncologist Lynn C. Hartmann, MD, coauthor of the study, says that the association of involution and cancer may be enough to consider involution as yet another in a series of factors that indicate the level of risk, some of which may be independent of others. It appears now that women in families with a history of breast cancer also have a lower rate of involution. On the other hand, one risk for breast cancer has been having had no children...and yet these women have greater involution. Clearly it is a complex puzzle and one that requires much more research.

For now, women can discover their degree of involution only through a biopsy because it takes place on a microscopic level. Dr. Hartmann says if a woman is having a biopsy for other reasons, she can certainly ask the lab to determine the amount of involution. However, be prepared to explain the reason for your request to the doctor because, as Dr. Hartmann notes, few people are as yet aware of this finding.

Experts Don't Acknowledge Cancer Risk

Norman F. Boyd, MD, senior scientist, Campbell Family Institute for Breast Cancer Research at the Ontario Cancer Institute at Princess Margaret Hospital in Toronto, Canada.

I t's not listed as a risk factor by the American Cancer Society, but extensive breast density—which relates to density of breast tissue on a mammogram, not how it feels to the touch—appears to be associated with an increase in the risk that a woman will develop breast cancer. This is according to a number of studies, including a Canadian one published in *The New England Journal of Medicine*. Researchers there said women (over age 40) with at least 75% breast density on a mammogram (three-quarters of the tissue qualifying as dense) were approximately five times more likely to develop breast cancer than women with less than 10% density.

EYE-OPENING STUDY

The study was led by senior scientist Norman F. Boyd, MD, of the Campbell Family Institute for Breast Cancer Research at the Princess Margaret Hospital in Toronto. Researchers compared records of patients from three Canadian mammogram screening studies, examining records of 1,112 women diagnosed with breast cancer between 1993 and 1999, along with an equal number of women who did not develop breast cancer. Compared with women with less than 10% density on their mammogram, women with density in at least 75% of the breast were three times more likely to have breast cancer found at the time of their screening, and 17 times more likely to have cancer diagnosed in the 12 months after a negative screening examination.

WHAT YOU NEED TO KNOW ABOUT BREAST DENSITY

Neither you nor your doctor can determine your breast density by visual or manual inspection, but a mammogram will show how much of the breast is made up of fat and how much is "dense," meaning made of milk gland and duct tissue, and fibrous tissue. Fat tissue is lucent (or dark on a mammography image), while dense tissue is light or white, as are cancers. With lots of fibroglandular tissue, it's less likely your mammogram will identify a growing cancer, as tumors may be masked or obscured.

Tumors don't typically grow in fat cells, but they do grow in the cells of other body tissue. The more fibroglandular tissue in the breast, the more cells capable of becoming cancerous. According to Dr. Boyd, though the BRCA1 and BRCA2 gene mutations, which appear among the American Cancer Society's risk factors for breast cancer, are associated with larger risks to individuals with these gene mutations, they actually account for a much smaller fraction of breast cancer cases overall than does high-density breast tissue.

345

MORE RESEARCH TO LEARN WHAT WE CAN DO

Researchers are now looking at what measures women with dense breasts can take to reduce their risk of getting breast cancer or it spreading, including having additional imaging methods used such as digital mammography, magnetic resonance and ultrasound that may detect tumors earlier, before cancer has spread. Another question being studied is if genes associated with dense breasts might be isolated and targeted for treatment. Further, Dr. Boyd notes that hormone therapy (HT), especially combined estrogen and progesterone, may cause an increase in density, so women on HT or considering it should discuss this finding with their doctor.

Catching Ovarian Cancer Before It Kills

Lloyd Smith, MD, chair of the department of obstetrics and gynecology, University of California, Davis, Women's Center for Health, Sacramento.

Ovarian cancer strikes fear in most women's hearts—with reason. It is the fifth-leading cause of cancer deaths among women, and it affects increasing numbers of them, from one in 70 several years ago to one in 57 now. With an aging population and the highest incidence of ovarian cancer occurring in women in their 60s, these numbers, unfortunately, may get worse. Without obvious early symptoms to alert them, the cancer diagnosis comes too late for survival for most patients.

EARLY SYMPTOMS

Fortunately, several new studies show there are indeed early symptoms after all, including...

- **Bloating, a feeling of fullness, gas**
- **Frequent or urgent urination**
- **Nausea, indigestion, constipation, diarrhea**
- **Menstrual disorders, pain during intercourse**
- **Fatigue, backaches.**

Admittedly, the list reads like symptoms of common gastrointestinal or menstrual problems. But when researchers from the University of Washington fine-tuned their data analysis, they found that far more women with undiagnosed cancer than others had a triad of symptoms—bloating, increased abdominal size and urinary urgency. Furthermore, the symptoms in women with cancer were persistent, recurring nearly every day, and more severe than in other women.

READING THE EARLY SIGNS

Researchers at the University of California, Davis, also studied possible early symptoms. Headed by Lloyd Smith, MD, chair of the department of obstetrics and gynecology, this study researched Medicare record codes of symptoms that brought women to their doctors months before actual diagnosis. Dr. Smith says that much to his surprise, the data demonstrated women who were later found to have cancer were seeing their doctor for four months to a year before diagnosis for symptoms of abdominal pain and swelling, gastrointestinal symptoms and pelvic pain. The records also showed that doctors routinely ordered abdominal imaging or gastrointestinal procedures, rather than any for ovarian cancer. Dr. Smith says this isn't surprising—the brain doesn't interpret the signals from pelvic nerves properly, so symptoms seem abdominal, not pelvic.

WHEN IN DOUBT, GET CHECKED

While this might seem confusing, Dr. Smith says there is a valuable message for all women. If you have any of the above symptoms on a persistent basis, get a routine medical evaluation. If no other cause is found, immediately get an ultrasound of the pelvis and the CA-125 blood test that measures cancer antigen-125, a protein produced in ovarian cancer cells. The CA-125 test is controversial because it is not dependable as a screening test. But Dr. Smith says that it is considerably better as a diagnostic tool than it is as a screening method, especially when used in combination with an ultrasound. Most important is to pay attention to the symptoms. If what you think is just gas or PMS doesn't get better, get checked.

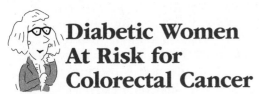

Diabetic Women At Risk for Colorectal Cancer

Jill E. Elwing, MD, is in private practice in St. Louis, Missouri.

There seems to be no end to the health risks associated with diabetes, a truly insidious disease that can lead to other serious health problems. Having diabetes increases risk for cardiovascular disease, kidney failure, hypertension, stroke and damage to the nerves and eyes. Research has also linked diabetes to a greater risk of certain cancers, including colorectal (colon or rectum) cancer. And a recent study from Washington University in St. Louis concludes that women with diabetes are at greater risk for developing colorectal adenomas—polyps that can turn into cancer. This is especially true for women who are diabetic and obese. Obesity is defined in this study as having a body mass index (BMI) of over 30.

The study compared the colonoscopy records of 100 women with type 2 diabetes with those of 500 nondiabetic women to evaluate the rate of adenomas in these women.

The results: Women with diabetes had a significantly higher rate of adenomas

compared with those who did not have the disease—37% versus 24%. Furthermore, women with type 2 diabetes were also more apt to have advanced adenomas —14% versus 6%. Apparently, at greatest risk of all are women who are obese and have diabetes. In fact, when compared with nonobese, nondiabetic women, these women faced nearly twice as high a risk of having any kind of adenoma and more than two times greater risk for having advanced adenomas.

THE INSULIN LINK

We spoke with the study's lead author, Jill E. Elwing, MD, about these results. She explains that insulin is in itself a growth factor and that might be what is behind the link between diabetes and colorectal adenoma—the growth factor could produce a pro-cancerous effect. The immediate take-away from this study, she says, is that medical professionals and this group of vulnerable women should have greater awareness and pay more attention to regular screening. Women of any age who have type 2 diabetes should discuss a colorectal screening schedule with their doctors. And because being over age 50 is also considered a risk factor for colorectal cancer, diabetic women over that age should be particularly careful to follow their doctor's advice about regular screenings, she says.

Startling Study Shows Osteoporosis Drug Bad for Some Bones

Salvatore Ruggiero, DMD, MD, formerly chief of oral and maxillofacial surgery at Long Island Jewish Medical Center, New Hyde Park, New York and currently in private practice in New York City and Long Island.

The drug *alendronate* (Fosamax) is one of the bisphosphonates developed to help prevent bone loss after menopause and treat it. Doctors assumed people could take the drug for life. Now, though, a startling study has cast long shadows on that assumption.

DETERIORATING JAW BONES

Salvatore Ruggiero, DMD, MD, formerly chief of oral and maxillofacial surgery at Long Island Jewish Medical Center in New Hyde Park, New York, and currently in private practice, was astonished to see a rare condition develop with the jaw bone in a particular set of female patients...the condition, called *osteonecrosis of the jaw* (ONJ), is a condition that tends to occur after dental work that causes trauma to the jaw. Doctors often detect it when the jawbone becomes exposed and sometimes an infection has set in. ONJ had been associated with bisphosphonates before Fosamax, but previous to this, patients were those who had been administered bisphosphonates as intravenously as a treatment for cancer. What Dr. Ruggiero observed was ONJ had also developed in another group of patients who had undergone oral surgery at his hospital over a three-year period. These women were taking bisphosphonates orally for the treatment of osteoporosis. (Besides Fosamax, other bisphosphonates for osteoporosis include Boniva and Actonel.)

BISPHOSPHONATES AND ONJ

Dr. Ruggiero stresses that while the US Food and Drug Administration (FDA) now requires that drug manufacturers add labeling stating that ONJ is a potential side effect of bisphosphonates, the condition as associated with osteoporosis is extremely rare. Of the 159 ONJ patients from his medical center, just 25 had taken the medication orally and the overall percentage of women on oral bisphosphonates who develop ONJ is much smaller than that—well under 1% of all patients, he says.

STEPS TO TAKE

Prior to this disclosure, the main reported side effects of bisphosphonates were a bevy of gastrointestinal problems. As long as women's "tummies didn't rumble" no one saw any reason to suspend use of the medication. Besides, *ibandronate* (Boniva), a newer bisphosphonate drug that requires taking just once a month rather than daily or weekly, as with Fosamax, seemed to help with GI side effects. However, Dr. Ruggiero feels it is time to rethink the length of time osteoporosis patients are allowed to stay on any of these drugs. He anticipates that the next step may be to have "drug holidays" in which women go off the medication for several years at a time, and then return to it for the same period before suspending its use once again. Women would need to be monitored in this period for any bone deterioration with bone density scans...and they must also be careful to continue vigilance about protecting their bone strength in more traditional ways, such as taking calcium and vitamin D, exercising regularly, limiting alcohol and not smoking.

ONJ AND DENTAL CARE

Dr. Ruggiero is extremely concerned about some of the over-reaction he is seeing among patients who are shying away from routine dental care and even among dentists who are reluctant to treat this group of patients. He stresses that routine dental care is not likely to open the gates to ONJ—it is bone that was once traumatized that fails to heal properly that causes the problem...for example, work that involves trauma to the jaw including extractions and implants. He says for those women who do have to have dental work that will involve jaw bone healing, information to date shows that there is nothing to worry about if they have been on oral bisphosphonates for up to five years.

The exception: For those patients taking steroids and a bisphosphonate, the time frame is much less, or as little as two years. For those who have taken them longer, he suggests going off the medication for at least a few months before elective dental work. Even though these drugs stay in the bones for an extremely long time, he says that a year off them does seem to make ONJ more manageable—assuming that normal bone cell function can be restored and metabolically supported, based on the ebb and flow of bone cell formation and resorption.

TELLTALE SIGNS OF ONJ

Symptoms of ONJ are pain and/or numbness in the jaw, swelling, loosened teeth, gum infections and exposure of bone within the oral cavity. Women who experience any of those should see their doctor right away.

Dr. Ruggiero says not to be alarmed about the possibility that problems like this could develop in other bones in the body, from bisphosphonates. To date, there have been no reports of this complication occurring anywhere other than the jaw, he added.

Constantly Cold? Here Are Some "Hot" New Healers

Erika T. Schwartz, MD, a New York City physician who specializes in women's hormones and author of *The 30-Day Natural Hormone Plan* and *The Hormone Solution*. Both from Grand Central.

Most midlife women are proactive about seeking relief from hot flashes, yet they seem resigned to accept chronic coldness as an inevitable part of getting older. However, constantly wearing extra layers to get warm isn't normal. A woman who's always chilled may have a hormone problem.

WHAT'S A WOMAN TO DO?

We spoke with Erika T. Schwartz, MD, a New York City physician who specializes in women's hormones, and author of *The 30-Day Natural Hormone Plan* and *The Hormone Solution* (both from Grand Central). She explains that feeling cold all over, or chilled to the bone, can signal a number of conditions…

• **An oncoming cold or flu.**

• **Depression** (which is often accompanied by hormonal problems).

• **Extremely low body fat** (such as in women who have eating disorders).

• **Premenstrual dips in estrogen and progesterone,** which can trigger sensitivity to cold.

A THYROID CHECK

"If sensitivity to cold is ongoing, it's usually an indicator of thyroid issues," Dr. Schwartz warns. The problem is, it's not unusual for women's thyroid tests to come back "normal," so many cases of subclinical hypothyroidism are missed and women often don't receive the treatment they need. According to Dr. Schwartz, many conventional doctors rely on an "antiquated" range of normal that was determined 50 years ago. Seeing an endocrinologist or a physician who is sensitive to hormone issues and treats a woman's symptoms, not her test results, can help.

WHY YOUR TEMPERATURE BAROMETER IS DROPPING

By midlife, the hormone levels begin to shift. As women approach menopause, estrogen and progesterone begin to diminish. Additionally, since all these hormones are integrated in a complex chain of events, the effect of thyroid hormone goes down too, Dr. Schwartz explains.

Bottom Line's Daily Health News consulting medical editor Andrew L. Rubman, ND, adds that taking cholesterol-lowering medications and/or following a restrictive cholesterol-lowering diet may add to the problem.

In addition to feeling cold, those with low thyroid levels may experience significant fatigue, weakness, mental sluggishness, low-back pain, muscle cramps, mood swings, weight gain or difficulty losing weight, and dry skin and nails. Dr. Schwartz points out that, there is a great deal of crossover, which is why it is important to work closely with a skilled physician to evaluate and diagnose."

To give your body the support it needs to continue making hormones, Dr. Schwartz recommends taking these steps…

•**Eat "hormone-friendly foods."** Skip coffee, alcohol, dairy foods, processed foods and foods with hormones in them, such as nonorganic meats. Dr. Rubman adds that while many people avoid eggs, they are actually an excellent source of hormone-making cholesterol.

•**Exercise regularly.**

•**Manage your stress as much as possible.** Every stressful event or period of stress affects your hormone balance. A stressful event can cause your thyroid levels to nosedive.

•**Use the right supplements.** Dr. Schwartz recommends women in midlife take L-carnitine, CoQ10, omega-3 fish oil, vitamin C, folic acid, all the B vitamins, calcium, magnesium, zinc, boron and alpha-lipoic acid. These nutrients boost the immune system, decrease inflammation, increase energy and support hormone balance. It is best to work directly with a trained physician who can prescribe the proper dosing and supplements specific to your needs.

If, despite living a hormone-friendly lifestyle, you still have the symptoms of low thyroid—the most significant symptom being exhaustion or severe fatigue—talk to your doctor. According to Dr. Schwartz, no over-the-counter supplement or herb will support your thyroid like thyroid medication. Untreated hypothyroidism can cause memory problems, lower your resistance to illness and lead to arthritis, high cholesterol, circulatory problems and arteriosclerosis.

Latest Lowdown on Vitamin D

Wendy Vannoy, ND, A Woman's Time, women's health care clinic in Portland, Oregon.

Vitamin D is increasingly being found on the list of vitamin powerhouses. Low levels of vitamin D may be behind susceptibility to multiple sclerosis, osteoporosis and even prostate cancer. Now there is evidence that vitamin D and calcium may help prevent premenstrual syndrome (PMS). In the Nurses' Health Study II (a large study of nurses that has been ongoing since 1989), women who consumed higher levels of these two nutrients faced a lower risk of premenstrual symptoms such as fatigue, irritability, mood swings and stomach cramps.

ABOUT THE STUDY

In the retrospective study, researchers from the University of Massachusetts, Harvard University and the University of Iowa examined the diets of 1,057 women who reported PMS symptoms and 1,068 who did not. *They found that...*

•**Women who consumed nearly twice the recommended daily allowance (RDA) of vitamin D** (the RDA for vitamin D is 400 international units, or IU)—the equivalent of seven or more cups of milk—were 40% less likely to experience PMS than women who consumed the vitamin D equivalent of one cup or less of milk daily.

•**Women who took in one-and-one-half times the RDA of calcium** (RDA is approximately 1,000 milligrams [mg] depending on your age) the equivalent of four-and-one-half or more cups of milk) were 30% less likely to experience PMS than women who consumed the calcium equivalent of less than half a cup of milk per day.

These results were reported in the *Archives of Internal Medicine.*

WHAT THIS MEANS TO YOU

While the study makes clear some kind of association between vitamin D, calcium, magnesium and PMS, the diary format of the study does not appropriately isolate each element to show causation. So what does that mean and what should you do?

According to Wendy Vannoy, ND, a naturopathic physician in Portland, Oregon, women often don't get enough calcium and vitamin D—two nutrients that are critical during the childbearing years.

Our consulting medical editor Andrew L. Rubman, ND, believes that milk and other dairy products are not necessarily the best sources of calcium. Instead, he recommends other good dietary sources of calcium, such as broccoli, spinach, collard greens and turnip greens. As far as vitamin D is concerned, it's actually one of the easiest vitamins to get, at least during nicer weather. Only 10 to 15 minutes a day outdoors in the sunshine will enable your body to manufacture all of this vitamin you need (people of color need longer exposure to sun).

In colder months, you will need to take a supplement. Dr. Vannoy recommends taking a good daily multivitamin along with a calcium/vitamin D/magnesium supplement. (The magnesium will help with the absorption of the calcium.) Dr. Vannoy finds that getting proper nutrition combined with regular sleep and exercise can significantly reduce PMS symptoms for many women.

Miss-Diagnosis: Why Weight Gain and More May Not Be Menopause

Kenneth Blanchard, MD, in private practice, Boston, and author of *What Your Doctor May Not Tell You About Hypothyroidism*. Grand Central.

Teenage girls used to blame a few extra pounds on their "slow metabolism"—they liked to think that they were suffering from *hypothyroidism*. Actually, the disorder isn't uncommon among females, but those who have it are usually middle-aged and older, not teenagers who are overly fond of pizza and french fries.

Hashimoto's disease, an autoimmune disorder, is the most common cause of hypothyroidism, resulting in a slowing of the body's metabolism and, in turn, a number of unpleasant symptoms, including weight gain, fatigue, constipation and difficulty concentrating. Diagnosing Hashimoto's disease is not easy. Its symptoms are often confused with symptoms of aging—menopause, specifically.

ABOUT HASHIMOTO'S DISEASE

Because the thyroid gland plays such an important role in the body, Hashimoto's symptoms can be extensive and, besides those mentioned above, can include intolerance to cold, dry skin, hair loss, joint stiffness and sometimes a puffy face. As a rule, symptoms develop so gradually that people may not realize anything is amiss...or women blame what they are experiencing on menopause.

The standard test for Hashimoto's disease measures the amount of thyroid-stimulating hormone (TSH) in the blood. Elevated amounts indicate that the pituitary gland is trying to get a sluggish thyroid to work harder and so is putting out extra hormone to push it. This high score suggests the presence of Hashimoto's disease. The diagnosis is confirmed if follow-up testing finds the presence of several different antibodies produced when the immune system malfunctions. Treatment today is usually with a synthetic form of a hormone called T4 (*levothyroxine*), although some doctors also supplement with a second hormone, T3 (*triiodothyronine*). Several studies in recent years, however, showed that adding T3 to the mix was not useful and might even make patients feel worse.

SORTING IT OUT

We called thyroid expert Kenneth Blanchard, MD, author of *What Your Doctor May Not Tell You About Hypothyroidism* (Grand Central) to find out more about this disorder that affects about 5% of Americans, most of them women. Dr. Blanchard explains that there currently are two major problems concerning Hashimoto's disease—one is how it is diagnosed and the other is a serious misunderstanding about the critical role of T3 in normalizing thyroid function.

DIAGNOSTIC CHALLENGE

The first issue is the diagnosis. The TSH test has been standard for about 30 years, but Dr. Blanchard explains that it is often not reliable. Numerous common medications, including Prozac, can suppress TSH in the bloodstream. Furthermore, if the pituitary gland is working less than optimally, also not that uncommon, the gland creates reduced levels of TSH. In both instances, the patient will have a normal TSH level even though hypothyroidism is present. Rather than rely on a shaky test, Dr. Blanchard reviews the person's history (including family predisposition, a frequent association) and evaluates the person's clinical symptoms. Because Hashimoto's disease symptoms can be confused with menopausal symptoms, Dr. Blanchard feels strongly that if there are any symptoms present, the patient should go through a therapeutic trial with thyroid hormones to see if symptoms abate. Side effects are usually minimal—the worst would be some short-term heart thumping, jumpiness and perhaps a small tremor, signals that either the person doesn't have hypothyroidism, or that the dosage is off.

USE OF T3/T4

The second issue is the use of T3, the active hormone. Contrary to common practice, Dr. Blanchard says T3 is mandatory for most patients. The standard treatment today of T4 hormone alone works well for a few people—generally those who are particularly active physically. Furthermore, almost all patients on T4 alone will enjoy a short period in which they feel much better.

The reason: T4 converts to T3. During the initial stages, there is what he calls a sweet spot when the balance is just right. But shortly thereafter, the amount of T4 starts to overwhelm that of T3 and patients begin to feel terrible again. The standard practice with many medications is that if the patient quits responding, the dosage is increased, and that's just what happens here. But it is exactly the wrong route for something as delicate as thyroid hormone balancing, says Dr. Blanchard. The goal is not to treat but to normalize. However, determining the dosage of medication and the balance of T3 to T4 isn't an easy process. This is where Dr. Blanchard says the doctor's artistry and persistence must come into play.

A BALANCING ACT

Dr. Blanchard supplements with T3 hormone for almost all patients, but with a tiny amount. The problem with T3 in most treatment plans and the reason the recent T3 studies had bad results, he says, is that the amounts of T3 given to patients is generally far too high. The lowest available standard dosage of T3 medication is 5 micrograms (mcg), but Dr. Blanchard says that patients should be on dosages much lower than that. This requires having a compounding druggist prepare the medication, and Dr. Blanchard advises getting it in time-release form. Even so, it generally takes three to five months to establish the balance that works best for a patient. After that, must see the doctor every six months or so to evaluate and adjust the medicine dosage and monitor for any symptom changes.

As with all hormone-based treatments, finding the right balance for your system is critical and time consuming. And finding a doctor who is willing to work with you to find that balance is likely to take time, but having good information will start you down the right road.

Hot Flashes May Be Warning Sign of High Blood Pressure

Linda M. Gerber, PhD, professor of public health and director of the biostatistics and research methodology core in the Department of Public Health at Weill Medical College of Cornell University, New York City. Dr. Gerber is the lead author of the study, "Hot flashes are associated with increased ambulatory systolic blood pressure," published in *Menopause: The Journal of the North American Menopause Society.*

Andrew L. Rubman, ND, consulting medical editor for *Bottom Line's Daily Health News* and director of the Southbury Clinic for Traditional Medicines in Southbury, Connecticut.

Most women know that simply reaching midlife puts them at greater risk for heart disease, since they tend to lose the protective effects of estrogen. While previous research has linked menopause to high blood pressure (a major risk factor for heart attack), a recent study also links one of its most irksome symptoms—hot flashes—to high blood pressure. With hot flashes—defined as being sudden feelings of intense heat that may include sweating and a rapid heartbeat, and lasting usually from two to 30 minutes—being one of the major hallmarks of menopause and perimenopause, this study may be a "red alert" to identify a danger signal for women at risk for future heart problems.

THE SYSTOLIC CORRELATION

Researchers at New York City's Weill Medical College of Cornell University found that women who had hot flashes tended to have higher systolic (top number) blood pressure compared with the lucky ones who didn't have hot flashes. In the study, 154 women aged 18 to 65 with no previous cardiovascular disease and who either had normal blood pressure or mild hypertension (high blood pressure) wore portable monitors that recorded their blood pressure while they were awake and asleep. Women who reported having hot flashes were found to have an age-adjusted average systolic blood pressure of 141 while awake, and 129 while they were asleep, compared with 132 and 119, respectively, for women who did not report hot flashes.

The blood pressure differences between these two groups remained statistically significant after controlling for high blood pressure risk factors including race/ethnicity, age and body mass index (BMI).

"One-third of the women we studied reported having had hot flashes two weeks prior to wearing a BP monitor," says Linda M. Gerber, PhD, the study's lead author, who is a professor of public health and director of the biostatistics and research methodology core in the Department of Public Health at Weill Medical College of Cornell University in New York City. "Among these women, systolic blood pressure was significantly higher—even after adjusting for whether they were premenopausal, menopausal or postmenopausal."

DO WOMEN WITH HOT FLASHES HAVE TO WORRY?

So does this study mean all women who get hot flashes should worry about their blood pressure? Do hot flashes cause high blood pressure, or does high blood pressure make you more vulnerable to hot flashes? And, does the blood pressure normalize in postmenopausal women?

"It's not a cause and effect," explains Dr. Gerber. "We can tell that hot flashes and blood pressure are associated with one another, but we can't tell the direction." She says that future research is planned to help better understand the mechanisms underlying this relationship. "We think it may be related to *norepinephrine* release that increases both blood pressure and the frequency of hot flashes, but we don't have data yet to show that," says Dr. Gerber.

"It's important to get an accurate representation of your blood pressure, but that is often difficult to get," says Dr. Gerber. "Blood pressure varies over the course of the day. Some people get the white coat effect, in which your blood pressure is high when you go to see your doctor. I don't want people to rush to see their doctors. Try getting a home monitor and check it on a frequent basis."

ABOUT THOSE FLASHES

And what about those pesky hot flashes? "You can do things that might be beneficial to limit the severity and frequency of your hot flashes," notes Dr. Gerber. "Keep your weight down, exercise regularly and eat a healthy diet."

Our consulting medical editor Andrew L. Rubman, ND, adds that the association between estrogen reduction and both hot flashes and increased systolic blood pressure may be due to concentrations of calcium within the tissue responsible for both. There are effective natural ways to modulate this, including black cohosh and soy isoflavones, but it's important to work with an experienced expert to ensure safety.

LOOK OUT FOR...

Most important, adds Dr. Gerber: "Be aware that if the frequency of hot flashes increases suddenly and if you have a lot of severe flashes when you didn't have them before, you should get your blood pressure checked."

New (and Better!) Fibroid Treatment

Susan D. Reed, MD, MPH, associate professor of obstetrics and gynecology and adjunct associate professor, department of epidemiology, University of Washington School of Medicine, Seattle. Her private practice is at the Harborview Medical Center, Seattle.

Fibroid treatment has historically involved the physical removal of fibroid tumors via such invasive procedures as myomectomy or hysterectomy.

The problem is that both procedures are complicated and risky. A noninvasive treatment for fibroids called *gonadotropin-releasing hormone* (GnRH) *agonist therapy*, which manipulates hormone secretion, could be a good option for many.

Our concern: Manipulating hormones is tricky business. Then again, is it worth riding the hormone roller coaster if it effectively stops fibroid growth and allows women in need to avoid surgery?

THE WHYS AND HOWS OF GNRH

Natural GnRH is a hypothalamic hormone that acts on the pituitary gland in the brain, causing actions that in turn trigger the ovary to secrete estrogen and progesterone. Susan D. Reed, MD, MPH, associate professor of obstetrics and gynecology at University of Washington School of Medicine in Seattle, explains that in the natural state, GnRH is released in a pulsing fashion, but when synthetic GnRH (GnRH agonist) is used therapeutically, it is administered in a continual stream. The difference in administration is key, says Dr. Reed, because continual administration has the opposite effect on hormone production, causing decreases in hormone secretion to menopausal levels or below.

Since fibroid growth is tied to estrogen production, diminished estrogen levels generally result in diminished fibroid growth.

WHO SHOULD TAKE GNRH AGONIST THERAPY?

"The ideal candidate for GnRH agonist therapy is a woman who is close to menopause," says Dr. Reed. "For example, a 49-year-old woman who comes into my office with increasing fibroid size and symptoms, who has skipped some periods, has been having some hot flashes, and whose mother went through menopause at age 50, is a perfect candidate for GnRH. I would prescribe it hoping that she would reach menopause soon, at which time her fibroids will shrink naturally. "

Is GnRH ever beneficial for younger women? Dr. Reed says yes. In younger women who are planning surgery, GnRH can shrink the tumor before surgery, which in turn decreases bleeding and need for transfusions during surgery. Also, GnRH therapy before fibroid-removal surgery might allow for a vaginal approach rather than an abdominal approach, which can mean quicker recovery time and less risk of complications from surgery.

Dr. Reed advises that GnRH is most effective in women with smaller fibroids. "If a woman has fibroids measuring 20 centimeters or more, I have found that it rarely works."

THE DOWNSIDE

The GnRH agonist *Lupron* is typically given for two to three months, at a dosage of 3.75 mg once a month. Therapeutic effects typically begin the second week after administration. During the first week of treatment, estrogen is actually increased. However, GnRH is not a long-term solution. Generally its effects don't last long, and it can result in bone loss.

OTHER SIDE EFFECTS

Other side effects include typical menopausal symptoms—hot flashes occur in 50% to 70% of women, and there is increased potential for mood changes, including depression. Dr. Reed says that it's not easy to predict depressive reactions to Lupron, but if a woman has already had a diagnosis of depression, her symptoms may worsen with treatment. What about fertility? Because Lupron causes a mock menopause, women can be rendered infertile during the treatment period.

The bottom line on GnRH therapy for fibroids? For women with small fibroids and who are very close to menopause, GnRH may be worth considering.

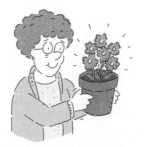

Get Rid of Fibroids—No Surgery Needed

Phyllis J. Gee, MD, obstetrician-gynecologist and medical director, North Texas Uterine Fibroid Institute, Plano, Texas.

InSightec, the privately held company that developed ExAblate 2000, *www.insightec.com.*

US Food and Drug Administration, *www.fda.gov.*

Some treatment options for fibroid tumors cause very troubling symptoms in some women. They include heavy or prolonged menstrual periods, pelvic pain and pressure on the bladder or bowel, to name just a few.

The problem is that none of the options—especially hysterectomy—are really "good." Hence, fibroid sufferers were fated to "pick their poison" with regard to the least unpleasant treatment option. The good news is that a noninvasive alternative to surgery, one that uses ultrasound, was approved by the US Food and Drug Administration (FDA).

AN INTERACTIVE COMBINATION—MRI AND ULTRASOUND

In October 2004, the FDA approved the first magnetic resonance-guided focused ultrasound surgery (MRgFUS)—the ExAblate 2000 System. To learn more about this innovative approach, we spoke with Phyllis J. Gee, MD, an obstetrician-gynecologist and medical director of the North Texas Uterine Fibroid Institute in Plano, Texas.

Dr. Gee says ExAblate combines magnetic resonance imaging (MRI) with focused ultrasound to seek out and destroy fibroid cells. For many women, this procedure represents a safe and effective alternative to invasive surgery such as hysterectomy (surgical removal of the uterus), myomectomy (surgical removal of the fibroids while leaving the uterus intact) and uterine artery embolization (blocking the arteries that carry blood to the fibroid).

The treatment, developed by the Israel-based firm InSightec, is available or will be available soon in Arizona, Georgia, California, Florida, Illinois, Massachusetts, Michigan, Minnesota, Nevada, New Jersey, New York, North Carolina, Texas and Washington. (Visit *www.insightec.com* for more details about locations.) So far, several hundred women in the US have been treated with ExAblate, and more than 1,000 women have been treated worldwide.

HOW IT WORKS

ExAblate is performed on an outpatient basis, and usually takes three to four hours. During the procedure, a woman lies inside an MRI scanner, which generates three-dimensional images of the fibroid and surrounding tissue. The role of MRI is to guide and monitor ultrasound treatment, allowing for precise targeting of highly focused waves to the fibroid. The high-intensity ultrasound energy waves raise fibroid tissue temperature sufficiently to coagulate it, in a process known as thermal ablation. Over time, the tumor continues to shrink and the body eventually reabsorbs it. Among the benefits of ExAblate is that it is not as "messy" as other fibroid procedures, which are more risky and invasive.

Throughout an ExAblate procedure, the patient is mildly sedated, so she is conscious but not fully alert. It is normal to experience a feeling of warmth in the abdomen. The treatment is generally well tolerated and the incidence of side effects is relatively low. So far, side effects do not appear to be severe or lasting. Possible risks of the procedure include skin burns, back or leg pain, abdominal cramping, nausea, vaginal discharge and urinary tract infection. However, Dr. Gee points out that as more procedures are done, there are fewer complications. For example, to prevent burns, practitioners have learned to make adjustments such as making sure the patient is well shaved, and the skin has been thoroughly cleansed with alcohol so that no oils or talc interfere with the passage of waves.

WEIGHING THE PROS AND CONS

ExAblate is not for everyone, including women who plan future pregnancies (since it may alter the composition and strength of uterine tissue)...women who have a large number of fibroids...and cases in which fibroids are close to vital organs such as the bowel or bladder. Like any medical procedure, ExAblate has both advantages and disadvantages.

Advantages...

• **Focused ultrasound is noninvasive,** so does not carry the risks of surgical procedures and general anesthesia.

• **No hospital stay is required.** (Traditional invasive surgeries require one to several days of hospitalization.)

• **Most women can resume normal activities within one to three days of treatment.**

Disadvantages...

• **There is always the risk of side effects** (listed above).

• **New fibroids can develop,** and more than two out of 10 women are likely to require additional treatment within a year either to treat new fibroids or to complete the destruction of the original one. Tumors that were treated will not regrow. However, problems can develop with new or untreated fibroids. This can occur with all fibroid treatments except, of course, hysterectomy.

• **Because focused ultrasound is so new,** it does not have a significant track record for safety, and insurance may not cover it. The average cost is several thousand dollars.

We asked Dr. Gee how claustrophobic women tolerated ExAblate, but she says that in her experience, this has not been a problem. Women are positioned stomach down, feet first in the MRI machine, so their heads are not actually in the tunnel. They're also medicated, and most women simply sleep through the procedure, says Dr. Gee.

LOOKING TOWARD THE FUTURE

Researchers are continuing to study ExAblate. The current trials are designed to include more African-American women, who have a greater incidence of fibroids and were under-represented in the original study. Additional trials are under way to explore the use of focused ultrasound in the treatment of breast, prostate, brain, liver and bone cancers.

Only time will tell whether ExAblate is a long-term, safe and effective answer to treating fibroids. In the meantime, it's a worthwhile option to explore with your physician.

Is HT Making You Fat?

Mark A. Stengler, ND, naturopathic physician in private practice, La Jolla, California...adjunct associate clinical professor at the National College of Natural Medicine, Portland, Oregon...author of many books, including *The Natural Physician's Healing Therapies* and coauthor of *Prescription for Natural Cures* (both from Bottom Line Books)...and author of the *Bottom Line/Natural Healing* newsletter.

Women often assume the change of life means a change in dress size. Even though research has proven that postmenopausal weight gain is not at all inevitable, the myth is so common many women don't question the pounds that pile up with the years. So it was with "Myrna," a 74-year-old woman who had gone through her menopause 25 years earlier. When she turned 70, she started to gain weight rapidly and inexplicably, even though she walked almost every day and watched her diet. Within four years, 20 pounds had piled on, mostly around her waist.

WHAT'S THE CULPRIT?

When Mark A. Stengler, ND, reviewed Myrna's health history with her, she told him she was taking several routine medications, including one for blood pressure, another for cholesterol and a daily one-milligram tablet of Estrace, an oral form of estrogen known as *estradiol*. This is a high estrogen dosage for a 74-year-old, but Myrna told Dr. Stengler that her doctor had prescribed it as hormone therapy (HT) when she was 50 to treat menopause symptoms. She had been taking the same dosage ever since. (Because she had had a hysterectomy, she did not take the combination therapy of estrogen/progesterone prescribed for women with an intact uterus to keep the endometrial lining from building up, a possible cancer risk.) The furor caused by the 2002 Women's Health Study demonstrating HT's negative implications for health had worried her, but Myrna's doctor had advised that she continue the estrogen regimen. Given this information and his patient's symptoms, including the rapid weight gain, Dr. Stengler ordered a saliva test to determine Myrna's current estrogen level. The results showed that it had soared, and was in fact, 10 times higher than it should have been.

ESTROGEN DOMINANCE

According to Dr. Stengler, Myrna had developed a condition known as "estrogen dominance." The body uses estrogen to promote growth of certain types of tissue but ordinarily natural levels of progesterone serve to prevent excessive estrogen growth effects. With age, however, the liver's elimination function begins to slow, making the body less efficient at metabolizing estrogen. Other reasons estrogen dominance can develop include obesity (the adipose tissue makes estrogen) and a low-fiber diet that results in improper elimination, along with a few other more obscure causes. In Myrna's case, the problem had caused water retention and fat deposition, especially in the abdomen. The excess estrogen can also suppress thyroid function...a poorly functioning thyroid can result in yet more weight gain, not to mention fatigue.

WEANING OFF HT

To resolve her problem, Dr. Stengler wanted Myrna to reduce her levels of estrogen. It's important to note that getting off HT is not something anyone should do cold turkey, says Dr. Stengler. For younger women, he prefers to wean them off over a period of one to two months, sometimes switching them first to bioidentical estrogen/progesterone and then starting the weaning process. But Myrna had such high levels of estrogen he took the unusual step of stopping estrogen right away, while starting her on a natural progesterone cream both to more efficiently offset the high estrogen levels and ease any withdrawal symptoms, including hot flashes and depression. Following Dr. Stengler's advice, Myrna continued eating carefully and exercising each day as she had been doing previously, and in three weeks she lost five pounds. Her bloating subsided, as did her abdominal protrusion.

POWERFUL HORMONES

Hormones are powerful chemicals, critical to many aspects of the body's proper function throughout life. Any kind of hormone treatment should therefore be evaluated and monitored with great care, says Dr. Stengler. *Before starting on hormones, discuss the following questions with your physician…*

•**Are your symptoms serious enough that you really need to take hormones?**

•**Are the hormones you will be taking the best form of them,** i.e., bioidentical hormones in the case of HT?

•**Are you taking the right dosage for you?**

The only safe way to take hormones is with careful supervision by a health-care professional thoroughly trained in, and experienced with, their use. HT can be valuable for some situations, but incorrect use of them can harm rather than enhance your health.

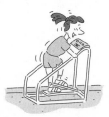

Shocking! Overweight Women Don't Get the Chemo They Need

Jennifer Griggs, MD, MPH, formerly at the University of Rochester School of Medicine and Dentistry and now director, Breast Cancer Survivorship Program, department of internal medicine, University of Michigan Health System.

If you are carrying excess pounds, finding clothes that fit may be the least of your problems. Besides the well-publicized increased risks of developing cardiovascular disease, diabetes and certain types of cancer, researchers now report that obese people may require different medication doses and are not necessarily getting them. This is leading to life-or-death consequences for some.

According to a study published in the *Archives of Internal Medicine*, some overweight or obese women receiving chemotherapy for breast cancer aren't getting doses of chemo that are appropriate for their size. That's because some doctors fear that using full doses (based on body size) of powerful chemo drugs could cause toxic side effects in these patients.

The researchers analyzed data from 9,672 breast cancer patients around the country who were treated with chemo after surgery. The heavier the woman, the greater the likelihood of receiving inadequate chemotherapy doses, the researchers found. And the women who received inadequate doses of chemo were more likely to experience poor outcomes.

DOSING CHEMO

Jennifer Griggs, MD, MPH, who was lead author of the study at the University of Rochester School of Medicine and Dentistry, explains that doctors currently base chemo doses on body surface area, which is calculated using a person's height and weight. But some physicians reduce that amount when treating heavier patients. Other doctors may reduce the dose during chemo and then add one or two more cycles. In the heavier patients, the total chemo doses may be the same, but these women don't receive the intensity of full doses. This practice is not supported by oncology specialty societies, hospitals, pharmaceutical manufacturers or, most importantly, by the studies used to prove efficacy. If doctors underdose or alter recommended frequency of administration, they are providing substandard, care and may be risking legal liability.

UNDERDOSING DILEMMA

Part of the problem is that current medical literature includes no information on dosing heavy patients, says Dr. Griggs, who is now director, Breast Cancer Survivorship Program, department of internal medicine, University of Michigan Health System. Since doctors are trained to "do no harm," many err on the side of caution. In reality, under-dosing may actually cause more harm than good. Full doses of chemo are safe, Dr. Grigg's study found. The severely obese women in her study who received a full chemo dose appropriate to their size were no more likely than leaner women to be hospitalized with side effects.

"Sixty-three percent of the women studied got the right doses, so a lot of doctors are confident that it's safe to give full doses. But 37% did not," says Dr. Griggs.

If you are overweight and you are beginning chemotherapy, Dr. Griggs advises you to be forthright and ask your doctor how he/she doses for heavy people, This issue applies to men with assorted cancers, as well.

Cancer treatment is traumatic enough. Be sure it is effective as well.

_____

16

Faster, Safer
Healing for Men

Is Saw Palmetto a Waste of Money?

Taken by more than two million men in the US for *benign prostatic hyperplasia* (BPH, an enlarged prostate), saw palmetto is among the top 10 most popular botanical remedies sold in the US. More than two dozen controlled human studies have demonstrated that this herbal supplement can help relieve uncomfortable symptoms such as nighttime urination, low flow and incomplete voiding. However, recently all this research was called into question when a study in *The New England Journal of Medicine* strongly suggested that saw palmetto was not an effective treatment after all.

NO CONTRADICTION

Mark Blumenthal, founder and executive director of the American Botanical Council (ABC), an independent, non-profit educational organization, says that the recent trial really did not contradict previous clinical research on saw palmetto for BPH. Earlier studies focused on men with mild to moderate symptoms...this study was conducted on men with more severe symptoms. The results were the same for all groups. According to Blumenthal, when researchers raised the bar on symptoms, they should have raised the dosage too, but they didn't. In his view, the body of scientific evidence overwhelmingly supports the notion that saw palmetto remains a safe and effective choice for BPH.

COMPARING APPLES AND ORANGES

Most previous trials were conducted on what would be termed either mild to moderate or stage 1 and 2 BPH, explains

Mark Blumenthal, founder and executive director of the American Botanical Council (ABC), Austin, Texas.

American Academy of Family Physicians, *www. aafp.org.*

Blumenthal. In contrast, the trial reported in *The New England Journal of Medicine* included men whose prostate symptom scores were in the moderate to severe category (sometimes referred to as stage 2 and 3, depending on which scale is used for measuring the symptoms).

Blumenthal emphasizes that a trial involving more advanced BPH does not compare directly with nor invalidate previous trials with a less advanced form. He adds that this is especially true given that the dosage was the same used in previous trials on the less advanced stages (160 milligrams [mg]—saw palmetto extract twice daily or 320 mg/day). In Blumenthal's opinion, it would have been preferable to also have tested a third arm—i.e., saw palmetto at 320 mg/day, placebo and saw palmetto at a higher dosage, e.g., 480 mg/day or 640 mg/day—to see if there was any trend toward symptom improvement at the higher dose. In other words, the trial should have been designed to see if there was a possible dose–response relationship, says Blumenthal.

MORE SERIOUS ADVERSE SIDE EFFECTS WITH PLACEBO

Another issue arises with the instance of side effects. If you look at the side effects carefully, there are more *serious* side effects in the placebo group than the test group, which normally would not make sense, observes Blumenthal. Saw palmetto is generally safe and very well tolerated, and the number of minor adverse effects in the saw palmetto and placebo groups were relatively equal (39 and 34, respectively) in the study. However, Blumenthal points out that there were nearly twice as many *serious* adverse effects in the placebo group. This suggests that the sample of men from the San Francisco Veterans Affairs Medical Center may have had other serious health issues.

A SAFE AND EFFECTIVE FIRST-LINE THERAPY

Blumenthal continues to recommend saw palmetto as a relatively safe, effective and inexpensive treatment for men with mild to moderate BPH. Before turning to aggressive alternatives such as drugs or surgery, he recommends that men try this herbal supplement.

Life-Saving Prostate Cancer Update

H. Ballentine Carter, MD, professor of urology and oncology, Johns Hopkins University School of Medicine, Baltimore.

I f a man lives long enough, he is likely to get prostate cancer. In spite of the high numbers of prostate cancer diagnoses—nearly 235,000 new cases are detected in this country each year—there is considerable confusion about appropriate treatment. Choices range from surgery... to implantation of radioactive pellets...to "watchful waiting." There is also a constant stream of new research, much of it with conflicting results.

THE LATEST STUDY OVERVIEWS

A study from Johns Hopkins University School of Medicine in Baltimore compared the results from two groups of men with small low-grade prostate cancer—one group had surgery within a few months of diagnosis, the other waited for more than two years on average before having surgery. In spite of the time lag, the chances for remaining disease-free 10 years post surgery were similar for both groups.

Implication: Immediate surgery may not be required.

Another study from the Fox Chase Cancer Center in Philadelphia was an observational study that investigated Medicare records of 49,375 older men who were diagnosed with prostate cancer, with the median age at diagnosis of 72. Median survival of those in the nontreatment group was 11 years. More than 50% of those receiving surgery or radiation therapy were still alive at the end of the study or after 12½ years.

Implication: Surgical and/or radiation treatment may be beneficial.

Finally, a Swedish research team gathered nearly 700 men who had been recently diagnosed and who were younger than 75 years of age and in good health other than the cancer. The men were randomly assigned to either surgery or watchful waiting. Ten years later, 10% of the surgical group had died versus 15% of those who did not have treatment.

Implication: Surgery is beneficial.

READING BETWEEN THE RESULTS

For clarification, we called H. Ballentine Carter, MD, professor of urology at Johns Hopkins University School of Medicine in Baltimore, and a coauthor of the Johns Hopkins study. Dr. Carter explains that the problem with the Philadelphia study is that its database was Medicare records. These records provide only a billing code, he says, and as such identify only the type of treatment the patient received. It tells you nothing about the health of the patient, or if the patient was too ill for other reasons to have surgery. Consequently, he says the findings of a Medicare observational study provide little insight in this case.

As for the Swedish study, the men in it were 10 to 15 years more advanced in their cancer at diagnosis than those in the Johns Hopkins study. Three out of four of the participants had tumors large enough to be felt, unlike the miniscule tumors in the Johns Hopkins study that had been detected by a *prostate-specific antigen* (PSA) examination.

IS SURGERY THE ANSWER?

Should you have surgery or not? Given the conflicting study results, the answer continues to be unclear. Best to talk through your individual situation, and the risk versus reward of having surgery, with your doctor.

So what about watchful waiting versus surgery? Dr. Carter explains that there are a number of considerations. First of all,

he says we should avoid use of the term "watchful waiting" because it implies not treating unless the cancer metastasizes. The preferred term today is "expectant management." *Doctors apply this concept to a carefully selected group of men whose cancer is within these boundaries...*

•**A low PSA density** (below 0.1 or less).

•**No more than two core needle biopsies** (or core biopsy) with cancer (typically 12 to 14 cores are taken), combined with a Gleason grade or score (a method to predict the cancer's aggressiveness) of 6 or less.

•**No biopsy core that shows more than 50% cancerous tissue.**

•**Cancer cannot be felt on a digital rectal examination.**

•**The patient is old or has a medical conditions.**

If a patient fits into this category, it is unlikely his disease will harm him. However, doctors continue to monitor these patients carefully and if they spot any change in the cancer, they treat it then while it is still considered curable, defined as having at least a 75% chance of remaining disease-free 10 years after surgery.

PSA OR NO PSA?

This brings us to the validity of the PSA test as a diagnostic tool, which has come under a cloud of suspicion in recent years. The problem, Dr. Carter says, is not the PSA test, but rather the way it has been applied. The value of the PSA level, he explains, is not the absolute number it shows but instead the rate at which numbers rise, called the PSA velocity. This is change that happens over a period of time, like years.

Consequently, men should have an original baseline screening at age 40 rather than at age 50 as is customary now. They should then be checked routinely to provide a history of PSA readings that would wave the red flag of a potentially dangerous cancer. Even a low PSA level—if it shows a consistent progression over the years—is an indicator of a problem that calls for investigation and, perhaps, treatment.

Prostate Danger For Overweight Men

Jonathan Bernie, MD, urologist based in Connecticut. He has published extensively on of urology and received numerous awards, including one for distinction in the study of prostate cancer. *www. urology-norwalk.com.*

The late Alan Mintz, MD, was medical director of Cenegenics Medical Institute, Las Vegas, Nevada. *www.cenegenics.com.*

Andrew L. Rubman, ND, consulting medical editor for *Bottom Line's Daily Health News* and director of the Southbury Clinic for Traditional Medicines in Southbury, Connecticut.

One frustrating thing about a lot of research studies is that they are observational; that is, they are really "correlation" studies. Scientists find that two factors (high cholesterol and heart disease, for example) occur together, but they aren't sure why. Is the relationship coincidental, causal or related to some completely different variable?

Example: Every time this country has experienced an invasion of the flying grasshopper since 1919, there has been a Republican president in office. Is there a connection just because the two occur together?

DOES OBESITY CAUSE CANCER?

So when a recent study linked obesity with an increased risk of prostate cancer, we decided to do a little digging. We already know that obese men are at greater risk for getting prostate cancer. Now a recent study from the National Cancer Institute based on more than 250,000 men reports that obesity vastly increases a man's risk of dying from the disease. Men with a body mass index (BMI) of 35 or more had double the risk of dying from prostate cancer, compared with men with

a BMI lower than 25. (A BMI of 30 or more is considered obese.)

But why? Is there a particular mechanism by which being very overweight puts you more at risk for prostate cancer, or does something about being overweight worsen the progress of the disease? Though it's unquestionably important to also consider the many other variables that may contribute (such as lifestyle, alcohol use, exercise and cardiovascular health, to name but a few) this particular study looked solely at BMI. And clearly, there is strong evidence correlating obesity with increased risk and prevalence of prostate cancer.

Correlation, yes. But they still don't know why.

MORE RESEARCH NEEDED

Further research will focus on understanding what, exactly, is different about the way the disease affects very overweight men. One theory from Jonathan Bernie, MD, a Connecticut urologist who studies prostate cancer, focuses on testosterone. "Obese men tend to have lower testosterone levels, and people with low testosterone oftentimes have a more aggressive cancer," explained Dr. Bernie. "Obese men also have higher levels of estrogen," said the late Alan Mintz, MD, from Las Vegas, who postulated that carcinogenic metabolites of estrogen might be at play, though he stresses that this is still in the realm of speculation.

Bottom Line's Daily Health News consulting medical editor Andrew L. Rubman, ND, has suggested a hypothesis of his own: "Obese folks frequently have hypertension, chronic inflammation and poor management of blood sugar. All are risk factors for assorted types of cancer…" But, still this does not quite explain the specific correlation with prostate cancer.

WHAT WE KNOW RIGHT NOW

Researchers don't yet know exactly why being significantly overweight increases your risk for prostate cancer, but they believe it does. While much is yet unproven, here is what we know for sure: Losing weight is critical to reducing all sorts of health risks, including cancer.

Early Weight Gain Means Bigger Prostate Problems

Sara S. Strom, PhD, assistant professor of epidemiology, M.D. Anderson Cancer Center, University of Texas, Houston.

Prostate cancer remains a disease of many mysteries. According to Sara S. Strom, PhD, assistant professor of epidemiology at the M.D. Anderson Cancer Center, University of Texas in Houston, autopsies of men who died from unrelated causes reveal the astonishing fact that even by age 35 nearly one-third of men have already begun to develop this cancer. While many men live with prostate cancer into old age, either unaware of its existence or unbothered by its presence, others are not so fortunate—prostate cancer kills nearly 30,000 men each year.

PATTERN OF WEIGHT GAIN

Patients and doctors face many questions about appropriate treatment, but Dr. Strom has recently published an important study that should guide men already treated for the cancer. Her study found that men's pattern of weight gain—including long before diagnosis—is closely linked with how prostate cancer progresses post-surgery. She followed 526 prostate cancer patients at M.D. Anderson for four and one-half years after they had surgical removal of the prostate (*prostatectomy*). Findings were that the disease was more apt to metastasize in men who had a BMI (body mass index) of at least 30 (30 or above is considered obese) and that those who were at that BMI or greater by age 40 had an even greater rate of progression.

Furthermore, in the group of men who had gained the greatest amount of weight

from age 25 to diagnosis, the disease progressed significantly sooner than it did in men who had gained less weight and more gradually over the years.

SCIENCE AND COMMON SENSE

No one really knows how weight gain relates to prostate cancer, though Dr. Strom speculates it might have to do with the estrogen that fatty tissue creates. Whatever the reason, because of this finding, doctors should consider patterns of weight gain in making treatment decisions and of course in tracking patients post treatment. Dr. Strom also says that this study is yet more evidence for the importance of exercise, good nutrition and maintaining an appropriate weight.

Amazing! Up to 47% of Men Have Bone Loss

Vonda Wright, MD, assistant professor, University of Pittsburgh School of Medicine, and specialist in sports medicine, UPMC Center for Sports Medicine, Pittsburgh.

Andrew L. Rubman, ND, consulting medical editor for *Bottom Line's Daily Health News* and director of the Southbury Clinic for Traditional Medicines in Southbury, Connecticut.

Many people think of bone-thinning osteoporosis solely as a disease of postmenopausal or elderly women. In reality, however, 4% to 6% of men over age 50 suffer from osteoporosis, and 33% to 47% have osteopenia (a less serious form of bone loss).

MEN VULNERABLE

Less common and less talked about, male osteoporosis often goes unrecognized and undiagnosed until a serious fracture occurs, says Vonda Wright, MD, a clinical instructor in the department of orthopedic surgery at the University of Pittsburgh School of Medicine. As with male breast cancer, men must be aware that they, too, are vulnerable to osteoporosis

...and when left untreated it can lead to more serious consequences.

HIP FRACTURES IN MEN: MORE COMMON THAN YOU THINK

It may surprise you to learn that three out of 10 hip fractures occur in men. The good news is that since men generally have greater bone mass, fractures typically occur 10 years later in men than in women. The bad news is that nearly twice as many men as women (31% of men versus 17% of women) die within one year following hip fracture, observes Dr. Wright. While no one knows why this is for certain, it may be due to a more advanced age at the time of fracture and/or the presence of other health problems.

MAJOR RISK FACTORS

According to Dr. Wright, major risk factors for osteoporosis in men include...

• **Age** (70 and older).

• **Low body mass index or BMI** (a number derived from height and weight that indicates whether weight falls in a healthy range).

• **Recent weight loss (more than 5% of body weight).**

• **Smoking.**

• **Physical inactivity.**

• **Loss of height.**

• **Family history of fractures.**

OTHER POSSIBLE FACTORS

Other possible contributing factors include excessive alcohol use, long-term treatment with steroids or anticonvulsant drugs, having arthritis, multiple myeloma or lymphoma, thyroid problems or conditions associated with an increased risk of falling (e.g., residence in a nursing home or dementia) as well as a vitamin D deficiency.

BENEFITS OF PREVENTION AND EARLY DIAGNOSIS

If you don't bring osteoporosis up with your doctor, chances are he/she isn't going to bring it up with you. Ask to be tested for osteoporosis, especially if you have one or more risk factors. According to Dr. Wright, prevention and early detection are the best forms of management.

Currently the most commonly prescribed conventional drug for osteoporosis is *alendronate* (Fosamax). However, *Bottom Line's Daily Health News* consulting medical editor Andrew L. Rubman, ND, points out that Fosamax has been shown to have a rare but dangerous side effect that actually involve the deterioration or death of bone (*osteonecrosis*) of the jaw. Dr. Rubman feels strongly that calcium and magnesium supplements are preferable.

LIFESTYLE CHOICES

Of course, smart lifestyle choices are also important for maintaining strong and healthy bones, and it's essential to eat well-balanced meals rich in calcium (e.g., heavy on the calcium-packed kale, turnip greens and okra)...engage in regular weight-bearing exercise (walking or running or lifting weights)...don't smoke...limit alcohol intake...and, Dr. Rubman adds, get sufficient nutritional support, including fiber.

Acupuncture Helps 70% of Infertile Men

Jian Pei, PhD, Christian-Lauritzen Institut in Ulm, Germany, and Longhua Hospital, Shanghai University of Traditional Chinese Medicine, Shanghai, People's Republic of China.

Mike Berkley, LAc, founder and director, The Berkley Center for Reproductive Wellness, New York City.

There's good news in the world of infertility. It seems that acupuncture could be an even bigger help to infertile men than was previously thought. According to a study published in the journal *Fertility and Sterility*, five weeks of acupuncture treatment improved the quality (meaning there were fewer anatomical defects) of sperm in 28 out of 40 (70%) infertile men. This adds yet another feather to the cap of acupuncture as an infertility treatment, which, previous to the study, was thought simply to boost overall sperm count and motility (the ability of the sperm to swim forward).

LATEST RESEARCH

Acupuncture has long been used to help increase sperm count and motility. It also prompts the release of endorphins that trigger relaxation and may improve the delivery and survival of viable sperm. The study, conducted at Christian-Lauritzen Institut in Ulm, Germany, looked beyond the quantity, to the *quality* of the sperm. After five weeks of treatments (two per week) researchers found that the physical structure of the sperm had significantly improved for the majority of study participants.

Note: Acupuncture for infertility places needles both on or around the male genitalia as well as in other locations along the energy meridians of the individual. Specific placement is tailored to the individual's energy needs.

Lead author of the study, Jian Pei, PhD, does not know *why* acupuncture improved the quality of the sperm. That will be the subject of studies that Dr. Pei and his associates plan to field in the near future.

OVERCOMING THE HURDLE FOR HELP

This study offers scientific evidence of the improvement that acupuncture can provide for men. But acupuncture faces a bigger hurdle than science—men need to start seeking treatment.

"There's this whole machismo thing attached to [infertility]—lack of manhood and all this nonsense," says Mike Berkley, LAc, founder and director of The Berkley Center for Reproductive Wellness & Women's Health in New York City. "My patients are mostly women, and I'll ask, 'Has your husband's sperm been analyzed?' and it's not uncommon for the woman to say no, her husband refuses to get his sperm checked."

So let's step back from the research and state the obvious: The first step for any infertile couple (meaning they've been trying, unsuccessfully, to get pregnant for one year) is to undergo testing—both the woman *and* the man—to find the underlying issues.

For the man, this includes sperm analysis as well as testing for varicoceles (varicose veins in the scrotum) which may be associated with increased testicular temperature and other physical problems. Only after those initial examinations is it possible to know if acupuncture is likely to be of help.

ACUPUNCTURE'S PLUSES

"If no specific physiological problem is found, then a man is a good candidate for acupuncture," says Dr. Berkley. Acupuncture is easy, noninvasive and virtually painless—and even more effective at helping male infertility than previously thought.

Kitchen "Cure" For Erectile Dysfunction

Arthur L. Burnett II, MD, professor of urology and director of the Male Consultation Clinic at the Johns Hopkins Medical Institutions, Baltimore, Maryland.

Many men look to viagra, the "little blue pill," to solve the problem of erectile dysfunction (ED), but according to a recent Italian study from the Seconda University of Naples, a better answer might not come from the medicine chest but the kitchen instead.

MEDITERRANEAN-STYLE EATING

The study investigated how following a Mediterranean-style diet (a diet rich in whole grains, fresh fruits/vegetables, dried beans and other legumes, olive oil, nuts and fish and a reduced intake of red or processed meat) would impact ED in men with metabolic syndrome, defined by a cluster of symptoms, including raised blood pressure, abdominal obesity, insulin resistance, blood lipid disorders and elevated markers for blood clotting and inflammation. Men with metabolic syndrome also have a higher incidence of ED—nearly 27% versus 13% of men without the syndrome.

ENCOURAGING RESULTS

For this study, researchers gathered 65 men with both ED and metabolic syndrome and put 35 of them on a Mediterranean diet. The 30 men in the control group received information about healthy eating practices, but they did not follow a specific food plan. At the end of two years, approximately one-third of the men on the Mediterranean diet regained normal sexual functioning versus just two men in the control group. And more good news—those following the Mediterranean diet had a significant decrease in blood glucose, insulin, low-density lipoprotein (LDL) cholesterol, triglycerides and blood pressure and a significant increase in high-density lipoprotein (HDL) cholesterol. Furthermore, their blood showed lowered measures of inflammation and improved endothelial function (having to do with the workings of blood vessels). Study authors speculate that the increased fiber and antioxidants in the diet, with its emphasis on whole foods and olive oil, may play a role in the men's improvement, though all elements acting together may have been even more important.

DIETARY CHANGES EFFECTIVE

Urologist and ED specialist Arthur L. Burnett II, MD, professor of urology and director of the Male Consultation Clinic at the Johns Hopkins Medical Institutions, says that this may be the first controlled study demonstrating how effective dietary changes can be. Dr. Burnett adds that we need more research to further confirm whether diet and modified lifestyle can limit or reverse the problem of ED, but it is obviously intuitive that eating healthfully as well as maintaining a normal weight and cholesterol levels and not smoking are, at the very least, important steps.

High-Tech Therapy For Impotent Men

George J. Christ, PhD, professor of urology and head of the program in cell, tissue and organ physiology, Wake Forest Institute for Regenerative Medicine, Wake Forest University School of Medicine, Winston-Salem, North Carolina.

Arnold Melman, MD, professor and chair of the Department of Urology at Albert Einstein College of Medicine/Montefiore Medical Center.

Creative thinking recently led researchers to explore gene therapy —also called "gene transfer"—as a potential treatment for erectile dysfunction (ED). Not only may their findings help severe ED, but perhaps also a variety of other maladies, including overactive bladder, irritable bowel syndrome and even asthma.

A BIT OF HISTORY

To understand why using gene transfer to treat ED is a creative leap, we need to look back to the early '90s, when gene therapy first became a viable, though cutting-edge, treatment. Even today, gene therapy (actual genetic manipulation of human cells) is often considered an experimental treatment to undo the effects of genetic mutations (such as one linked to Parkinson's disease), replace missing or faulty genes (such as with *phenylketonuria* or PKU) and potentially treat deadly diseases. Using gene therapy for non-life-threatening problems like ED seems frivolous, maybe even unethical. That's because aggressive genetic treatments can have risky consequences such as sparking cancer growth or triggering a severe immune system reaction.

LESS RISKY GENE TRANSFER

For ED, however, the type of gene transfer used does not appear as risky, since it doesn't affect the DNA of all the cells in the body. Also, it isn't particularly aggressive—the substances used (at least in this particular application) are only actually taken up and used by less than 10% of the cells, and the intended effects are short-lived because of its delivery method into the body.

That's where the creativity came in. Where most researchers saw those characteristics of this type of gene transfer as inefficiencies, rendering it less effective than other forms of gene therapy, it occurred to George J. Christ, PhD, and Arnold Melman, MD, that the limitation of this type of therapy might be useful in some circumstances. Dr. Christ is head of the cell, tissue and organ physiology program at the Institute for Regenerative Medicine at Wake Forest University School of Medicine, and Arnold Melman, MD, is professor and chair of the Department of Urology at Albert Einstein College of Medicine/Montefiore Medical Center (both are cofounders of Ion Channel Innovations, the sponsor of the clinical trials).

DIFFERENT PERSPECTIVE LEADS TO SUCCESS

In the study, 11 men with moderate to severe ED (none had performed sexual intercourse successfully for at least six months, and their ED was not age-related) were given one shot of a plasmid DNA hMaxi-K (also called naked DNA) modified so that it would stimulate the body to over-express a protein that relaxes smooth-muscle cells. (To achieve erection, the smooth-muscle cells in the penis must relax, which enables blood to flow in—hence the expansion.) The plasmid DNA was injected directly into the *corpus cavernosum* (the expandable tubes that run the length of the penis) where it would then be taken up by various cells, theoretically stimulating production of the necessary protein.

Because this was primarily a "phase I" safety trial, focused on testing the safety of gene transfer rather than its efficacy, varying amounts of the plasmid DNA were tested—three subjects received 500 micrograms (mcg)...three received 1,000 mcg...three received 5,000 mcg...and two received 7,500 mcg. Clinical evaluations and laboratory tests were done over the next six months to check that the plasmid DNA had no lasting ill effects, and that it had not migrated to organs other than the penis. The surprise payoff? Not only did the DNA not cause unwanted effects, but in two of the patients (one from the 5,000 mcg group and one from the 7,500 mcg group), the treatment had restored their ability to achieve an erection for the duration of the study.

WHY IT WORKED

Dr. Christ postulates that the small percentage of cells that take up the DNA "express it at a high level," meaning they work overtime and produce lots of the helpful protein. "Those cells work as a battery, powering the rest of the tissue," he says. "They provide the relaxing current that runs through the tissue from a few point sources."

POSSIBILITIES BEYOND THE BEDROOM...

Since this was only a phase I safety study, the researchers are quick to point out that more testing needs to be done before we can truly judge the effectiveness of gene transfer as an ED treatment and put it to work. The fact that it appears to work well with low risk is encouraging. But what is generating even more excitement is that, given how the gene transfer helps smooth-muscle relaxation in the penis, it may also be helpful to treat irritable bowel syndrome, asthma, benign prostatic hyperplasia (BPH), and other ailments involving smooth-muscle disorders.

In fact, Drs. Christ and Melman found that in preclinical studies it appears this treatment can temporarily abate undesired, nonproductive bladder contractions without interfering with the bladder's normal urinary function, so it may be useful in treating overactive bladder syndrome. A Phase I multicenter clinical trial to examine this possibility has recently been completed (*www.ionchannelinnovations.com* for more information).

Warning: ED Drugs May Cause Vision Problems

Jacqueline M. Winterkorn, MD, professor of neuro-ophthalmology, Weill Cornell Medical College, New York City.

There are old wives' tales about certain personal behaviors causing blindness. However, it was no laughing matter when a study from the University of Alabama at Birmingham showed a strong association between the two most popular erectile dysfunction (ED) drugs—*sildenafil* (Viagra) and *tadalafil* (Cialis)—and an increased risk in men with a history of heart attack or high blood pressure for a type of vision loss.

A SMALL STUDY

The study was small—just 78 men being treated for ophthalmologic care. Nonetheless, it found that men taking ED drugs who had a history of heart attack were 11 times more likely to develop *nonarteritic anterior ischemic optic neuropathy* (NAION), which normally affects two to 10 people per 100,000 men and women age 50 and over. Men on the drugs who had high blood pressure were at seven times at risk.

WATCH OUT FOR NAION

Jacqueline Winterkorn, MD, professor of neuro-ophthalmology, at the Weill Cornell Medical College in New York City, says it is well-known that ED drugs can have a temporary effect on vision—causing a bluish tinge in the visual field—but that it is nothing to worry about. The effect generally wears off as the medication wears off. NAION, though, damages the optic nerve head and is not reversible. There is no warning of its onset, rather it appears one day as a big blur or cloud in the visual field of one eye. While NAION is not necessarily debilitating, says Dr. Winterkorn, it is certainly an annoyance. About 15% to 20% of people with NAION go on to develop it in the other eye in the next 10 years.

WHO'S AT RISK FOR NAION

Risk factors for developing NAION include high blood pressure (HBP), especially recently treated, when medication doses are still being adjusted. Blood pressure normally spikes in the morning to get the body up to speed, but HBP medication not yet properly adjusted is sometimes too much and can prevent pressure from spiking. The result might be a spasm in the blood vessels that feed the optic nerve and this, or a brief blockage, can trigger a small-vessel stroke and NAION, says Dr. Winterkorn.

Other risk factors include having had a mild heart attack, diabetes and smoking. About half of NAION patients, however, have no apparent risk factors. The likely contributing factor of ED drugs to NAION is reduced blood flow, and the reduced blood flow might be due to more blood being directed to the penis. More study is needed to determine the pathophysiology of this.

GET EYES CHECKED FIRST

Dr. Winterkorn says she has some concern about NAION and ED drugs, but the numbers are so small given the universe of users that it is not alarming at this point.

Her advice: Before using an ED drug, men who have hypertension or a history of heart attack should have an ophthalmologic exam. The ophthalmologist can look at the optic nerve and determine whether it is at risk for NAION. This knowledge allows patients to make an informed decision, including considering more natural options to help overcome ED.

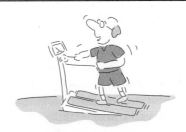

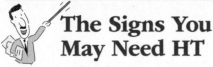

The Signs You May Need HT

Boyer B. Cole, NMD, treats many men with hypogonadism in his practice in San Anselmo, California.

The changes men experience with aging sometimes mirror those experienced by women. Energy often ebbs, there are night sweats, belly fat that won't go away and breasts that are looking womanly. There's also increased irritability, memory trouble, decreased libido and erection problems, indecision, and, sometimes, depression.

HYPOGONADISM/ANDROPAUSE

Understandably, men attribute these and other symptoms to getting older, but many doctors believe, and studies are confirming, that the cause is often more than age alone. Found in men under age 45, these changes can be symptoms of "hypogonadism" (lower than functional levels of various hormones, including testosterone). When they develop as part of the normal aging process in many men, the more accurate term for an older population would be "hypogonadic syndrome" or "andropause." Estimates of its prevalence vary widely, ranging from a low of three million to as many as 19 or 20 million men age 45 or older.

RESEARCH FINDINGS

Researchers were surprised by the finding of a recent study based on blood tests taken of 2,162 male patients age 45 or older who were making a standard visit to their primary care physician—38.7% had suboptimal levels of serum testosterone, which was not in line with earlier expectations. (Though it should be noted that as men get older, this becomes a less reliable measure, due to natural changes that occur with aging.) These men also had a higher incidence of history of hypertension, high cholesterol, diabetes and obesity. Given that the study specifically focused on average men making a routine visit to their doctor, these findings are surprising. It is important to note that Solvay Pharmaceuticals, makers of a testosterone gel, provided funding for this multicenter study.

According to Boyer B. Cole, NMD, who treats many men with hypogonadism in his practice in San Anselmo, California, the study's findings are not out of line.

IT'S HORMONAL

He explains that the reason men usually don't realize the extent of these changes is that they typically evolve slowly over time, and there is no clear marker for them (as there is for women, whose periods become erratic and eventually came to a halt). Both genders experience hormone changes with age, but not in the same way. The gradual lowering of testosterone in men may eventually cause a shift toward estrogen, as body fat starts producing increasing amounts of it. When this occurs, it may cause enlarged breasts, night sweats, and, to some degree, excess abdominal fat.

CONSIDER AN EVALUATION

But the imbalance is not just testosterone—it's also related to other hormones, including estradiol, progesterone, DHEA, cortisol and more. Dr. Cole says that all men over 45 or so who show these symptoms should consider being evaluated for low-functional testosterone and hormonal imbalance. Since hormones function in concert, not as disparate elements, Dr. Cole gives patients a complete hormone evaluation before considering treatment. Depending on the results of the hormone analysis, Dr. Cole may prescribe bioidentical testosterone replacement therapy and he may prescribe other hormones also, when indicated.

THE HORMONE THERAPY (HT) OPTION FOR MEN

Over the years, there has been considerable concern about testosterone therapy and the possibility of associated prostate cancer, although research results have been conflicting, with no definitive resolution as yet. As a precautionary step, Dr. Cole includes a *prostate-specific antigen* (PSA) test to determine the status of the prostate before starting treatment. After three months he does another PSA test to see if there is any change. (Some researchers now believe that estrogen metabolites, rather than testosterone, may be what fuels cancerous prostate changes.) Should signs of cancer emerge, Dr. Cole points out that it would have been there before replacement therapy began, and that having it surface means the patient can be treated for early-stage cancer rather than down the line when it would have grown. He continues to closely monitor hormone levels and symptoms of all patients on hormone treatment to watch the effect of the hormones and their balance relative to one another, and adjusts dosage according to need.

WHAT WILL IT DO?

Though the study found a higher than expected incidence of the aforementioned diseases with low testosterone, it's not at all clear whether andropause has a role in causing them, or whether the diseases lead to hypogonadism. It's an intriguing question, agrees Dr. Cole, noting that supplementing with testosterone when clinically indicated has been shown to improve blood sugar regulation and reverse heart disease. Supplementation can also increase bone growth, increase lean muscle mass, improve mood and memory, improve energy, reduce cholesterol and improve libido.

Dr. Cole advises plenty of protein and avoidance of dairy products, alcohol and caffeine because even two cups of coffee can adversely affect dehydroepiandrosterone (DHEA) production, and two drinks a day can adversely affect testosterone levels. Regular exercise is also beneficial, but he recommends moderate exercise such as walking, hiking, yoga, swimming and biking, which is less taxing on the body, rather than intense forms of it.

TESTOSTERONE THERAPY DOCTORS

Many physicians, both conventional and naturopathic, are prescribing testoster-

one therapy, says Dr. Cole. Our consulting medical editor Andrew L. Rubman, ND, agrees that many men likely don't realize their hormone levels are not where they should be, and would benefit from making changes in lifestyle, nutrition and diet, sometimes along with bioidentical hormone therapy (usually for multiple hormone replacement). It is important for men who are interested in hormone therapy to seek out a doctor who works with bioidentical hormones, rather than injections of synthetic ones.

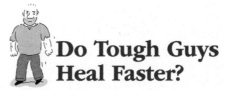

Do Tough Guys Heal Faster?

Glenn E. Good, PhD, professor in the department of educational, school and counseling psychology, University of Missouri-Columbia.

Although the media has reported widely on a recent study showing that macho guys bounce back from serious injury better, when analyzed more closely it turns out that the findings were not quite so clear-cut. The study, conducted at the University of Missouri-Columbia, found that certain attributes of the "strong, silent type" were beneficial when it came to recovering from traumatic brain and spinal cord injury.

THE STUDY'S FINDINGS

To understand the findings, we contacted Glenn E. Good, PhD, professor in the department of educational, school and counseling psychology at the University of Missouri-Columbia and lead researcher of the study which was published in the journal *Psychology of Men & Masculinity*. For this research, Dr. Good surveyed 52 men with traumatic brain injuries or spinal cord injuries in order to measure their beliefs about gender roles, attitudes toward seeking psychological help and overall satisfaction with life, among other things.

Rehabilitation professionals rated the functional independence of those men—such as how well they could get around, communicate and take care of themselves.

What the researchers found: While some traditional masculine traits (including restrictive emotionality and a reluctance to seek professional psychological help) were not beneficial to recovery, other masculine ones—including a desire for status, success, power and competition—turned out to be quite helpful. "When the rehabilitation specialists rated their improvements, the guys who were more oriented toward success and status regained more of their function," explains Dr. Good.

DOUBLE-EDGED SWORD

Even so, according to Dr. Good, by solely focusing on the idea that macho men bounce back better than others, you miss another key idea about the complex relationship between masculinity and injury. "The often-overlooked part is that macho guys do stupid things and get hurt more," Dr. Good explains. So, though a macho attitude may (or may not) help you deal with the rigors of rehabilitation, that same attitude is often what leads to injury in the first place.

So…what does this study really show? Along with providing reinforcement for the fact that avoiding unnecessary risks is good advice for everyone, it comes down to common sense. For injured "manly" men, setting realistic goals, working hard toward those goals and focusing on success can have a significant impact on the outcome. Is there anything about that idea that doesn't work for women too?

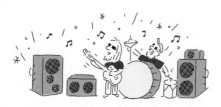

How Friends Can Help Your Heart

Linda Sapadin, PhD, clinical psychologist in private practice, Valley Stream, New York, and author of *Master Your Fears*. Wiley.

Paul Wright, PhD, professor emeritus of psychology, University of North Dakota.

A woman's tendency to socialize when under stress is an important survival technique that is not just behaviorally based, but chemically driven. So what about the men? Are they doomed to death because they lack the levels of the "befriending hormone" oxytocin?

No—while men's friendships seem different from women's, they actually are similar in many important respects.

RETHINKING MEN'S FRIENDSHIPS

The classical view of friendship has been that women's friendships are richer than men's because they are communal and involve an inward-looking personalized interest and concern, while men's are more outward-looking, involving tasks, projects and depersonalized topics having nothing to do with their feelings or relationships. For example, women will go out for lunch with their female friends and discuss the problems they are having with their children or their anxiety about a visit to the doctor. Men will go out to lunch and discuss the error made by a first baseman or how to sand the hull of a boat.

This characterization of friendship comes from Paul Wright, PhD, a professor emeritus of psychology at the University of North Dakota, who spent his entire career studying this very topic. In a chapter he contributed to *Sex Differences and Similarities in Communication* (Lawrence Erlbaum), he describes women's friendships as "face-to-face" while men's are "side-by-side." But that doesn't mean they aren't rich…or close.

He also points out that women have friendships just like men's as well—they get together to discuss books, for instance.

How different is that from talking about football?

The key here is what *kind* of friends we're talking about—casual, good or "supergood." By supergood, Dr. Wright is referring to the kind of friend who'll be at your side in an instant if needed in an emergency. And men and women both have these kinds of friends.

WOMEN GET ALL THE CREDIT

Linda Sapadin, PhD, a psychologist in private practice and author of *Master Your Fears* (Wiley), says unequivocally that in the area of friendship research, there is a bias toward women today. Women use intimacy and emotional closeness as the defining factors for friendship, and that automatically puts women's friendships in a brighter light since they are so much better at it.

But the fact is, there is no real test of what constitutes a friendship—it can only be defined as a "voluntary relationship of relatively equal status." In a recent survey, Dr. Sapadin learned that both men and women ranked intimacy and trust as most important in a friendship. Also on that list for both sexes were sharing, enjoyment, caring and acceptance.

THE FEMININE EDGE

Both men and women suffer from stress, but each gender deals with it differently— and this is where friendship comes in. In her book, *The Tending Instinct*, Shelley E. Taylor, PhD, noted that both men and women release a hormone called oxytocin into the bloodstream when they are under stress, but it only benefits women.

Called the "tend and befriend" hormone, it "directs" women to seek protective and nurturing communal experiences, such as talking with a close friend to help alleviate the stress, which in turn reduces the onset of stress-based disease. However, it does not have this effect on men, primarily because their testosterone interferes with the positive effect of the hormone. So instead of turning to a friend for help, a man might go to a sports bar, have a beer and watch some football, or head to the gym and play racquetball—not a bad thing, but not as good for his health as talking about his problem.

WHAT CAN MEN DO?

Dr. Wright suggests that men should consider using some of women's stress-coping strategies. Women have the wonderful advantage of not needing to be told to look to their friends because oxytocin directs them there. Men, on the other hand, might try to leverage their oxytocin by becoming more aware that they are holding stress in, say, the stomach or muscles of the shoulders or neck and, instead, making a conscious decision to deal with stress in a more social way.

For instance, if men are having problems at work or at home, they should consider turning to a sympathetic and supportive supergood friend who's a good listener to talk the problem out. Both Drs. Wright and Sapadin noted in their research into cross-gender friendships that for many men, their best friend often is their wife.

WORTH TRYING NEW BEHAVIOR

Whether this new behavior will positively impact men's health as it does women's, however, is something that has yet to be studied. But given the longer average life expectancy for women, it's probably worth a try. Practicing a conscious stress-reducing activity, such as the mindful breathing taught in Hatha yoga, makes a great difference for many men.

17

Super-Healthy Children

Today's Kids: Eating Themselves to Death

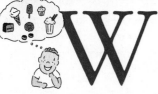

We're killing our children. According to the Centers for Disease Control and Prevention (CDC), 17% of American children and teens ages six to 19 are overweight. Since 1980, the number of overweight children between ages six and 11 has more than doubled, and the rate of overweight teens has more than tripled. This means more young people are at risk for developing potentially life-threatening type 2 diabetes, high blood pressure, sleep apnea, asthma and psychological issues, such as low self-esteem and depression.

To make matters worse, according to a recent report in the *British Medical Journal*, children don't tend to outgrow their "baby" fat. Researchers found that children

who were overweight at 11 were just as likely to be overweight at 16.

For advice to parents and caregivers on how to deal with this problem, we spoke with obesity and nutrition expert William Dietz, MD, PhD, at the Centers for Disease Control and Prevention…

THE PROBLEM

Dr. Dietz says that the problem can't be chalked up to any one cause. There are many contributing factors…too many soft drinks and junk foods…less opportunity for active play inside school and out…far too much TV and computer games.

The schools are finally stopping the sale of soft drinks, thanks to an agreement between former President Bill Clinton's Clinton Foundation, the American Heart Association and the American Beverage

---

William Dietz, MD, PhD, director, Division of Nutrition, Physical Activity and Obesity, Centers for Disease Control and Prevention, Atlanta, Georgia.

Centers for Disease Control and Prevention, *www.cdc.gov.*

Association. Even so, in some schools, Snapple soft drinks, which contains high-fructose corn syrup, are still available, and breakfast options continue to include sugar-sweetened cereals, such as Froot Loops and Cinnamon Toast Crunch.

More meals eaten outside the home, the easy availability of inexpensive fast food, larger portion sizes and aggressive TV advertising of junk foods all add up to overweight children.

But in the long run, as usual, it boils down to this: Most children are getting fatter because they're moving less and eating more.

THE SOLUTION

The solution for children is the same as for adults—exercise more and eat less. Children are coping with all sorts of complicated and confusing messages and issues, and it's up to us as parents and caregivers to guide them through this thicket and get them back in shape.

Grandparents can help, too. While part of the fun of being a grandparent is "spoiling" your grandchildren, spoiling them with unhealthy food choices contributes to the problem. There are many other ways to shower grandchildren with love—play a game…teach them to knit…show them old family photos…buy a pet goldfish that lives at grandma and grandpa's house, etc. Be creative.

According to Dr. Dietz, early parenting decisions set the stage, for better or worse. He points out that breastfeeding reduces the child's risk for obesity later in life.

Other things to think about: Do you put water in the bottle or sippy cup instead of juice? How much TV are you going to allow your toddler to watch? You don't need to put him/her in an exercise program, says Dr. Dietz, but you should provide ample opportunity for active play.

ADDITIONAL STRATEGIES…

•**Be a good role model.** Parents who watch more TV have children who watch more TV, and children eat the way their parents eat, observes Dr. Dietz. If you dine on chicken nuggets and french fries, your child is likely to do the same. Instead, opt for baked chicken and salad, and whenever possible make it yourself at home.

•**Always have healthy snacks on hand.** Welcome your hungry kids home from school with a colorful plate of baby carrots, sliced red peppers, nuts, sunflower seeds and celery filled with peanut butter.

•**Don't keep unhealthy foods in the house.** If there are no soft drinks, potato chips, bologna or white bread available, your child can't snack on them. (And neither can you.)

•**Emphasize whole foods rather than processed foods or beverages.** A piece of fruit contains more fiber and nutrients than fruit juice. If your child insists on fruit juice, dilute it by half with water.

•**Turn off the TV.** On average, children watch three to four hours of television daily, and the more TV, the more obesity. Dr. Dietz points out that 50% of American families have the TV on during meals, and studies in adults have shown that this leads to higher calorie intake.

•**Eat meals as a family.** Getting together at the table and sharing the day's news is not only nurturing, it's also likely to add fewer calories than mindlessly shoveling in food in front of the TV, says Dr. Dietz.

•**Never use food as a reward or punishment.** Don't offer candy or cookies as bribes for good behavior, or withhold dessert when your child is acting up.

•**Avoid fad diets.** They usually don't work anyway, and can do far more harm than good.

•**Build more activity into family time.** Instead of going out to a movie, go for a bike ride or a swim or simply a walk in the woods.

•**Support your child.** Overweight kids already feel bad about themselves, so make sure you let your children know you love them unconditionally no matter how much they weigh.

•**Consult your physician.** If your child is overweight, it is especially important to get regular medical care, advises Dr. Dietz. He/she needs to be monitored for possible problems such as high blood pressure and/or diabetes. Additionally, your doctor can help you devise a safe exercise program and refer you to a nutritionist if necessary.

WORTH THE EXTRA TIME AND EFFORT

Helping your child with weight management may seem like a daunting task. Keep in mind, however, that the extra time and effort you put into raising your child now will make for a happier and healthier life in the long run.

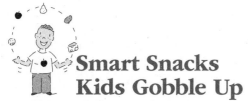

Smart Snacks Kids Gobble Up

Shereen Jegtvig, chiropractic physician, and a certified nutrition specialist located in Albuquerque, New Mexico. She has more than 15 years of professional experience providing chiropractic health care and nutritional consultation. She is the nutrition guide at About.com.

Childhood obesity is making headlines all over—so a mailer from a children's pediatric practice regarding the importance of healthy snacks for kids caught our attention.

Our hope for answers dissipated quickly as we scanned: Fat-free ice cream, baked tortilla chips, gelatin, low-fat pudding, animal crackers, baked potato chips were all on the list. The doctors took the time to single out five different types of cookies and crackers but lumped "fruit" and "fresh vegetables" into one category each. No mention of nuts, raisins or more nutritious whole foods. If pediatricians don't know nutrition, how can parents?

FOOD MARKETING AND SNACKS

"Everyone gets caught up in trendy food marketing, even medical professionals," says Shereen Jegtvig, chiropractic physician, mother of two and certified nutrition specialist in Albuquerque, New Mexico. "Though many newly formulated snack foods are better than their predecessors, that doesn't mean they're the healthiest snack choices. Personally, I recommend keeping most chips and candy out of the house because, as shown in a study from Oxford, England, high glycemic index foods just make kids hungrier," says Jegtvig, who also works as the nutrition guide for About.com.

NUTRITION ADVICE HELPS

Perhaps the most frustrating aspect of all this is that research shows that if you teach kids to eat right, they'll really do it—on their own. In a study published in the *Journal of Pediatrics*, researchers tracked 595 children, half of whom had received, along with their parents, education on making healthy food choices. Three years later, kids who attended the nutrition classes were still eating healthier than those who didn't receive such education.

SMARTER SNACKS

The key to creating healthy snacks your kids will crave is making them as fun and engaging as the glitzy commercial stuff—a challenge, considering that most moms and dads don't have multimillion-dollar marketing budgets. What's more, these foods are perfect for parents, too. *Here's what Jegtvig and other snack-savvy experts recommend...*

•**Fruit kabobs.** Buy some shish kabob skewers and create colorful strawberry, pineapple and mandarin orange kabobs kids can grab and go. Kids enjoy making them, too.

•**Frozen grapes.** They have the consistency of mini-popsicles, yet no added sugar and plenty of flavonoids. Just pop a bowlful of grapes in the freezer for a sweet treat anytime.

•**Ants on a log.** Part craft project, part after-school treat. Get your kids involved in making their own snacks. Take celery sticks, smear them with light cream cheese or natural peanut butter and sprinkle with a line of raisins.

•**Seasoned nuts.** Nuts, especially walnuts, which are rich in omega-3 fatty acids, are a perfect snack. Sprinkle with a bit of cinnamon sugar and bake in a 350°F oven for 10 to 15 minutes.

•**Veggie chips and dip.** There is no excuse for not having fresh vegetables on hand. Buy prechopped, prewashed bagged veggies. "Then give your kids a little bit of whatever dip they want," says Jegtvig. "Kids need a little fat, and fat helps you absorb many of the nutrients in vegetables, so a little ranch dip or chip dip is fine."

•**Smoothies.** Mix half a banana, a fistful of grapes, some berries and some plain yogurt in a blender and make a smoothie. In the summertime, freeze the mixture to make a cool dish that's as sweet as ice cream but much more nutritious.

•**Rainbow melons.** Slice honeydew, cantaloupe and watermelon to make a candy-colored natural treat.

•**Carrots and hummus.** You can buy hummus in most grocery stores today, and baby carrots are sold practically everywhere. This spicy snack is rich in protein, so it's filling and helps stave off hunger.

•**Star fruit sandwiches.** Place banana slices between sliced star fruit for funky, filling sandwiches.

•**PB&J.** Don't shy from the classics. "Traditional kid favorites like peanut butter and jelly are still better choices than processed snacks," says Jegtvig. Just choose whole grain bread and natural peanut butter, and go light on the sugary jelly.

•**Nuked sweet potatoes.** Thinly slice a sweet potato, spread it out on a plate, sprinkle with a little salt and pepper and microwave for three to five minutes. These "potato chips" are more filling than the fried, bagged kind, and they're chock-full of beta-carotene.

•**Berry blends.** "Anything with berries is great," says Jegtvig. Mix a bowlful of berries in season, including blueberries, blackberries, raspberries and strawberries.

•**Assorted seeds.** Seeds are a rich source of vitamin E and some, like pumpkin seeds, have omega-3 acids. Roast seeds for extra crunch and deeper flavor.

•**Make a mix.** In a Tupperware container, mix whole grain cereal, such as multigrain Cheerios, dried fruit, seeds and nuts, for a trail mix that satisfies indoors, too.

•**Roll ups.** For a heartier snack, layer thinly sliced turkey breast, spinach leaves and a light spread on a whole-wheat tortilla. Roll up and slice into tasty disks. Roll ups also work with tuna salad, refried beans and spreads such as hummus.

THINK SMALL

"Sometimes you want a cookie and that's fine. The most important thing is portion control," says Jegtvig. "We all ate cookies growing up. There's nothing inherently bad about cookies. What's gotten out of control is the size of these and frequency of snacks." As a rule, buy single servings of snacks like crackers, pretzels, and baked chips. Reserve these foods for special occasions rather than daily indulgences.

Sleeping Their Way To Slim

Emily Snell, lead researcher on the Northwestern University sleep study published in the journal *Child Development*. Snell was a graduate student in the School of Education and Social Policy at Northwestern University, Evanston, Illinois.

A recent study has added to the mounting evidence that there's a connection between sleep and weight. Several major studies have already linked the sleeping habits of adults to how much they weigh and now it turns out to be true for kids as well. Using data from the decades-long Child Development Supplement of the Panel Survey of Income Dynamics, researchers at Northwestern University analyzed information on 2,281 children, looking for a connection between sleep and weight. The main finding was that "children who don't get enough sleep tend to be overweight five years later," said Emily Snell, who was lead researcher on the study.

BEDTIME A KEY PREDICTOR

Early to bed may not always mean early to rise, but it does mean a smaller number on the bathroom scale. "For children ages three to seven, bedtime was key to predicting weight gain five years later," Snell said. According to the researchers, even another hour of sleep made a difference, reducing a child's chance of being overweight from 36% to 30%. "Those three- to seven-year-olds who went to bed at 8 pm, for example, were significantly less likely to be overweight than those who went to bed by 9 pm," she notes.

KIDS AND ADULTS: SAME MECHANISM

Why? The research on causality is further along for adults, but the same mechanisms hold true for children, according to Snell. "Adults who are sleep-deprived tend to produce different levels of hormones that affect appetite," she explained. When you sleep less, you produce more of an appetite-stimulating hormone called *ghrelin*, which might account for why people who burn the midnight oil walk around hungry the next day. Conversely, the less you sleep, the less *leptin* (the hormone that sends a message of satiety to your brain after eating) is produced. And insufficient sleep of the deepest and most restful kind (known as stages three or four, the stages before REM sleep) inhibits production of *human growth hormone*, which helps you gain muscle and lose fat.

STRESS, ACTIVITY, BAD HABITS

Finally—as we adults well know—not sleeping enough affects our ability to process stress, leading to higher production of the stress hormone *cortisol*, which contributes to weight gain particularly around the middle. Also, people of any age who don't get enough sleep are tired and less likely

to be active, another factor that leads to weight gain, Snell pointed out. Not to mention that many kids who aren't going to bed at a reasonable hour are watching TV and snacking. "The research is very clear that for kids, the more hours of television you watch, the more likely you are to be overweight," said Snell.

RECOMMENDED AMOUNTS OF SLEEP

It should be non-negotiable. Kids need to go to bed at a decent hour. The National Sleep Foundation recommends 11 to 13 hours a night for preschoolers (three- to five-year-olds)…nine to 11 hours for kids ages five to 12…and eight-and-a-half to nine-and-a-half hours for teens. That gives us adults an hour or two for ourselves before we turn in for our own recommended seven to nine hours a night.

Making Medicines Safer for Kids

Lisa Mathis, MD, associate director, pediatric and maternal health staff, Center for Drug Evaluation and Research, US Food and Drug Administration, Rockville, Maryland.

It is relatively easy to speak with your doctor about getting the lowest dose possible for a prescription if you are small or drug-sensitive, and how best to adjust for over-the-counter (OTC) products. But it's not so easy with children's medications. It's not simply a matter of adjusting for body weight. When it comes to metabolizing medications, kids are not just like adults, but smaller.

WHAT'S BEEN GOING ON

When a drug company makes a children's version of an adult medication, its primary concern is that the medication be easy to take. The company, therefore, adjusts the dose based on a child's weight and size, and creates a flavored liquid formula that is both easy to swallow and palatable enough that a child will actually take it. The problem is that children's bodies are continually growing and changing. They have different metabolisms than grown-ups and their organs are not fully developed, so medications that work on adults may have a very different impact on children. The drug companies do not generally adjust the medications for a child's metabolism.

Lisa Mathis, MD, associate director of the US Food and Drug Administration's (FDA) pediatric and maternal health staff at the Center for Drug Evaluation and Research (CDER), says that based on MedWatch reports and results from studies conducted in pediatric patients, the percentage of total children's reactions to drugs is similar to that of adults. Children, however, are more likely to experience specific adverse events, such as seizures and skin rashes—and it is more common for them to be overdosed. But adverse reactions to medication in both children and adults may be mild enough to go unnoticed. It may even go unreported.

DRUG TESTING—CATCHING UP

Until recently, drug testing on children was not a priority for the government and for drug companies. (The exceptions are for treatments of common childhood conditions such as attention deficit hyperactivity disorder, ear infections, asthma and eczema.) Then, in an effort to correct the problem, Congress passed the Food and Drug Administration Modernization Act (FDAMA) in 1997...and in 2002, it passed the Best Pharmaceuticals for Children Act (BPCA). Under these acts, companies that agreed to research an approved drug for the effects it had on children were given six months of marketing exclusivity. There now are more than 100 labels under the BPCA and FDAMA.

In 2003, Congress passed the Pediatric Research Equity Act, which requires the study of the effects of drugs on children prior to approval. If there are *significant* safety concerns, the drug is not authorized for prescription to children. If there are no significant concerns initially identified, then formal studies on children are then instituted. Drugs must be clearly labeled if they are marketable for treating adults but not safe for children.

PROGRESS SLOW

While these new laws are spurring an increase in research on children, progress is slow due to special rules that must be followed and special equipment needed to measure the reduced quantity of blood collected from children. Plus, there's the matter of consent. Parents must give their consent for any minor to participate in medical trials, but children over age seven can assent or dissent, meaning that even if a parent gives his legal consent, if a child of seven or older does not agree to participate in a study, he/she is not eligible.

SAFETY STRATEGIES

Given that you can't simply assume a drug to be safe for your child, what should you do to keep your child safe? Here, Dr. Mathis recommends drug do's and don'ts.

Do...

•**Double check with your pediatrician as to whether or not the drug being prescribed has been tested on children.**

•**Read all labels carefully.** Different medications provide different dosing guidelines. Be sure to follow label instructions carefully.

•**Give the drug to your child at the appropriate time of day** and at the appropriate intervals.

•**Pay attention and follow the directions on how the drug needs to be taken.** Some drugs need to be taken on an empty stomach, while others should be taken with special food such as peanut butter (which contains fat).

•**Ask your pediatrician what side effects the drug has** so you can keep an eye out for them.

•**Also ask your pediatrician what to look for to make sure the medication is working.** And be sure that you know how long it will take. Some drugs may take 24 to 48 hours (or longer) before you see results, while others should begin to work immediately. If you know what to look for and when, you can go back to your pediatrician if there is a problem with the medication or the dose.

●**Give your sick child plenty of fluids to drink.**

●**Be conservative.** For example, you don't need to medicate a mild fever unless your child is experiencing discomfort. Keep in mind that all drugs have side effects, and they should not be used frivolously.

Don't…

●**Overdose your child.** Know the ingredients of the drugs you are giving. If your cold medicine has a fever reducer like acetaminophen (Tylenol) already in it, make sure you don't give another fever reducer on top of that.

●**Give antibiotics (or any medication) if your child does not really need them.** Antibiotics are only helpful for bacterial infections…and taking antibiotics can create resistant bacterial strains.

●**Don't use Tylenol and Children's Advil/Motrin as psychological support for a boo-boo.** They are "real" medicines. Try ice, a big hug or a rest on the couch first.

●**Don't forget that prescription and OTC creams are still medications.** Topical drugs are absorbed by the skin and, like drugs that are taken by mouth, they have side effects.

●**Don't assume you can cut a pill to adjust the dose of the medication.** You should never cut a pill that is an extended release form of a medication (for a child or an adult). Note that most pills that can be safely cut are scored.

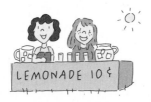

Flu Meds May Not Be Safe for Children

Mark A. Stengler, ND, naturopathic physician in private practice, La Jolla, California…adjunct associate clinical professor at the National College of Natural Medicine, Portland, Oregon…author of many books, including *The Natural Physician's Healing Therapies* and coauthor of *Prescription for Natural Cures* (both from Bottom Line Books)…and author of the *Bottom Line/Natural Healing* newsletter.

Once flu season is in full swing, it's not surprising to open the newspaper or go on-line and be greeted with the latest news about influenza.

Of course, that news is not always good…or clear cut. The latest reason to be on guard: The US Food and Drug Administration (FDA) says patients (including children) taking the flu drug *oseltamivir* (Tamiflu) should be closely monitored. There have been reports of abnormal behavior in people who take this medicine.

NEW WARNING LABEL

Tamiflu is used to prevent the flu and lessen the length and severity of its symptoms. It is much more commonly prescribed in Japan than in the US, and the more than 100 new cases of bizarre behavior occurred primarily in Japanese children. Tamiflu is indicated for patients one year and older. Adverse effects reported in Tamiflu users included disturbances in consciousness, delirium, hallucinations, confusion, delusions, convulsions and an increased risk of self-injury, including three deaths from falls.

The Japanese Tamiflu already carries a strong warning label. In view of these possible risks, an FDA advisory committee proposed adding a stronger, more specific warning label to the US-prescribed Tamiflu, recommending that close monitoring—especially in children—begin immediately after beginning treatment. Meanwhile, the FDA acknowledges that it has not definitively established if the drug causes the bizarre behavior, and acknowledges that the flu virus itself might be responsible in at least some cases...the warning, however, could "...mitigate a potential risk associated with Tamiflu."

BETTER SAFE THAN SORRY

Mark Stengler, ND, author of *Bottom Line Natural Healing* newsletter (*www. DrStengler.com*) and author of *The Natural Physician's Healing Therapies* (Bottom Line Books) says that with any medication, there is always the risk of side effects, and—as with the flu vaccines—there are no long-term studies documenting the safety and effectiveness of Tamiflu. With Japanese health-care officials documenting serious side effects involving the nervous system, Dr. Stengler believes that it is important for Americans to be aware of these risks and take them into consideration before using the drug.

The bottom line: If someone taking Tamiflu shows any signs of unusual behavior, contact a health-care professional immediately. And, as always, keep in mind that pills are not the only answer. There are many natural ways to boost immunity and cope with symptoms during flu season.

FDA Warning—Ritalin May Raise Heart Risk

Steven E. Nissen, MD, FACC, chairman of the department of cardiovascular medicine at the Cleveland Clinic, Cleveland, Ohio and past president, American College of Cardiology, Bethesda, Maryland.

It seems as if more and more kids are being put on *methylphenidate* (Ritalin) for so-called behavioral disorders. But in a dramatic reminder that Ritalin and related attention deficit hyperactivity disorder (ADHD) medications are potent drugs with dangerous side effects, a US Food and Drug Administration (FDA) advisory panel has recommended that they carry a "black box warning"—the FDA's highest level warning—that they may increase the risk of death from heart attack and other cardiovascular problems. This advice came after 25 deaths and 54 serious cases of cardiovascular problems among children and adults taking these stimulants (methylphenidate or amphetamines) between 1999 and 2003.

TOO MANY DRUGS FOR TOO MANY CHILDREN

In recent years, there has been growing concern that too many children are being put on ADHD medications. Once reserved for kids with obvious and major symptoms (hyperactivity, impulsivity and inattention), there seems to have been a kind of trickle-down effect. Now children who would formerly have been considered merely fidgety, impatient or inattentive are being pumped full of powerful drugs.

Are parents using drugs to medicate behavioral and discipline issues? To learn more about this dilemma, we consulted advisory panel member Steven E. Nissen, MD, chairman of the department of cardiovascular medicine at the Cleveland Clinic in Ohio and past president of the American College of Cardiology. He says that he hopes the new awareness of the risks will slow down the escalating number of prescriptions for ADHD.

All drugs have side effects, and should be prescribed only when absolutely necessary. This is especially true when it comes to powerful stimulants like Ritalin, which can cause adverse cardiovascular effects including high blood pressure, a racing heart, abnormal heartbeat or stroke.

TRY NONDRUG APPROACHES FIRST

In Dr. Nissen's opinion, while there are still some children who need and benefit from Ritalin, this drug should be prescribed only after other approaches have been exhausted. Be certain that it truly is real ADHD and not just a child overwhelmed by his/her overscheduled world or in desperate need of parental attention. Psychotherapy, behavior modification, social skills training and nutritional guidance have all met with some degree of success in controlling ADHD symptoms.

Often a combination of strategies is best, along with a team approach ensuring that parents, physicians, therapists and teachers are all on the same page.

The bottom line: If you're the parent of a child with behavioral difficulties, you're not alone, and there are many helpful treatment options. Don't let yourself be talked into giving your child powerful drugs with powerful side effects until you explore more healthful alternatives.

When Vaccines Backfire

Barbara Loe Fisher, President, National Vaccine Information Center.

Jeanne Marconi, MD, pediatrician in private practice in Norwalk, Connecticut.

Centers for Disease Control and Prevention, *www.cdc.gov.*

National Vaccine Information Center, *www.nvic.org.*

US Food and Drug Administration, *www.fda.gov.*

According to Jeanne Marconi, MD, a pediatrician in Norwalk, Connecticut, there appears to be some fallout from the chicken pox vaccine, which was licensed by the US Food and Drug Administration (FDA) in 1995. She is seeing fewer cases of chicken pox (*varicella*), but the cases that do show up in her office tend to be far worse than they used to be in children. Instead of 100 or so lesions or blisters that used to develop during a typical case of chicken pox, there are now hundreds of blisters or lesions on unvaccinated children and adults who get this once fairly benign childhood disease.

ACQUIRED IMMUNITY DECREASING

These more severe cases of chicken pox can lead to potentially life-threatening complications such as pneumonia, warns Dr. Marconi. Her theory for the change—acquired immunity, a passive immunity that we develop from being part of a general population in which viruses and bacteria exist, has decreased. This is in part due to antiseptic, germ-free environments and mass vaccination programs. Unvaccinated people are getting more severe chicken pox than they would have before the chicken pox vaccine started being widely used. This is because they are less likely to be continually exposed to the varicella zoster virus that causes chicken pox, says Dr. Marconi. Lacking exposure and reexposure, they don't have the opportunity to develop even low-level antibodies to chicken pox, she adds.

CONCERNS WITH THE CHICKEN POX VACCINE

The Centers for Disease Control and Prevention's (CDC) Advisory Committee on Immunization Practices (ACIP) now recommends two-dose chicken pox vaccinations for children, taken three to five years apart for children under 13 and at least 12 weeks apart for those age 13 and above. All states require certain vaccines to attend school. However, depending upon the state, there are medical, religious and philosophical exemptions that parents may be able to obtain for their children to opt out of one or more vaccines. According to a 2002 CDC study, the "effectiveness of the vaccine was 44% against disease of any severity and 86% against moderate or severe disease." The remaining 15% failed to respond to the first chicken pox vaccination, leaving them susceptible to a mild case of the disease at some point.

However, there are lingering questions about the vaccine. Barbara Loe Fisher, president of the National Vaccine Information Center (NVIC), a national, nonprofit, educational organization dedicated to the prevention of childhood vaccine injuries and deaths, has safety concerns about the vaccine, and believes that it should not have been mandated.

ADVERSE EVENTS

According to the federal Vaccine Adverse Event Reporting System (VAERS), there were 67.5 adverse events per 100,000 doses of varicella vaccine reported between 1995 and 1998. In some cases, these were severe, including shock, encephalitis (brain inflammation), Guillain-Barré Syndrome, herpes zoster (shingles), cellulitis (serious bacterial skin infections) and death. From March 1995 to December 2001, according to VAERS, there were 15,180 reports of adverse events—759 of which were considered serious. While the CDC's position is that the benefits of vaccination outweigh the risks for most people, Fisher points out that there are many questions about the true adverse event profile. In particular, the numbers of adverse events may be understated since events such as seizures and other signs of brain inflammation following vaccination are often dismissed as coincidental, she says. Additionally, chicken pox is generally mild in vaccinated children, and most children who have chicken pox develop lifelong immunity to it. The chicken pox vaccine, like all vaccines, gives only temporary immunity. This means that as adults, vaccinated individuals could still be vulnerable to chicken pox—and in adults, chicken pox can be a far more serious disease.

THE SHINGLES ISSUE

There is also concern that despite the drop in the incidence of chicken pox, there will be a corresponding rise in shingles, or herpes zoster. This acute viral infection—characterized by numbness, burning and tingling on parts of the body—can cause a searingly painful, blistering rash. Shingles is most common in the elderly or adults over 50 and is caused by the same varicella zoster virus that causes chicken pox. The theory is that adults receive natural, asymptomatic immune boosting against shingles by occasional contact with children who have chicken pox. Because shingles usually strikes decades after chicken pox, and the vaccine was only approved in 1995, it is not known how long the temporary immunity associated with the vaccine will last.

WHAT YOU CAN DO

The NVIC recommends that you address these eight questions before vaccination:

•**Is my child sick right now?** If so, you may want to hold off on vaccination, since adverse effects can be more likely to occur in ill people having a coinciding viral or bacterial infection at the time of vaccination can affect the ability of the vaccine to stimulate the desired immune reaction.

•**Has my child had a bad reaction to a vaccination before?** According to the CDC, people who have had a life-threatening allergic reaction to chicken pox vaccine, neomycin or gelatin should not receive the chicken pox vaccine. The NVIC advocates caution if a child has previously had a bad reaction to any vaccination.

•**Does my child have a personal or family history of vaccine reactions...** convulsions or neurological disorders...severe allergies...immune system disorders? According to the CDC, people should consult with their doctor about whether or not they should get the chicken pox vaccine if they have any kind of cancer or are receiving cancer treatment with X-rays or drugs...a disease that affects immune function...are receiving treatment with drugs such as long-term steroids (as in some cases for asthma, for example)...or have recently gotten blood products (or a transfusion). In addition, the NVIC advocates caution if a child has had a personal or family history of convulsions, neurological disorders, severe allergies or immune system disorders.

•**Do I know if my child is at high risk of reacting?** NVIC urges caution if a child is sick at the time of vaccination, or has a personal or family history of vaccine reactions, convulsions or neurological disorders, severe allergies or immune system disorders. Discuss the risks versus benefits of vaccination with your physician.

•**Do I know how to identify a vaccine reaction?** The most common reaction is soreness, redness or swelling at the shot site, which occurs 20% of the time... chicken pox lesions on the body within one to four weeks of vaccination...and fever over 102°F. In the case of more serious reactions, signs of brain inflammation such as a seizure, confusion or strange behavior, seek immediate medical attention. Children should be monitored for at least four weeks following vaccination for signs of serious changes in physical, mental or emotional health and all symptoms of health deterioration reported to a doctor.

•**Do I know how to report a vaccine reaction?** The federal Vaccine Adverse Event Reporting System (VAERS) monitors adverse effects of vaccines. Ask your physician or health department to file a Vaccine Adverse Event Report System form, or call 800-822-7967.

•**Do I know the vaccine manufacturer's name and lot number?** Get this information from your physician at the time of vaccination.

•**Do I know I have a choice?** Most states require the chicken pox vaccine for child care and school entry. However, there are possible medical, religious and philosophical exemptions depending upon the vaccination laws in your state. If you have concerns about vaccination, check with your state health department to learn more about them.

THE VACCINATION DILEMMA

Because of the reduction in naturally acquired immunity to chicken pox due to mandatory vaccination policies, we are now in a difficult spot regarding whether or not to vaccinate ourselves or our children. Should we get the vaccine and risk future wellness from vaccine side effects or increased risk of shingles? Should we skip the vaccine, and risk a potentially severe case of chicken pox? Should we get one dose of the vaccine but skip the booster?

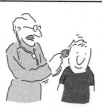

Medicines that Make Your Child Sick

Andrew L. Rubman, ND, consulting medical editor for *Bottom Line's Daily Health News* and director of the Southbury Clinic for Traditional Medicines in Southbury, Connecticut.

Drugs like *lansoprazole* (Prevacid), a high-powered acid-suppressant known as a proton-pump inhibitor (PPI) are increasingly being used to deal with pediatric gastroesophageal reflux (GER), also known as GERD in children. We've come a long way from the standard dose of Pepto Bismol from years past.

But are the newer drugs better than the stand-by tummy tamers of old? *Bottom Line's Daily Health News* consulting medical editor Andrew L. Rubman, ND, lays out the differences between the medications.

A WARNING

Dr. Rubman says that acid suppressants (such as PPI drugs Prilosec [*omeprazole*] and Prevacid) relieve heartburn by decreasing stomach acid production. Antacids (such as Mylanta and Maalox) neutralize stomach acid.

These drugs should rarely be taken by children, he says, just as they should rarely be taken by adults. It's all marketing, hucksterism and salesmanship, now at the cost of even our children's health and well-being, warns Dr. Rubman. He adds that not only are these drugs often unnecessary, they are actually harmful to our health—and our children's health. Digestive difficulties are actually more likely to develop due to insufficient rather than excess stomach acid, says Dr. Rubman.

ACID SUPPRESSANTS AND CHILDREN

Acid suppressants like Prevacid suppress normal digestive function, explains Dr. Rubman. He points out that whenever you tinker with the natural processes of the body, you are asking for trouble. *In this case, when you limit a child's ability to digest food by giving him or her an acid suppressant, there are a number of negative consequences in the body...*

•**Greater susceptibility to germs and disease.** Not for digestion alone, germ-killing stomach acid is also part of the body's natural defense system against microbial invaders such as bacteria, viruses, yeast and mold, says Dr. Rubman. When you disarm this system, invaders are left free to colonize the stomach and digestive tract. The immune system counters with an inflammatory response, damage to stomach cells ensues, and the door is open to diseases such as gastritis, Crohn's disease and asthma, Dr. Rubman believes.

Although some children actually take GER drugs for uncontrolled or poorly controlled asthma, Dr. Rubman says that they might be helpful in the short run (asthma drugs can cause or worsen reflux) but in the long run drugs that reduce gastric acid negatively impact the body.

•**Bloating, gas, bad breath, rashes.** A child taking antacids or acid suppressants can get away with eating greasy, fatty foods—just the sort of foods you want him/her to avoid—without getting a tummy ache. However, Dr. Rubman warns that this is not a free pass, and the body's digestive discomfort may manifest itself elsewhere, as in skin rashes or passing gas.

•**Suppressed liver function.** When you suppress stomach acid, you also suppress liver function, cautions Dr. Rubman. This means that fat can no longer be as efficiently excreted with bile. Additionally, acid suppressants reduce the body's ability to thoroughly digest proteins, which reduces its ability to manufacture "the good cholesterol," high-density lipoprotein (HDL), says Dr. Rubman. Young developing bodies with developing hormones are especially vulnerable to damage due to suppressed liver function, he says. Additionally, suppressing the liver's ability to produce HDL can create a cholesterol problem that would not have existed without the acid suppressants, according to Dr. Rubman.

•**Increased risk of acid reflux "disease."** Ironically, antacids and acid suppressants can contribute to the very problem they are designed to treat, says Dr. Rubman. When there is insufficient stomach acid, the stomach cannot properly break down food. This can lead to inadequate sterilization of food content allowing microbes present in the meal to survive and colonize the stomach lining. For example, food-borne *H. pylori*, a cause of chronic gastritis and an established cause of stomach cancer, may be more likely to survive in an acid-suppressed stomach, says Dr. Rubman.

Note: In rare cases, as when children have ulcers, antacids may be taken on a short-term basis (no longer than 14 days), if not caused by *H. pylori*, which would need to be treated separately.

A SAFE AND EFFECTIVE ALTERNATIVE

Fortunately, Dr. Rubman offers many safe and natural ways to address heartburn and other digestive disturbances in children...

•**Lose weight.** Obesity is a growing problem in children and more often than not, heartburn and GER are due to excess pounds from overeating.

•**Look at simpler ways to control heartburn.** Instead of turning to acid suppressants, try an antacid. Add a half teaspoon of pure baking soda to a glass of cold water. Do this only on an empty stomach. Suppressing acid in the absence of ulcer only perpetuates the symptoms, says Dr. Rubman.

•**Chew food thoroughly.** Tell your child to slow down while eating. Chewing stimulates enzyme activity, and the more food is broken down in the mouth, the more readily the nutrients in the food are absorbed and utilized.

•**Eat three meals a day.** While popular thinking holds that small, frequent meals are less likely to cause indigestion, Dr. Rubman disagrees. With three reasonably-sized meals a day, stomach acid can efficiently dissolve food and extract nutrients when a child eats, and the stomach can rest between meals. So, watch the snacking as well if your child is having stomach upsets. Ripe fruit that is not citrus is the best bet for a snack because it tends to digest quickly in a compromised environment. Avoid offering snacks within an hour of bedtime.

•**Limit fluids with children's meals.** Fluids dilute stomach acid, leaving more work for the stomach to do. Dr. Rubman advises that children cease drinking one-half hour before eating, and refrain from drinking for an hour afterward.

•**Monitor food combinations.** It's unwise to combine foods that digest quickly (sugar, white flour products, white potatoes, etc.) with highly saturated fats (such as red meat or dairy), cautions Dr. Rubman.

Another good rule of thumb: No fruit with meals. Either eat the fruit one-half hour before the meal or wait at least an hour to an hour and a half after the meal to eat the fruit depending on the size and complexity of the meal.

•**Consider digestive enzymes or herbal remedies.** When stomach acid levels are low, Dr. Rubman recommends digestive aids such as DuoZyme (Karuna) and Gastri-Gest (Priority One). These supplements stimulate hydrochloric acid release. Check with a trained professional regarding the proper dosage for your child's age and weight.

ACID SUPPRESSANTS ARE NO ANSWER

Acid suppressants that limit a child's natural ability to digest food are no answer to heartburn, indigestion or GER, says Dr. Rubman. Instead, take simple steps to support the body's natural ability to heal itself, keeping a closer eye on what your child eats and when, and make sure food is chewed thoroughly instead of gulped.

If necessary, your doctor might want to consider tests that measure low stomach acid, such as a stool analysis or the Heidelberg gastrogram.

18

Today's Biggest Health Myths

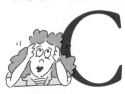

Supplement Savvy— What's Really Best for Your Health

Confused about vitamin and mineral supplements? How can a consumer be sure that a product really contains what's on the label? Or that the manufacturer is using the best form of a substance, since research has shown that not all types of vitamins or parts of plants are equally effective.

We spoke with Tod Cooperman, MD, president of *ConsumerLab.com* to get some perspective on the issue. ConsumerLab.com has been conducting quality-control testing on vitamins, minerals, protein drinks, energy bars and the like for years and reporting its findings on its information-packed site. It is one of the most respected companies in the country when it comes to product quality evaluation of this kind.

PRODUCT TESTING

"We've tested 1,300 products in the last six years," Dr. Cooperman says, "and we've found that one out of four has some type of problem. The product might be missing an ingredient, or it might be contaminated. For example, we test most supplements for lead. And if we're testing a fish oil, we'll check for rancidity, mercury and PCBs. Rancidity in particular is a potential problem with fish oil."

MOST COMMON PROBLEMS

Problems with supplements run a very wide spectrum, ranging from too little of an ingredient, too much of another or even to some kind of contamination.

In many cases, a product will not acquire an "approved" rating—not because it has too little of a compound it's supposed to

---

Tod Cooperman, MD, researcher, writer and speaker on consumer health-care issues and president, ConsumerLab.com, White Plains, New York.

have, but because it has too much of something that's not supposed to be there. One startling finding was that *Weil Balanced Cal-Mag* contained 2.3 micrograms (mcg) of lead per daily serving. *Theragran-M Advanced Formula High Potency* multiple vitamin also contained lead—3 mcg per serving. Both of these amounts are more than the amount allowed by the state of California without a warning label! And *Lil Critters Gummy Bears Vites*, a vitamin marketed for children, contained a high amount of lead and was missing half of the folic acid content claimed on the label.

And what about vitamin tablets that are found completely unabsorbed, intact in toilet bowls? Dr. Cooperman explains that it's very important to find out if a product breaks apart properly. "We'll do a disintegration test in which we drop the tablet or capsule in a solution at the correct acidity and temperature to simulate what happens to it in the body," he tells us.

According to Dr. Cooperman, the top problems with supplements are…

- **Too little of the active ingredient**
- **Too much of the active ingredient**
- **Wrong ingredient**
- **Contamination**
- **Misleading or unsupported health claims** (especially with herbal products).
- **Dangerous or illegal ingredients** (sometimes found in bodybuilding supplements).
- **Poor disintegration** (product is not digested properly or fully).

WHAT'S IN A NAME

In the absence of more knowledge, consumers often assume that a well-known brand will mean better quality. As was seen with Weil's Balanced Cal-Mag, this is not necessarily the case. Similarly, consumers assume that a generic product from a discounter will be of lower quality. According to Dr. Cooperman, Wal-Mart supplements are actually higher quality than other mass brands. "I'm much more comfortable with Wal-Mart's Spring Valley

line than I am with many other drugstore brands, such as Rite-Aid's." Dr. Cooperman also says that he'd put more faith in a Costco or a Sam's Club than a supermarket brand because of the pressure they are placing on manufacturers.

Dr. Cooperman says it's impossible to say which brands are the very best. *However, some companies choose to participate in programs, such as Consumerlab. com's Voluntary Certification Program, on a regular basis, so consumers are more likely to find product information on the following brands…*

- **Nutrilite**
- **Nature Made**
- **Nature's Resource**
- **Puritan's Pride**
- **Vitamin World.**

Multilevel marketing companies, such as Usana and Shaklee, do a surprisingly good job of quality control and produce excellent products in spite of their high prices. "Every company makes mistakes from time to time, but in general, the multilevels do a very good job. Their supplements are correctly labeled, they go out of their way to give you good information and they recommend a dose that's appropriate. They break apart, they're pure and they have all the ingredients on the label," says Dr. Cooperman.

NATURAL VS. SYNTHETIC

Are "natural" products better than "synthetic?" *Bottom Line's Daily Health News* consulting medical editor Andrew L. Rubman, ND, says that synthetic is often the same as natural and points out that if you eat well with lots of fresh whole foods and simply use supplements to augment your nutrition, then either version will usually provide support.

What are the most important things you need to know when buying nutritional supplements? *Here are Dr. Cooperman's top recommendations…*

1. Know what ingredient you're looking for. "If you're told to take an herb, understand that there are different species and parts of plants known to be effective. Know which one you're looking for—it should be clearly marked on the label." For example, if you are told to get "dandelion root," make sure what you buy says "dandelion root" on the package.

2. If you're buying an herbal, know what form you're looking for. "Is it an extract or a powder?" asks Dr. Cooperman. Extracts can be 10 times as strong as the whole powder!

3. Read labels carefully. "With, for example, soy isoflavones, manufacturers can label them in different ways that can be misleading," says Dr. Cooperman. For example, "genistin" is isoflavone and sugar, and "genistein" is just the isoflavone. "Genistein" contains about 50% more soy.

4. Ask your doctor. A holistic physician probably has brands that he/she prefers for different items.

Finally, and most important...

"Buy brands that have been independently tested," Dr. Cooperman says. *ConsumerLab.com* is a reliable source for product testing, and now the US Pharmacopeia tests products as well.

Do Chemo-Vitamins Really Work?

Timothy Birdsall, ND, vice president, integrative medicine, Cancer Treatment Centers of America. He was a member of the board of directors for the American Association of Naturopathic Physicians. He was also the founding editor-in-chief of *Alternative Medicine Review*. Cancer Treatment Centers of America can be reached at 800-615-3055 or *www.cancercenter.com*.

A common challenge for people battling cancer is how to stay strong and healthy while subjecting their bodies to the toxins of chemotherapy and radiation treatments. Although some research has shown that vitamins—and antioxidants in particular—may help prevent cancer, other studies show that antioxidants' protection of cells against damage actually can work against chemotherapy's intentionally destructive actions. So, what's the truth?

To learn more, we spoke with Timothy Birdsall, ND, a naturopathic physician who is vice president of integrative medicine at the Cancer Treatment Centers of America, a hospital-based program that blends conventional treatment with integrative medicine.

TARGETING WHICH CELLS TO KEEP OR KILL

According to Dr. Birdsall, "The essential issue here is that many chemotherapy drugs attack cancer cells through the mechanism of oxidation, which is precisely the mechanism that antioxidants defend against. However, most chemotherapy drugs have multiple agents of action, not just oxidation. And the flip side of the coin is that many studies have shown that malignant cells metabolize the typical dietary antioxidants very differently from normal cells." Dr. Birdsall explains that studies have shown that more antioxidants wind up in healthy cells than in the cancer cells. "The cancer cells appear to metabolize antioxidants a bit differently from healthy cells," he said. "This would appear to be a good thing, but there is very little clinical data to support either side."

COMPLEX ISSUES

Dr. Birdsall notes the very special challenges presented in treating cancer patients. Cancer is a very complex disease. It's an umbrella term that refers to more than 200 different diseases. Because something is effective for prostate cancer does not mean that it's effective for breast cancer. Furthermore, there are no "intermediate markers" for cancer to see if a treatment is working.

EXTRAPOLATING IS DIFFICULT

Cancer is also a disease in which it is extraordinarily difficult to extrapolate from cell studies and animal studies to humans. "If we could extrapolate from those studies, we would have known how to cure cancer 20 years ago. We can do it in cells, and with cancers created in the laboratory. But ultimately, we have to track the results in people, not in Petri dishes," says Dr. Birdsall.

ANTIOXIDANTS AND CHEMO SIDE EFFECTS

"There is clear evidence of protection by antioxidants against some side effects of chemotherapy—in particular the protection of the liver and gastrointestinal tract as well as reduction in malaise, nausea and diarrhea," Dr. Birdsall says. "But just because something lowers side effects does not mean that it's necessarily good for that patient. We have to know that it reduces side effects without interfering with the treatment."

Dr. Birdsall poses the question: "What if a patient using antioxidants and chemo together gets 50% tumor shrinkage? At first you think that's great. But the underlying question is, might she have gotten 75% shrinkage without the antioxidants? We just don't know."

WHAT'S A PATIENT TO DO?

"The general advice that most patients are given—don't use any antioxidants—is a blanket condemnation often used by people who don't know or don't understand them," Dr. Birdsall says. "If people are interested in using antioxidants, there are safe ways to do it—and questionable ways as well. It's a complex area, and one that is changing so fast."

This leaves a puzzling dilemma, but one in which there is still a hopeful message. "The appropriate thing to do is to find a naturopathic physician who is well trained in oncology," Dr. Birdsall recommends.

"In most situations I think a daily multiple vitamin is absolutely safe during chemo," Dr. Birdsall concludes. "And in most situations 1,000 milligrams (mg) of vitamin C and 400 international units of vitamin E are safe as well. But each situation needs to be evaluated by someone who does this every single day. That's where a naturopathic oncologist can really be of service."

info Visit these Web sites for more on integrative treatments for cancer: The Oncology Association of Naturopathic Physicians (*www.oncanp.org*)…and the Cancer Treatment Centers of America (*www.cancercenter.com*).

Natural Cholesterol Reducer Doesn't Work (But What Does)

Eric Yarnell, ND, RH, a practitioner at Northwest Naturopathic Urology, Seattle. Dr. Yarnell is the author of numerous books including *Clinical Botanical Medicine*. Mary Ann Liebert. He is president of Healing Mountain Publishing and vice president of Heron Botanicals. *www.dryarnell.com*.

Jay S. Cohen, MD, adjunct (voluntary) professor of family and preventive medicine, University of California, San Diego. Dr. Cohen is author of *What You Must Know About Statin Drugs & Their Natural Alternatives* (Square One) and *Over Dose: The Case Against the Drug Companies* (Tarcher/Putnam). *www.medicationsense.com*.

According to a recent German study, the popular supplement *policosanol* may not be effective after all in reducing cholesterol. Earlier research had suggested significant health benefits in taking this natural sugar cane derivative—so now what are we to believe? Does it work or doesn't it? Should we take it or shouldn't we?

To get to the bottom of the matter, we called on two experts in botanicals and cholesterol-lowering drugs—Eric Yarnell, ND, RH, author of *Clinical Botanical Medicine* (Mary Ann Liebert, Inc.) and Jay S. Cohen, MD, author of *What You Must Know About Statin Drugs & Their Natural Alternatives* (Square One). They told us that the research on policosanol has been shaky all along, and neither was particularly surprised to hear the results of the German study.

Fortunately, there are plenty of safe and effective natural alternatives with a better track record in supporting cardiovascular health.

POLICOSANOL: A BRIEF HISTORY

Policosanol was originally developed from sugar cane in Cuba. In the US, it is commonly derived from sugar cane and rice bran. Other possible sources are wheat germ and beeswax. More than 80 studies have suggested that policosanol at doses from 5 milligrams (mg) to 40 mg could lower low-density lipoprotein (LDL) cholesterol (the bad kind) as effectively as statin drugs. The cumulative research indicated that 10 mg to 20 mg daily lowered LDL by 21% to 29%...lowered total cholesterol by a slightly lower amount... and raised high-density lipoprotein (HDL) (the good cholesterol) by 8% to 15%. Side effects were minimal.

So far, so good. But upon closer examination, it turns out that the majority of the early research was underwritten by Cuba's National Center for Scientific Research. In addition, this research group founded the company Dalmer Laboratories, which supported the studies to market policosanol. A conflict of interest?

ABOUT THE GERMAN RESEARCH

In the recent German study, 143 people were randomly assigned to take 10, 20, 40 or 80 mg of Cuban sugar cane-derived policosanol or a placebo. As the study was double-blind, neither the participants nor the health-care professionals knew who was taking what. After 12 weeks, there was no significant difference between the LDL levels of volunteers in any group—even though some were taking twice the normal dose or more of policosanol. There were also no significant differences in related risk factors, including total cholesterol, HDL, VLDL (very low-density lipoprotein), LDL, triglycerides, lipoprotein (a), and the ratio of total or LDL cholesterol to HDL cholesterol.

This was a very well-designed study, observes Dr. Yarnell. He also points out that unlike the majority of previous research, it was not backed by a Cuban company or research group. The results were published in the *Journal of the American Medical Association*.

HEART-HEALTHY ALTERNATIVES

Fortunately, policosanol is far from the only cholesterol-lowering supplement. According to Drs. Yarnell and Cohen, there are a number of natural alternatives that have been researched more thoroughly and objectively. *Among the many available options are...*

•**Garlic.** Tasty and inexpensive, garlic has a modest effect on lowering LDL, total cholesterol and triglycerides. Simply incorporate a clove or two in your meals, or take a supplement.

Caution: If you take blood thinners or have a bleeding disorder, consult your physician before taking garlic supplements.

•**Niacin.** Niacin helps keep bad cholesterol from circulating through the body. There are two types of niacin—Niaspan, the pharmaceutical form that is FDA-approved and is preferred by mainstream physicians...and the niacin derivatives that are more commonly recommended by natural practitioners. Dr. Cohen notes that Niaspan can cause uncomfortable side effects such as flushing, nausea, vomiting and palpitations, and can cause serious side effects such as hepatitis. He recommends *inositol hexaniacinate.* Consult your health-care practitioner about dosage, and have regular blood tests when you take any niacin preparation. Talk to your health-care provider before taking if you have liver disease, diabetes, ulcers or gout.

Note: Niacinamide supplements are a different form of niacin and have not been shown to lower cholesterol.

•**Omega-3 fatty acids.** Omega-3 fatty acids in ocean fish such as wild salmon, halibut and tuna boost beneficial HDL, lower harmful triglycerides, keep a lid on inflammation and enhance blood vessel health. If you're not a fish eater, you can take fish oil capsules instead.

Caution: If you take blood thinners or have a bleeding disorder, consult a physician trained in nutritional supplementation before taking fish oil supplements.

• **Plant sterols.** The American Heart Association recommends plant sterols as one of the ways to reduce LDL cholesterol. Small amounts are naturally present in vegetable oils, seeds, nuts and various vegetables or fruits. In addition, you can buy plant sterol esters in supplement form. They are also available in spreads such as Benecol, which you can use in place of butter, and enriched orange juice.

• **Red yeast rice.** This supplement contains the same active ingredient as the statin drug *lovastatin* (Mevacor). Like Mevacor, red yeast rice lowers LDL, total cholesterol and triglycerides. An additional benefit is that it may also reduce elevated C-reactive protein (CRP), another marker of cardiovascular disease risk. Because of its statin-like effects, Dr. Cohen recommends that red yeast rice be used under medical supervision. People should not take red yeast rice if they are also on statin drug therapy.

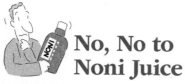

No, No to Noni Juice

David Winston, founding member of the American Herbalists Guild (AHG) and coauthor of *Herbal Therapy and Supplements: A Scientific and Traditional Approach*. Lippincott.

US Food and Drug Administration (FDA), *www.fda.gov*.

Might noni juice be the next big thing on the super fruit horizon? Apparently not. According to our experts, noni juice does not measure up to its claims.

While there may be interesting compounds in noni juice and some benefit to drinking it, there is little information or evidence to back up the extravagant health claims being made by marketers, says David Winston, founding member of the American Herbalists Guild and coauthor of *Herbal Therapy and Supplements: A Scientific and Traditional Approach* (Lippincott). In fact, multiple noni juice purveyors on the Web have been sent letters from the US Food and Drug Administration (FDA), warning them to tone down their reckless, hyped-up claims.

NOTHING CAN DO EVERYTHING

Noni juice comes from the *Morinda citrifolia* fruit, which is grown in the South Pacific in exotic locales such as Tahiti. Its boosters assert that noni juice is a miracle tonic that lowers cholesterol, cures headaches, relieves arthritis pain, lessens the symptoms of cancer, boosts energy and improves allergy and asthma symptoms.

Other ailments marketers claim are helped by noni: High blood pressure, artherosclerosis, fibromyalgia, multiple sclerosis, drug addiction, AIDS and pain. The list goes on and on.

But nothing can do everything, observes Winston. And when sales materials state or imply that a product can do just that, you should take pause. He adds that most traditional uses of noni juice were actually as an external, topical treatment for cuts, wounds and the like.

IF IT SOUNDS TOO GOOD TO BE TRUE...

To add insult to injury, noni juice is expensive and has an unpleasant odor and flavor, which Winston compares with rancid cheese. As for safety concerns, two cases of liver toxicity were attributed to noni juice in a study reported in the *World Journal of Gastroenterology*. Because the juice is high in potassium, it should not be used by people with kidney disease or those taking potassium-sparing diuretic drugs. This could result in a dangerous buildup of potassium in the body.

The bottom line: If it sounds too good to be true, it probably is. In this case, the claims for noni juice are definitely too good to be true.

How Colon Cleansing *Harms* Your Health

Andrew L. Rubman, ND, consulting medical editor for *Bottom Line's Daily Health News* and director of the Southbury Clinic for Traditional Medicines in Southbury, Connecticut.

Colon cleansing for good health traces back to the ancient Egyptians (between the 15th-and 17th-century BC), with records of their use of enemas (cleansing of part of the colon). Colon hydrotherapy—the practice of flushing water through the entire colon or large intestine—was all the rage in Europe in the late 1800s and early 1900s and was popular in the US in the 1920s and 1930s...and recently has increased in popularity once again. The theory behind "colonics" or colonic irrigation, then and now, is the same: the cleaner the colon is kept from toxins and waste, the less opportunity there is for disease to develop.

But this is not the case. In fact, it couldn't be more incorrect, says *Bottom Line's Daily Health News* consulting medical editor Andrew L. Rubman, ND. "The truth is that colonic irrigation can be harmful, and the unscrupulous hucksters who regularly tout its virtues on the Internet are, by and large, out to make a fast buck," says Dr. Rubman. While Dr. Rubman is normally open-minded about many sorts of traditional treatments, this is one he strongly feels he must warn people about. He outlined why colonics are harmful to digestion and dangerous to your overall health.

HOW COLONIC IRRIGATION WORKS...AND WHY IT DOESN'T

On-line and in many alternative health publications, colonic irrigation is heralded as the solution to problems ranging from constipation to weight loss, skin problems, arthritis, asthma and chronic fatigue. It is likened to a super-enema, even a "car wash" for the large intestine.

In the procedure, a plastic or rubber tube is passed through the rectum into the colon, and large amounts of warm water are pumped in to flush the contents out and remove buildup from the large intestine. Proponents claim that colonic irrigation works by boosting immunity through the removal of accumulated toxins.

But, says Dr. Rubman, it's important to understand that "cleaning out" the colon is counterproductive because proper digestive function depends upon a colony of friendly bacteria (approximately three to four pounds' worth in a healthy adult) that lives in a delicate state of balance in the large intestine. In fact, Dr. Rubman refers to the large intestine as the body's "disease-fighting control center" since its role in immune function is so important to our health. The beneficial bacteria in residence keep intestinal walls healthy and intact, working together to prevent dangerous bacteria in what we eat (and the toxins that they produce) from leaking out of the intestine and migrating elsewhere to cause inflammation and disease. By flushing out these helpful bacteria, colonic irrigation interferes with efficient digestion and immune function.

WHY IT'S SO DANGEROUS

In addition to not being helpful, Dr. Rubman outlined very specific hazards relating to colonic irrigation...

•**Disruption of normal balances.** The colon normally absorbs water and sodium to maintain a proper balance of fluid and electrolytes. When colonic irrigation disturbs this balance, dangerous, sometimes even life-threatening salt loss and dehydration can follow.

•**Introduction of contaminants.** Colonic irrigation can also introduce contaminants via equipment that has not been properly sanitized.

•**Unqualified practitioners can cause serious injury.** While regulations vary from one state to another, few require certification or licensure, so colonics are sometimes performed by individuals with little or no formal training or medical qualifications. According to Dr. Rubman, having a colonic irrigation at the hands of an unskilled practitioner is akin to having an intravenous (IV) drip administered by a person with no training—it's hit or miss. One improperly executed colonic can cause serious damage, such as a perforated colon.

•**High cost.** To add insult to injury, the potential risks and dangers of colonic irrigation come hand-in-hand with a steep price. A brief on-line search reveals price tags ranging approximately $75 to $800 (the latter figure for a series of multiple treatments).

HERE'S THE SAFE WAY TO ENSURE OPTIMAL COLON HEALTH

What is correct about the health claims of the colonics movement is that the health of the large intestine is essential to our well-being, even if colonic cleansing is the wrong way to achieve this goal. Dr. Rubman points out that the place to start is at the other end of the body, by eating healthy foods. In other words, for optimal digestion, follow an optimal diet.

If you regularly consume large quantities of difficult-to-digest saturated fat and red meat, you'll likely suffer intestinal disturbances. For optimal digestion, eat lean proteins including skinless turkey or chicken breast...healthy fats from foods such as olive oil, avocado and wild, cold-water fish like salmon and mackerel... foods that boost intestinal health, such as nutrient-packed, fiber-rich steamed veggies, fruits, bran, beans, nuts and seeds. In particular, fiber helps food move efficiently through the digestive tract, and binds and transports cholesterol-rich bile acids out of the body.

Other tried and true recommendations from Dr. Rubman...

•**Pay attention to salt intake.** Sodium is an important mineral that helps regulate the body's fluid balance. Don't assume it's best to consume as little as possible.

Instead, discuss proper salt intake levels with your physician.

•**Drink to satisfy thirst.** Water needs vary among individuals and Dr. Rubman disagrees with the often-cited recommendation that we all need to drink eight 8-ounce glasses of water daily. Again, when in doubt, consult your physician about proper intake levels.

•**Chew food thoroughly.** The more you break down food in your mouth, the less work the rest of the digestive system has to do.

Dr. Rubman acknowledges that on rare occasions, depending on a person's individual digestive issues, colonic irrigation by a highly trained health-care professional may serve a valid medical purpose. In that case, however, it should only be performed by an experienced, skilled medical professional such as a naturopathic doctor (ND).

info To locate a naturopathic doctor in your area, visit the Web site of the American Association of Naturopathic Physicians (AANP) at *www.naturopathic.org*.

Cardiac Calcium Score—Medicine or Marketing?

Kelly Anne Spratt, DO, clinical associate professor of medicine, University of Pennsylvania Health System, Philadelphia.

In the last few years you may have seen ads for hospitals or private clinics offering an electronic-beam CT scan (EBCT) to determine your coronary artery calcium score. This is one of the newest screenings available, supposedly useful in determining a person's level of risk for coronary artery disease (CAD) and heart attack. It does its magic by imaging and measuring the calcium deposits in the coronary arteries and then assigning a score, based on the amount of total calcium.

While the ads often imply that knowing your score is a must, others—including some cardiologists—have asked if this is good medicine or merely good marketing.

CHANGE OF HEART BY HEART ASSOCIATION

In 1999, the American Heart Association (AHA) did not recommend calcium screening for diagnosing obstructive CAD. But the AHA did an about-face and began to advocate it for some people, such as those with an intermediate risk of CAD. Cardiovascular specialist Kelly Anne Spratt, DO, clinical associate professor of medicine at the University of Pennsylvania Health System in Philadelphia, explains that plaque is made of fat, cholesterol and calcium. When calcium becomes more dense as plaque hardens, it shows up on EBCT scans. While imaging can't show cholesterol, it can show calcium deposits. Though some plaque formation is inevitable as we age, the assumption here is that a higher calcium score indicates a higher likelihood of underlying coronary disease or future CAD event risk.

The test, Dr. Spratt says, is not appropriate for people at low risk for CAD (having few risk factors) or those at high risk who are already being treated. Calcium scoring can be useful, she says, for people who have more than one risk factor and are therefore at "intermediate risk" for developing CAD. The major risks include high blood pressure, high cholesterol levels and a strong family history of cardiac disease. Calcium scoring is another tool to help doctors better manage treatment for such people, including lifestyle recommendations as well as, perhaps, daily aspirin or cholesterol or blood pressure medications.

The test is also useful for one other group, says Dr. Spratt. These are people who experience unexplained chest pains. A calcium score screening can calm fears and concerns about the cause of the pain, providing insight and sometimes reassurance that their heart is fine.

CT Scans Show Up to 69% False Positives

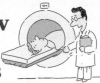

Stephen J. Swensen, MD, chair, department of radiology, Mayo Clinic, Rochester, Minnesota.

Technology can be great, but it can also create new problems or challenges to cope with.

Example: The debate over mammograms, which can improve early detection of breast cancer for some while increasing anxiety for many others who fall victim to "false positives" that require further testing. Not surprisingly, a similar debate rages with computed tomography (CT) scans. These special X-rays are produced with an X-ray machine hooked up to a computer to generate cross-sectional images of the body, which can help detect tissue abnormalities, tumors and other conditions. Unfortunately, one concern that keeps popping up is the high rate of false positives (results that mistakenly identify disease when none is present), generating concerns about over-diagnosis and the high cost for additional testing.

To learn more about this problem, we talked to Stephen J. Swensen, MD, chair of the department of radiology at the Mayo Clinic in Rochester, Minnesota. He was the lead researcher in a recent study last year on using CT scans to detect early-stage lung cancer. According to Dr. Swensen, CT scanning catches more early-stage lung cancers, but does not necessarily reduce death from the disease. So, is it worth it?

CT SCANNING FOR LUNG CANCER

In the Mayo Clinic study involving 1,520 current or former smokers, an astounding 69% had false-positive findings, meaning that nodules originally identified as cancerous turned out to be benign. Among the possible consequences of these false positives are unnecessary and potentially risky biopsy procedures, unnecessary medical expenses and impaired quality of life. Moreover, the average death rate from lung cancer surgery is 3% to 5%—this mortality rate would generally be acceptable in operations for a deadly condition, but not for a benign condition.

Even when growths are not benign, CT scanning detects more early-stage tumors that are sometimes so slow-growing they are unlikely to cause death. This raises the question of whether or not detection by these methods is valuable for the population at risk. Dr. Swensen adds that other cancers are so lethal and fast-growing that there are not a lot of ways to effectively treat them, even when they are detected early.

IMPLICATIONS FOR FURTHER TESTING

We asked Dr. Swensen if this and similar studies mean that we should reconsider early CT screening for disease. Not yet, was his response, but he pointed out that large, multi-center trials should give us definitive answers in two to three years. As for now, he advises people at risk (for example, smokers) undergo early screening for lung cancer only after being informed about the pros and cons of the procedure by a physician who is not an owner or part-owner of the screening facility. You want to be sure that the physician making the recommendation is focused solely on what is best for the patient, not financial gain.

Index